Frontiers of Cognitive Therapy

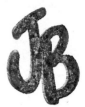

Frontiers of Cognitive Therapy

Paul M. Salkovskis
Editor

Foreword by S. Rachman

The Guilford Press
New York London

Printed in the United States of America

This book is printed on acid-free paper.

Last digit is print number: 9 8 7 6 5 4 3 2

Library of Congress Cataloging-in-Publication Data

Frontiers of cognitive therapy / Paul M. Salkovskis, editor.
        p.   cm.
   Includes bibliographical references and index.
   ISBN 1-57230-112-0 (hard) — 1-57230-113-9 (pbk.)
   1. Cognitive therapy. I. Salkovskis, Paul M.
RC489.C63F76 1996
616.89'142—dc20

96-22618
CIP

To Aaron T. Beck

Contributors

Arthur Auerbach, MD, Department of Psychiatry, University of Pennsylvania School of Medicine, Philadelphia

David H. Barlow, PhD, Department of Psychology, State University of New York at Albany

Aaron T. Beck, MD, Department of Psychiatry, University of Pennsylvania, Philadelphia; Beck Institute for Cognitive Therapy and Research, Bala Cynwyd, Pennsylvania

Judith S. Beck, PhD, Beck Institute for Cognitive Therapy and Research, Bala Cynwyd, Pennsylvania; Department of Psychiatry, University of Pennsylvania, Philadelphia

Ivy-Marie Blackburn, PhD, Newcastle City NHS Trust, Newcastle upon Tyne, U.K.; Department of Psychiatry, University of Newcastle, Newcastle upon Tyne, U.K.; Department of Psychology, University of Durham, Durham, U.K.

David D. Burns, MD, Department of Psychiatry and Behavioral Science, Stanford University School of Medicine, Palo Alto, California

Dianne L. Chambless, PhD, Department of Psychology, University of North Carolina at Chapel Hill

David A. Clark, PhD, Department of Psychology, University of New Brunswick, Fredericton, New Brunswick, Canada

David M. Clark, PhD, Department of Psychiatry, Warneford Hospital, University of Oxford, Oxford, UK

Robert D. DeRubeis, PhD, Department of Psychology, University of Pennsylvania, Philadelphia

Mark D. Evans, PhD (deceased), Department of Psychology, University of Minnesota, Minneapolis

Rober A. Franz, MA, Department of Psychology, University of Kansas, Lawrence

Robert A. Franz, MA, Department of Psychology, University of Kansas, Lawrence

Steven D. Hollon, PhD, Department of Psychology, Vanderbilt University, Nashville, Tennessee

Debra A. Hope, PhD, Department of Psychology, University of Nebraska, Lincoln

Philip C. Kendall, PhD, Department of Psychology, Temple University, Philadelphia, Pennsylvania

Bruce S. Liese, PhD, Department of Family Medicine, University of Kansas Medical Center, Kansas City

Lata K. McGinn, PhD, Department of Psychiatry, Albert Einstein College of Medicine/Montefiore Medical Center, Bronx, New York

Stirling Moorey, MRCPsych, Department of Psychology, St. Bartholomew's Hospital, London, U.K.

Christine A. Padesky, PhD, Center for Cognitive Therapy, Newport Beach, California; Department of Psychiatry and Human Behavior, University of California, Irvine

A. John Rush, MD, Department of Psychiatry, University of Texas Southwestern Medical Center, Dallas, Texas

Paul M. Salkovskis, PhD, Department of Psychiatry, Warneford Hospital, University of Oxford, Oxford, U.K.

Tracy Sbrocco, PhD, Department of Medical and Clinical Psychology, F. Edward Hébert School of Medicine, Uniformed Services University of the Health Sciences, Bethesda, Maryland

Robert A. Steer, EdD, Department of Psychiatry, School of Osteopathic Medicine, University of Medicine and Dentistry of New Jersey, Camden

John D. Teasdale, PhD, Applied Psychology Unit, Medical Research Council, Cambridge, U.K.

Kelly M. Vitousek, PhD, Department of Psychology, University of Hawaii at Manoa, Honolulu

Melissa J. Warman, MS, Department of Psychology, Temple University, Philadelphia, Pennsylvania

Marjorie E. Weishaar, PhD, Department of Psychiatry and Human Behavior, Brown University, Providence, Rhode Island

Jan E. Weissenburger, MA, Psychology Service, Audie L. Murphy Department of Veterans Affairs Medical Center, San Antonio, Texas

J. Mark G. Williams, DPhil, School of Psychology, University of Wales, Bangor, U.K.

Jesse H. Wright, MD, PhD, Department of Psychiatry and Behavioral Sciences, University of Louisville School of Medicine, Louisville, Kentucky; Norton Psychiatric Clinic, Louisville, Kentucky

Jeffrey E. Young, PhD, Cognitive Therapy Centers of New York and Fairfield County, Connecticut; Department of Psychiatry, College of Physicians and Surgeons, Columbia University, New York, New York

Foreword

The exhilaration that ensued from the early advances of behavior therapy, between 1954 and 1965, was followed by a period of worthy consolidation during which these techniques were refined and the therapeutic claims evaluated. The successes of behavior therapy in treating anxiety disorders, however, were not accompanied by comparable advances in dealing with depression, and when Aaron Beck began reporting on the effectiveness of cognitive therapy applied to depression, he found a ready audience. His inclusion of behavioral concepts and techniques added the touch of respectability that enabled behavior therapists to absorb, unseen or unnoticed, many of Beck's ideas and later apply them in an innovative cognitive analysis of panic and other anxiety disorders. As a result, we now have a greatly improved understanding of panic disorder, obsessional disorders, hypochondriasis, and social phobia.

The originality and value of these fresh ideas is evident in this rich collection, edited by one of the leading contributors to the advance of cognitive-behavioral therapy. There are excellent and up-to-date chapters on the full range of psychological problems, which give one a keen sense of irresistible forward movement. The collection gives weight to Martin Seligman's observation that this is indeed the golden age of cognitive therapy.

A welcome feature of many of the chapters is the generous acknowledgment given to Beck for his inspiring contributions, and I take this opportunity to add my own gratitude to him. His opening chapter is a timely and welcome report on the progress of his thinking.

It is also fitting that Paul Salkovskis should be the editor of a book marking out the frontiers of cognitive therapy because his own work is so characteristically novel and original, and also because so much of the scientific inspiration for cognitive-behavioral therapy originated in the Oxford department of which he is a distinguished member.

These are indeed the frontiers of cognitive therapy, and beyond the frontiers we can expect intensive attempts to evaluate its newer applications, incisive examinations of its theoretical basis, and a steady absorption of the concepts of nonconscious processing into the overall theory.

S. Rachman
The University of British Columbia

Preface

In 1976, Aaron T. Beck published a book entitled *Cognitive Therapy and the Emotional Disorders*. In it he described a theory of emotion and emotional disorders, and a new psychotherapeutic approach with an emphasis on the treatment of depression. Twenty years later, in 1996, cognitive therapy has become the single most important and best validated psychotherapeutic approach. It is the psychological treatment of choice for a wide range of psychological problems. Clinical and experimental research has resulted in the theory being enlarged and developed, but has left the fundamentals unchanged. Month by month, new applications of cognitive therapy are developed. There can be no doubt that Beck's cognitive approach to the understanding and treatment of emotional problems represented a paradigm shift, and that the paradigm has truly shifted.

This book describes the present status of cognitive theory and therapy as applied to a range of psychological problems. It is not exhaustive, otherwise this book would have had to be an encyclopedia. Prominent omissions are work on psychosis (including bipolar disorder) and couples therapy. It does represent much of what is best in current thinking and practice in this field, and in this sense highlights the frontiers of cognitive therapy. This includes new developments and areas where the cognitive approach to emotion and emotional problems links with cognitive and biological sciences.

The book begins with a chapter by Beck himself, in which he describes his present thinking on the relationship between mood, beliefs, and personality and how these relate to psychopathology. John Teasdale then highlights the crucial influence of clinically relevant theorizing in the past, present, and future development of cognitive therapy approaches. In my own chapter, I show how the original statement of the cognitive theory of emotional problems continues to bring new insights to the development of such clinical theories. Next, David A. Clark and Robert Steer show how the research findings in the fields of anxiety and depression have resulted in validation of the fundamental premises of cognitive theory, and in their refinement. In their chapters, Mark Williams, Jan Weissenburger, and John Rush describe important features of the relationship between the cognitive approach and cognitive science and neuroscience.

Taking a more directly clinical approach, David Burns and Arthur Auerbach clearly articulate the importance of empathy in cognitive therapy, and show not only that empathy is important, but also that it can be taught and that the characteristics of cognitive therapy make it possible to maximize its therapeutic impact. In the next two chapters, Judith Beck, Lata McGinn, and Jeffrey Young focus on pervasive and long-term psychological difficulties (i.e., personality disorders) and show how there is at last real hope of change in this most difficult group of problems. Jesse Wright shows that the cognitive approach can be readily adapted to make a major impact on the most traditional of psychiatric settings, the inpatient unit. Suicide is a particular problem in which cognitive theory has made crucial contributions; these are summaraized by Marjorie Weishaar. Vulnerability to depression is addressed by Ivy-Marie Blackburn, showing how work on depression has progressed even as it has retained the fundamental ideas generated by Beck in his original work in this area.

Contrary to the beliefs of its critics, cognitive therapy is not an assembly of techniques applied mechanically. Christine Padesky highlights the importance of ensuring therapist competency in the full range of psychotherapeutic skills involved in cognitive therapy, dispelling any crude notions that this approach is prescriptive. The chapters that follow hers, on specific disorders, show just how important the combination of focused interventions are, and how these are invariably based on idiosyncratically derived formulations. Steven Hollon, Robert DeRubeis, and Mark Evans extend previous work on the treatment of depression and cast important new light on the issues of treatment maintenance. David M. Clark describes the current status of work on panic disorder: cognitive treatment in panic is groundbreaking both in the precision of theoretical predictions and in the remarkable demonstration of high-end state functioning in an unprecedentedly high proportion of patients at the end of treatment and at follow-up. Social phobia is a further rapidly developing area; Dianne Chambless and Debra Hope show the way in which theoretical development has been matched by improvements in treatment. Kelly Vitousek also highlights the key interactions between theory, experimental research, and treatment outcome, and shows how the cognitive approach helps focus on key clinical concepts in ways that facilitate the development and implementation of effective treatment. Tracy Sbrocco and David Barlow describe the experimental foundations for new developments in the cognitive approach to the understanding of sexuality and its problems. The development of cognitive approaches to medical problems is well represented by Stirling Moorey's work on helping people deal with the psychological consequences of cancer. Substance abuse is a problem with a particularly poor prognosis, not least due to the complex interactions between psychological, biological, and social factors; Bruce Liese and Robert Franz describe the newly developed and validated cognitive treatment approach. Philip Kendall and Melissa Warman describe cognitive treatment of emotional disorder in youth; clearly, cognitive development is likely to feature more and more prominently not only in this area of work, but across the entire lifespan. The final chapter examines one lifespan in particular, that of the founder of cognitive therapy, Aaron T. Beck, by identifying his achievements and influence. This chapter casts some light on how and why cognitive therapy developed in the way that it did.

Finally, I would like to thank the many people who made this book possible. Judith Sumida kept things shipshape in my office. Seymour Weingarten, Anna Brackett, and others at The Guilford Press were unfailingly patient, helpful, and encouraging when I faltered. Barbara Marinelli helped in a variety of ways, not least in providing a laugh or two. David M. Clark was, as ever, a rock. My wife, Lorna, and daughter, Cora, helped in more ways than I can describe. And Tim Beck was and is both an inspiration and a support.

Paul Salkovskis
University of Oxford

Contents

Frontiers of Cognitive Therapy

Chapter 1

Beyond Belief: A Theory of Modes, Personality, and Psychopathology

Aaron T. Beck

first applied the concept of negative cognitive schemas to explain the "thinking disorder" in depression over 30 years ago (Beck, 1964). Borrowing from the cognitive constructs of Kelly (1955) and drawing on the vocabulary of Bartlctt (1932) and Piaget (1947/1950), I proposed that the activation of certain idiosyncratic cognitive schemas represented the core problem in depression and could be assigned a primary role in the production of the various cognitive, affective, and behavioral symptoms. I also proposed that interventions aimed at moderating or modifying the dysfunctional interpretations and predictions as well as the underlying dysfunctional beliefs (incorporated into the dysfunctional schemas) could ameliorate the clinical disorder.

Since my first forays into the domain of depression and subsequently other clinical disorders (Beck, 1964, 1976; Beck, Emery, & Greenberg, 1985; Beck, Freeman, & Associates 1990; Beck, Wright, Newman, & Liese, 1993), much of the theorizing about the role of schemas in depression and other disorders has been supported by clinical and experimental studies (for a review, see Haaga, Dyck, & Ernst, 1991). Although the clinical formulation has been useful in understanding and treating psychopathology, it has become apparent over the years that the theory does not fully explain many clinical phenomena and experimental findings.

Specifically, a number of psychological problems are not adequately addressed by the model of individual schemas (linear schematic processing) and, thus, warrant attention. This chapter is an attempt to take them into account by expanding my original model. Among those problems are the following:

1. The *multiplicity* of related symptoms encompassing the cognitive, affective, motivational, and behavioral domains in a psychopathological condition.

2. Evidence of *systematic bias* across many domains suggesting that a more global and complex organization of schemas is involved in intense psychological reactions.
3. The findings of a *specific vulnerability* (or diathesis) to specific stressors that are congruent with a particular disorder.
4. The great *variety* of "normal" psychological reactions evoked by the myriad life circumstances.
5. The relation of content, structure, and function in *personality*.
6. Observations of the variations in the *intensity* of an individual's specific reactions to a given set of circumstances over time.
7. The phenomenon of *sensitization* ("kindling phenomenon"): successive recurrences of a disorder (e.g., depression) triggered by progressively less intense experiences.
8. The *remission* of symptoms by either pharmacotherapy or psychotherapy.
9. The apparent *continuity* of many psychopathological phenomena with personality.
10. The relevance of the model to normal "*moods.*"
11. The relationship among consciousness and nonconscious processing of information.

Although the current model of schematic processing still seems valid and useful for clinical interventions, it is apparent that these and related problems call for more global constructs and additional refinements related to progress in the field. A number of writers have shown a gradual convergence toward the integrative model in this chapter (Bandura, 1986; Bargh & Tota, 1988; Bower, 1981; Dweck & Leggett, 1988; Epstein, 1994; Higgins, 1996; Kihlstrom, 1990; Mischel & Shoda, 1995; Williams, Watts, McLeod & Matthews, 1988; Segal & Ingram, 1994; Teasdale & Barnard, 1993; Rachman, 1990).

In this chapter, I will attempt to present two main additions to the theory of simple schematic processing. First, I invoke the notion of modes, a network of cognitive, affective, motivational, and behavioral components. The modes, consisting of integrated sectors or suborganizations of personality, are designed to deal with specific demands or problems. The "primal modes" of most interest for the study of psychopathology include the derivatives of ancient organizations that evolved in prehistoric circumstances and are manifested in survival reactions, but also, in an exaggerated way, in psychiatric disorders. Second, I propose the use of the concept of charges (or cathexes) to explain the fluctuations in the intensity gradients of cognitive structures. This concept can be applied to the phenomena of sensitization, extinction, and remission.

The concept of "energetics" (charges or cathexes) provides an explanatory model for the instigation of, and changes in, normal and abnormal states. For example, it helps to account for the clinical observation that at the onset of a particular clinical disorder (e.g., anxiety, panic, or depression), various systems (cognitive, affective, motivational, and behavioral) shift from a relative quiescent state to a highly activated state. Further, the concept of modes encompasses clinical conditions characterized by the prepotence (or hypercathexis) of a conglomerate of related or contiguous dysfunctional beliefs, meanings, and memories that influence, if not control, the processing of information. The model also accounts for the observation that when the clinical syndrome remits, the characteristic dysfunctional interpretations and beliefs become less salient—or even disappear.

CASE ANALYSIS

Consider a relatively simple clinical example: A young man, Bob, suffers from an elevator phobia. As he approaches a tall office building containing an elevator he will be using, he starts to feel anxious—even though he is involved at the time in discussing routine business affairs with a colleague. As they come closer to the building, his anxiety increases. Although he has not been thinking about taking the elevator, obviously some kind of preconscious processing of the anticipated event is occurring and producing anxiety. The implicit knowledge that he will be taking an elevator to reach a top floor has already set in motion cognitive, affective, behavioral, and physiological processes.

Although Bob may not be consciously thinking about the elevator (and may be absorbed in his business discussion), a "cognitive probe" at this point would elicit the same information as if he were actively ruminating about the elevator ride: If asked to introspect—to explore all of his thoughts about his anticipation—he would acknowledge that he was fearful about taking the elevator. He might initially, perhaps, be more worried about the unpleasant anxiety he would feel in the elevator than about the presumed physical danger associated with a malfunctioning elevator. As he enters the lobby, however, the specific fear of catastrophe becomes salient. He becomes conscious of the fear that the elevator will crash or get stuck: He will get killed, suffocate, or faint. He is also fearful that his distress will accelerate to the point that he will start to yell uncontrollably and will be humiliated.

Later when Bob is no longer confronted with the threat of taking an elevator, he is no longer fearful of these erstwhile "dangers." The distance from the source of danger represents a safety zone or a "safety signal" (Woody & Rachman, 1994). But when the same situation arises again, the same pattern of fears is repeated.

Let us examine this phobic reaction pattern. The *activating circumstances* revolve around the anticipated event of riding in the elevator. These circumstances are processed through the orienting component of the primal mode relevant to danger—the imagined risk of being killed, suffocating, fainting, and losing control. As this specific fear is activated, the various component systems of the mode are energized. We then see the manifestation of the activation of the mode: Bob becomes pale, sweaty, and shaky; his heart races; he feels faint; and he has a "squishy feeling" in his abdomen.

The progression of events may be analyzed as follows. Initially, as Bob approaches the building, his *orienting* schema signals that there is danger ahead. This signal is sufficient to activate all the systems of the *mode*: the *affective system* generates rapidly increasing levels of anxiety; the *motivational system* expresses an increasing intensity of the impulse to escape; and the *physiological system* produces an increased heart rate, a lowered blood pressure resulting in a faint feeling, a tightening of the chest muscles, and a cramping of the abdomen.

At this point, Bob becomes fully aware of his unpleasant feelings and wishes to escape, but he is able to activate his *voluntary controls* to override this "primal" reaction and to force himself into the elevator. He manages to stay in the elevator, albeit with considerable anxiety, until it reaches the desired floor. As he steps out, his anxiety recedes.

We should note the importance of Bob's interpretation of his physiological sensations in adding to his fear of a physical or psychological disaster. Through feedback from his bodily sensations to his cognitive processing system, the faint feeling elicits a powerful fear of passing out; the tightening of his intercostal muscles leads to a fear of not being able to breathe; and the feeling of turbulence produced by his increased heart rate and abdominal distress intensify his desire to escape and his fear of uncontrollable yelling and banging on the walls of the elevator. This imagined sequence of events leads to another fear—that of feeling humiliated by his loss of control in the presence of other people. Having analyzed Bob's elevator phobia, we can now turn to a presentation of the concept of the mode and its application to clinical disorders and normal affective states.

DEFINITION AND DESCRIPTION:
STRUCTURE AND FUNCTIONS

Modes are specific suborganizations within the personality organization and incorporate the relevant components of the basic systems of personality: cognitive (or information processing), affective, behavioral, and motivational. I conceive of each of these systems as composed of structures, labeled "schemas." Thus the cognitive system consists of cognitive schemas, the affect of affective schemas, and so on. I also include the peripheral physiological system as a separate component insofar as it contributes a unique dimension to the function of the mode.[1] The mode by virtue of the integrated cognitive–affective–behavioral network produces a synchronous response to external demands and provides a mechanism for implementing internal dictates and goals.

Some modes are more "primal" in the sense of embodying more immediate and basic patterns relevant to crucial evolutionary derived objectives (e.g., survival and procreation). The content of these modes—for example, fears, anxiety, impulse to run away—is experienced as though they are reflex reactions to vital situations. Other models are less peremptory and are activated by less compelling circumstances, including such prosaic situations as studying or watching television.

I assume that each of the systems participating in a mode has a specific individual function, but that they operate in synchrony to implement a coordinated goal-directed strategy. For example, the fight flight mode is composed of a perception of threat (cognitive system), feelings of anxiety or anger (affective system) that prod the individual to do something, the creation of an impulse to act (motivational system), and the action itself (behavioral system). The physiological component consists of the physical mobilization for fight or flight. Thus it is possible to describe each system (cognitive, affective, etc.) separately, as though autonomous, or in terms of its synchronous interactions with the other systems.

The *cognitive system*[2] accounts for the functions involved in information processing and assignment of meanings: selection of data, attention, interpretation (meaning assignment), memory, and recall. This system is composed of a variety of cognitive structures relevant to persons' constructions of themselves and other people, their goals and expectations, and their storehouse of memories, previous learning, and fantasies. The processing often extends to the secondary elaboration of complex meanings relevant to abstract themes such as self-worth, social desirability, and causal attributions. The processing generally proceeds out of awareness (Kihlstrom, 1990) but the content can be consciously accessed. The basic structures of this system have been labeled "cognitive schemas" (see Beck, 1967, for a review). The schemas involved in inferences and interpretations are consolidated into a "meaning assignment" subsystem.

Memories have an important place in the cognitive system. Even though memories of past events may not be conscious, they can help to mold reactions of present events (Williams, Watts, McLeod, & Matthews, 1988). Experiences are abstracted and organized in memory around specific themes. When a particular mode is activated, the memories congruent with the theme of the mode are also activated. Reactions labeled as "conditioned reflexes" have such memories at their core.[3]

The *affective system* produces the various feeling states and their shadings and combinations (sadness, joy, anxiety, anger). An affective reaction is not simply an emotional experience devoid of any vital function. It is an integral part of psychobiological strategies concerned with survival and procreation. Through pleasure (positive affect) and dysphoria (negative affect), the affects reinforce adaptive behavior (Beck, Emery, & Greenberg, 1985). My conception of negative affect assigns it a specific role, namely to engage the attention of individuals and to prod them to focus on a particular circumstance that diminishes them in some way. Positive affect functions to reinforce goal-directed activity by "rewarding" goal attainment.

The operation of this system may be analogized to the perception of physical pain designed to elicit corrective actions and sensory pleasure that rewards adaptive experiences. This system also is composed of defined structures—the affective schemas—that produce affect when activated.

The *motivational and behavioral systems* provide the mechanism for the automatic mobilization (or inhibition) of the organism for action (or into inaction). These systems include the various emergency strategies, such as fight, flight, and freeze (Beck et al., 1985). The term "motivation," used here as opposed to "conscious intention," applies to the automatic involuntary impulses and inhibitions that are tied to the primal strategies. The construct of motivation includes the biological "drives," such as appetite and sexuality, the spontaneous urges to attack or flee, and the "involuntary" pressures to avoid or suppress "risky" action. The motivational and behavioral systems, also, are composed of structures, labeled respectively "motivational schemas" and "behavioral schemas." These structures are triggered automatically and rapidly.

Although automatic, these motivational–behavioral patterns can be brought under conscious control in many instances. The behavioral activations may arise independently of conscious intention and, indeed, may precede conscious awareness of the impulse to fight or flee, for example. The automatic mobilization and conscious impulse to flee or to fight are often contrary to the superordinate conscious control wishes. Bob, for example, desired strongly to be able to ride in the elevator without experiencing anxiety and an impulse to escape. He was able to express his conscious desire by overriding the unpleasant anxiety and automatic impulse through the application of his "conscious control system" (described below).

The *physiological system* is generally involved whenever a mode relevant to threat has been activated. In this discussion, I am referring not to the central nervous system activation (or inhibition) that underlies all psychological processes but to the innervation of the peripheral systems such as the autonomic nervous system, the motor systems, and the sensory systems. The physiological symptoms, accompanying anxiety or anger, for instance, are important not only because they enhance the impulse to flee or fight but also because of the interpretations ("I'm going to faint," "I can't stand this") placed on them. The physiological feedback from the muscles when the person is mobilized for action add to the feeling of being "charged up" (see Figure 1.1).

The *conscious control system* is the instrument of the more reflective, deliberate, conscious, and less automatic desires, goals, and values; for example, to be free of unreasonable fears, to set and attain reasonable goals, to solve problems. In contrast to the automatic reflexive impulses in the motivational and behavioral systems, these desires and goals are flexible and are not so peremptory. The system is also involved in procedural process-

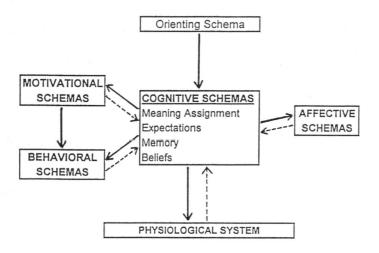

FIGURE I.I. Activation of the mode.

es such as applying logic to problems and engaging in long-term planning. This system is involved in setting controls on the primal systems, by, for example, correcting the "automatic thoughts" emanating from the primal cognitive system, withdrawing attention from unpleasant thoughts or memories, inhibiting dysfunctional impulses, or ignoring unpleasant affect. A major function is gaining perspective over the basic cognitive reactions.

This system allows the individual to form conscious intentions as well as to override primal thinking, affect, and motivation. Bob, for example, was able to force himself to enter the elevator despite his discomfort and powerful urge to escape. Through a therapeutic intervention, he could consciously reframe the threatening situation (i.e., the inferred danger) into a relatively innocuous encounter. The control system, thus, plays the role of evaluating the products of the primal cognitive processing (automatic fears, self-criticisms, blaming, etc.) by applying more adaptive, flexible, and mature thinking. The operation of this system has sometimes been labeled "metacognition," since it involves "thinking about thinking."

Activation of the numerous primal modes depends on the "demand characteristics" of a situation (e.g., a defensive mode, anxiety mode, evaluative mode, attacking or aggressive mode). The arousal of a particular mode is generally predictable from the presenting circumstances or, more precisely, the person's constructions or image of these circumstances.

The integrated systems of the primal modes are fashioned to achieve particular primal goals—in the example of Bob's phobia, survival. These particular modes are primal in the sense that they are oriented towards crucial goals such as survival, safety, and security and are essentially reflexive in nature. They also involve primal thinking, such as selective abstraction, dichotomous inferences, and overgeneralization (Beck, 1967). The interconnections of the systems in the "vulnerability mode," for example, lead to a buildup of anxiety and either inhibition or an impulse to avoid or escape from the threatening situation. Paradoxically, a pattern that is activated to *insure* safety often produces discomfort and possibly *threatens* safety by immobilizing the individual.

The concept of the mode has several advantages in explaining complex reactions such as an elevator phobia. This concept can account for the following: the regularity and homogeneity of an individual's specific phobic reactions and other dysfunctional reactions; the consistency in the cognitive content of these reactions; the multiplicity of symptoms across all systems; the low threshold for formation of symptoms in susceptible individuals; and the progressive sensitization to activating events.

NORMAL AND EXCESSIVE REACTIONS

Each of the clinical disorders can be characterized in terms of a specific primal mode that, when activated, draws on congruent systems to implement the "goal" of the mode. Consider the following observation: People experience discriminable, well-defined reactions that can be regarded as logical consequences of the activating circumstances. For example, a serious loss generally leads to a composite of sadness, memories of past losses, and, perhaps, some passivity and retardation.[4] A threat of impending disaster evokes a variety of symptoms such as catastrophic thinking, anxiety, and sleep disturbance. These reactions, with a characteristic individual flavor, are generally consistent when they are aroused. The broad symptom picture of the psychiatric disorder—or primal mode—can be understood in terms of the activation of the component of the various systems including cognition, affect, motivation, and behavior.

The specific primal reactions of a given patient, although consistent in form and content, vary in intensity and threshold. A severe reaction, for example, may follow a relatively mild stressful experience if there has been a previous succession of stressors. This phenomenon can be explained as a buildup of the charge (or energy) of the mode. A particular mode is generally silent or latent at first, but through successive relevant experiences can receive incremental charges until it reaches the threshold for full activation. In some psychopathological conditions—for example, recurrent depression—the mode is chronically but subliminally charged so that it can become fully activated after a comparatively minor stressful event (the kindling phenomenon). In some conditions, there may be a temporary reduction of the intensity of the charge through a conscious strategy; for example, panic attacks may be interrupted by distraction.[5]

The concept of the mode can also help to explain feelings of anxiety or distress that occur when the person is not consciously concerned about a particular threat. In Bob's case, for example, the impending encounter with an elevator activated the danger–vulnerability mode, accounting for his vague anxiety, but the cognitive content (i.e., fear of crashing, etc.) did not fully reach consciousness until he prepared to enter the elevator. The present model asserts that much data is processed implicitly (out of awareness) by the mode while those data requiring conscious implementation become conscious.

MODAL PROCESSING VERSUS SIMPLE SCHEMATIC PROCESSING

The cognitive component of the mode consisting of a number of interrelated elements such as core beliefs, compensatory rules, and behavioral strategies is more complex than the original simple linear model. The relevant visual, auditory, and other sensory data are processed simultaneously through multiple channels, as it were. In the primal mode, the highly focused information processing results in biased cognitive products.[6] A phobic mode, for example, by virtue of the dominant focus on the concept of danger, selectively abstracts and interprets data relevant to a specific danger. This biased cognitive processing is reflected in dichotomous thinking, overgeneralization, catastrophizing, and personalizing. Attentional resources are locked onto the specific content of the mode (e.g., in panic, on somatic or physiological experiences; in paranoia, on possible signs of personal abuse). In other words, the cognitive processes are driven by the activated cognitive schemas. As Epstein (1994) points out, however, these primal reactions are not necessarily dysfunctional and, indeed, may be lifesaving in certain situations.

The difference between simple schematic processing and modal processing is illustrated in the following example: A student arrives late to a classroom. The specific reactions of the other students are shaped by their idiosyncratic schemas; for example, concern for the late student, annoyance for the interruption, or gloating over the fact that he had missed some important instruction. These specific interpretations, as well as the affect, are usually transient. There is no mobilization to action and the students' attention can again be switched onto the lecture. The myriad of brief reactions like this can be explained by the simple schematic processing model.

When we analyze the scenario from the standpoint of the experience of the late student, however, a more complex model of cognitive processing is needed to account for the observations. On his way to class our student is determined to arrive on time because the lecture material will be covered in an examination. However, he is delayed because his automobile is in a traffic jam due to an accident on the highway and he realizes that he could miss the entire class.

These are the activating circumstances for the instigation of a fearful mode. Its orienting mechanism, related to the concept of vulnerability and danger, is a vital part of the cognitive organization. When a situation or circumstance is perceived as threatening physical or psychological security, the orienting mechanism activates the primal mode. The student starts to visualize a flood of terrible consequences of his being late: He will fail the examination, flunk out of school, be humiliated by the other students, end up in skid row. Memories of other students who failed accentuate his fears.

When a primal mode is activated, all of the systems (cognitive, affective, behavioral, physiological) remain energized for a period of time after the activating circumstances have disappeared. Thus, the tardy student remains anxious for a prolonged period of time even after he gets to class and is able to retrieve the material he missed. Similarly, the major dysfunctional modes like depression remain operative long after the precipitating event (e.g, a failure or a breakup in a relationship) has passed. The patient remains sad and withdrawn and the mode also continues to mold the patient's interpretations of his experiences according to its own negative content.

"CONSTRUCTIVE" OR "POSITIVE" MODES

Productive activities directed toward increasing vital resources may also be manifestations of primal modes. A very obvious example is the state of infatuation that facilitates fulfilling the evolutionary imperative of intimate bonding. Other expansive modes may be expressed in expanding resources through activities such as acquiring wealth and property. The *total engagement* in enhancing interpersonal and material resources is characteristic of the manic mode and is reflected in a bloated self-concept. In depression, the productive mode is de-energized and the self-concept is impoverished; part of treatment is directed toward priming this mode (either through pharmacotherapy or cognitive-behavioral intervention). Also included in the constructive mode is the kind of constructive thinking described by Epstein (1992).

Minor Modes

Until now, I have been discussing the major or primal modes, concerned with vital issues (such as danger, failure, and rejection). For most of our waking life, however, we experience minor modes in more prosaic activities such as our involvement in reading, conversing with others, or working. Our attention is focused on the immediate situation and the cognitive, affective, behavioral, and motivational systems are mobilized at a level sufficient to satisfy the demands of the situation. In contrast to the major or primal modes, these minor modes are not highly energized and are under flexible conscious control; for example, it is comparatively easy to switch from the studying or conversational mode to another (say, recreational) mode. This easy switch is not available in depression and other serious disorders.

RELATION OF MODES TO MOODS

The concept of mode may be used to replace the traditional concept of mood. Although there are similarities in these two constructs, I believe that the construct of the mode incorporates the main features of mood and has greater explanatory value than do the standard formulations.[7] Although some descriptions of mood allude to a cognitive component, the defining characteristic has been the presence of affect (sad, glad, scared, etc.). Further, moods have been viewed as transient states that simply have no specified function. In contrast, the concept of mode includes the specific functions not only of information processing but also of the other psychological systems in providing a specific integrated response to external demands as well as a mechanism for implementing one's goals.

The theory of mode also includes the concept of structure and charge (or energy) to explain the regularity with which specific states are aroused and their activation after intervals by progressively less intense stimuli (sensitization or kindling). In accordance with the concept of mode, a person in a "bad mood" (or mode) would not only feel angry but would perceive events as intrusive and offensive and would be disposed to snap at people without ostensible provocation.

In keeping with this present formulation, terms such as "mood disorders" would be translated into "mode disorders"; "mood induction experiments" become "mode induction"; and sayings such as "I'm in a bad mood" would become "I'm in a bad mode." This formulation does not preclude biological explanations for the instigation of the moods or mood disorders but would broaden their characterization as including the basic systems of the modes.

ACTIVATION OF THE MODES

In my earlier theorizing, I postulated a simple pathway from cognition to affect, motivation, and behavior (Beck, 1967, 1976). I proposed that a stimulus situation activated a cognitive schema, which then simultaneously activated motivation, affect, and behavior. According to my current formulation, the initial formation and development of the mode depends on the interaction of innate patterns ("protoschemas") and experience. These protoschemas simply provide the basic structures that respond selectively to congruent experiences and evolve into cognitive schemas in a way analogous to the development of specific language structures from the undifferentiated primitive language structures (Pinker, 1994). Thus, learning how to recognize and respond to real threats depends on the availability of the protoschemas and their exposure to relevant life experiences which then interact to produce differentiated schemas. Thus the preliminary framework of a dysfunctional mode is already in place *prior* to the onset of psychological disorders—for example, depression—and is then triggered by a congruent event such as a loss.

How is a particular mode activated by a congruent situation? When the individual perceives the relevant stimulus situation (the elevator, in Bob's case), or is in geographical or temporal proximity to it, an orienting schema assigns a preliminary meaning to the stimulus situation and activates the rest of the relevant mode (in this case, the "danger mode,") which is manifested clinically by the phobic reaction to the elevator. The matching of the orienting schema to the situation is an intricate process that occurs rapidly and, in the case of the danger situations, practically instantaneously.

The content of the orienting schemas may be likened to an algorithm that stipulates the necessary conditions for a "match." The terms of the algorithm are not applied in a stepwise progression but operate simultaneously in a global way as though fitted into a template. When these conditions are fulfilled, the schema is activated and, in turn, triggers the rest of the mode to which it is attached. The excitation spreads through the cognitive system of the mode to the affective, motivational, behavioral, and physiological systems (see Figure 1.1). This formulation has some similarities to Bower's network theory (1981)—especially in regard to the spread of excitation across the network—but is much more closely related to Mischel's and Shoda's (1995) formulation of cognitive–affective networks.

The "conscious control system" is separate from, and relatively independent of, the mode. When activated, this control system has the potential to override, or, more precisely, to de-energize the mode.

What is the role of the orienting schemas when the person is already in a clinical state (e.g., depression)? The orienting schema is still operating but requires much less "evidence" in order to make a match with (i.e., assign a meaning to) a stimulus situation. For example, in depression events that are either ambiguous or irrelevant may be interpreted in a negative way. The hypercharged negative schemas preempt the more normal schemas and stamp their own meaning on the event (see Beck, 1967, p. 285). Thus a depressed person may interpret a smile as patronizing, an expression of empathy, or a sign of disdain, and a transient separation from a significant person as an abandonment.

It should be emphasized that the primal modes are not necessarily dysfunctional. The mobilization of the entire psychobiological organization in time of real danger can be very adaptive, even lifesaving. Since the primal modes evolved in ancient environments, they can cause problems because they are not necessarily adapted to modern circumstances. The "niche" has changed and many of the derived strategies were better adapted to solving the crude primeval problems than the more complex problems of contemporary life. The danger mode, for example, originating in the dangerous conditions in prehistoric wilds, becomes mobilized when a threat is symbolic—for example, being negatively evaluated—but is experienced as though there is a serious threat to life (as might have been the case at one time).

MODES AND PSYCHIATRIC DISORDERS

The various psychopathological disorders can be conceptualized in terms of the primal modes. There are, for example, anxiety, depressive, hopeless-suicidal, panic, obsessive–compulsive, and specific phobic modes corresponding to each of the disorders or clinical problems (see Table 1.1). Also, the operation of modes may be observed in compulsive behaviors such as substance abuse, overeating, anorexia nervosa, compulsive hair pulling, or wrist slashing. Also, modes are obviously involved in paranoia and homicidal behavior (see Table 1.1).

Even the personality disorders can be formulated in terms of modes (Beck et al., 1990). When persons with dependent, histrionic, avoidant, or narcissistic personality disorders decompensate, they may slip into a hostile, depressive, anxious, or other mode. Personality disorders may also be characterized in terms of their habitual or prevailing modes that play an ongoing role in the patient's daily life. Thus dependent, avoidant, and histrionic personality disorders are characterized by persistent dependent, avoidant, and histrionic modes. In these disorders, the modes are operational most of the time and do not require a strong stimulus to activate them.

TABLE 1.1. Typical Cognitive, Affective, Behavioral, and Physiological Systems associated with Specific Diagnostic Categories

| Disorder | Primal systems | | | |
	Cognitive	Affective	Behavioral impulse	Physiological
Specific phobia	Specific danger	Anxiety	Escape or avoid	Autonomic nervous system activation
General fear	Generalized danger	Anxiety	Escape, avoid, inhibit	Same
(Hostility)[a]	Threatened, wronged	Anger	Punish	Same
Depression	Loss	Sad	Regress	Parasympathetic activation

[a]Although hostility has not been listed as a "mental disorder" in the current classifications, I believe that it should be included in order to account for individuals' excessive reactions leading to violence and homicide.

The cognitive organization within the various Axis I disorders may be analyzed in terms of major modes. These modes have the same cognitive structures as the conceptual formulations currently used in formulating a case. The cognitive organizations are composed of a hierarchy of beliefs labeled the "controlling cognitive constellation" (Beck et al., 1985) that form the framework for assigning meanings, interpretations, explanations, and expectations.

The *core beliefs* consist of the most sensitive component of the self-concept (e.g., vulnerable, helpless, inept, loveless, worthless) and the primitive view of others (rejecting, hostile, demeaning). The *conditional rules* (embedded in the "orienting schema") stipulate the conditions under which the core belief is applicable and, thus, becomes operative. The orienting rules correspond to the "if . . . then" behavioral rules described by Mischel and Shoda (1995). When the criteria for these rules have been fulfilled, the core belief or its derivative is either activated or enhanced. For example, Bob's conditional rule was: "If I take the elevator, I am likely to get killed." Thus, the decision to take the elevator fulfilled the conditions of the rule and activated the phobic mode centered in the core belief "I am vulnerable to physical disaster." Other examples of the conditional rules are:

"If I mingle with others, I will be rejected" (social anxiety).
"If I have an inexplicable sensation, it is a sign of a catastrophic internal danger" (panic).
"If I attempt to do anything, I will certainly fail at it" (depression).

The therapist can infer the unconditional *core beliefs* underlying those conditional rules: "I am friendless, unlovable," "physically vulnerable," and "useless, worthless"; other people are "rejecting," "critical," or "dangerous." (These core beliefs become fully conscious and often are experienced as ruminations when a person has a clinical depression but are more subtle in other conditions.)

The core beliefs are generally balanced by *compensatory rules*:

"If I avoid others, I can avoid rejection" (social anxiety).
"If I get medical attention right away, I can be saved" (panic).
"If I keep achieving, I am not worthless" (depression).

The compensatory rules lead to imperatives, injunctions, and prohibitions, such as "Work as hard as you can," "Don't stick your neck out," "Don't leave a safe haven."

In obsessive–compulsive disorder there are at least two core beliefs. First, "I (or other individuals linked to me in a causal pathway) am vulnerable to some external toxic condition." These threats are usually invisible, such as pathogenic microbes, radar, thought rays, toxic fumes, or even "evil thoughts," which can (according to the patient) cause disease, damage, or death. Allied to these threats is a second core belief: "I am responsible if I don't prevent the disaster."

The negative conditional rules in obsessive–compulsive disorder are (1) "If I (or someone linked to me) am exposed, then grave consequences will occur"; (2) "If I do not act to prevent the damage from any of these noxious or lethal agents, I am responsible (and blameworthy)." The *compensatory conditional rule* is "If I take appropriate measures, I can prevent the disaster from occurring." The *imperative rule* is "I must do everything I can to prevent this disaster from occurring."

The mode in obsessive–compulsive disorder may not be operational all the time. Nonetheless, the mode always carries some subthreshold charge until an additional charge provided by a stimulus situation (e.g., exposure to dirt) raises the charge above the threshold and the mode becomes fully operational. Thus when the conditions of the negative conditional rules are fulfilled, the mode is activated and the specific symptoms of obsessive–compulsive disorder become apparent. The same dynamics occur in other disorders such as generalized anxiety disorder and depression.

THERAPY: DISCHARGING AND MODIFYING THE MODES

There are three major approaches to "treating" the dysfunctional modes: first, deactivating them, second, modifying their structure and content, and third, priming or "constructing" more adaptive modes to neutralize them. In actual practice, the first and third procedures are carried out simultaneously for example, demonstrating that a particular belief is wrong or dysfunctional and that another belief is more accurate and adaptive. In addition, priming dormant problem-solving strategies (Nezu & Nezu, 1989) helps to activate the more "normal" adaptive mode.

The primal modes, particularly those corresponding to disorders such as panic, social anxiety, depression, and obsessive–compulsive can be discharged—that is, reduced to a quiescent level—through a variety of methods. In a normal adaptive reaction, the primal danger mode is activated when individuals perceive a set of conditions that seem to represent a real danger. If they recognize that their interpretation of "danger" was wrong, or when they determine the danger has passed, the primal mode is deactivated.

Suppose you are awakened from your sleep by strange noises that sound like an intruder in your bedroom. You become instantly mobilized to protect yourself. You then discover that the sounds are caused by the flapping of your venetian blinds. You calm down and go back to sleep: The danger mode activated by your interpretation of the sounds was discharged by your reinterpretation, based on more accurate information.

A somewhat different sequence occurs in the experience of patients with psychological disorders. For example, panic disorder patients learn that their panic attacks can be interrupted by distraction, by the transfer of their attention to some external stimulus. The charge of the panic mode is temporarily reduced below the threshold for activation and the symptoms subside. It should be noted, however, that in contrast to the normal reaction when a presumed danger has passed, the panic mode still carries a subthreshold (subliminal) charge and can be readily reactivated—that is, reach threshold—under the conducive circumstances; for example, experiencing an "unnatural sensation," such as a sudden chest pain.

The fluctuations in the charge of the mode are particularly obvious in phobic disorders, such as Bob's elevator phobia. When exposed to the problem of riding in the elevator, his danger mode becomes more highly charged (cathected) and he becomes anxious. If he chooses to use the stairs (i.e., he escapes from the phobic situation) the charge is reduced below threshold and he is no longer symptomatic. However, even thinking about riding the elevator can increase the charge of the mode above its activation threshold and produce anxiety, rapid breathing, and sweaty palms.

Other methods besides distraction can be temporarily effective in reducing the supraliminal charge of the primal mode. For example, the cathexis of the activated panic mode can be reduced to a subthreshold level during a panic attack by reassurance from a physician or other professional. The confident communication of corrective information leads to a more benign interpretation of the unnatural sensation and lowers the modal charge below the activation threshold. Depending on the source of anxiety or phobia, the persuasive information may simply be the assurance that there is no danger of suffocating in a tunnel, or losing control in a supermarket, or fainting on top of a tall tower.

The corrective information from an acknowledged authority not only contradicts the content (e.g., the fear) embodied in the mode but also activates a "safety mode," incorporating a more realistic belief (see Rachman, 1990). As this adaptive mode becomes cathected, it draws some of the charge away (temporarily) from fixation on the danger. However, the charge or safety mode is generally unstable and when the patient is exposed once again to the threatening stimuli, the danger mode becomes recharged above the activation threshold and the patient will experience his or her typical anxiety complex.

How does a therapist achieve a more durable modification of the content or structure of a mode? It seems that for such a lasting change to occur, it is necessary to achieve a substantial change in the underlying absolute and conditional rules that shape the individual's interpretations. For example, treatment studies have demonstrated that as the panic-prone patients' conditional rules regarding the explanation for their unnatural bodily sensations or psychological experiences are substantially and repeatedly repudiated, *and* a more credible explanation for these sensations is incorporated, they no longer experience panic attacks.[8]

The durable change in beliefs, for example, from "My mild chest pain is probably a heart attack" or "My faint feeling means I'm dying" to "This kind of transient chest pain is due to innocuous spasm of chest muscles" or "The faint feeling is a result of hyperventilation," not only produces rapid relief from panic attacks but also produces a kind of "immunity" from future attacks. The solid learning involved in a convincing demonstration of the unrealistic nature of the fears *plus* the incorporation of a more realistic belief form a solid protective wall against subsequent panic attacks.

This kind of corrective learning becomes "structuralized," that is, embodied in an adaptive mode. A crucial change occurs in the orienting schema. The formerly provocative conditions (e.g., lightheadedness or chest pain) no longer produce panic but evoke an adaptive meaning (such as, "My lightheadedness is a normal physiological reaction to overbreathing" or "My chest pain is simply tension in my chest muscles"). As the orienting schema (or rule) is changed, the infrastructure of absolute beliefs is modified. This modification is probably the paradigm for most corrective learning. In addition, the implicit knowledge embedded in the new adaptive mode inhibits the activation of the old dysfunctional beliefs that become inoperative, although not totally deleted. They can become charged again under uniquely stressful circumstances.

Modifying the depressive mode follows a route similar to that of phobias and panic disorder. Standard supportive interventions, for example, may defuse the core belief, "I am helpless" or "I am unlovable" (Beck, Rush, Shaw, & Emery, 1979). The therapist's interest and guidance transfers some of the cathexis from the "helpless" or "unlovable" belief to a more adequate, "likable" belief. Since this process does not, in itself, permanently change the dysfunctional beliefs, however, the disorder is subject to recurrence. Similarly, pharmacotherapy can neutralize the charge of the depressive mode but, since it does not alter the structure of the mode, it does not prevent recurrence of the disorder. The most durable change follows from changing the meaning assignment rules that equate, for example, a failure or a disappointment with being unlovable or powerless and substituting more precise rules regarding the meaning of a rebuff or a failure.

The basic cognitive–behavioral approaches to depression, consisting of assigning a structured activity program and emphasizing "mastery" and "pleasure" (Beck et al., 1979), help to prime the productive or adaptive mode that has been dormant during the depression. The priming of specific problem-solving and productive schemas counteract the regressive passivity. Activities such as graded task assignment, confronting and solving practical problems (including those created by the depression), demonstrate to the patients that they can do more than they believed and that they have more control over themselves than they realized. Thus, the core "inadequacy belief" is partially deactivated. The recognition, review, and reframing of the "automatic negative thoughts" also helps to energize reality testing as well as to modify the negative self-image.

Other cognitive skills, such as examining the evidence for an interpretation, exploring alternative explanations, and reinforcing (and recharging) reality testing, are also crucial in reducing the cathexis of the depressive mode. While applying these skills may be effective in interrupting the progression of depression and promoting recovery, it does not necessarily change the predisposition to depression. In order to forestall recurrence, it is necessary to modify the content of schemas and to apply the cognitive skills when dysfunctional interpretations arise. Barber and DeRubeis (1989) assert that the protection against recurrence of depression following successful cognitive therapy may be ascribed to the patients' learning the basic cognitive skills during therapy and then applying them when adverse circumstances arise.

The approach to modifying the *predisposition* to depression consists of changing the specific structural characteristics of the depressive mode. First, the kind of negative evaluations, originating in the orienting schemas, that trigger the mode and indeed are a component of the depressive mode are evaluated and modified. For example, if patients believe that their happiness and worth depend on continued success and recognition, they are is prone to overinvest in goal seeking. The more they value this attainment and equate their self-worth with achievement, the more vulnerable they are to any reversal or setback. Modifying the meaning assignment rules involves clarifying the role of personal success, for example, as only one part of living and not as *the* measure of the individual's worth. These changes in the patients' value systems lead to a stabilization of their self-esteem and self-image. By reducing the degree of ego-involvement in proving themselves successful, for example, they find that events become less important.

The fact that drugs appear to have the same impact as psychotherapy on the functioning of the modes is a problem that needs to be addressed. For example, improvements in depressive beliefs are observed following successful treatment by *either* cognitive therapy or pharmacotherapy (Simons, Garfields, & Murphy, 1984). Just as experiences such as gains, losses, or threats can activate an expansive, depressive, or vulnerable mode and psychological interventions can deactivate these modes, so pharmacological agents, such as amphetamines, tricyclics, and barbiturates, can have similar effects in charging, discharging, and inhibiting specific modes. With deference to the quandary of the mind–body problem, it is still possible to encompass these observations within the present theory: The modes are conceptualized as unitary structures. From a psychological perspective, they have the characteristics (structures, content, level of activation) already described. From a neurochemical perspective, the modes can be viewed as consisting of patterns of neural networks, as yet undefined. The activation of the psychological phenomena and the neural substrates occur as a unitary process, the psychological and neural aspects simply representing different perspectives of the same phenomenon.

The point of entry into the central nervous system and the *pathway* for activation (or deactivation) of the mode differs for drugs and life experience (including psychotherapy): Drugs affect the mode through direct entry into the brain via the bloodstream and modify neural activity. External events are funneled through sensory channels, such as vision and hearing, and after preliminary processing are transformed into the neural activity that culminates in the modal activation or deactivation. Irrespective of the point of entry—whether through sensory channels or through introduction of psychotropic materials into the brain—the effect is the same: The mode is deactivated.

The drawback to pharmacotherapy is that, although it can discharge or inhibit the dysfunctional mode, it does not produce any durable changes in the meaning assignment beliefs. Thus, at a later date, the confluence of predisposing and precipitating conditions can once again produce a recrudescence of the symptoms.

The therapeutic implications of the present discussion are relevant to the duration of therapy and the impact on the belief systems. In clinical practice, it is important to concentrate on modifying the dysfunctional beliefs as well as inculcating cognitive skills. Since patients vary in their "learning curves," the duration of therapy should be adapted to the individual requirements, particularly as indicated by changes in dysfunctional and constructive beliefs. Booster sessions following the completion of the formal course of therapy would also be indicated as a way of reinforcing the adaptive learning.

SUMMARY

The formulation of the theory of modes was prompted by my difficulty in accommodating various psychological and psychopathological phenomena to the simple schematic model of *stimulus → cognitive schema → motivation, affect,* and *behavior.* The notion of mode can provide a more complete explanation of the complexity, predictability, regularity, and uniqueness of normal and abnormal reactions. A model that encompasses a composite of cognitive, affective, and behavioral structures addresses the clinical phenomena and at the same time preserves the essential psychobiological unity of the organism. This new model, moreover, can clarify not only the form and content of psychiatric disorders but also their precipitation, oscillation, and remission.

The concept of modes represents a global expansion of simple schema theory and provides the scaffolding for an integrated theory of personality and psychopathology. Modes are conceived of as structural and operational units of personality that serve to adapt an individual to changing circumstances. The modes consist of a composite of cognitive, affective, motivational, and behavioral systems. The relevant components of these systems are unified within the mode and function synchronously as adaptational strategies. The modes can account for a variety of functions ranging from the relatively brief reactions in emergency situations to the more diverse and enduring phenomena such as affection, clinical depression, and prejudice.

It is clear that the cognitive organization in depression, for example, cannot be reduced to a few simple schemas, but consists of a complex array of schemas that vary along a number of dimensions such as accessibility (explicit or implicit) and potency or intensity (e.g., prepotent or latent). The conglomerate of schemas also includes broad belief categories such as self-image, expectations, imperatives, and memories. The content of these beliefs vary according to certain characteristics such as absolute or relative and conditional or unconditional.

As circumstances and demands change, a mode relevant to the changing situation is instigated. Although a mode is viewed as being generally activated by relevant external circumstances, some modes may be instigated by biological factors such as hunger or sexual arousal or by abnormal conditions such as bipolar affective disorders. Moods—reformulated as modes—may also be instigated by endogenous factors.

From a functional standpoint, it is more economical for an organism to have immediate access to a suborganization drawing on the relevant cognitive, affective, and motivational systems in a global fashion than to have to rely on a linear process of individual schemas and beliefs triggering congruent affect and motivations. Further, the availability of clusters of beliefs and memories facilitates parallel (i.e., global) processing so that the organism can respond almost instantaneously to all the relevant variables in a particular situation.

A new contribution to the theory is the concept of the "orienting schema." The orienting schema consists of a kind of algorithm that sets the conditions or circumstances necessary for activating the mode. Thus, a single glance at a threatening figure can set in motion a simultaneous evaluation of the personal relevance, context, risks, coping strategies, and prediction of outcome for a given strategy. As the mode is activated, the relevant coordinate schemas come into play and the affective motivational and behavioral systems are energized. Almost simultaneously, the organism becomes prepared for action that sets the conditions or circumstances necessary for activating the mode. Once the mode is activated, the variety of coordinate schemas come into play. The affective, motivational, and behavioral systems are activated simultaneously.

Irrespective of whether they are triggered by environmental events or by internal neuroendocrine factors, the modes operate as information processors of ongoing situations. Individuals continuously scan their internal and external milieu and when a particular set of conditions "fits" the algorithm or template of the orienting schema attached to a mode, the cognitive composite of the mode becomes charged. As the meaning is assigned to the situation by the cognitive schemas, the congruent affective, motivational, and behavioral systems become charged. The *content* of the cognitive schemas consists of rules, beliefs, and memories that mold the flow of information into the cognitive *products*: interpretation, predictions, and images. The initial cognitive *process* is generally outside of awareness but the products frequently proceed into awareness.

A fight (or hostile) mode, for example, may be activated by another person brandishing a club. The orienting belief attaches the label of "threat" and almost instantaneously energizes the fight mode: The initial impression includes a global representation of the risk, seriousness, and imminence of the threat and the individual coping resources (Beck et al., 1985). The appropriate components of the mode are activated—meaning: "being attacked"; affect: anger; motivation: urge to fight; behavior: mobilization for counterattack. There is also a physiological component to this kind of mode, specifically an activation of the autonomic nervous system, manifested by increased blood pressure, heart rate, and sweating.

Much of the cognitive processing in emergency situations occurs out of awareness, but generally there is a conscious cognitive product in the form of an image of the potential danger of being attacked. In general, the nonconscious processes occur as an automatic, practically reflex, immediate response to a threat and the conscious processing occurs as a slower response.

The conscious system registers the derivatives (thoughts, feelings, and wishes) of the reflexive components of the modes as well as the more reflective components. This component also consists of important phenomena such as the conscious sense of identity ("I" or "me"), choice, will, values, aesthetics, and curiosity. The conscious system is the most flexible and adaptable of the personality systems and functions (1) to override the automatic operations of a mode when it conflicts with conscious values and plans, (2) to provide more perspective on a situation, (3) to "reality test" the products (automatic inference and predictions), and (4) to provide for longer-term planning, changes in strategies, and goal setting. Thus, the interplay between the conscious system and the mode can proceed in a "top-down" as well as a "bottom-up" direction.

The notion of "energetics" (cathexis, charge) can explain the phenomena of activation and deactivation, lowering and raising of thresholds, and sensitization and desensitization. The concept of charge or cathexis can explain how a particular mode becomes more active with successive stimulus situations until it dominates the individual's functioning. This buildup can occur in "normal" circumstances, such as a profound hostile reaction after repeated insults, or abnormal reactions, such as clinical depression.

The concept of de-energizing and modifying the dysfunctional modes and constructing or reinforcing more adaptive modes can clarify such problems as remission and relapse and the appropriate choice of intervention. The model can also provide some insight into the relative value and specific applications of various therapeutic interventions such as distraction, skills training, and restructuring basic beliefs. The model also underscores the importance of a multifaceted approach to complex disorders such as depression, which requires a combination of interventions consolidated by "booster sessions" in order to defuse the dysfunctional mode and reinforce the adaptive mode. This construct also provides an explanation for the similarity and difference between cognitive therapy and pharmacotherapy. Cognitive therapy is more effective in protecting against relapse because it modifies the structure of the mode.

The content of a particular mode provides a clue as to whether an individual is experiencing a normal reaction or a clinical disorder. A prolonged state characterized by an extreme content out of proportion to provoking circumstances, and which fails to recede with a change in circumstances, suggests that a clinical disorder is present.

Each of the clinical disorders can be described in terms of a specific mode with idiosyncratic cognitive, affective, motivational, and behavioral properties. The symptoms are manifestations of these properties; for example, in the depressive mode there is preoccupation with loss (cognitive), sadness (affective), and general inertia and passivity (behavioral). A function of the depressive mode is conservation of resources and a function of the anxiety mode is immediate self-preservation. The other clinical disorders can also be understood in terms of the components of the specific mode. Their function can generally be viewed as an aberration or exaggeration of a normal adaptive process. Obsessive–compulsive disorder, eating disorder, or panic disorder, for example, may be viewed in this way.

In essence, the formulation of the concept of mode can provide an approach to a number of questions regarding the relation of the various psychological systems to each other, the relation of nonconscious to conscious functions, reactions to situational or endogenous variables, changes in the intensity and quality of feeling states, and relation of personality to psychopathology and the differential responsiveness of psychological disturbances to pharmacotherapy and cognitive therapy. This addition to the present cognitive theory can provide further clarification of normal and abnormal processes and can facilitate the refinement of intervention strategies.

ACKNOWLEDGMENTS

I am grateful for the very valuable feedback on earlier drafts of this chapter from Judith S. Beck, David A. Clark, David M. Clark, Cathy Flanagan, Robert Leahy, James Pretzer, Paul Salkovskis, John Teasdale, Jeffrey Young, and Larry Weiss.

NOTES

1. The physiological system is not so isomorphic with (i.e., it is at a different level of abstraction than) the other systems. However, in order to account adequately for the phenomena, it is necessary to mix physical constructs with the psychological.

A somewhat similar problem is posed with the concept of charge or cathexis of the schemas.

2. Teasdale's conceptual framework of Interacting Cognitive Subsystems (ICS), described in Chapter 2 (this volume), presents a far more detailed description of the various cognitive units, codes, and patterns than I present here. In this sense, his formulations are complementary to mine and provide a rich lode of testable hypotheses derived from cognitive science. Further, by drawing on the language as well as the concepts of cognitive psychology he helps to bridge the gap between the clinically derived formulations and those of the experimental disciplines.

3. The memories ascribed to the mode have been described in the literature as a specialized system recording "emotional events"; that is, the original experiences were associated with affect (McGaugh, Introini-Collison, Cahill, & Castellano, 1993).

4. Of course, in the final analysis, the *interpretation* of the event and the relevant circumstances determine the response. For a religious person, the death of a loved one, for example, may be framed as a happy event, as an entry into an eternally blissful afterlife.

5. The use of terms such as "charge," "cathexis," and "energy" should not be confused with the same words used in psychoanalytic theory. Freud conceived of hysteria, for example, as an expression of damned up energy attached to repressed ideas or memories. The symptomatic derivation of this repressed energy could be relieved through catharsis or abreaction of the affect. I use the terms in much the same way as Floyd Allport (1955, pp. 48–415) in his description of the activation and deactivation of sets. Although these terms have fallen into disuse, they add substantial explanatory power to structural models of personality and psychopathology. In a sense, the charging of modes may correspond to the neuronal activity of specific brain areas that have been demonstrated to correlate with mental functions such as energy, memory, and ruminations.

6. Biased thinking is not necessarily dysfunctional. In certain dangerous conditions, it is better to overreact than to underreact, to overinterpret danger, and to personalize certain threats.

7. English and English (1958) define mood as "a relatively mild emotional state, enduring or recurrent, . . . an internal state of readiness for a specific kind of emotional response; excited, joyful, depressed." The concept of mode covers both definitions.

8. An Oxford study showed that changes in health–disease rules were correlated with enduring cessation of attacks as well as recovery from the current period of multiple attacks (Clark et al., 1994).

REFERENCES

Allport, F. H. (1955). *Theories of perception and the concept of structure.* New York: Wiley.

Bandura, A. (1986). *Social foundations of thought and action: A social cognitive theory.* Englewood Cliffs, NJ: Prentice Hall.

Barber, J. P., & DeRubeis, R. J. (1989). On second thought: Where the action is in cognitive therapy for depression. *Cognitive Therapy and Research, 13,* 441–457.

Bargh, J. A., & Tota, M. E. (1988). Context-dependent automatic processing in depression: Accessibility of negative constructs with regard to self but not others. *Journal of Personality and Social Psychology, 54,* 925–939.

Bartlett, F. C. (1932). *Remembering*. Cambridge, UK: Cambridge University Press.

Beck, A. T. (1964). Thinking and depression: 2. Theory and therapy. *Archives of General Psychiatry, 10*, 561–571.

Beck, A. T. (1967). *Depression: Causes and treatment*. Philadelphia: University of Pennsylvania Press.

Beck, A. T. (1976). *Cognitive therapy and the emotional disorders*. New York: International Universities Press.

Beck, A. T., Emery, G., & Greenberg, R. L. (1985). *Anxiety disorders and phobias: A cognitive perspective*. New York: Basic Books.

Beck, A. T., Freeman, A., & Associates. (1990). *Cognitive therapy of personality disorders*. New York: Guilford Press.

Beck, A. T., Rush, A. J., Shaw, B. F., & Emery, G. (1979). *Cognitive therapy of depression*. New York: Guilford Press.

Beck, A. T., Wright, F. D., Newman, C. F., & Liese, B. S. (1993). *Cognitive therapy of substance abuse*. New York: Guilford Press.

Bower, G. H. (1981). Mood and memory. *American Psychologist, 36*, 129–148.

Clark, D. M., Salkovskis, P. M., Hackman, A., Middleton, H., Anastasiades, P., & Gelder, M. (1994). A comparison of cognitive therapy, applied relaxation and imipramine in the teatment of panic disorder. *British Journal of Psychiatry, 164*, 759–769.

Dobson, K. F., & Kendall, P. (1993). *Psychopathology and cognition*. New York: Academic Press.

Dweck, C. S., & Leggett, E. L. (1988). A social-cognitive approach to personality and motivation. *Psychological Review, 95*, 453–472.

English, H. B., & English, A. C. (1958). *A comprehensive dictionary of psychological and psychoanalytical terms*. New York: Longman.

Epstein, S. (1992). Constructive thinking and mental and physical well being. In L. Montada, S. H. Filipp, & M. J. Lerner (Eds.), *Life crises and experiences of loss in adulthood*. Hillsdale, NJ: Erlbaum.

Epstein, S. (1994). Integration of the cognitive and psychodynamic unconscious. *American Psychologist, 49*, 709–724.

Haaga, D. A., Dyck, M.J., & Ernst, D. (1991). Empirical status of cognitive theory of depression. *Psychological Bulletin, 110*, 215–236.

Higgins, E. T. (1996). Knowledge activation: Accessibility, applicability, and salience. In E.T. Higgins & A. W. Kruglanski (Eds.), *Social psychology: Handbook of basic principles* (pp. 133–168). New York: Guilford Press.

Kelly, G. (1955). *The psychology of personal constructs* (Vols. 1 & 2). New York: Norton.

Kihlstrom, J. F. (1990). The psychological unconscious. In L. A. Pervin (Ed.), *Handbook of personality: Theory and research* (pp. 445–464). New York: Guilford Press.

McGaugh, J. L., Introini-Collison, I. B., & Cahill, L. F., Castellano, C. (1993). Neuromodulatory systems and memory storage: Role of the amygdala. Special issue: Emotion and memory. *Behavioral Brain Research, 58*, 81–90.

Mischel, W., & Shoda, Y. (1995). A cognitive–affective system theory of personality: Reconceptualizing the invariances in personality and the role of situations. *Psychological Review, 102*, 246–248.

Nezu, A. M., & Nezu, C. M. (1989). *Clinical decision making in behavior therapy: A problem-solving perspective*. Champagne, IL: Research Press.

Pervin, L. A. (1994). A critical analysis of current trait theory. *Psychological Inquiry, 5*, 103–113.

Piaget, J. (1950). [*Psychology of intelligence*] (M. Piercy & D. E. Berlyne, Trans.). New York: Harcourt, Brace. (Original work published 1947)

Pinker, S. (1994). *The language instinct: How the mind creates language.* New York: Morrow.

Rachman, S. (1990). The determinants and treatment of simple phobias. *Advances in Behaviour Research and Therapy, 12*, 1–30.

Segal, Z., & Ingram, R. E. (1994). Mood priming and construct activation in tests of cognitive vulnerability to unipolar depression. *Clinical Psychology Review, 14*, 1033.

Simons, A., Garfields, S., & Murphy, G. (1984). The process of change in cognitive therapy and pharmacotherapy for depression. *Archives of General Psychiatry, 41*, 45–51.

Teasdale, J. D., & Barnard, P. J. (1993). *Affect, cognition, and change: Re-modelling depressive thought.* Hove, UK: Erlbaum.

Williams, M. G., Watts, F. N., McLeod, C., & Matthews A. (1988). *Cognitive psychology and emotional disorders.* New York: Wiley.

Woody, S., & Rachman, S. (1994). Generalized anxiety disorder (GAD) as an unsuccessful search for safety. *Clinical Psychology Review, 11*, 743–753.

Chapter 2

Clinically Relevant Theory: Integrating Clinical Insight with Cognitive Science

John D. Teasdale

"What kind of theory will improve psychological treatment?" This question provided the title and focus of a book chapter that I wrote in the early 1980s (Teasdale, 1982). In that chapter, I looked at the initial rapid success and development of behavior therapy and argued that this was the result, in no small measure, of the fruitful interaction that existed between behavioral formulations and treatments of problems, on the one hand, and the experimental paradigms of learning and conditioning on the other. The existence of a shared conceptual framework across these two domains allowed clinicians to draw on the theoretical models, empirical findings, and methods of measurement developed by experimentalists, to the mutual benefit of both parties. At the time I wrote the chapter, I argued that, in the case of depression, there was nothing that quite corresponded to a shared conceptual framework, or paradigm, that could act as a fruitful interface between the clinical and experimental domains.

Much the same might be said of the situation today. Beck and his colleagues have made truly great advances in developing the cognitive approach to understanding and treating depression. Future historians of the field will undoubtedly single out this work as one of the most important turning points that revised, radically, our approach to this disorder. Nonetheless, the cognitive model underlying cognitive therapy is expressed in essentially lay, or everyday, terms, rather than within the terms of any of the conceptual frameworks developed within cognitive psychology or cognitive science. In many ways this has been a strength rather than a handicap; the ready communicability and commonsensicality of aspects of the cognitive model have probably been one factor contributing to the dramatically successful rise of cognitive therapy. However, commonsensical versions of the cognitive model are not without their problems. At one level, such accounts strain to give convincing accounts of key phenomena, such as the fact that measures of dysfunctional attitudes, often assumed to represent stable underlying cognitive vulnerabilities, are very powerfully influenced by mood states (e.g., Haaga, Dyck, & Ernst, 1991). At another level, everyday language is not a suitable vehicle for expressing some of the subtleties of the working hypotheses, often implicit, that guide successful and creative cognitive therapists. There often seems to be a danger, using everyday concepts such as rules and beliefs as approximate tags to refer to more subtle and complex underlying concepts, that our theories may get trapped and limited by the language in which we express them. Further, such accounts do not provide a particularly permeable interface through which the findings and concepts of cognitive science can fruitfully interact with those of clinicians.

I shall describe a conceptual framework, rooted in cognitive psychology and cognitive science, that may go some way to meeting the need for more precise articulation of the insights and ideas that have so fruitfully guided the development of the clinical cognitive movement to date. The framework is not as closely bound to particular experimental phenomena as the paradigms that guided the initial development of behavior therapy. However, it shares with them the advantage over more "everyday" conceptual schemes of more precise articulation and specification of constructs in a way that facilitates interaction with experimental disciplines and allows us to frame alternative explanations of complex phenomena. Equally, it can do justice to the richness of clinical hunch and observation, often providing an analysis of phenomena that comes closer to the "working models" that guide clinicians than theories expressed in more everyday language. Most importantly, it provides a fresh view of phenomena that, with a suitable admixture of clinical insight and inspiration, can lead to the development of novel approaches to treatment and prevention.

In this chapter, I shall concentrate on communicating ideas. The empirical basis for those ideas is presented at length by Teasdale and Barnard (1993).

THE INTERACTING COGNITIVE SUBSYSTEMS (ICS) FRAMEWORK

Interacting Cognitive Subsystems (ICS) comprises a comprehensive conceptual framework, within which, in principle, accounts of all aspects of information processing can be developed. Originally developed by Barnard (1985), this framework has recently been extended and elaborated specifically to incorporate emotion and has been applied to the analysis of emotional disorders, notably depression (Teasdale & Barnard, 1993).

ICS is based on a few, basically simple, ideas. The first is that, in order to do justice to what we know about the way the mind works, we have to recognize that there are qualitatively different kinds of information, or mental codes. Each of these codes represents a distinct aspect of experience.

So, in ICS, certain codes represent the information of relatively "raw," "un-digested" sensory experience, such as patterns of light, shade, and color; the pitch, timbre, and temporal patterns of sounds; and the patterns of propri-oceptive stimulation arising from the musculature and other internal sen-sory organs. Other codes represent recurring regularities that have been extracted from the patterns of sensory codes created by individuals over the course of their life experience. So, for example, a speech-level code cap-tures the features that are common to particular words, irrespective of the loudness or accent with which they are spoken, so that only the essential "wordness" is retained, and other, more superficial, sensory features are discarded. Similarly, a visual object code captures underlying patterns that have recurred in the patterns of visual sensory codes. This code would represent, for example, "sphericity" or "behindness." Recurring patterns in speech-level and visual object codes are, themselves, represented by codes that represent meanings. ICS distinguishes two kinds of meaning, a rela-tively specific and a more generic. As this distinction is particularly impor-tant for the present discussion, it will be considered in greater detail shortly.

The second basic idea of ICS is that there are processes that transform information from one kind of code to another. The conversions performed by these transformation processes are "learned" on the basis of regularities and covariations in the patterns of information codes previously encoun-tered in the system's experience. So, for example, one process, when it receives a particular pattern of sound sensory information as input, will produce a pattern of speech-level code corresponding to the word "good" as output. The same process, on receiving a different pattern of sound sensory infor-mation, will produce as output a pattern of speech-level code correspond-ing to the word "live." Similarly, another process, when it receives a pattern typical of previous loss-related situations in the information code representing high-level meanings, will produce, as output, patterns of effector code that will produce components of the depressive emotional reaction.

The final basic idea of the ICS approach is that all the patterns of in-formation codes created are stored in memory, with separate memory sys-tems for each of the different mental codes. For example, following a conversation, multiple records of that event will exist—in the speech-level store will be representations corresponding to the words uttered during the conversation, in the specific meaning store will be representations correspond-ing to the specific meanings derived during the conversation from sentences including those words, and in the high-level meaning store will be represen-tations corresponding to the high-level interpretations (e.g., of threat, at-traction, or "hidden agendas") created in relation to the total conversation experience. The information stored in memory records is accessed not only at times of obvious "remembering," but also in the course of extended process-ing operations, such as those involved in understanding a current situation or in predicting future states of affairs.

In the ICS cognitive architecture, the transformation processes that convert patterns of information in one code to patterns of information in another code, and the code-specific memory stores, are arranged in nine cognitive subsystems. Each subsystem is specialized for processing input in a given information code; all the transformation processes that take input in that code are included in the subsystem, as are the memory records that store representations of all the information entering the subsystem in that code.

Within ICS, information processing involves the transformation of patterns in one information code into patterns in another information code. Extended information processing involves a continuing flow and exchange of data between subsystems, in the course of which the nature of the information processed is repeatedly modified as a result of the actions of transformation processes and the contributions from memory stores. Such processing will often involve reciprocal transformations that, for example, create high-level meanings from patterns of low-level meanings and then create new low-level meanings from those high-level meanings. Information processing can take as input either "externally" derived patterns of sensory information originating in environmental events or "internally" derived patterns of information arising from previous processing or from access to memory.

MEANING IN ICS

ICS recognizes *two* levels of meaning, a specific and a more generic level. Patterns of *Propositional* code represent specific meanings in terms of discrete concepts and the relationships between them, for example, the specific meaning behind the speech form "Roger has brown hair." Meaning at this level can be grasped relatively easily as there is a fairly direct relationship between language and concepts at this level. Propositional meanings have a truth value that can be assessed. That is, they convey information about specific states of the world that can be verified by reference to evidence.

Patterns of *Implicational* code represent a more *generic, holistic* level of meaning. Meaning at this level is difficult to convey because it does not map directly onto language. Traditionally, attempts to convey such holistic meanings by language have taken the form of poems, parables, and stories. This generic level of representation encodes recurring very high-order regularities across all other information codes. ICS proposes that only this generic level of meaning is directly linked to emotion. Implicational meanings cannot be evaluated as simply true or false in the same way that more specific Propositional meanings can. ICS suggests that, subjectively, synthesis of generic meanings is marked by experience of particular holistic "senses" or "feelings" with implicit meaning content: "something wrong," "confidence," "on the right track," "hopelessness."

Reflecting the fact that patterns of Implicational code represent recurring patterns extracted across *all* other codes, sensory features, such as tone of voice or proprioceptive feedback from facial expression or bodily arousal, make a *direct* contribution to Implicational meanings, together with patterns of specific meanings. So, the higher-order meanings we derive from the specific meanings conveyed in what someone is telling us may be directly influenced by the actual sounds of the words, whether the speaker's voice tone is tense and strained rather than warm and relaxed, and whether, at a bodily level, we are calm and alert rather than tired and uncomfortable.

Coherent patterns of Implicational code represent schematic models of experience. Mental models, in general, represent the interrelationships between semantic elements (Johnson-Laird, 1983). *Schematic* models represent inter-relationships between *generic* features of experience, capturing very high-level recurring regularities in the world, the body, and "the mind." These models are about what goes with what at a high level of abstraction. Just as mathematical models, provided with the input of a given set of values on a number of variables, will compute a particular set of output values, so schematic models produce outputs that reflect the implications computed from the state of the information that they have taken as input.

The knowledge in schematic models is implicit rather than explicit. For example, presented with a text conveying the specific meanings "John knocked the glass off the table. Mary went to the kitchen to fetch a broom," the ["brokenness"][1] schematic model will be synthesized. This model encodes all the high-order recurring regularities that have previously been extracted from experiences involving breakage of fragile objects. The implicit knowledge inherent in this schematic model allows us to immediately infer the specific meaning that the glass was broken, without recourse to any explicit rules such as "If something is knocked, and someone goes for a cleaning implement, then the thing must be broken."

Some "feel" for representations at the Implicational level can be gained by considering the analogy between a sentence and a poem. A sentence conveys one or more specific meanings by appropriate arrangements of letters or phonemes in the appropriate sequence. A poem conveys "holistic" meanings that cannot be conveyed by single sentences by arranging sentences in appropriate sequences, together, very importantly, with appropriate direct sensory contributions from the sounds of the words, the rhythms, and meters of the whole, and from the visual imagery elicited.

The total meaning conveyed by a poem is qualitatively different from the sum of the separate specific meanings, just as the meaning of a sentence is qualitatively different from that of its component letters or words. This is illustrated in Table 2.1, where an extract of a poem is presented. The holistic meaning created by the poetry is marked by a "sense" of melancholy and abandonment. Table 2.1 also includes a prose version that retains the same sequence of specific level meanings, but the ways in which they are expressed lack the coherence, evocative sound qualities, and imagery of the poem. The total effect of the prose version is quite different!

Table 2.1 can also be used to illustrate the implicit knowledge inher-

TABLE 2.1. Poetry as Implicational Meaning

"O what can ail thee, knight-at-arms,
Alone and palely loitering?
The sedge has wither'd from the lake,
And no birds sing."

"What is the matter, armed old-fashioned soldier,
standing by yourself and doing nothing with a pallid expression?
The reed-like plants have decomposed by the lake
and there are not any birds singing."

Note. The original poem in the upper part of the table and the alternative version in the lower part have the same sequence of propositional meanings. However, only the original version conveys a coherent Implicational "sense." From Teasdale and Barnard (1993, p. 73). Copyright 1993. Reprinted by permission of Erlbaum (UK) Taylor & Francis, Hove, UK.

ent in the schematic models created by the poem. If one reads the poetry aloud, gets the "sense" that it conveys, and then answers the question "Would he be fun to meet at a party?," one can answer the question very directly and immediately by consulting the implicit knowledge of the schematic model constructed. By contrast, if one reads the prose version and then answers the question, most likely one will have to do this piecemeal, considering each of the propositions in turn and arriving at a judgment more slowly and "rationally."

ICS AND EMOTIONS

How, within the ICS framework, are emotions produced? According to ICS, affect-related schematic models play a central role in the production and maintenance of emotional states. In the same way that Implicational schematic models, in general, encode the features extracted as prototypical from classes of experience, emotion-related schematic models encode features extracted as prototypical of previous situations eliciting a given emotion. When, subsequently, in the course of information processing, patterns of Implicational code corresponding to such models are synthesized, the corresponding emotion is produced. So, for example, synthesis of schematic models encoding themes extracted as prototypical of previous depressing situations, such as ["globally negative view of self"] or ["hopeless, highly aversive, uncontrollable situation that will persist indefinitely"], will lead to production of a current depressed emotional state.

Within ICS, the ability to elicit directly an emotional response is restricted to affect-related schematic models; emotion-related representations in other information codes only contribute to emotion production to the extent that they feed the production of such models. Relatedly, ICS restricts the capacity to elicit emotion to the more generic of the two levels of meaning that it recognizes (Teasdale, 1993). Meanings at this level may include substantial contributions from sensorily derived elements. Consequently, sensory inputs can make a *direct* contribution to the synthesis of high-level affect-related meanings, and so to the production of emotion. For example, patterns of loss-related low-level meanings that may create depressogenic ["hopeless–self-devaluative"] schematic models in conjunction with bodily feedback indicating sluggishness, bowed posture, and frowning expression might create more acceptant or coping models (meanings) in conjunction with feedback indicating bodily alertness, erect, dignified posture, and half-smiling expression.

Although based on a few simple principles, the ICS approach, in application, can become quite complex, reflecting the intricacies and subtleties of human information processing (Teasdale & Barnard, 1993). The basic account just presented will be elaborated as I consider the maintenance and treatment of depression. Application of ICS yields an analysis that retains the centrally important insights of the original clinical cognitive model, but expresses them in a more systematic framework that also suggests the importance of factors emphasized in more recent developments of cognitive therapy. ICS has the further advantage that accounts of depression are expressed in terms of a general-purpose information-processing explanatory framework, so allowing us to draw on more general conclusions and findings from cognitive psychology.

ICS AND DEPRESSION

Maintenance of Depression

As already noted, ICS suggests that synthesis of an emotion-related schematic model is the immediate antecedent to the production of an emotional response. If that emotional response is to be sustained, the relevant emotion-related schematic model has to be repeatedly resynthesized. It follows that maintenance of a depressed state depends on the continuing production of depressogenic schematic models from patterns of specific meanings and patterns of sensorily derived input. The ICS account is essentially dynamic; if the production of depressogenic models ceases (e.g., as a result of the production of alternative, nondepressogenic schematic models), then the depressed state will lift.

What keeps the production of depressogenic models going? One obvious possibility is that a continuing stream of severe loss events or difficulties from the environment will be sufficient to provide a flow of externally derived information that will lead to repeated synthesis of depression-maintaining schematic models. However, it often appears that depression is maintained by more minor negative events that, if encountered in a nondepressed state, would not elicit much of a depressive response. At other times, depression seems to be maintained, not so much by negative environmental events, as by persistent streams of negative, ruminative thoughts. ICS suggests that, in all these situations, any contribution to the production of depressogenic schematic models from environmental events is substantially enhanced, prolonged, or even supplanted by cognitive processes that support the "internal maintenance" of depression. The ICS analysis suggests that such internal maintenance depends, to a considerable extent, on the establishment of self-perpetuating processing configurations that continue to regenerate depressogenic schematic models. Figure 2.1 illustrates such a configuration. For simplicity, the contributions to model synthesis from concurrent environmental events have been omitted from this figure.

In the configuration shown in Figure 2.1, the outputs generated from depressogenic schematic mental models "feedback" to regenerate schematic models similar to those from which the outputs were derived. Feedback loops involving contributions to model synthesis both from patterns of specific meanings and from proprioceptive, sensory input form parts of this self-maintaining configuration.

The "cognitive loop" shown in Figure 2.1 depends on the reciprocal relationship that exists, within ICS, between generic, Implicational representations, and specific, Propositional representations. On the one hand, Implicational schematic models produce, as outputs, specific Propositional

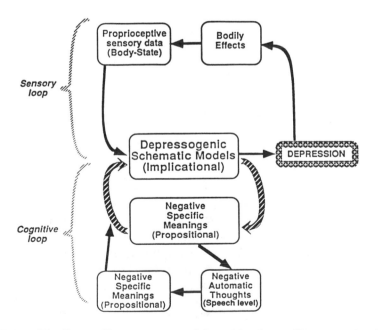

FIGURE 2.1. The "internal" maintenance of depression by a self-perpetuating "interlocked" processing configuration. The central engine of cognition (Implicational–Propositional–Implicational cycles) is shown as broad, hatched arrows.

meanings; on the other hand, patterns of specific meanings provide one of the major sources of input from which Implicational schematic models are synthesized. Given such a reciprocal relationship, there is an inherent possibility that the exchange of information between the Propositional and Implicational subsystems can "settle" into a pattern in which only a narrow range of thematically related cognitive contents are processed. It is suggested that such a situation arises in the cognitive loop of the depression-maintaining configuration illustrated in Figure 2.1. Here, depressogenic schematic models output negative specific meanings (negative predictions for the future, attributions of failures to personal inadequacy, negative evaluations of interpersonal interactions, retrieval cues to access memories of previous failures or difficulties, etc.). These outputs will often be components of motivated processing routines, directed (ineffectually) at obtaining highly valued goals that can neither be attained nor relinquished (see Teasdale & Barnard, 1993, Chap. 14; and cf. Pyszczynski & Greenberg, 1987). Because they encode specific negative meanings, these outputs, after further processing, may act to regenerate further depressogenic schematic models, similar to those from which the outputs were derived. For example, a schematic model related to the theme ["self as a worthless, useless, incompetent person whose actions will probably fail but who has to keep seeking others' approval"] might output specific meanings related to attributions of personal inadequacy for a particular recent failure experience. Such specific meanings (e.g., "It's because I'm no good as a person that I failed at X [or that Y dislikes me]") are, of course, likely to fuel further synthesis of "globally negative self" models on the next processing cycle. These negative specific meanings may also (but not necessarily) be experienced, downline, as streams of "negative automatic thoughts" as a result of the operation of transformation processes that generate patterns of speech-level code from patterns of specific meanings (Figure 2.1).

The cognitive loop shown in Figure 2.1 becomes established when the reciprocal interaction between the cognitive subsystems handling generic (Implicational) and specific (Propositional) levels of meaning becomes "locked" onto processing a limited range of thematically related negative contents. This locked processing, supplemented to a greater or lesser extent by information arising from concurrent environmental input, acts to maintain synthesis of a class of related, depressive, Implicational schematic models, and to perpetuate the depressed state. Such a locked configuration is particularly likely to become established with globally negative schematic models of self (["self as totally worthless, useless, helpless person"]) or future (["future totally hopeless, devoid of any satisfaction or relief"]). Such global models, as well as producing depressed states of considerable intensity, can also be reinstated by inputs corresponding to a wide range of negative specific meanings. Consequently, considerable variations in the specific content of the negative information circulating round the cognitive loop can still lead to continued maintenance of the locked configuration, and of the depressed state. Consistent with this analysis, depression is, of course, associated with the experience of negative thoughts reflecting globally negative views of self, world, and future (Haaga et al., 1991); Beck's negative cognitive triad.

Figure 2.1 also shows a sensory loop. Here, depressogenic schematic models produce the bodily components of a depressive emotional response, such as reduced arousal and activation; bowed and stooped posture; tearful, sad, frowning expression; and so forth. These responses lead to sensorily derived (*Body-state*) informational elements that, because they have been associated with the synthesis of depressogenic schematic models and the production of depression in the past, can contribute to the current synthesis of further depressogenic schematic models. These models will again produce depressive responses in the body. In this way, the sensory loop, in conjunction with the cognitive loop, can act to perpetuate the "depressive interlock" configuration maintaining the production of depression.

The ICS analysis suggests that vulnerability to onset or relapse of severe or persistent depression will depend on the ease with which interlocked configurations, of the type illustrated in Figure 2.1, will develop in situations of mild negative affect. It is also suggested that the risk of interlock is particularly high for globally negative models of the self or future. Consistent with these suggestions, vulnerability to disabling depression is associated with elevated scores on measures of global negative self-view, administered in mildly depressed mood (Teasdale & Dent, 1987). Similarly, vulnerable individuals score higher than normal controls, when both groups are tested in states of mild depression, on measures of dysfunctional attitudes indicating a dependence of global personal worth on specific approval- or achievement-related events (Miranda & Persons, 1988; Miranda, Persons, & Byers, 1990).

The ICS analysis of the internal maintenance of depression provides a basis from which we can now consider, in more detail, aspects of the ICS approach to understanding and treating depression.

ICS and the Role of Negative Thoughts in the Maintenance and Treatment of Depression

Within the ICS framework, the subjective experience of thoughts in verbal form is associated with production of corresponding patterns in speech-level mental code. Subjective experience of thoughts in visual image form is associated with production of corresponding patterns in visual object code. In both cases, subjectively experienced thoughts will have been created as "downline" products of related specific meanings. These specific meanings, in turn, will have been derived either as outputs from schematic models encoding high level meanings, or from the processing of inputs in speech-level or visual object codes.

Some earlier statements of the clinical cognitive model implied that depression was a consequence of the experience of negative automatic thoughts. By contrast, the ICS analysis, summarized in Figure 2.1, sees surface-level negative thoughts, available to awareness, as having no *direct* or necessary role in the production of depression. Such thoughts may give conscious access to the information circulating around the depression-maintaining configuration, and may contribute, indirectly, via the production of negative specific meanings, to the synthesis of depressogenic schematic models. However, in the ICS analysis, the primary antecedent to the production of a depressed emotional response is the synthesis of depressogenic schematic models, rather than the experience of negative thoughts or the production of negative specific meanings.

In many situations, of course, depression will be maintained by an integrated self-perpetuating processing configuration that includes important components at the levels of depressogenic schematic models, depression-related specific meanings, and negative automatic thoughts, as in Figure 2.1. However, from the ICS perspective, it is not surprising that, in cognitive therapy for example, it may sometimes be difficult to identify any negative thoughts preceding the onset of depressed feelings (or, any thoughts with content consistent with the severity of the emotional response). Depression can be maintained by the continuing synthesis of depressogenic schematic models without the processing of those models being necessarily reflected in awareness of corresponding content at the level of consciously accessible negative automatic thoughts.

Relatedly, the ICS analysis has implications for the significance of consciously accessible thoughts in psychological treatment. This analysis suggests that the primary goal of treatment should be to replace synthesis of the depressogenic schematic models maintaining depression with the synthesis of alternative, nondepressogenic models. On the ICS view, there is a place for modifying thoughts and images, but only if, in doing so, one achieves change at the level of higher-order meanings:

First, it may be that procedures that successfully modify negative thoughts also modify the "parent" schematic models from which the thoughts were derived. In this situation, the thoughts and images act as useful "markers" of the state of the target of ultimate interest.

Second, just as making small changes to the sequence of letters making up a sentence can radically alter the specific meaning it represents ([The man said "GO ON"] vs. [The man said "NO GO"]), so changing just a small portion of a total pattern of Implicational code may be sufficient to alter radically the high-level meaning represented. In this way, the effect of changing a thought and its related specific meaning may, by changing a discrete corresponding section of an affect-eliciting Implicational code pattern, be sufficient to change emotional response. For example, for someone who has synthesized the high-level meaning ["self-as-a-total-failure"] following failure on an examination, helping him or her discover that 95% of other candidates also failed may create changes in the related parts of the total Implicational pattern that, although limited, are sufficient to create a radically different higher-order meaning.

Third, the very action of attempting to deal with negative thoughts, in common with other active coping procedures, may lead to the synthesis of schematic models related to "taking control." These would replace the schematic models related to themes of helplessness and hopelessness that otherwise maintain depression (see Teasdale & Barnard, 1993, Chap. 16, for a fuller discussion of these issues). Further implications of the ICS analysis for psychological treatment of depression are discussed in a later section.

"Emotional" versus "Intellectual" Belief

Depressed patients will often say something like "I know, rationally, that I'm not worthless but I don't believe it emotionally." In discussing this question, the standard text on cognitive therapy of depression advises: "Patients often confuse the terms 'thinking' and 'feeling' . . . the therapist can tell the patient that a person cannot believe anything 'emotionally' . . . when the patient says he believes or does not believe something emotionally he is talking about *degree of belief*" (Beck, Rush, Shaw, & Emery, 1979, p. 302, italics in original). Such statements of the clinical cognitive model appear to reject any distinction between *kinds* of meaning; it is suggested that, in the contrast of "intellectual" versus "emotional" belief, we are dealing simply with *quantitative* variations of a single level of meaning. Further, it often seems that the level of meaning that the clinical model has in mind is specific — propositional statements that have a truth value that can be determined. The goal of therapy is then to invalidate the truth value of specific depressive meanings.

By contrast, the ICS analysis proposes a *qualitative* distinction between two kinds of meaning and suggests that only the more generic, holistic level of Implicational meaning, corresponding to "emotional" or "intuitive" belief, is directly linked to affect. ICS suggests that change at the level of Implicational schematic models should be the prime target of therapy. We noted earlier that the contrast between Propositional and Implicational meaning was analogous to the contrast between a sentence and a poem. Applying this analogy to the task of therapy, we can see that, according to ICS, the goal should be to help the patient to write a different poem, rather than merely to rewrite single sentences of his or her existing poem. However, as noted in the preceding section, there will also be situations in which, by rewriting one or more single sentences, we effectively write a different poem.

By articulating the difference between two kinds of meaning, ICS provides a perspective on the difference between "hot" and "cold" cognition more generally. Propositional representations of emotion-related information cannot, alone, elicit emotion. Processing of such specific Propositional representations would be associated with cold consideration of emotion-related material. Hot processing of emotion-related material depends on the synthesis of appropriate generic level meanings in Implicational code. Relatedly, intellectual belief or "knowing with the head" is equated with agreement or disagreement with specific Propositional meanings, whereas emotional or intuitive belief, "knowing with the heart," is related to the state of holistic Implicational representations.

Dissociations between "head"-level Propositional knowledge and "heart"-level Implicational knowledge are wholly consistent with the ICS analysis. A given specific meaning is only one of a potentially large number of contributors to the synthesis of a schematic model. Consequently, in Figure 2.1, for example, it is quite possible for the left-hand lower box to contain Propositional representations indicating that there is evidence logically inconsistent with the proposition "I am a total failure as a person" without this necessarily having much impact in preventing the subsequent synthesis, from a much wider array of information, of a ["self-as-total-failure"] depressogenic schematic model.

Competition for Limited Cognitive Resources: ICS, Distraction, and Depressive Cognitive Deficits

One advantage of expressing clinically relevant theory in terms compatible with the concepts used in more experimentally oriented cognitive theories is that insights and conclusions can be transferred more readily between clinical and laboratory domains of investigation. ICS incorporates, in its basic operating principles, one of the best established conclusions of experimental cognitive psychology; there is a limit to the amount of information that any one specialized cognitive processing resource can handle at a time. In ICS, this generalization is embodied in the principle that each of the processes that transform information from one mental code to another can only handle one coherent data stream at a time.

If we consider this principle in relation to the dynamic view of the "internal" regeneration of the depressed state, illustrated in Figure 2.1, a number of insights emerge. First, we have an explanation for the effects of distraction in producing immediate short-term alleviation of depression (e.g., Fennell, Teasdale, Jones, & Damlé, 1987). The cognitive loop of the depressive interlock configuration (illustrated in Figure 2.1) involves repeated cycles in which specific meanings are derived from schematic models, and schematic models are synthesized from patterns of specific meanings. Similar reciprocal cycles of Propositional–Implicational processing lie at the heart of many other processing configurations supporting a wide range of "controlled processing" tasks, often involving the processing of information unrelated to depression. For that reason, such cycles have been termed the "central engine" of cognition (Teasdale & Barnard, 1993, pp. 76–81). Within the central engine, the processes that transform, respectively, specific meanings into schematic models, and schematic models into specific meanings, represent two potential processing "bottlenecks." The limited transformation capacity available at each of these points means that, frequently, there will be a need to select between alternative data streams competing for access to the same processing resources; processing of one data stream necessarily means that other streams cannot also be processed at the same time. From this analysis, it follows that distraction tasks that successfully compete for limited central engine resources will make those resources unavailable to the depressive interlock configuration. Consequently, depression should immediately begin to lift. Further, this analysis indicates that the most effective distraction tasks will be those that make the greatest demands on central engine resources. These will generally be novel or complex tasks that make great demands on controlled processing resources for task coordination and control.

The ICS analysis suggests that, in depressed states that have already existed for some time, the effects of brief distraction tasks alleviating depression may not persist long, once the demand to process task-related information has been withdrawn. Each ICS subsystem has a memory that stores copies of all the patterns of information that it takes as input. It follows that, where the depressive interlock configuration has been operating for some time, the recent sections of the Implicational subsystem's memory store will contain many representations of depression-related schematic models. Once the distraction task is complete, these models will be easily accessed, effectively "leaking back" into the data stream circulating round the central engine, and so restarting the depressive interlock configuration. More enduring alleviation of depression requires changes to the depression-related schematic models maintaining depression.

Competition for limited central engine resources also explains the cognitive deficits associated with depression. Where the depressive interlock configuration maintaining depression wins the competition for resources, fewer resources will be available for cognitive task performance and deficits may be expected. Further, this account suggests that these deficits will be most pronounced on tasks that require substantial central engine resources of control and coordination for successful execution. This is exactly the conclusion emerging from empirical studies, which consistently point to much greater deficits on tasks involving substantial controlled processing than on tasks that can be performed more "automatically," that is, with few demands on central engine resources (Hartlage, Alloy, Vasquez, & Dykman, 1993; Watts, 1993).

Logical Distortions and the State
Dependency of Dysfunctional Attitudes

Early statements of the clinical cognitive model suggested that vulnerability to depression depended on possessing, as a relatively enduring, trait-like, cognitive predisposition, certain dysfunctional basic assumptions or attitudes. Repeated failures to find elevated scores on measures of such attitudes in depressed patients, once they have recovered from episodes of depression (reviewed by Haaga et al., 1991), have posed a considerable challenge to this view. Equally, it is not at all clear how this view explains the well-established mood-state dependency of such attitudes; studies investigating effects of both short-term (Miranda et al., 1990) and long-term (Haaga et al., 1991) changes in mood have convincingly demonstrated that scores on measures of dysfunctional attitudes are powerfully influenced by mood state. Recently, Persons and Miranda (1992), in their "mood-state" hypothesis, have attempted to account for the mood-state dependency of dysfunctional attitudes and beliefs by proposing that dysfunctional beliefs are always present in the cognitively vulnerable, but that, in positive mood, they are "unavailable for report" (Persons & Miranda, 1992, p. 497).

The ICS analysis provides a radically different perspective to the view that dysfunctional assumptions and attitudes exist as relatively enduring "beliefs" that can be adequately expressed as verbalizable rules. Equally, so-called "logical distortions," such as overgeneralization, are not seen as the result of logical operations working on "faulty premises" (cf. Kovacs & Beck, 1978, p. 528). Rather, the ICS analysis suggests that the concepts of dysfunctional attitudes and logical distortions provide approximate descriptions of the results of the tendency to synthesize particular types of schematic models in situations of depressed mood or loss-related events. Before presenting this analysis, it is necessary to describe more fully the nature of Implicational representations.

Words consist of arrangements of letters, differences in the letters and their sequence encoding particular words. Sentences consist of arrangements of words, the nature and sequences of the words encoding particular specific meanings. Analogously, Implicational schematic models are composed of informational elements, or variables, each element corresponding to a high-order feature or dimension extracted from experience. These variables can take different values, corresponding to the current state of the underlying dimensions of experience that they represent. We can think of the high-order meanings of schematic models in terms of patterns of values across variables. We can use the convention of representing a schematic model by a pattern of values (arbitrarily indicated by closed and open circles in Figure 2.2) across variables, each of which represents a high-order dimension of experience. These patterns will be constantly made, remade, and varied according to the shifting state of the underlying dimensions, as reflected in changes in the patterns of lower-level codes from which the models are synthesized. The figure reminds us that those inputs include contributions based not only on patterns of lower-level, specific meanings, but also on patterns derived directly from sensory elements. It is the total pattern, derived from both kinds of source, that determines high-level meaning and emotional response.

We are now in a position to consider the ICS analysis of dysfunctional attitudes, logical distortions such as overgeneralization, and the mood-state dependency of these phenomena. As illustrated in Figure 2.1, the maintenance of depression depends on the continuing regeneration of depressogenic Implicational schematic models. These models may include patterns of values on variables indicating a range of negative characteristics of the self, future,

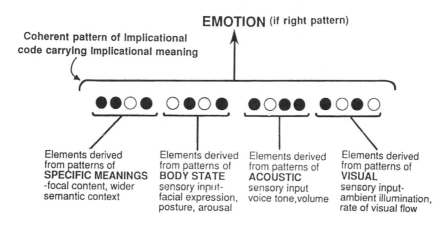

FIGURE 2.2. A diagrammatic representation of an emotion-related schematic model, showing contributions from inputs derived both from patterns of specific meanings *and* from patterns of sensory information. The schematic model is represented as a pattern of values (○ or ●) across a range of variables, each variable corresponding to a higher-order dimension of experience. From Teasdale (1993). Copyright 1993 by Pergamon Journals, Ltd. Reprinted by permission.

or world, together with variables indicating proprioceptive sensory input reflecting depressive bodily effects. The patterns of values on these variables provides an implicit informational context within which the "generic meanings" of particular incidents or pieces of information are evaluated. The results are characteristic patterns of depressive thinking. We can use analogies with lower-level mental codes to illustrate this point.

At the word level, presenting the letter *E* has very different consequences if it occurs following the context of the letters *WIS* rather than *DUNC*. Similarly, at the sentence level, the word "silence" has very different implications if it occurs in the context: "His joke was followed by total _____" than if it occurs in the context: "The sun was setting, a warm breeze stirred the palm leaves, otherwise there was utter _____."

Figure 2.3 illustrates how, at the Implicational level, comparable effects of differences in context can produce "overgeneralization" from a specific failure experience in a depressed patient, but a quite different response in the same person when nondepressed.

The figure uses the convention of representing schematic models in terms of patterns of values (arbitrarily indicated by closed and open circles) across variables, each of which represents a high-order dimension of experience. The figure illustrates fragments of the total pattern of information, at the schematic model level, assumed to be present in a depressed patient immediately before and after a specific failure experience. The response of the same person when recovered is also shown. The difference in prevailing mood state between the depressed and recovered condition is reflected in differ-

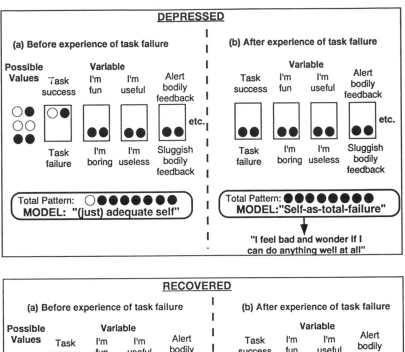

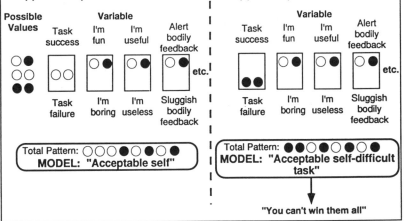

FIGURE 2.3. The ICS analysis of "overgeneralization" from a specific failure experience. The different responses in the depressed and nondepressed states reflect differences in the preexisting semantic contexts at the generic level of representation. From Teasdale and Barnard (1993, p. 158). Copyright 1993. Reprinted by permission of Erlbaum (UK) Taylor & Francis, Hove, UK.

ences in the pattern of values on variables that provide the semantic context prior to the experience of failure.

In the depressed person, the [○ ● ● ● ● ● ● ●, etc., "(just) adequate self"] pattern is already present as a result of depressogenic schematic models previously created. This pattern corresponds to a model that is sufficient to maintain some level of depression, but that is "saved" from "completing"

to the pattern characteristic of the ["self-as-total-failure"] model (● ● ● ●
● ● ● ●) by the value on the variable related to recent experiences of suc-
cess/failure. If this person now experiences a specific failure, the value of
the related variable will change from ○ to ●, the schematic model will
become [● ● ● ● ● ● ● ●, etc., "self-as-total-failure"], and the person
will have a "sense" of themselves as a total failure as a person.

The clinical cognitive model explains such "overgeneralized" responses
to specific failure experiences by suggesting that those vulnerable to depression have dysfunctional "beliefs" or "attitudes" such as "If I fail at my work,
then I am a failure as a person." On this account, both the excessive affective
response to failure and the "logical error" of overgeneralization result from
the "faulty premises" underlying depressive thinking. From the ICS perspective, postulating such beliefs can be seen as an attempt to describe effects
that are actually mediated by quite different mechanisms, namely, changes
in the contexts provided by patterns of generic informational elements.

The ICS account explains the change from the "dysfunctional" response
of the depressed person to the "functional" response of the same person after recovery in terms of changes in preexisting generic semantic context.
The recovered depressed person's prevailing schematic model is
[○ ○ ○ ● ○ ● ○ ●, etc., "Acceptable self"]. Given this preexisting context,
a change in value on the single variable related to a specific failure will not
disturb the total pattern sufficiently to create a ["self-as-total-failure"] model.
Consequently, in contrast to the situation when depressed, a functional
response is observed.

Differences between the depressed and nondepressed states reflect differences in the schematic models maintaining these moods. Unlike the situation at the word or sentence level, we are not explicitly aware of the state
of the semantic elements that constitute the preexisting context at this level
of representation. The implicit and highly abstract nature of the contextual
elements at the generic level may lead us to regard the depressed person's
response to failure as some special form of "logical distortion," based on
the "rules" embodied in dysfunctional "beliefs" or "attitudes." However, the
ICS analysis suggests that both the catastophic response to failure of the
depressed person and the mood-state dependency of this response, and of
measures of related "dysfunctional attitudes," are simply further examples
of the effects of context.

THE ICS PERSPECTIVE ON PSYCHOLOGICAL
TREATMENT FOR DEPRESSION

The consequences of the ICS analysis for understanding and improving the
effectiveness of cognitive therapy for depression, and of psychological treatments for depression more generally, are discussed in some detail by Teasdale and Barnard (1993, Chap. 16). Here I shall summarize the main
implications.

The ICS analysis suggests that the task of therapy is to replace the schematic models maintaining depression with more adaptive alternative schematic models. In many situations, maintenance of depression will depend on the integrity and persistence of interlocked processing configurations similar to that illustrated in Figure 2.1. Because maintenance of such configurations depends on a number of interlinked feedback loops, the total configuration is vulnerable to attack by interventions that create changes at a number of "peripheral" points, in addition to interventions specifically targeted on the "central" goal of changing schematic models. We noted earlier the potential contribution of interventions directed at changing specific meanings and related negative automatic thoughts. The ICS analysis suggests that interventions targeted at creating changes at the bodily level (e.g., by physical exercise, changing posture, facial expression, etc.) also have a contribution to make. For example, by changing the information circulating around the sensory loop shown in Figure 2.1 so that it is no longer congruent with a depressive bodily state, such interventions may alter the sensorily derived contribution to synthesis of depressogenic schematic models sufficiently to disrupt the integrity of the self-perpetuating processing configuration.

Changing schematic models requires attention to a wider semantic context than invalidating specific meanings. In suggesting a primary focus on creating whole, coherent, alternative views at a schematic level, the ICS analysis is consistent with a range of developments within cognitive therapy. For example, the highly successful cognitive therapy for panic (Clark & Salkovskis, 1991) aims to do just this by creating whole alternative "views" or models of anxiety and panic, rather than by serially invalidating specific negative beliefs (D. M. Clark, personal communication, July 1991). Similarly, Padesky (1993) has drawn a very useful distinction between "changing minds" (getting patients to admit that the specific negative thoughts or beliefs that they hold are inconsistent with available evidence) and "guiding discovery" (helping patients gain alternative, wider perspectives on problematic situations). On the basis of extensive clinical experience, Padesky has argued forcefully for the advantages of the second of these strategies, focusing, in ICS terms, on the creation of alternative schematic models, rather than the invalidation of specific thoughts or meanings. Interestingly, Padesky has pointed out that the majority of therapy vignettes available in published texts of cognitive therapy actually focus primarily on "changing minds."

In contrast to more purely "cognitive" models and treatments of depression, the ICS analysis suggests that the high-level meanings derived from situations can be powerfully influenced by techniques that modify purely sensory elements. As Figure 2.2 reminds us, direct contributions from sensory sources may form components of affect-related schematic models that are as important as the contributions derived from patterns of specific meanings. For example, the higher-order meaning that I create following a failure experience may be quite different if I combine the specific failure-related meanings with the elements related to the sensory feedback from a smiling facial expression rather than a frown, or from high bodily arousal and an erect posture rather than from a sluggish body-state and bowed, stooped posture.

Also consistent with the general treatment strategy indicated by the ICS analysis, recent developments in the treatment of long-standing depressions and personality disorders (e.g., Beck, Freeman, & Associates, 1990; Young, 1990) have focused on change at a schematic level, albeit using a somewhat different formulation of schematic processing than that described by ICS. Some of these approaches have incorporated treatment approaches from Gestalt therapy, such as guided imagery or enactive procedures. Although of little value in providing evidence to discredit specific negative thoughts or meanings, such interventions can be seen as ways to alter coherent packages of meanings and sensory contributions at the schematic level. For example, "replaying" in guided imagery scenes of childhood abuse, incorporating elements of the control and power that the patient now has as an adult but lacked as a child, can be seen as a powerful method of introducing new elements into patterns of Implicational code related to themes of helplessness, domination, betrayal, and suffering.

As well as providing a systematic conceptual framework that allows us to refocus the emphasis of cognitive therapy in a way that is wholly consistent with recent clinically inspired developments in treatment, the ICS framework can also provide the basis for radically new developments in treatment. For example, the ICS information processing analysis of depressive relapse and its prevention by cognitive therapy has led to exploration of a novel approach to preventing depressive relapse, integrating aspects of cognitive therapy with aspects of attentional control (mindfulness) training in a cost-efficient format (Teasdale, Segal, & Williams, 1995).

CONCLUDING COMMENTS

The development of the cognitive approach to understanding and treating depression by Beck and his colleagues represents one of the major clinical advances of the century in this field. It has been an invaluable and natural part of this highly successful enterprise that the underlying ideas guiding therapy should evolve in the light of experience, systematic investigation, and feedback from patients. It is a delight to me to know that the perspective on cognitive approaches to understanding and treating depression that emerges from the ICS analysis is wholly consistent with the current state of the clinically derived cognitive model, as described in Beck's chapter in the current volume. In particular, there are striking parallels between the concept of the mode, which now occupies a central place in Beck's theorizng, and essential features of the ICS analysis. The distributed, self-perpetuating cycles of cognitive–affective interaction that, in the ICS analysis, play such an important role in the maintenance of certain affective states, seem intriguingly close to Beck's concept of mode. Indeed, in previous accounts (Teasdale & Barnard, 1993), I have actually described these states as "modes of mind."

The cognitive approach to clinical problems inspired by Aaron T. Beck has been enormously and impressively successful. I hope that the ICS framework, by providing a vehicle for interchanges between those working clinically and those working more experimentally, will contribute to the further growth of the work that has been fathered and nurtured so effectively in its development by this remarkable and generous man.

NOTE

1. Following the convention used by Teasdale and Barnard (1993), square brackets are used to denote schematic models. The contents of the brackets indicate the thematic content of the model.

REFERENCES

Barnard, P. (1985). Interacting cognitive subsystems: A psycholinguistic approach to short-term memory. In A. Ellis (Ed.), *Progress in the psychology of language* (Vol. 2, pp. 197–258). London: Erlbaum.

Beck, A. T., Freeman, A., & Associates. (1990). *Cognitive therapy of personality disorders.* New York: Guilford Press.

Beck, A. T., Rush, A. J., Shaw, B. F., & Emery, G. (1979). *Cognitive therapy of depression.* New York: Guilford Press.

Clark, D. M., & Salkovskis, P. M. (1991). *Cognitive therapy with panic and hypochondriasis.* Oxford: Pergamon Press.

Fennell, M. J. V., Teasdale, J. D., Jones, S., & Damlé, A. (1987). Distraction in neurotic and endogeneous depression: An investigation of negative thinking in major depressive disorder. *Psychological Medicine, 17,* 441–452.

Haaga, D. A. F., Dyck, M. J., & Ernst, D. (1991). Empirical status of cognitive theory of depression. *Psychological Bulletin, 110,* 215–236

Hartlage, S., Alloy, L. B., Vasquez, C., & Dykman, B. (1993). Automatic and effortful processing in depression. *Psychological Bulletin, 113,* 247–278.

Johnson-Laird, P. N. (1983). *Mental models.* Cambridge, UK: Cambridge University Press.

Kovacs, M., & Beck, A. T. (1978). Maladaptive cognitive structures in depression. *American Journal of Psychiatry, 135,* 525–533.

Miranda, J., & Persons, J. B. (1988). Dysfunctional attitudes are mood-state dependent. *Journal of Abnormal Psychology, 97,* 76–79.

Miranda, J., Persons, J. B., & Byers, C. N. (1990). Endorsement of dysfunctional beliefs depends on current mood state. *Journal of Abnormal Psychology, 99,* 237–241.

Padesky, C. A. (1993, September 24). *Socratic questioning: Changing minds or guiding discovery?* Keynote address delivered at the European Congress of Behavioural and Cognitive Therapies, London.

Persons, J. B., & Miranda, J. (1992). Cognitive theories of vulnerability to depression: Reconciling negative evidence. *Cognitive Therapy and Research, 16,* 485–502.

Pyszczynski, T., & Greenberg, J. (1987). Self-regulatory perseveration and the depressive self-focusing style: A self-awareness theory of reactive depression. *Psychological Bulletin, 102,* 122–138.

Teasdale, J. D. (1982). What kind of theory will improve psychological treatment? In J. E. Boulougouris (Ed.), *Learning theory approaches to psychiatry* (pp. 57–66). Chichester, UK: Wiley.

Teasdale, J. D. (1993). Emotion and two kinds of meaning: Cognitive therapy and applied cognitive science. *Behaviour Research and Therapy, 31,* 339–354.

Teasdale, J. D., & Barnard, P. J. (1993). *Affect, cognition and change: re-modelling depressive thought.* Hove, UK: Erlbaum.

Teasdale, J. D., & Dent, J. (1987). Cognitive vulnerability to depression: an investigation of two hypotheses. *British Journal of Clinical Psychology, 26,* 113–126.

Teasdale, J. D., Segal, Z. V., & Williams, J. M. G. (1995). How does cognitive therapy prevent depressive relapse and why should attentional control (mindfulness) training help? *Behaviour Research and Therapy, 33,* 25–39.

Watts, F. N. (1993). Problems of memory and concentration. In C. G. Costello (Ed.), *Symptoms of depression* (pp. 113–140). New York: Wiley.

Young, J. (1990). *Cognitive therapy for personality disorder.* Sarasota, FL: Professional Resource Exchange.

Chapter 3

The Cognitive Approach to Anxiety: Threat Beliefs, Safety-Seeking Behavior, and the Special Case of Health Anxiety and Obsessions

Paul M. Salkovskis

The basis of Beck's (1976) cognitive model of emotion is now almost universally accepted and understood. The fundamental idea is that emotions are experienced as a result of the way in which events are interpreted or appraised. It is the meaning of events that triggers emotions rather than the events themselves. The particular appraisal made will depend on the context in which an event occurs, the mood the person is in at the time it occurs, and the person's past experiences. Particular types of emotions depend upon this specific interpretation. Effectively this means that the same event can evoke a different emotion in different people, or even different emotions in the same person on different occasions. The idea of cognition–emotion specificity is well illustrated by a story:

> As I left for work this morning, three other men set out at the same time. By coincidence, the same thing happened to each of us. As each walked out of his house, he had the misfortune to stand directly in some dog mess. The first person has a tendency to feel depressed. His immediate reaction was typical: "I am a failure. I used to be successful, but now something as simple as leaving my own house becomes a disaster. There is no point in my continuing; this is just typical of what the rest of the day is going to be like." Feeling very depressed, this person went back to bed.
>
> The second person had the same unpleasant experience. His reaction, however, was quite different. Being prone to anxiety, this person's reaction was: "What am I going to do? If I go back in the house and wash this off I will be late for work and lose my job. On the other hand, if I don't, then people at work will believe I have a personal hygiene problem, the word will get around, and I will lose my job anyway."

We leave this person in a state of indecision and find that the third person has also encountered the dog mess. Now this person tends to have a problem with anger, and this occasion is no exception. His immediate thought is, "WHOSE DOG DID THIS! HOW MANY TIMES MUST I TELL MY NEIGHBORS NOT TO ALLOW THEIR DOG TO STOP OUTSIDE MY HOUSE BUT, OH NO, DO THEY LISTEN? YOU WAIT 'TIL I CATCH WHO'S RESPONSIBLE FOR THIS, THEY'RE IN REAL TROUBLE!"

This story neatly encapsulates the principle of specificity, with feelings of depression associated with ideas of loss, feelings of anxiety associated with ideas of personal danger or threat, and feelings of anger associated with ideas that someone has been unfair or broken one's personal rules. In the story there is, of course, a cognitive therapist as well.

The cognitive therapist leaves his house (and it is important to note that proficiency in this area doesn't protect you from unpleasant events such as a foot in dog mess). However, the cognitive therapist's reaction is quite different from that of the others. Looking down at his shoes, he smiled broadly, mopped his forehead, and said to himself, "Well, isn't it good that I remembered to put my shoes on this morning."[1]

There is a serious point here concerning the nature of cognitive interventions. Cognitive therapy is not necessarily about thinking more rationally, nor is it necessarily about thinking more positively. The fundamental idea is that there may be several alternative ways of looking at a particular situation. People suffering from emotional problems are often trapped by a particularly negative or unhelpful way of looking at their situation and can only see this way of interpreting it. Being told to think more rationally is dangerously close to being told to pull oneself together. The role of the cognitive therapist is to help persons explore whether or not there might be alternative ways of appraising their situation. Once other options are considered, therapy continues by helping persons check the relative merits and accuracy of these alternatives against their past, present, and future experience. Therefore, the aim is *not* to persuade persons that their current way of looking at the situation is wrong, irrational, or too negative; instead, it is to allow them to identify where they may have become trapped or stuck in their way of thinking and to allow them to discover other ways of looking at their situation.

Once this is done, the therapist helps the person identify any obstacles to thinking and acting in this new, more helpful way. Thus, cognitive therapy aims to free patients to choose other ways of interpreting and reacting to their situation drawing from the fullest possible range of alternatives available (including their current negative account). In this way, the therapist seeks to empower patients by broadening the choices they can make about the way they react to their situation and by helping them to discover information that allows them to decide between the available choices in an informed way. The chosen alternative may be more rational or more positive, but it does not have to be. This philosophy highlights the importance of guided discovery where the therapist helps the patients themselves to explore alternative ways of looking at their situation. By definition this style of therapy means that the alternatives arrived at are acceptable to the patients and consistent with their beliefs and values. It also means that there is no place in the theory or the therapy for the idea of therapist-defined "wrong thinking," which is inappropriately judgmental.

Having highlighted some of the fundamental normalizing notions of Beck's approach to cognitive therapy, the rest of this chapter will examine the way in which the cognitive model deals with anxiety in general and, more specifically, the maintenance of anxiety in people who have persistent anxiety disorders. I will pay particular attention to a new and specifically cognitive perspective on the link between cognition and "avoidance" behaviors in the maintenance of anxiety problems. Arising from this discussion will be the consideration of ways in which the cognitive hypothesis can be used to deal more effectively with the special case of health anxiety and obsessive–compulsive problems.

THE ROLE OF APPRAISAL OF THREAT OR DANGER

The cognitive theory proposes that people experiencing anxiety *believe* that they are threatened with either physical or social harm. Whether or not the harm they fear is objectively present is immaterial to the *experience* of anxiety. Thus, it is the interpretation of a situation or stimulus as a sign of personal threat that is essential to the experience of this emotion. By implication, the experience of the panic patient who erroneously believes that he or she is having a heart attack is very similar to that of the person who really is having a heart attack. The person who mistakenly believes that he or she has been scorned and mocked by a group of acquaintances reacts similarly to the person who was truly subjected to this experience. This normalizing view can be actively used in therapy to "empower" patients; a cognitive account can have the effect of reducing the low self-esteem that often accompanies a psychiatric diagnosis which can carry the implication of "mental illness." By the same token, adoption of this normalizing approach can release the patient from the helplessness he or she feels in the face of an uncontrollable "disease" explanation on the one hand and the insidious implication of moral or personal weakness because of "irrational" sensitivity on the other. The cognitive therapist and patient agree that anyone (including the therapist) who held the same beliefs would react in a similar way.

The way in which the cognitive model can be applied to both accurate and mistaken threat perceptions therefore becomes an important component of therapy itself. Cognitive approaches can readily be applied to situations where an objective stressor is present (e.g., see Moorey, Chapter 19, this volume, for a discussion of the use of cognitive therapy in cancer patients).

In depression, negative life events are often a major and continuing stress. As Clark and Wells (1995) point out in the context of social phobia, for some anxious patients the feared catastrophe may actually happen *at some level.* For example, the person really is unable to speak or really does tremble, others really see that he or she is anxious, and so on.

Although not espousing a pathological (disease) view of anxiety, the cognitive hypothesis does specify circumstances under which otherwise normal cognitive processes can become "stuck," resulting in the excessive and disabling levels of anxiety experienced by people who suffer from anxiety disorders. The factors involved in the occurrence of more severe and persistent anxiety can be divided into two categories: (1) factors that lead people to experience relatively greater levels of anxiety, and (2) factors involved in the maintenance of high levels of anxiety.

Factors That Increase the Degree of Anxiety Experienced

Fundamental to the cognitive theory of the development of emotional disorders (Beck, 1976) is the notion that people are more likely to interpret situations as more dangerous than they really are *because of particular assumptions or beliefs they learned during an earlier period in their life.* Such beliefs may have been useful during that earlier stage, but may become problematic when new situations arise that call for a different type of understanding. Examples of this kind of belief would be, "It is important to be perfectly calm at all times"; "If I don't control myself then I am in danger of losing control"; "I must not show my feelings"; "If I don't worry about things, then everything will go wrong for me." Apart from general assumptions about anxiety itself, other types of assumptions characterize different disorders such as panic, social phobia, obsessive–compulsive, hypochondriasis, and so on. Life events or other "critical incidents" can cause in the activation of this type of assumption resulting in a more or less continuous interpretation of a range of situations in an unduly threatening way (Beck, 1976).

A second related factor involved in the production of excessive anxiety concerns the specific appraisal of threat itself. Most commonly, the cognitive model is viewed as specifying that people who suffer from anxiety tend to *overestimate* the likelihood of threat. However, Beck, Emery, and Greenberg (1985) describe a much broader and more useful conceptualization of the cognitive component of anxiety. This can be summarized by the following equation:

$$\text{Anxiety} \propto \frac{\text{Perceived probability of threat} \times \text{Perceived cost/Awfulness of danger}}{\text{Perceived ability to cope with danger} + \text{Perceived "rescue factors"}}$$

According to this view, an increased perception of likelihood of danger would result in an increase in anxiety. However, perceived probability interacts with the specific meaning the person assigns to the danger concerned. For example, some people may believe it is very likely they will faint in a given situation but would not feel unduly anxious *unless they felt that fainting was a particularly bad or dangerous thing to do* (e.g., resulting in other people rejecting them or in them choking on their own vomit). These two factors are regarded as multiplicative and synergistic. This conceptualization of cognitive factors in anxiety also accounts for the situation where the person believes that a specific negative outcome is extremely unlikely but nevertheless shows extreme fear of it. Such a pattern is particularly likely when the person believes that, although unlikely, the threat is too awful to risk. This combination is prominent in many instances of both severe health anxiety and obsessional problems, where persons recognizes that their concerns are probably senseless but would be utterly devastated if the unlikely were to happen.

The combination of risk and cost is further modulated by the extent to which people feel they would be able to cope or not cope with the danger should it materialize and the extent to which factors extraneous to their own coping (e.g., helpful reactions from other people) would be involved. Clinical and research evidence suggests that people who suffer from anxiety problems can show distortions involving each of these factors singly or in combination. Different combinations are likely across individuals and probably between disorders. For example, patients suffering from panic may show elevations in all aspects. Patients suffering from obsessive–compulsive disorder and hypochondriasis often report relatively low probabilities of danger but unusually high levels of perceived cost or awfulness. Assessment of anxiety disorders should focus on all of the components described.

Factors Involved in the Maintenance of Anxiety

Persistence of overly negative interpretations of stimuli, events, or situations is regarded as crucial to the understanding of anxiety disorders. According to the cognitive theory, the maintenance of negative thinking and anxiety have at least three major components (Beck, Emery, & Greenberg, 1985; Clark, 1986b; Clark & Beck, 1988). Figure 3.1 illustrates the three principal vicious circles believed to be involved in the maintenance of anxiety. These are as follows:

1. *Selective attention.* Those who believe themselves to be in danger tend to become sensitive to noticing stimuli consistent with that perceived danger. Although it seems likely that this is to some degree an automatic response (closely akin to the way in which people who have discovered that they or their partner is pregnant begin to notice other pregnant women), at least some of the selective attention observed in anxiety is a deliberate scanning for danger. Thus, spider phobics check the room for signs of spider webs, people anxious about their health read medical books, and panic pa-

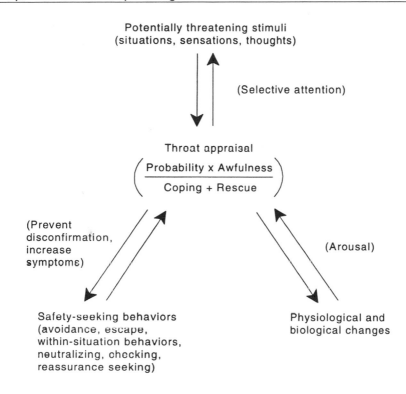

FIGURE 3.1. An illustration of the way in which psychological factors can perpetuate threat cognitions and therefore maintain anxiety problems.

tients focus their attention on (and as a result often find) sensations that may originate from their cardiac region. The anxious person who *notices* more signs of danger may then erroneously interpret that as a sign that danger has really increased, thus increasing their concern and further reinforcing that interpretation.

2. *Physiological change.* Anxiety has direct and indirect physiological effects. Persons who perceive themselves as being in danger may experience the effects of adrenaline being released. If the source of danger is perceived as being linked to bodily sensations then the perception of danger is heightened, spiraling up into a panic attack (Clark, 1986a, and Chapter 15, this volume). Socially anxious patients who are afraid that other people will see their anxiety and think them foolish may as a result of this idea begin to sweat, flush, and shake. Obsessional patients who have the idea of being contaminated despite having washed their hands repeatedly start to sweat more and experience the sensation of their hands becoming "dirty"; this may actually be because their hands have become very dry and are moistened by sweating in response to anxiety. In each instance, the vicious circle results in an increased perception of threat.

3. *Changes in behavior.* The perception of danger is known to increase avoidance behavior. Avoidance behavior increases preoccupation with threat and as such constitutes a third vicious circle involved in the maintenance of anxiety according to the cognitive model. However, at this stage a reappraisal of the role of behavior in the maintenance of anxiety is needed. Typically, cognitive theorists and therapists have tended to regard anxiety-related behaviors from a perspective largely influenced by behavioral theory. While this has allowed the adoption of techniques such as exposure by cognitive therapists,, it has also had the effect of distracting from a fuller cognitive analysis of the role of behavior in the maintenance of anxiety.

A Cognitive Perspective on Anxiety-Related Behavior

For most of this century the "neurotic paradox" has vexed anxiety researchers and clinicians. Put at its simplest, the paradox is this: Why do people suffering from anxiety fail to benefit from the repeated experience of surviving anxiety-provoking situations unharmed? In behavioral terms this has been framed as the failure of phobic reactions to extinguish in the face of unreinforced presentations of the conditioned stimulus (Eysenck, 1979). For the cognitive theorist it revolves around the question of why someone continues to fear a catastrophe that repeatedly fails to materialize (Seligman, 1988).

This represents a serious challenge for cognitive theory and therapy given the clear normalizing philosophy. If the logic of anxiety disorders is as clear as is supposed, why does the logic of disconfirmation not hold equally? In other words, why does the panic patient who believes that she will faint still believe this after approximately 2,000 attacks where fainting did not occur? The same could be said of obsessional patients and the range of other anxiety disorders.

Fortunately the theoretical and practical logic is clear and can readily be identified if the anxious patient is asked the appropriate questions. Panic patients who are asked why they did not die in the supermarket will tell you it is because they left *just in time.* Social phobics who are not laughed at will tell you it is because they remained silent in the group of people having a conversation. Obsessional patients will tell you that they did not act impulsively because the violent thought was resisted and then neutralized by a "good" thought. Far from being pathological, such "avoidance" responses are characteristic of normal anxiety. The behavior of anyone who believes him- or herself to be in danger will usually focus on anything that he or she believes may reduce the danger or otherwise make them safe. Safety-seeking behavior is a highly adaptive type of response where real threat is concerned. People leave a burning building as quickly as they possibly can. However, if the perception of danger is based on a misinterpretation then the safety-seeking behavior can have an unfortunate side effect. Inappropriate seeking of safety can prevent anxious persons from discovering that their fears are groundless. After an episode that should have established that the

feared consequence did not happen, persons engaged in active safety behaviors may believe they had a lucky escape because they did things that
prevented the feared catastrophe from occurring. From this perspective, panic
patients who have had 2,000 attacks where they did not faint perceive themselves as having had more than 2,000 attacks where they were on the verge
of fainting and were only just able to prevent it from happening. Safety-
seeking behaviors can be global behaviors, such as avoidance and escape,
or more subtle forms of avoidance occurring within a situation that the person
feels prevented a danger from materializing.

Safety-seeking behavior tends to fall into three main categories: (1)
avoidance of situations that the patient believes *might* provoke panic (e.g.,
avoiding supermarkets); (2) escape from a situation *when* a panic attack
occurs (e.g., leaving a shop once the symptoms of panic begin); and (3) safety-
seeking behaviors carried out during panic with the intention of actively
preventing the feared catastrophe (e.g., when dizziness leads to the thought
"I'll faint," holding onto another person or shopping trolley or sitting down).
Previously we have described this later category as "subtle avoidance behaviors." Each of these behaviors can have the effect of maintaining the
panic-related beliefs; the patients logically infer that they have prevented
the occurrence of feared catastrophes by their behavior (e.g., "If I had gone
to the supermarket yesterday, then I would have passed out"; "If I had not
left immediately I would have fainted"; "If I had not sat down then I would
have fainted"). Thus, behavior of the type described above prevents disconfirmation of the feared catastrophes and transforms potential disconfirmations into "near misses."

Treatment Implications

This specifically cognitive analysis of the role of safety-seeking behavior in
the maintenance of anxiety has a number of important implications both
for the understanding of existing treatments and the development of further and more effective interventions. From the cognitive perspective, it is
possible to argue that exposure treatments work by allowing anxious patients to repeatedly experience entering the feared situation and thereby eventually learning that the things they are afraid of do not actually happen—that
is, they experience a disconfirmation of their fears. However, this redefini-
tion of the effects of exposure is of little value unless it makes empirically
testable predictions that go beyond those generated by the exposure approach
itself. It is clear that there are a number of predictions about (1) ways of
optimizing the effects of exposure and (2) behavioral experiments that have
no clear elements of exposure per se. Both types of procedure would be
predicted to reduce anxiety in proportion to the extent to which they have
the effect of reducing key threat beliefs; this association would be stronger
than that between the amount of exposure and degree of fear reduction.

Exposure in the purely behavioral tradition is relatively "hit or miss" in this respect. Eventually the patient may indeed receive disconfirmation if he or she stays in the situation for long enough. However, most patients in exposure use subtle avoidance behaviors, such as distraction, if they believe that the anxiety itself may cause them harm if it were to go too high—for example, walking close to walls if they feel they are going to lose their balance, neutralizing an obsessional thought when they are no longer able to wash their hands in response to it, and so on. The cognitive approach, on the other hand, emphasizes the value of interweaving initial discussion aimed at reducing the patient's belief in the particular negative appraisal he or she makes of the feared situation with behavioral experiments explicitly designed to provide people with a direct disconfirmation of their fears. Thus persons who are afraid that their legs might give way are encouraged to relax their legs then stand on one leg to see if they do fall. The person who is afraid that they will act on having thoughts about cutting someone with a sharp knife is asked to think these thoughts while holding such a knife in the presence of the therapist. Analysis in terms of safety seeking behavior allows behavioral experiments to be devised to test negative ideas about the consequences of anxiety itself. Rather than attempting to control anxiety, patients are asked to focus on frightening thoughts in such a way as to increase their anxiety level beyond those they would regard as safe in order to test their beliefs. Our group's experience has been that procedures such as these and those described in Salkovskis, Clark, and Gelder (in press) can be used to bring about extremely rapid changes in anxiety within sessions (usually very brief, often less than an hour) and that such anxiety reductions can be persistent, and generalize with little or no further work. However, it is important to note that effects of safety behaviors sometimes go beyond disconfirmation itself.

Safety-Seeking Behaviors Can Increase Symptoms

Experience in working with safety-seeking behavior suggests that many such behaviors may have a further unwanted effect. Not only can a safety-seeking behavior prevent disconfirmation but, in some circumstances, it can also increase the symptoms that were the initial source of misinterpretation and therefore anxiety. This type of effect is most obvious in obsessive–compulsive disorder. By definition, obsessional patients experience intrusive thoughts that they "attempt to suppress or neutralize by some other thought or action" (American Psychiatric Association, 1994, p. 418). The deliberate attempt to suppress naturally occurring intrusive thoughts demonstrably increases the occurrence of these thoughts (Salkovskis & Campbell, 1994; Trinder & Salkovskis, 1994). If the reader were to attempt to exclude thoughts of giraffes from the mind at this moment it is almost inevitable that such thoughts or images would occur more frequently throughout the time that the active attempts of suppression were taking place. This is almost certainly due, in at least part, to the fact that the person is paying attention to the idea of giraffes. It is also self-evident from the exercise itself why the "unwanted" thoughts are occurring. However, in the case of an obsessional patient who is experiencing blasphemous or other types of unwanted thoughts, it is considerably less obvious. Such patients often think that the unwanted thoughts are occurring at an alarmingly high frequency when he or she tries not to think them; it therefore follows that thoughts would occur yet more frequently and in a more uncontrolled way if he or she were to cease attempts at suppression.

It is not only in obsessional problems that safety behaviors increase the symptoms that have a focus of anxiety. In patients anxious about their health it is not uncommon for lumps to be palpated or rubbed until they are painful and swell more, for medical tests to be sought with such determination that enough tests are conducted to give several false positive results, and so on.

When this type of pattern occurs, as it seems to in both obsessive–compulsive disorder and severe health anxiety, the therapeutic strategy needs to involve (1) the provision of a comprehensible and comprehensive cognitive formulation and (2) a clear and unambiguous demonstration of the way in which misinterpretation-maintaining factors (including safety-seeking behaviors) are tending to increase both the misinterpretation and the symptoms. Precisely why this is so is discussed next.

When Disconfirmation Is Not an Option

As described above, the cognitive hypothesis allows a clear understanding of both the origin and the maintenance of anxiety problems. A particularly powerful component of therapy involves techniques directed at bringing about disconfirmation of danger (Salkovskis, 1991). However, obsessive–compulsive disorder and severe anxiety about health (hypochondriasis) pose some special difficulties in this latter respect. Attention to the details of the beliefs characteristic of these two problems illustrates where the difficulty lies and how it may best be resolved. In both obsessions and hypochondriasis the danger that is feared is most commonly judged as likely to occur *at some relatively distant future time*. For example, obsessional patients may believe that their failure to control their blasphemous thoughts means that they will suffer eternal torment after their death. Hypochondriacal patients may believe that the tingling they are experiencing in their fingertips is an early sign of multiple sclerosis that will progressively worsen, eventually becoming severely symptomatic then crippling in only 10–15 years time. In both instances, maneuvers intended to show the person that his of her feared consequences did not come about are likely to fail. It has long been known that obsessional problems and hypochondriasis do not respond to reassurance. Indeed, part of the definition of hypochondriasis is the failure to respond to reassurance, namely, "The preoccupation persists despite appropriate medical evaluation and reassurance."

It is clear, then, that the emphasis in treatment requires close attention. Even in anxiety problems where the feared catastrophe is regarded as imminent, the idea that treatment should exclusively focus on helping people to understand what *isn't* going to happen is problematic. Fundamental to the practice of cognitive therapy is the therapist and patient working together to reach a shared understanding (conceptualization) of the way the patient's problem works. The most effective way of changing a misinterpretation (whether it be of a symptom, a situation, or a thought) is to help the person come up with an alternative, less threatening interpretation of his or her experience. Subsequent therapy (including discussion, behavioral experiments, and exercises in disconfirmation) is then all directed at helping the person distinguish between the different interpretations that he or she has. In every instance the alternative explanation is going to be highly idiosyncratic, based on the particular pattern of symptoms and interpretations experienced by each person.

The cognitive hypothesis also specifies that different types of psychological problems will show certain broad consistencies within categories. Thus the concerns of the person experiencing repeated panic attacks are particularly likely to focus on the way in which that person interprets bodily and mental sensations as a sign of *imminent* catastrophe (see Clark, Chapter 15, this volume); the social phobics' concerns are particularly likely to focus on ideas of being humiliated, scorned, or rejected. The more specific models of particular psychological problems provide the clinician and researcher with general guidance that allow them then to focus their interventions in a more accurate way. Cognitive treatment thus emphasizes the negotiation of a shared understanding of the patient's problems combined with subsequent maneuvers designed, where possible, to help the patient achieve a disconfirmation of his or her negative interpretation as well as bolstering the less threatening alternative. Because the feared catastrophes in health anxiety and obsessive–compulsive disorder lie further in the future than in other problems, disconfirmation is much less useful as a strategy. This increases the relative importance of both the patients' and the therapist's understanding of the nonthreatening explanation of their problem, that is, the cognitive model as is idiosyncratically applied to the patients' symptoms and situation. The features of the cognitive account of obsessive–compulsive disorder and hypochondriasis that tend to play an important role in such an account will be described next.

THE COGNITIVE HYPOTHESIS
OF OBSESSIVE–COMPULSIVE DISORDER

For many years the idea that any kind of verbally based procedure would be helpful in obsessional problems was regarded with great doubt. Even advocates of the psychodynamic approach, who are not noted for their responsiveness to whether the patient's symptoms improve or not, regarded obsessive–compulsive disorder as a problem not particularly amenable to psychotherapy. This is scarcely surprising, given that almost by definition, obsessional patients regard their intrusive thoughts as senseless. Any therapy aimed at convincing patients that their obsessional thoughts were not true would therefore be unlikely to be succeed. The success of behavior therapy involving exposure to feared stimuli and response prevention of compulsive and neutralizing behavior resulted in a change in emphasis in the way that obsessional problems were seen (Salkovskis & Kirk, 1989).

The foundations of the cognitive theory are easily understood. Rachman (1971) made the crucial observation that obsessional thoughts could probably be best regarded as conditioned stimuli. Beck (1976) had previously observed that emotional responses occurred as a result of the way in which particular stimuli were interpreted in a negative fashion. Salkovskis (1985) drew upon these ideas, and the observation that intrusive thoughts indistinguishable from obsessional thoughts occurred in the majority of the population (Rachman & de Silva, 1978; Salkovskis & Harrison, 1984), in the development of a specific cognitive hypothesis of obsessional problems.

The cognitive-behavioral theory of obsessive–compulsive disorder starts with the proposition that obsessional thinking has its origins in normal intrusive cognitions. Intrusive cognitions are ideas, thoughts, images, or impulses that intrude in the sense that they interrupt the person's current stream of consciousness and the person also finds them upsetting, unacceptable, or otherwise unpleasant. The difference between normal intrusive cognitions and obsessional intrusive cognitions lies not in the occurrence or even the (un)controllability of the intrusions themselves but rather in the interpretation made by obsessional patients of the occurrence and/or content of the intrusions. If the appraisal is entirely focused upon harm or danger on the one hand or loss on the other, then the emotional reaction is likely to be anxiety or depression respectively. Such evaluation of intrusive cognitions and consequent mood changes may become part of a mood-appraisal spiral (Teasdale, 1983; Rachman, 1983), but would not necessarily be expected to result in compulsive behavior, neutralizing, and clinical obsessions. According to the cognitive hypothesis, an obsessional pattern *would* occur if intrusive cognitions were interpreted as an indication that the person may be, may have been, or may come to be responsible for harm or its prevention (Salkovskis, 1985, 1989; Salkovskis, Richards, & Forrester, 1995; Rachman, 1993). It is this specific interpretation in terms of responsibility for harm to oneself or other people that is believed to link intrusive cognitions with both the discomfort experienced and neutralizing (compulsive) behaviors, whether overt or covert.[2]

The structure of this conceptualization closely parallels the cognitive approach to other types of anxiety disorder in that a particular nonthreatening situation becomes the focus of concern as a result of beliefs concerning danger or threat. The way in which anxiety manifests therefore depends on the focus of threat perceptions and the consequences that this perception has for subsequent reactions. For example, in the cognitive hypothesis of panic (Clark, 1986a; Salkovskis, 1988), panic attacks are said to occur as a result of the misinterpretation of normal bodily sensations, particularly the sensations of normal anxiety. Most normal people experience such sensations, but only people who have an enduring tendency to interpret them in a catastrophic fashion will experience repeated panic attacks. This is probably as a result of the tendency for catastrophe-focused anxiety to result in (1) a perceived increase in the symptoms that were the original focus of concern and (2) in safety-seeking behaviors that have the effect of preventing persons from discovering that the things which they are afraid of do not happen and sometimes increasing the symptoms themselves (Clark, 1986a; Salkovskis, 1991). By the same token, intrusive thoughts, impulses, images, and doubts are part of normal everyday experience, but only people who have an enduring tendency to interpret their own mental activity as indicating personal "responsibility" will experience the pattern of discomfort and neutralizing characteristic of obsessive–compulsive disorder. The effects of the emotion aroused and the safety-seeking behaviors will be to maintain and increase the pattern of concern.

For example, an obsessional patient may believe that the occurrence of a thought such as "I might kill or molest my baby" means that there is a risk that she will succumb to the action unless she does something to prevent it, such as avoiding being left alone with her child. She would seek reassurance from people around her and try to prevent or escape from her intrusive thoughts, or try to think positive thoughts to balance the negative ones (neutralize them). Thus, the *interpretation* of obsessional intrusions as indicating increased responsibility has a number of important and interlinked effects: (1) increased discomfort, anxiety, and depression; (2) increased focused attention on these intrusions; (3) greater accessibility of the original thought and other related ideas; (4) active and usually counterproductive attempts to reduce the thoughts and decrease or discharge the responsibility that is perceived to be associated with them, including behavioral and cognitive "neutralizing" responses. These may include compulsive behavior, avoidance of situations related to the obsessional thought, seeking reassurance (having the effect of diluting or sharing responsibility), and attempts to get rid of or exclude the thought from the mind (see below).

Each of these effects contributes not only to the prevention of extinction of anxiety but also to increased preoccupation and a worsening spiral of intrusive thoughts leading to maladaptive affective, cognitive, and behavioral reactions. In some instances, where a feared consequence is seen as *imminent,* behavioral responses can have the additional effect of preventing disconfirmation of the person's negative beliefs (Salkovskis, 1991). For example, a patient may believe that failing to wash his hands vigorously for 15 minutes could lead to severe illness in his family. Having washed in this way, none of his family become ill, providing him with confirmation of his initial belief, and leaving the belief intact (or even strengthening it) for subsequent occasions when the thought of contamination occurs again.

Obsessional patients thus tend to *interpret* aspects of their own mental functioning—such as intrusive (obsessional) thoughts, images, impulses, doubts, and memories—differently from nonobsessionals. A major and counterproductive result is that obsessionals try too hard to exert control over their own cognitive function, over the occurrence of thoughts, over their memory, over the details of how they perform everyday actions, and so on. The *discomfort* experienced is due to the patient's appraisal of the content and occurrence of intrusive thoughts. The increased *frequency* of intrusions relative to nonobsessionals may in large part be directly due to the behaviors (overt and covert) that are motivated by the appraisal made, as described below.

The cognitive hypothesis proposes that inflated responsibility appraisals can focus on either the occurrence or the content of intrusive cognitions or on both. Emotional significance is a result of the particular idiosyncratic pattern of appraisal. It therefore follows that intrusions are initially emotionally neutral, but are like other potentially emotional stimuli in that they can take on positive, negative, or no emotional significance, depending on the person's prior experience and the context in which intrusions occur (Beck, 1976; Edwards & Dickerson, 1987; England & Dickerson, 1988). As described above, a crucial part of the appraisal of an intrusion will concern the implications of an intrusion and the need for further action. If the intrusion is appraised as having no implications, processing priority will tend to be diminished.

Appraisal of responsibility arising from the *occurrence* and *content* of intrusions can be at least partially independent, although often linked. A patient who was unable to get rid of bizarre and unpleasant thoughts and images interpreted this apparent resistance to his efforts at control as a sign that he was in danger of losing control and behaving in some unpredictable and violent way. He became preoccupied with efforts intended to prevent unwanted thoughts from coming into his mind and attempted to regiment his thinking. In this instance, it was primarily the *occurrence* of intrusions that was misinterpreted. In another example, a patient experienced repeated and vivid images of herself lying dead in front of her local shop, and of her family assembled around a coffin in which she lay. She interpreted the occurrence of *these particular images* as a prediction of the future and was especially disturbed by the fact that the images represented real places and people and that they were vivid and detailed. Here, the *particular content* of the intrusions was of relatively greater importance. Although these two facets of appraisal are most commonly linked in obsessional problems ("Having *these* thoughts means that I am a danger to my family"), this is not necessarily obvious in every instance. For example, a positive thought might be negatively appraised if it occurs incongruously on a sad occasion. When the *meaning* of the particular thought occurring is taken into account, however, the link between occurrence and content is usually evident.

When appraisal of occurrence and content of intrusions suggests a specific voluntary reaction (including attempts to neutralize, suppress, or avoid the intrusion, or even to monitor its occurrence carefully) processing priority will inevitably be increased. Intrusions interpreted as relevant to responsibility will therefore tend to persist and become the focus of further thought and action; irrelevant ideas can be considered but no further thought or action will ensue. However, sometimes unpleasant or upsetting cognitions cannot be resolved and become more persistent, as in depression, anxiety, and worry. In instances where *the occurrence of a particular type of thought* is appraised as an indication that the individual has become responsible for averting harm to him- or herself or others, then the occurrence and content of the thought becomes both a source of discomfort and an imperative signal for action that is intended to neutralize the thought and its potentially harmful consequences as well as to prevent or control its further occurrence.

In order to prevent the occurrence of intrusions and/or be aware of and limit the implications for responsibility, the obsessional patient often feels it necessary to pay close attention to his or her mental processes. The deployment of effortful strategies and attention towards the *control of mental activity* involves a variety of phenomena that all may contribute to the experience of obsessional symptoms and their maintenance. These may include, for example, attempts to be sure of the accuracy of one's memory, to take account of all factors in one's decisions, to prevent the occurrence of unacceptable material, to ensure that an outcome has been achieved when the difference between achieving it and not achieving it is imperceptible (e.g., deciding that one's hands are properly clean after washing in order to remove contamination). The precise strategies will be determined by the person's idiosyncratic beliefs about their impact. The choice of strategies is best understood from a safety-seeking perspective; the patient will react in ways that he or she believes are most likely to effectively reduce the threat of responsibility for avoidable harm. Safety behaviors can thus be directed at either *preventing harm* or *preventing responsibility for harm*. However, if one accepts the possibility of being able to prevent even potential harm, then perceived responsibility may be increased by this knowledge, on the basis that if one can influence an event then one assumes some responsibility for the possible outcomes. That is, by acting to reduce one's responsibility, one implicitly accepts the implication of being responsible in the first place. The short-term "evasion" or transfer of responsibility therefore has the additional unwanted effect of strengthening more enduring beliefs concerning the extent to which one is responsible in the first place and in the future.

Assumptions

The cognitive theory proposes that people are predisposed to making particular appraisals because of assumptions that are learned over longer periods from childhood onwards or that may be formed as a result of unusual or extreme events and circumstances. Some assumptions that characterize patients with obsessive–compulsive disorder are described in Salkovskis (1985) and include the following:

> "Having a thought about an action is like performing the action."
> "Failing to prevent (or failing to try to prevent) harm to self or others is the same as having caused the harm in the first place."
> "Responsibility is not reduced by other factors such as something being improbable."
> "Not neutralizing when an intrusion has occurred is similar or equivalent to seeking or wanting the harm involved in the intrusion to happen."
> "One should (and can) exercise control over one's thoughts."

If someone holds these attitudes very strongly, then the overt and covert behaviors characteristic of people suffering from obsessional problems tend to follow naturally.

The effects of these types of assumptions are often described in terms of "thinking errors" (Beck, 1976); thinking errors are characteristic distortions that influence whole classes of reactions. Thinking errors are not of themselves pathological; in fact, most people make judgments by employing a range of "heuristics," many of which can be fallacious (Nisbett & Ross, 1980).

The cognitive hypothesis suggests that patients with obsessive–compulsive disorder show a number of characteristic thinking errors that link to their obsessional difficulties; probably the most typical and important is the idea that "any influence over outcome = responsibility for outcome." A particularly interesting possibility is the relationship between responsibility through action as opposed to inaction. As outlined above, Salkovskis (1985) suggests that the belief that "failing to prevent (or failing to try to prevent) harm to self or others is the same as having caused the harm in the first place" may be a key assumption in the generation of obsessional problems. Recently, Spranca, Minsk, and Baron (1991) demonstrated what they refer to as "omission bias" in nonclinical subjects. They showed that normal subjects judge responsibility for negative consequences to be diminished when an omission is involved as opposed to when some specific action was involved in bringing about the negative consequence. This is true in normal subjects even when the study controls for the element of intention (i.e., the extent to which the person wishes the "negative" outcome to occur). Thus, most people appear to regard themselves as more responsible for what they actively do than what they fail to do. Clinical experience (and recent pilot work by our group) suggests that obsessional patients do not seem to show evidence of this type of omission bias. If this observation is experimentally validated, it opens up a range of new possibilities for the understanding of obsessional behavior.

The general belief that *"any* influence over outcome = responsibility for outcome" could be expected to increase concern with omissions; consideration of the phenomenology of obsessional problems suggests several other more specific ways in which omissions may become relatively more important to a vulnerable individual. An important factor in judgments concerning responsibility is the perception of "agency," meaning that one has chosen to bring something about. Particular importance is usually given to *premeditation* in the sense of being able to foresee possible harmful outcomes. Attribution of responsibility in this sense depends on what we believe to have been the person's mental state before or during the time of the act or omission, with some degree of premeditation or foresight tending to make an objectionable action (or intentional inaction) seem more a sign of responsibility or blame. *If a real possibility of causing avoidable harm is actually foreseen,* an act or omission is more likely to be seen as blameworthy and a source of guilt. That is, the person's state of mind at the time of the act determines the degree to which he or she is regarded as blameworthy. If an act or omission was quite accidental and unforseen, the person is unlikely to be blamed, unless we think that the person should have been aware of the possible harmful outcome. Believing that one has an implicit or explicit *duty* to foresee harm would have the effect of increasing perceived responsibility for possible omissions.

One of the problems experienced by obsessional patients is that it is often in the nature of the condition that they frequently foresee a wide range of possible negative outcomes. That is, the intrusive thoughts often concern things that could go wrong unless dealt with (such as passing on contamination, having hurt someone accidentally, having left the door unlocked or the gas turned on). Sometimes it is not even permissible for an obsessional to try not to foresee problems/disasters, because this would mean that he or she had deliberately chosen this course, which again increases responsibility. When aware of this, some patients regard it as a *duty* to try to foresee negative outcomes. However, if in any case a negative outcome *is* foreseen even as an intrusive thought, responsibility is established, because to do nothing the person would have to decide not to act to prevent the harmful outcome. That is, deciding *not* to act despite being aware of possible disastrous consequences becomes an active decision, making the person a causal agent in relation to those disastrous consequences. Thus, the occurrence of intrusive/obsessional thoughts transforms a situation where harm can only occur by omission into a situation where the person has "actively" chosen to allow the harm to take place. This might mean that the apparent absence of omission bias in obsessionals is mediated by the occurrence of obsessional thoughts.

Deciding not to do something results in a sense of "agency"; thus, patients will not be concerned about sharp objects they have not seen and will not be concerned if they did not consider the possibility of harm. However, if something is seen and it occurs to them that they could or should take preventative action, the situation changes because *not* acting becomes an active decision. In this way, the actual occurrence of intrusive thoughts of harm and/or responsibility for it come to play a key role in the perception of responsibility for their contents. Suppression, as described above, will further intensify this effect by increasing the thoughts in precisely the situations that the obsessional most wishes to exclude any intrusion. Thus, having locked the door, the person tries not to think that it could be open, experiences the thought again, and is therefore constrained to act or risk being responsible through having chosen not to check. Interestingly, checking and reassurance seeking are prominent in both obsessive–compulsive disorder and in hypochondriasis, and it may be reasonable to suppose that decision making in health anxiety can be governed by similar considerations.

SEVERE ANXIETY ABOUT HEALTH (HYPOCHONDRIASIS)

In its most severe form, anxiety about health is known as hypochondriasis. Hypochondriasis is defined in DSM-IV (American Psychiatric Association, 1994, p. 462) as "preoccupation with fears of having, or the idea that one has, a serious disease based on the person's misinterpretation of bodily symptoms." The definition of severe anxiety about health therefore depends on the presence of threat misinterpretations. The cognitive hypothesis of health anxiety again starts with innocuous stimuli that are, *by definition,* misinterpreted as a sign of some serious threat to illness.

The cognitive theory states that, in severe health anxiety and hypochondriasis, bodily signs, symptoms, variations, and medical information tend to be perceived as more dangerous than they really are, and that a particular illness is believed to be more probable than it really is (Salkovskis, 1989; Salkovskis & Warwick, 1986; Warwick & Salkovskis, 1990). At the same time, the patient is likely to perceive him- or herself as unable to prevent the illness and unable to affect its course, that is, as having no effective means of coping with the perceived threat.

Knowledge of and past experiences of illness (in self or others) leads to the formation of specific assumptions about symptoms, disease, and health behaviors. These are learned from a variety of sources, particularly from early experience, but also from events in the patient's social circle or the mass media. Previous experience of physical ill health in patients and in their families and previous experience of unsatisfactory medical management may be important (see Bianchi, 1971). A further factor is the information carried by the media. A striking example is provided by the influx of cases of "AIDS phobia" noted after the publicity campaign on this topic.

Examples of potentially problematic assumptions are "Bodily changes are usually a sign of serious disease, because every symptom has to have an identifiable physical cause" and "If you don't go to the doctor as soon as you notice anything unusual then it will be too late." Some assumptions concern health worries, for example, "If I don't worry about my health then I could get sick." In this instance, it can be that persons believe that worrying about health keeps them safe in some direct superstitious way (as in not tempting fate) or that worrying about health means they remain vigilant for symptoms that they may otherwise neglect until they are too strong (and it is therefore too late). Other types of belief relate to specific personal weaknesses and particular illnesses; for example, "There's heart trouble in the family"; "I've had weak lungs since I was a baby." Such beliefs may be a constant source of anxiety and/or may be activated in vulnerable individuals by critical incidents. Assumptions can also lead the patient to selectively attend to information that appears to confirm the idea of having an illness and to selectively ignore or discount evidence indicating good health. Thus, particular assumptions often lead to a *confirmatory bias* in the patient's thinking once a critical incident has resulted in the misinterpretation of bodily symptoms and signs as being indications of serious illness. Situations that constitute critical incidents and activate previously dormant assumptions include unfamiliar bodily sensations, hearing details of illness in a friend of a similar age, or new information about illness. Further bodily sensations may then be noticed as a consequence of increased vigilance arising from anxiety. In patients who become particularly anxious about their health, such situations are associated with thoughts that represent personally catastrophic interpretations of the bodily sensations or signs.

Catastrophic interpretations can in turn lead to one of two patterns of anxiety. If the sensations or signs are *not* those that increase as a result of anxiety (as a consequence of autonomic arousal), or the patient does not regard the feared catastrophe as immediate, then the reaction will be hypochondriacal anxiety about health, with the cognitive, behavioral, physiological, and affective correlates as detailed above (e.g., "The pains in my stomach mean I have an undetected cancer"). On the other hand, if the symptoms that are misinterpreted are those that occur as part of anxiety-induced autonomic arousal and the interpretation is that the symptoms are the signs of *immediate* catastrophe (e.g., "These palpitations mean that I am having a heart attack right now"), a further immediate increase in symptoms will result. If this process continues, then a panic attack is the more likely response (Clark, 1988; Salkovskis, 1988). Despite the differences in type of symptoms and time course of feared illness, the ideation in panic and hypochondriasis is similar and the two presentations often overlap (see Noyes, Reich, Clancy, & O'Gorman, 1986).

Factors Directly Involved in Maintaining Preoccupation with Worries about Health

Figure 3.2 illustrates the main ways psychological factors operate to maintain anxiety and preoccupation with health. It is important to remember that, in many patients, these physical and psychological factors interact with other mechanisms involved in the maintenance of somatic changes, interacting with the factors described here rather than overriding them.

1. *Increased physiological arousal.* This stems from the perception of threat and leads to an increase in autonomically mediated sensations; these sensations are often interpreted by the patient as further evidence of illness. For example, a patient noticed an increase in sweating and had the thought that this was a sign of a serious hormonal imbalance; sweating increased when this thought occurred, which provided further evidence of "disturbance." This factor is important in determining the high comorbidity rates of hypochondriasis with panic (Salkovskis & Clark, 1993); illness-based panic-type misinterpretations are common in hypochondriasis, such as interpreting palpitations as a sign that something is wrong with one's heart, dizziness as a sign of a stroke, and so on. (Salkovskis and Clark [1993] discuss the similarites and differences between panic and hypochondriasis in greater detail.)

2. *Focus of attention.* Normal variations in bodily function (including those that give rise to bodily sensations) or previously unnoticed aspects of appearance or bodily function may come to patients' attention and be perceived as novel. Patients may conclude that these perceived changes

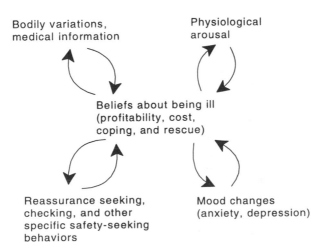

Bodily variations, medical information

Physiological arousal

Beliefs about being ill (profitability, cost, coping, and rescue)

Reassurance seeking, checking, and other specific safety-seeking behaviors

Mood changes (anxiety, depression)

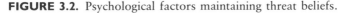

FIGURE 3.2. Psychological factors maintaining threat beliefs.

represent pathological departures from "normal." For example, a patient noticed that the roots of his fingernails looked pale and that he had white spots on his nails and interpreted this as a sign of a "hormone problem." He found this observation extremely upsetting and could not believe that he could have missed something so significant in the past, which meant it must be a new phenomenon. Focus of attention may also lead to actual changes in physiological systems where both reflex and voluntary control is involved (e.g., breathing, swallowing, muscular activity, etc). For example, a patient may notice difficulty in swallowing dry foods and interpret this as a sign of throat cancer. Focusing on swallowing can then lead to undue effort and increased discomfort and difficulty. The experience of pain is increased by focus of attention (Melzack, 1979) independently of the way in which pain is interpreted.

3. *Avoidant behaviors.* Unlike people with phobias, patients with worries about their physical condition are primarily anxious about threats posed by internal situations or stimuli (bodily sensations such as stomach discomfort or pains, bodily signs such as lumps under the skin). However, their attention can be focused on to these internal stimuli by external factors such as reading about a particular disease, or the inquiries of a concerned spouse. Patients seldom have the option of completely avoiding anxiety-provoking stimuli, so they resort instead to behaviors designed to minimize bodily discomfort and to behaviors they believe may prevent feared disasters. The belief that danger has been averted sustains the patients' beliefs; for example, "If I hadn't used my inhaler, I would have suffocated and died"; "I never exercise because it might kill me."

In some patients prone to anxiety about their health, behaviors such as bodily checking and reassurance seeking are reinforced by a temporary reduction of anxiety; as with obsessional patients, this is at the expense of a longer-term increase in anxiety and preoccupation. In reassurance seeking, the patient's intention is to draw the attention of others to his or her physical state so that any physical abnormality would be detected (and hence decrease long-term risk). In fact, checking and reassurance seeking focus patients' attention on their fears and prevent habituation to the anxiety-provoking stimuli. In some instances, persistent distress, impairment of normal behavior, and frequent requests for medical consultation, investigations, and reassurance persuade sympathetic physicians to opt for more drastic medical interventions. These can sometimes include surgery or powerful medication, which patients may take as confirmation of their fears, thereby worsening their symptoms and complaints, and sometimes adding new iatrogenic symptoms to those already present (e.g., side effects from the medication).

Some behaviors have a more direct physical effect on the patient's symptoms. For example, a patient who noticed persistent weakness reduced his activities, stopped playing sports, and reduced the amount he walked. After some months, he noticed that the weakness was getting worse (actually due to unfitness), which confirmed his initial fears that he was suffering from multiple sclerosis. Pain patients frequently reduce the amount they exercise and adopt exaggerated postures in attempts to moderate their pain. As a result of this behavior, the pain (which may originally have been muscular) worsens, and the patient begins to experience pain from other muscles persistently held in awkward positions. A patient with pains in his testicles frequently pressed them to check whether the pain was still there; he did this for periods of up to 15 minutes, sometimes with only 2 or 3 minutes between. Not surprisingly, the pain increased, and his disability with it. Other common behaviors include excessive use of things such as inappropriate medication (prescribed or not), corsets, sticks, crutches, and so forth.

4. *Beliefs and misinterpretation of symptoms, signs, and medical communications.* The most important aspect of health anxiety and a crucial component in the complaints of many patients with somatic problems is the misinterpretation of innocuous bodily changes, or of information provided by doctors, friends, or the media. Patients take these changes and communications as evidence that they are suffering from a more serious problem than is really so. This is especially likely when exaggerated beliefs that patients have about the nature of symptoms or illness result in a *confirmatory bias* with respect to illness-related information. As a result, such patients selectively notice and remember information consistent with their negative beliefs about their problems. For instance, a patient saw a neurologist about headaches and dizziness; the neurologist told him that if he had a brain tumor it would have worsened and then killed him. The patient, who believed that any sensations in the head were a sign of something internally wrong, later told his therapist that the neurologist had said that he had a fatal brain tumor, because he was noticing his symptoms more which he thought meant that his tumor was getting worse. He believed that the neurologist saying that he had nothing seriously wrong with him was an example of "breaking it gently."

The specific identification of factors such as these in any individual patient is crucial to the strategy used in cognitive therapy, which focuses on reaching a shared understanding of psychological processes that might account for the patient's problems. This general strategy, as applied to both health anxiety and to obsessional problems, will be discussed next.

TREATMENT IN HEALTH ANXIETY
AND OBSESSIVE–COMPULSIVE DISORDER

It follows from the preceding discussion that treatment of obsessional problems and severe anxiety about health needs to involve reaching a shared understanding with the patient concerning the psychological basis of their problem. This is crucial because at the beginning of therapy, these patients believe that their problem is that they are in danger of some terrible catastrophe. If this belief is held very strongly, the patient is unlikely to engage in psychologically (or psychiatrically) based treatment. The obsessional patient believes that he or she is a child molester or is contaminated, the hypochondriacal patient believes that he or she has heart disease or cancer. Patients at that stage, therefore, seek to solve their problems by being cleaner, by ensuring that they are not responsible for harm, by getting the appropriate medical help, and so on. It is therefore necessary that in the early stages of treatment patients are helped to see that there may be an alternative explanation for the difficulties they are experiencing. Patients are introduced to an idiosyncratically based cognitive model that offers a quite different and less threatening account of their problems. That is, it is not that they are a child molester or that they have cancer but that they are *worried about and believe* that they might be a child molester and that they are *worried about and believe* that they might have cancer. For treatment to be effective, it follows that it is crucial that the patient agrees therapeutic strategies should be aimed at reducing such worries rather than the fruitless attempts to reduce risk.

At this stage of treatment (engagement) the two possible explanations for the patient's problems are considered alongside each other rather than as mutually exclusive alternatives. The patient is invited to consider how the two alternative views match up to his or her experience. Once therapist and patient agree on the two alternatives, therapy proceeds as an evaluation of the relative merits of these two views. Evidence for and against each is reviewed and discussed in detail (see Salkovskis, 1989, for a more comprehensive clinical description of how this can be done).

Often, discussion reaches the point where further information not currently available to the patient has to be sought. This is where behavioral experiments come in; they are information-gathering exercises that help persons reach conclusions about their beliefs. For example, a patient may have noticed that his chest pain tends to worsen around the time that he exercises. During the discussion he is not certain whether this is before, during, or after exercise. In order to test this out therapist and patient go for a brisk walk around the hospital, taking repeated ratings of chest pain intensity. The obsessional patient can see that trying not to think a thought might increase the frequency of that thought. However, she also considers it possible that her thoughts of harming her children may not follow this pattern and it may be that she is only managing to hold them at bay by pushing them away and distracting herself. To test this out the patient keeps a diary record of the frequency of the thoughts' occurrence and on some days attempts to distract herself from them as hard as she possibly can and on other days tries to allow the thoughts to come and not fight them. In doing so she discovers that the thoughts occur more frequently and upset her more on those days when she chooses to resist them. In this way there is a constant interplay between the cognitive behavioral formulation drawn up by patient and therapist, discussion of how the patient's experience fits with that formulation, and generation of new and informative experience using behavioral experiments to further illuminate the model. Cognitive and behavioral elements are interwoven, but the guiding principle is always enabling the patient to consider and adopt a more helpful and less frightening belief than the one they have been stuck with previously.

The main elements of treatment are as follows:

1. Working with patients to develop a comprehensive cognitive-behavioral model of the maintenance of their obsessional problems. This involves identifying key distorted beliefs and the collaborative construction of a nonthreatening alternative account of their obsessional experience to allow patients to explicitly test beliefs about responsibility.

2. Detailed identification and self-monitoring of obsessional thoughts and patients' appraisal of these thoughts combined with exercises designed to help patients to modify their responsibility beliefs on a minute-by-minute basis (e.g., by using the Daily Record of Dysfunctional Thoughts).

3. Discussion techniques for challenging appraisals and basic assumptions upon which these are based. The aim is modification of the patients' negative beliefs about the extent of their own personal responsibility (e.g., by having the patient describe all contributing factors for a feared outcome and then dividing the contribution in a pie chart).

4. Behavioral experiments to directly test appraisals, assumptions, and processes hypothesized to be involved in the patients' obsessional problems (e.g., demonstrating that attempts to suppress a thought lead to an increase in the frequency with which it occurs, or showing that beliefs such as "If I think it I therefore want it to happen" are incorrect). Each behavioral experiment is idiosyncratically devised in order to help patients test their previous (threatening) explanation of their experience against the new (nonthreatening) explanation worked out with their therapist.

5. Helping patients to identify and modify underlying general assumptions (such as "Not trying to prevent harm is as bad as making it happen deliberately") that give rise to their misinterpretation of their own mental activity.

In the treatment of both obsessional problems and health anxiety the idea is that the factors that previously triggered anxiety and discomfort may continue to occur. However, therapy has the effect of modifying the meaning of physical variations or intrusive thoughts to the level experienced by most other people who do not suffer from an anxiety disorder of this type. No direct attempt is made to decrease the number of bodily sensations or variations experienced, and any intention on the part of the patient to bring about such a reduction is challenged on the basis of the beliefs that drive it. However, a fortunate and desirable side effect of cognitive therapy is that there is usually an actual decrease in such symptoms. Note that the "normal" person does not constantly seek to control symptoms or thoughts;

control tends to be indirect, because there are no serious negative consequences of failing to control symptoms.

CONCLUSION

In this chapter I have tried to show the way in which the cognitive hypothesis deals with the relationship between normal emotional responding and emotional problems or disorders. Experiencing anxiety is a normal phenomenon and the factors involved in generating and maintaining severe anxiety problems are also fundamentally normal. In emotional disorders a resonance or interlock is set up between beliefs concerning threat and the way in which the person responds to that perceived threat. In the course of therapy a *new*, nonthreatening pattern of meaning is established or reestablished. The aim is to have the nonthreatening beliefs become a relatively automatic way of responding to situations that would previously have triggered anxiety-maintaining reactions. Such reactions should be self-maintaining, removing the need for constant vigilance and control attempts that characterize more behavioral approaches to the management of anxiety. The analysis of anxiety-related efforts to control or prevent negative outcomes in terms of safety-seeking behaviors allows a clear theoretical and clinical distinction to be made between adaptive coping as opposed to avoidance. This, then, is part of the legacy of Aaron T. Beck; a flexible, empirically based view of emotions and emotional problems with a unique normalizing and empowering emphasis.

NOTES

1. This story is borrowed with permission from Philip Kendall (Kendall, 1992). Phil, have you heard the one about swearing?

2. Responsibility is used in this context in a specific way. The responsibility appraisal that is hypothesized as characterizing obsessional problems is operationally defined as "the belief that one has power which is pivotal to bring about or prevent subjectively crucial negative outcomes. These outcomes may be actual, that is, having consequences in the real world, and/or at a moral level" (Salkovskis, Rachman, Ladouceur, & Freeston, 1992).

REFERENCES

American Psychiatric Association. (1994). *Diagnostic and statistical manual of mental disorders* (4th ed.). Washington, DC: Author.

Beck, A. T. (1976). *Cognitive therapy and the emotional disorders*. New York: International Universities Press.

Beck, A. T., Emery, G., & Greenberg, R. L. (1985). *Anxiety disorders and phobias*. New York: Basic Books.

Bianchi, G. N. (1971). The origins of disease phobia. *Australia and New Zealand Journal of Psychiatry, 5,* 241–257.

Clark, D. M. (1986a). A cognitive approach to panic. *Behaviour Research and Therapy, 24,* 461–470.

Clark, D. M. (1986b). Cognitive therapy for anxiety. Behavioural Psychotherapy, 14, 283–294.

Clark, D. M. (1988). A cognitive model of panic, In S. J. Rachman & J. Maser (Eds.), *Panic: Psychological perspective.* Hillsdale, NJ: Erlbaum.

Clark, D. M., & Beck, A. T. (1988), Cognitive approaches. In C. G. Last & M. Hersen (Eds.), *Handbook of anxiety disorders.* New York: Pergamon.

Clark, D. M., & Wells, A. (1995). A cognitive model of social phobia. In R. G. Heimberg, M. R. Liebowitz, D. A. Hope, & F. A. Schneier (Eds.), *Social phobia: Diagnosis, assessment and treatment.* New York: Guilford Press.

Edwards, S., & Dickerson, M. (1987). On the similarity of positive and negative intrusions. *Behaviour Research and Therapy, 25,* 207–211.

England, S. L., & Dickerson, M. (1988). Intrusive thoughts: Unpleasantness not the major cause of uncontrollability. *Behaviour Research and Therapy, 26,* 279–277.

Eysenck, H. J. (1979). The conditioning model of neurosis. *Behavioral and Brain Sciences, 2,* 155–166.

Kendall, P. C. (1992). *Anxiety disorders in youth: Cognitive behavioral interventions.* Boston: Allyn & Bacon.

Melzack, R. (1979). Current concepts of pain. In D. J. Oborne, M. M. Gruneberg, & J. R. Eiser (Eds.), *Research in psychology and medicine: 1.* London: Academic Press.

Nisbett, R. E., & Ross, L. (1980). *Human inference: Strategies and shortcomings of social judgement.* Englewood Cliffs, NJ: Prentice Hall.

Noyes, R., Reich, J., Clancy, J., & O'Gorman, T. W. (1986). Reduction in hypochondriasis with treatment of panic disorder. *British Journal of Psychiatry, 149,* 631–635.

Rachman, S. J. (1971). Obsessional ruminations. *Behaviour Research and Therapy, 9,* 229–235.

Rachman, S. J. (1983). Irrational thinking, with special reference to cognitive therapy. *Advances in Behaviour Research and Therapy, 5,* 63–88.

Rachman, S. J. (1993). Obsessions, responsibility and guilt. *Behaviour Research and Therapy, 31,* 149–154.

Rachman, S. J., & de Silva, P. (1978). Abnormal and normal obsessions. *Behaviour Research and Therapy, 16,* 233–238.

Salkovskis, P. M. (1985). Obsessional-compulsive problems: A cognitive-behavioural analysis. *Behaviour Research and Therapy, 25,* 571–583.

Salkovskis, P. M. (1988). Phenomenology, assessment and the cognitive model of panic. In S. J. Rachman & J. Maser (Eds.), *Panic: Psychological perspectives.* Hillsdale, NJ: Erlbaum.

Salkovskis, P. M. (1989). Somatic problems. In K. Hawton, P. M. Salkovskis, J. Kirk, & D. M. Clark (Eds.), *Cognitive behaviour therapy for psychiatric problems: A practical guide.* Oxford: Oxford University Press.

Salkovskis, P. M. (1991). The importance of behaviour in the maintenance of anxiety and panic: A cognitive account. *Behavioural Psychotherapy, 19,* 6–19.

Salkovskis, P. M., & Campbell, P. (1994). Thought suppression in naturally occurring negative intrusive thoughts. *Behaviour Research and Therapy, 32,* 1–8.

Salkovskis, P. M., & Clark, D. M. (1993). Panic and hypochondriasis. *Advances in Behavior Research and Therapy, 15,* 23–48.

Salkovskis, P. M., Clark, D. M., & Gelder, M. G. (in press). Cognition-behaviour links in the persistence of panic. *Behaviour Research and Therapy.*

Salkovskis, P. M., & Harrison, J. (1984). Abnormal and normal obsessions: A replication. *Behaviour Research and Therapy, 22,* 549–552.

Salkovskis, P. M., & Kirk, J. (1989). Obsessional disorders. In K. Hawton, P. M. Salkovskis, J. Kirk, & D. M. Clark (Eds.), *Cognitive-behavioural treatment for psychiatric disorders: A practical guide.* Oxford: Oxford University Press.

Salkovskis, P. M., Rachman, S. J., Ladouceur, R., & Freeston, M. (1992). *Proceedings of the Toronto cafeteria.* Unpublished manuscript.

Salkovskis, P. M., Richards, C., & Forrester, G. (1995). The relationship between obsessional problems and intrusive thoughts. *Behavioral and Cognitive Psychotherapy, 23,* 281–299.

Salkovskis, P. M., & Warwick, H. M. C. (1986). Morbid preoccupations, health anxiety and reassurance: A cognitive behavioural approach to hypochondriasis. *Behaviour Research and Therapy, 24,* 597–602.

Seligman, M. E. P. (1988). Competing theories of panic. In S. Rachman & J. D. Maser (Eds.), *Panic: Psychological perspectives.* Hillsdale, NJ: Erlbaum.

Spranca, M., Minsk, E., & Baron, J. (1991). Omission and commission in judgment and choice. *Journal of Experimental Social Psychology, 27,* 76–105.

Teasdale, J. D. (1983) Negative thinking in depression: Cause, effect or reciprocal relationship? *Advances in Behaviour Research and Therapy, 5,* 3–25.

Trinder, H., & Salkovskis, P. M. (1994). Personally relevant intrusions outside the laboratory: Long term suppression increases intrusion. *Behaviour Research and Therapy, 32,* 833–842.

Warwick, H. M. C., & Salkovskis, P. M. (1990). Hypochondriasis. *Behaviour Research and Therapy, 28,* 105–118.

Chapter 4

Empirical Status of the Cognitive Model of Anxiety and Depression

David A. Clark
Robert A. Steer

BASIC ELEMENTS OF THE COGNITIVE MODEL

Cognitive Theory and Therapy: A Case of Shared Identity

From its inception, the cognitive therapy that was developed and advanced by Aaron T. Beck has established a strong link between theory and research on cognitive factors in psychopathology (Beck, 1967, p. 318). According to a monograph based on his Malcolm Miller Lecture in Psychotherapy at Aberdeen University, Professor Beck described cognitive therapy as a direct outgrowth of his observations and research about cognitive factors in depression (Beck, 1988). In fact, he (Beck, 1976) argued that a psychological treatment approach can only qualify as a system of psychotherapy if it provides "(a) a comprehensive theory or model of psychopathology, and (b) a detailed description of and guide to therapeutic techniques related to this model" (pp. 306–307). Thus over the years Beck has repeatedly emphasized a close link between cognitive theory and practice in his research and writings (Beck, 1976, 1991).

Empirical research about the cognitive model underlying psychopathology is important for the practice of cognitive therapy for two primary reasons. First, the distinctiveness of cognitive therapy as a system of psychotherapy does not depend on the particular therapeutic techniques employed by cognitive therapists (many of these are borrowed from other therapy schools), but upon the fundamental cognitive constructs and propositions that guide the implementation of therapy (Beck, 1991). Consequently, research testing the validity of these assumptions is highly relevant to the veracity of the cognitive treatment approach.

Second, research on the cognitive model may help to elucidate possible change mechanisms that may account for the effectiveness of cognitive therapy. Understanding such mechanisms may, in turn, lead to improvements in the cognitive treatment of various disorders. Obviously, the efficacy of cognitive therapy can only be determined by the results of treatment outcome and process studies. However, after 30 years of theory, research, and practice, Beck's cognitive therapy has been described by Dobson (1994) as "an internally consistent model with proven outcome effectiveness." This optimistic conclusion can be partly attributed to the interdependence between cognitive theory and practice, making research about cognitive theory directly relevant for the cognitive treatment of psychopathological disorders.

Basic Assumptions of the Cognitive Model

The cognitive theory of psychopathology is based on an information-processing perspective (Beck, 1987). According to Beck, systematic information-processing biases are evident in all psychopathological states (Beck, 1967, 1976, 1987). The faulty information processing is an integral part of the emergent symptom complex and functions to maintain psychological disorders (Beck, 1991; Clark & Beck, 1989). In addition to biased information processing, the cognitive model states that psychopathological conditions represent streams of consciousness dominated by negative automatic thoughts and images that are, in turn, derived from enduring, latent cognitive structures or schemas with a dysfunctional or maladaptive orientation (Beck, 1976, 1987; Clark & Beck, 1989). Based on this model, four intrinsic assumptions can be identified that guide cognitive theory and treatment:

    1. *Individuals actively construct their reality.* The core tenet of the cognitive model is that individuals are not passive receptacles of environmental stimuli or physical sensations, but are actively involved in constructing their own realities (Beck, 1967, 1987). All perception, learning, and knowing are the products of an information-processing system that actively selects, filters, and interprets environmental and other sensory stimuli that impinge on the individual. Consequently, individuals attach highly personal, idiosyncratic meanings to events, and these meanings may subsequently lead to maladaptive emotional or behavioral responding if such meanings reflect inaccurate representations of events (Beck, 1991). For example, in depression individuals tend to interpret personally significant negative experiences as supporting their beliefs about being a failure.

    2. *Cognition mediates affect and behavior.* Cognitive content, processes, and structures are assumed to influence or mediate behavior and emotion (Dobson & Block, 1988). At the descriptive level, the model views cognitive factors as mediators or concomitants of psychological disorders, rather than as causal agents (Beck, 1987; Haaga, Dyck, & Ernst, 1991). The cognitive model does not postulate a sequential unidirectional relation-

ship in which cognition always precedes emotion, but assumes that cognition, emotion, and behavior are reciprocally determining and interactive constructs (Beck, 1991). Negative automatic thoughts and biased cognitive processes do not play a causal role in depression but instead are cardinal symptoms of the depressive disorder that play a primary mediating role in maintaining other emotional, behavioral, and motivational symptoms of the disorder (Beck, 1987, 1991).

3. *Cognition is knowable and accessible.* Beck's cognitive model proposes constructs that can be operationally defined and empirically tested. The measurement of cognition has played an important role in Beck's research over the years, and development of such instruments as the Beck Depression Inventory (Beck & Steer, 1993c), the Beck Anxiety Inventory (Beck & Steer, 1993a), the Beck Hopelessness Scale (Beck & Steer, 1993b), and Cognitions Checklist (Beck, Brown, Steer, Eidelson, & Riskind, 1987) indicates his level of commitment to the measurement of cognitive constructs. However, the cognitive model does not assert that all cognitive processes are conscious, controlled, or effortful. The model recognizes varying levels of accessibility (Beck, 1976). In fact, the definition of negative *automatic thoughts* assumes that the thoughts associated with psychological disorders are quite spontaneous and just on the fringe of consciousness (Beck, 1988). One of the basic assumptions of cognitive theory and treatment is that individuals can be trained to gain access to the products of their faulty information processing (Beck, 1991).

4. *Cognitive change is central to the human change process.* This assumption, which is the cornerstone of cognitive therapy, is a logical extensive of cognitive theory to the treatment of psychological disorders. If cognitive dysfunction is crucial for the maintenance of anxious and depressive symptoms, then change across a broad range of behavioral, emotional, and somatic symptoms can only be achieved by modifying the cognitive symptoms. In other words, behavioral and emotional improvement is possible only if the mediating cognitive products, processes, and structures change. This may be achieved directly by a cognitive therapeutic technique, such as cognitive restructuring, or indirectly by a behavioral intervention, such as graded *in vivo* exposure or activity schedules.

Descriptive Level of the Cognitive Model

At the descriptive level, the cognitive model proposes a number of hypotheses about the role of cognition in depression that are derived from the basic assumptions of the model (Haaga et al., 1991). These hypotheses are testable and have been, to varying degrees, investigated in a number of studies.

The first, labeled the "negativity hypothesis," states that in all types of depression one will find a significant increase in negative self-referent thinking concerning the self, future, and world (Beck, 1976, 1987, 1988, 1991). Considerable empirical support has been found for the negativity hypothesis in both clinical and nonclinical samples (Clark & Beck, 1989; Engel & DeRubeis, 1993; Haaga et al., 1991). These studies suggest that negative cognitions are associated with depression at the syndrome, symptom, and mood-state levels. However, there have been challenges to the "universality" of negative thinking in depression. The hopelessness theory of depression, for example, asserts that only a subtype of depression will present with the *negative cognitive triad* (Abramson, Metalsky, & Alloy, 1989; Engel & DeRubeis, 1993). Based on their own research findings and those of Hamilton and Abramson (1983), Miller and Norman (1986) concluded that approximately 50% of depressed patients have high levels of cognitive distortion. Thus, cognitive negativity bias may not be found in all depressed persons.

Second, the *primacy hypothesis* states that biased cognition or information processing will critically influence the other symptoms of anxiety and depression. Beck (1987) considers *primacy* to mean that biased cognitive processing will lead to a corresponding change in the individual's emotional and behavioral responding. This suggests that negative cognition may be so integral to the depressive experience that cognitive symptoms should be targeted in the treatment of depression, rather than "noncognitive" depressive symptoms. In a footnote, Beck (1987) clarifies this point by noting that primacy does not mean that biased cognitions cause the other symptoms of depression. In their review, Haaga et al. (1991) consider the primacy "hypothesis" as a convenient strategy for helping clinicians understand and organize their patients' problems rather than as a construct that can be empirically tested. Despite this misgiving about the *primary* role of negative cognitions in depression, evidence from the mood induction and psychophysiological literature suggests that the production of negative self-referent thoughts and images can lead to affective, behavioral, and physiological responses characteristic of depression (D. M. Clark, 1983; Martin, 1990; Sirota & Schwartz, 1982; Teasdale & Bancroft, 1977; Teasdale & Rezin, 1978). However, no prospective clinical studies have yet investigated the temporal sequence of cognitive and noncognitive symptoms.

The third hypothesis relevant to the descriptive level of the cognitive model is referred to as the *cognitive content–specificity* hypothesis. This is one of the central hypotheses of the cognitive model and has been subjected to considerable research over the last few years. The hypothesis states that every psychological disorder has a distinctive cognitive profile which is reflected at all levels of cognitive functioning (Beck, 1967, p. 270; Beck, 1987). In depression, the predominant cognitive theme is about personal loss or deprivation, whereas in anxiety the main theme is about physical or psychological threat or danger. Thus, the specific cognitive content associated with a disorder is considered to be critical for the differential diagnosis of anxiety or depression.

Table 4.1 summarizes the main characteristics that distinguish nega-

TABLE 4.1. Comparison of Cognitive Profile in Anxiety and Depression

Depression	Anxiety
Cognitive structures	
Maladaptive beliefs focused mainly on personal loss and failure in interpersonal and achievement domains	Maladaptive beliefs focused on physical or psychological threat to self or significant others with an increased sense of personal vulnerability.
Cognitive processing	
Enhanced processing of negative and exclusion of positive self-referent information	Selective processing of threat cues with an overestimation of vulnerability.
Appraisals are pervasive, global, absolute, and exclusive.	Appraisals are selective, tentative, and specific to a fear situation(s).
Increased self-focused attention may reduce responsiveness to external stimuli.[a]	Increased self-focused attention reflects attempts to control stimuli.[a]
Negative cognitions	
Thoughts of personal loss and failure.	Thoughts of threat and danger.
Thoughts take the form of past-oriented self-statements.	Thoughts take the form of questions ("what if") involving possible harm and danger.

[a]See Kendall and Ingram (1987, pp. 94–98).

tive thinking in anxiety and depression (see also Beck & Clark, 1988). Negative thinking in depression stresses past losses and failures, and a patient describes such thoughts in terms of global, absolute, and exclusive self-statements (Beck & Clark, 1988). Anxiety disorders, on the other hand, are characterized by future-oriented automatic thoughts about potential physical or psychological threats and these thoughts express an increased sense of vulnerability (Beck & Clark, 1988). Anxious thoughts tend to be more selective, tentative, and anticipatory in nature, usually taking the form of a question, such as "what if" (Beck & Clark, 1988; Kendall & Ingram, 1987, pp. 94–98).

Research on the cognitive content–specificity hypothesis addresses the validity of the cognitive model for the following reasons. First, cognitive content–specificity is one of the main tenets of the cognitive model. If negative cognitive content found in anxiety is similar to that found in depression, then Beck's cognitive model is questionable. It would lead one to question the efficacy of focusing on negative thinking in the treatment of anxiety and depression, and instead suggest that other noncognitive symptoms may be more critical to psychopathological states (Ingram, 1990). Although one should not discount the importance of nonspecific variables in psychopathological research, nevertheless it is the unique or specific elements that establish the pathognomic nature of the disorder and suggest possible points of intervention (Garber & Hollon, 1991).

Second, cognitive content–specificity research has important implications for the diagnosis of psychological disorders (Garber & Hollon, 1991). A viable classification system of psychopathology must include symptoms with high sensitivity and/or specificity (Frances, Pincus, Widiger, Davis, & First, 1990). The classification system must describe both the essential and discriminating features of the disorders. Research into specificity can indicate whether cognitive content is useful for arriving at a differential diagnosis of anxiety and depression. However, it should be noted that DSM-IV (American Psychiatric Association, 1994) considers affective and motivational, rather than negative cognition symptoms, to be the critical core features of a major depressive episode. On the other hand, cognitive symptoms, such as worrying about the consequences of a panic attack or apprehensive expectation, are critical defining symptom features of panic disorder and generalized anxiety disorder, respectively.

Finally, cognitive content–specificity research has implications for the measurement of psychological disorders, such as anxiety and depression. Review articles have consistently reported a high correlation (average r's of .62–.70) between anxiety and depression instruments (L. A. Clark & Watson, 1991a; Dobson, 1985; Gotlib & Cane, 1989). If psychopathological states have a distinct cognitive profile, then one should be able to improve the discriminant validity of symptom measures by increasing the number of cognitive items contained in anxiety and depression instruments. In the following section we shall review the empirical literature about the cognitive content–specificity of anxiety and depression at the symptom, syndrome, and measurement levels. However, before reviewing this literature, we briefly describe a second level of conceptualization in the cognitive model: cognitive vulnerability or causality.

Causality and the Cognitive Model of Anxiety and Depression

Beck's model does not limit cognitive theory to the description of symptom patterns. There is a causal level in the model that considers certain cognitive constructs crucial in the etiology of some depressions (Beck, 1987, 1991). Before describing these constructs, it is important to consider two qualifications often overlooked in critiques of the causal status of cognitive variables or cognitive vulnerability as it is commonly referred to in the literature. First, Beck (1987, 1991) clearly states that cognitive structures, such as latent maladaptive beliefs or schemas, are distal predisposing factors that may contribute to the onset of a depressive episode. The maladaptive schemas are neither necessary nor sufficient causes of depression. Second, the interaction of a predisposing cognitive vulnerability with a precipitating life event will be evident in only some depressions, possibly only those of a "reactive" nature (Beck, 1991; Clark, Beck, & Brown, 1992). Thus, the cognitive vulnerability hypothesis is not considered to be applicable universally to all cases of depression.

In his earlier cognitive theory of depression, Beck (1967, 1976) emphasized the role of latent, maladaptive schemas in the etiology of depression. In recent years, the emphasis in Beck's cognitive vulnerability hypothesis has shifted away from idiosyncratic negative schemas to broader, superordinate schematic constellations that reflect personality orientations or modes (Beck, 1983, 1987). Beck (1983) postulated sociotropy and autonomy as two possible vulnerability factors involved in the predisposition to reactive depression or other psychopathological conditions, such as anxiety.

According to Beck (1983), the *sociotropic* personality orientation places a high value on having close interpersonal relations, with a strong emphasis on being loved and accepted by others. On the other hand, the *autonomous* personality orientation reflects a high investment in personal independence, achievement, and freedom of choice. From a vulnerability perspective, a highly sociotropic or autonomous individual may be equally at risk for either depression or anxiety. Sociotropic or socially dependent individuals try to satisfy their needs for security and self-worth by pleasing others and avoiding others' disapproval by maintaining close interpersonal attachments (Beck, 1983; Beck, Epstein, Harrison, & Emery, 1983). In contrast, the highly autonomous person derives self-worth from mastery and achievement and so can make excessive personal demands for self-control and accomplishment. Autonomous individuals tend to be less sensitive to the needs of others, preferring solitude and privacy instead of the company of others (Beck, 1983; Beck et al., 1983).

In recent years, Beck (1983, 1987, 1991) has argued that depression does not occur in isolation, even in cognitively vulnerable individuals. He recognizes that an acute or chronic environmental stressor or strain is usually involved in the onset of depression. In his reformulated cognitive theory, Beck (1987) postulated a *cognitive diathesis–stress* model to account for the etiology of reactive depressions and other clinical disorders. Sociotropy and autonomy are considered distal personality diatheses that interact with congruent or matching life events to precipitate a depressive reaction. Sociotropic persons are more likely to become depressed if they experience an event perceived as a loss of social resources, whereas an autonomous person is more likely to become depressed in response to events perceived to involve defeat or loss of personal independence, control, or mobility (Beck, 1987, 1991). According to this hypothesis, we would expect the precipitants of depression to reflect a specific congruence between (1) sociotropy and negative interpersonal events and (2) autonomy and negative achievement events.

EMPIRICAL SUPPORT FOR COGNITIVE SPECIFICITY

Cognitive Symptom Specificity

Numerous studies have demonstrated that thoughts of personal loss and failure are more highly associated with depression at the mood, symptom, and syndrome levels, whereas thoughts of harm and danger tend to be more highly associated with anxious symptoms and syndromes (for reviews see Clark & Beck, 1989; Engel & DeRubeis, 1993; Haaga et al., 1991; Ingram, 1990). Early studies testing about cognitive content–specificity tended to associate cognitive measures with their corresponding mood states, thereby producing inconclusive results about cognitive-symptom specificity (Clark, 1988). However, recent studies have compared different diagnostic groups, such as major depression and panic disorders, on measures of negative cognitions. Other studies using either clinical or nonclinical samples have examined the pattern of correlations between measures of cognitive content and different mood or symptom states. Overall, these more recent studies have supported the cognitive content–specificity hypothesis, although the data appear to be more supportive for the specificity of loss and failure cognitions in depression than they are for threat and danger cognitions in anxiety (Ambrose & Rholes, 1993; Beck et al., 1987; Clark, 1986; Clark, Beck, & Brown, 1989; Clark, Beck, & Stewart, 1990; Garber, Weiss, & Shanley, 1993; Harrell, Chambless, & Calhoun, 1981; Hollon, Kendall, & Lumry, 1986; Ingram, Kendall, Smith, Donnell, & Ronan, 1987; Jolly & Dykman, 1994; Jolly & Kramer, 1994; LaPointe & Harrell, 1978; Laurent & Stark, 1993; Rholes, Riskind, & Neville, 1985; Thorpe, Barnes, Hunter, & Hines, 1983; Wickless & Kirsch, 1988). Furthermore, there is some evidence that cognitive content–specificity may not be as consistent in certain populations, such as children, adolescents, or nonclinical college students (Garber et al., 1993; Laurent & Stark, 1993; Steer, Beck, Clark, & Beck, 1994).

Two recent issues about cognitive-symptom specificity center on (1) whether specificity may be stronger in positive rather than negative cognitions, and (2) whether cognitive-symptom specificity is consistent across various levels of disturbance. L. A. Clark and Watson (1991a, 1991b) have proposed a tripartite model to account for the relationship between anxiety and depression. According to their model, anxiety is distinguished from depression by symptoms of physiological hyperarousal, whereas depression is differentiated from anxiety by symptoms of loss of interest, low motivation, and anhedonia which reflect low positive affect (PA). General distress or high negative affect (NA) is considered to be a nonspecific symptom common to both psychological states. In the tripartite model, negative cognitions are characteristic of NA and nonspecific to anxiety and depression. On the other hand, low frequency of positive cognitions is expected to be specific to depression because depression reflects an absence of positive affect. Studies assessing the frequency of positive cognitions have found that depression is associated with a significantly lower rate of positive thinking (Burgess & Haaga, 1994; Ingram, 1989; Kendall, Howard, & Hays, 1989). However, it has not been shown that low frequency of positive thinking is *more* specific to depressive symptomatology than a high frequency of negative cognitions. Two studies found that there was decreased positive thinking in both anxiety and depression (Ingram, 1990; Ingram & Wisnicki, 1988).

Recently, Ambrose and Rholes (1993) reported that cognitive content–specificity may vary according to the frequency levels of the negative cognitions. Based on a large sample of nonclinical children and adolescents, they found a curvilinear relationship between threat cognitions and anxious symptoms, instead of the usual linear relationship that has been found between thoughts of loss and failure and depressive symptoms. At low levels of negative cognitions, loss cognitions were associated with both anxious and depressive symptoms (nonspecificity), whereas threat cognitions were related only to anxious symptoms (specificity). At the higher levels of negative thinking, both loss and threat cognitions were more positively associated with depressive than anxious symptoms. The authors concluded that a modification should be made to the cognitive content–specificity hypothesis to account for these differences in cognitive-symptom relationships with different frequency levels of negative thinking. They also suggested that the curvilinear relationship for threat cognitions indicated that anxiety may predominate at low levels of distress and depression may be dominate at high levels of disturbance. In a recent study by Clark, Steer, Beck, and Snow (1996), the relationship between loss and threat cognitions and anxious and depressive symptoms was investigated in psychiatric patients, chronic medically ill individuals, and normal controls. A strong linear relationship was evident in most of the regression analyses between cognition and symptom measures, with the curvilinear component making only a minimal contribution to the association. Moreover, cognitive content–specificity did vary with level of symptom severity. Specificity was found more consistently in the psychiatric inpatient and outpatient samples and, to a lesser extent, in the medical subjects than in the nonclinical control group. In sum, these findings suggest that future research on cognitive-symptom specificity must take into account sample characteristics, level of disturbance, and whether the cognition measures assess frequency of positive and/or negative cognitions.

Cognitive Specificity and Diagnosis

Few studies have investigated whether cognitive variables significantly improve upon the differential diagnosis of mood and anxiety disorders. In a discriminant analysis of patients with "pure" generalized anxiety disorder (GAD) and dysthymia (DD), Riskind et al. (1991) found that hopelessness and thoughts of loss and failure differentiated the DD group from the GAD group, but that anxious cognitions related to worry and apprehensive expectation did not distinguish the GAD group from the DD group. In a review of the literature on syndrome and symptom co-occurrence in anxiety disorders, Di Nardo and Barlow (1990) concluded that cognitive variables, such as excessive worry, attributional style, perception of control, and interpretation of symptoms, may differentiate anxiety and depressive disorders. Watson and Kendall (1989) also concluded in their review that the content of negative thinking and differences in biased information processing may differentiate anxious and depressive disorders.

In a study by Clark, Beck, and Beck (1994), affective, behavioral, motivational, cognitive, and somatic symptoms were measured in four diagnostic groups drawn from outpatients at the Philadelphia Center for Cognitive Therapy: (1) major depressive disorder (MDD; $n = 262$), (2) DD ($n = 82$), (3) panic disorder with or without agoraphobic avoidance (PD; $n = 156$), and (4) GAD ($n = 79$). The diagnoses were made by trained psychologists using the Structured Clinical Interview for DMS-III/DSM-III-R (Spitzer, Williams, Gibbon, & First, 1990). The Beck Depression Inventory (BDI), Beck Anxiety Inventory (BAI), Cognitions Checklist (CCL), and Hamilton Psychiatric Rating Scales for Anxiety and Depression were administered at the intake evaluation to assess depressive and anxious symptoms and cognitions. A principal components analysis (PCA) using a Varimax rotation was performed on the combined items of these instruments. Two of the components that emerged were particularly relevant with respect to cognitive content–specificity. The first component, labeled *Negative Self-View,* included all 14 CCL Depression items, as well as BDI items dealing with "sense of failure," "self-accusations," "self-dislike," "punishment," and "guilt." The second component, *Threat Cognitions,* included all 12 anxiety items of the CCL, as well as the BAI "fear of dying" item and the BDI "loss of libido" item. To determine the relative importance of the symptom dimensions in differentiating the four diagnostic groups, the 12 symptom components were entered into a standard discriminant function analysis. The first bipolar function differentiated depression and anxiety, and separated the MDD and DD groups from the PD and GAD groups. The second function represented a severity dimension and separated the MDD and PDD groups from the DD and GAD groups. Inspection of the standardized discriminant function coefficients and loading matrix indicated that negative self-view, anhedonia, and dysphoria distinguished depression, whereas presence of panic symptoms, threat-related cognitions, and subjective anxiety distinguished anxiety. These results, then, indicated that thoughts of loss and failure (negative self-view) had emerged as one of the best symptom variables for differentiating depression from anxiety, whereas cognitions of threat and danger, along with panic symptoms (physiological hyperarousal) and tension, were the best symptoms for distinguishing panic. Interestingly GAD was not well differentiated by these symptom measures. The findings thus supported cognitive content–specificity and indicated that the assessment of negative thought content may be useful in the differential diagnosis of anxiety and depression.

Cognitive Specificity and Measurement Issues

Various reviews of the psychometric literature on anxiety and depression have concluded that self-report and clinical rating scales of anxious and depressive symptoms and mood state are highly correlated (L. A. Clark & Watson, 1991a; Dobson, 1985; Gotlib & Cane, 1989). Reviewers have consistently recommended that the discriminant validity of anxiety and depression measures could be improved by including more items that assess unique or specific symptoms. According to Beck's cognitive content–specificity hypothesis, anxiety and depression measures that emphasize distinct cognitive content should have higher discriminant validity than measures that do not emphasize cognitive differences. L. A. Clark and Watson (1991a), on the other hand, argue that instruments which emphasize negative cognitions should have reduced discriminant validity because negative cognitions are characteristic of general distress which is common to both anxiety and depression.

To address this issue, we performed a series of factor analytic analyses on the 42 items of the revised BDI and BAI to determine the relative percentage of common and specific variance evident in these two self-report measures (Clark, Steer, & Beck, 1994). Separate factor analyses were conducted with 844 psychiatric outpatients and with 439 undergraduate students. Principal factor analyses using an oblique Promax rotation found two correlated factors in both samples, a Depression factor and an Anxiety factor. Using a Schmid–Leiman transformation (Gorsuch, 1983, pp. 248–254), it was discovered that the second-order factor accounted for over 40% of the shared variance in the BDI and BAI for both the outpatient and student samples. However, after partialing out the effects of this general second-order factor, the first-order Depression and Anxiety factors continued to explain over 20% of the common variance for the BDI and BAI in both samples. Our results are thus consistent with other studies suggesting that the BDI and BAI assess distinct symptom dimensions (Endler, Cox, Parker, & Bagby, 1992; Hewitt & Norton, 1993). Therefore, symptom measures of anxiety and depression which include cognitive symptoms in their item pool do assess specific anxiety and depression dimensions, even though a large nonspecific general distress or NA component may also be present in the measures (see also Jolly & Kramer, 1994). In contrast, researchers using a variety of traditional anxiety and depression measures have concluded that these instruments merely assess general distress (Feldman, 1993; Gotlib, 1984). Thus the inclusion of cognitive items may improve the specificity of anxiety and depression symptom measures.

EMPIRICAL STATUS OF COGNITIVE DIATHESIS–STRESS

During the last few years, a number of studies have tested the cognitive diathesis–stress hypothesis of depression. Different personality diatheses have been examined, such as negative attributional style (Metalsky, Halberstadt, & Abramson, 1987; Metalsky & Joiner, 1992), hopelessness (Metalsky & Joiner, 1992), perfectionism (Hewitt & Flett, 1993), interpersonal dependency, and self-criticism (Blatt & Zuroff, 1992; Zuroff & Mongrain, 1987). A few studies have investigated sociotropy and autonomy using either the Sociotropy–Autonomy Scale (SAS; Beck et al., 1983) or Approval by Others and Performance Evaluation subscales of the Dysfunctional Attitude Scale (DAS; Weissman & Beck, 1978). Generally, the findings have been equivocal. Analogue studies employing nonclinical subjects have tended to find a significant interaction between sociotropy and negative interpersonal event and no significant interaction between autonomy and negative achievement events (Clark et al. 1992; Robins & Block, 1988; Robins, 1990, Study 1; Nietzel & Harris, 1990; Rude & Burnham, 1993) . Prospective studies with remitted depressives have reported significant autonomy × negative achievement interactions, but the results have tended to be inconsistent (Hammen, Ellicott, Gitlin, & Jamison, 1989; Hammen, Ellicott, & Gitlin, 1989; Hammen, Ellicott, & Gitlin, 1992; Segal, Shaw, & Vella, 1989; Segal, Shaw, Vella, & Katz, 1992). It has been suggested that the inconsistent results with autonomy may be attributable to the psychometric limitations of the SAS Autonomy scale (Barnett & Gotlib, 1988; Robins & Block, 1988). In addition, Rude and Burnham (1993) concluded that there may be conceptual shortcomings with the achievement or autonomy vulnerability construct. They conclude that autonomy is a less coherent construct than sociotropy or interpersonal dependency, and so achievement vulnerability measures display low concurrent and predictive validities.

We recently completed two analogue studies on Beck's cognitive diathesis–stress hypothesis with undergraduate student samples. Students are an appropriate subject group for studying depression vulnerability because they tend to have higher rates of dysphoria and experience a greater number of stressful interpersonal and achievement events (Vrendenburg, Flett, & Krames, 1993). As well, vulnerability factors must be investigated in nonclinical samples if one's purpose is to identify the temporal antecedents to depression.

Using a cross-sectional design that involved 438 students who completed the BDI, the 60-item SAS, and a 104-item self-report life event inventory, Clark, Beck, and Brown (1992) recently tested the cognitive diathesis–stress hypothesis. Three independent raters categorized the life event items into 44 negative interpersonal events and 46 negative achievement events. Subjects rated each of the endorsed life events on three 5-point scales for degree of upset, perceived loss of interpersonal resources, and perceived loss of goals and independence. Subjects scoring above 16 on the BDI (n =

64) were classified as dysphoric, and a random sample of 64 nondysphoric individuals were selected from subjects scoring below 10 on the BDI. Using hierarchical multiple regression analysis, the main effects for personality, number of negative interpersonal events, and ratings of social and goal loss were evaluated on the first three steps. The interaction terms of personality with life event frequency and ratings of social and goal loss were entered on the final step of the analysis. The sociotropy × negative interpersonal event interaction was significant ($p < .05$) at the final step of the equation, whereas the incongruent interaction failed to attain significance (i.e., sociotropy × negative achievement events). The SAS Autonomy scale failed to have any significant main effects or interactions with negative life events. Personality diathesis also did not interact significantly with appraisals of loss associated with the events. Thus, the results were consistent with previous findings and partially supported the cognitive diathesis–stress hypothesis. However, cross-sectional designs cannot assess causality, but rather prospective research designs are needed to establish the temporal antecedence of the diathesis (Barnett & Gotlib, 1988; Garber & Hollon, 1991; Haaga et al., 1991; Hammen, 1985).

A more stringent study of the cognitive diathesis–stress hypothesis was next conducted (Clark, Purdon, & Beck, 1994). A prospective research design was employed in which 176 undergraduates completed the BDI and Extended SAS (Clark & Beck, 1991) at time 1 (T1), followed 3 months later by a retest on the BDI and the student version of the Negative Life Experiences Inventory (NLEI). The Extended SAS consisted of the 60 items of the original SAS (Beck et al., 1983) as well as 33 new autonomy items written to provide a more accurate assessment of the autonomous personality as described by Beck (1983). A series of item and factor analyses on successive samples of undergraduates yielded three scales for the Extended SAS (Clark & Beck, 1991; Clark, Ross, Beck, & Steer, 1995). The first scale, Sociotropy, consisted of 29 items with all but two taken from the original SAS, whereas two new autonomy dimensions also emerged, Solitude and Independence.

Separate hierarchical multiple-regression analyses were performed for each of the three SAS personality constructs. In each analysis, T1 BDI was entered on the first step as a covariate with BDI at time 2 (T2) as the dependent variable. The main effects for personality and number of negative interpersonal and autonomous events were entered on the second step, and the congruent and incongruent interaction terms were entered as the last step. Analysis of SAS Sociotropy and number of negative interpersonal events revealed a significant incremental R^2 ($R^2 = .03$; $F(6, 169) = 4.03$, $p < .02$) for the interaction terms. The congruent interaction of Sociotropy with negative interpersonal events was significant ($F(6, 169) = 4.82$, $p < .03$), whereas the incongruent interaction (Sociotropy × negative achievement events) emerged was a suppressor variable ($F(6, 169) = 7.61$, $p < .01$). The Sociotropy × negative achievement event interaction was not directly related to the prediction of BDI change scores ($r = -.03$), but rather suppressed the variance that detracted from the relationship between the congruent interaction and the dependent variable. The significance of the Sociotropy × negative interpersonal interaction held even when the suppressor variable was entered separately on a previous step. A plot of the regression lines revealed that only the high sociotropic subjects who experienced more negative interpersonal events had an increase in BDI scores from T1 to T2.

Analysis of Solitude and negative autonomous events revealed a significant incremental R^2 of .03 ($F(6, 170) = 3.11$, $p < .05$) for the interaction terms. The Solitude × negative autonomous event interaction was significant ($F(6, 170) = 4.80$, $p < .03$) and the incongruent interaction emerged as a suppressor variable ($F(6, 170) = 4.98$, $p < .03$). A plot of the regression slope suggested a different interpretation of the Solitude × negative achievement interaction. The significant interaction was attributable to high Solitude subjects with a lower number of negative achievement events showing the largest *decrease* in BDI scores from T1 to T2. Thus, the presence of negative achievement events reduced the degree of *invulnerability* to depression that was associated with high Solitude. The SAS Independence subscale failed to reveal any significant main effects or interactions.

Further analyses were conducted on subjects' single most distressing life event, appraisal ratings on this event, and coping strategies. The combination of high Sociotropy and a congruent life event remained a significant predictor of depression even when the unit of analysis was subjects' single most distressing life event. However, the combination of high Solitude and a negative achievement event was no longer significant. In addition, high Sociotropy subjects reporting a negative interpersonal event rated themselves as having less control over the event and poorer overall coping abilities. Ironically, these subjects also scored significantly higher on the adaptive coping subscales of the Cope Scale (Carver, Scheier, & Weintraub, 1989), but did not differ significantly from other subjects on the maladaptive subscales. Thus the findings from this study provide only partial support for Beck's cognitive diathesis–stress hypothesis. The interaction of Sociotropy and negative interpersonal events was significant in both cross-sectional and prospective studies. However, there was no significant interaction between SAS Autonomy (i.e., Solitude and Independence) and negative achievement events.

CONCLUDING REMARKS AND FUTURE DIRECTIONS

Research about Beck's cognitive model of anxiety and depression is crucial for establishing the empirical basis of cognitive therapy. In the last decade, considerable research has focused on two primary hypotheses of the cognitive model, the *cognitive content–specificity hypothesis* and the *cognitive diathesis–stress hypothesis*. To date, research addressing the model at the descriptive level has been more supportive than studies investigating cognitive constructs at the causal level of analysis (Haaga et al., 1991).

Cognitive Content–Specificity Hypothesis

Studies on the relationship between cognitions and symptoms have consistently found a specific relationship of thoughts of loss and failure with depressive disorders, symptoms, and mood state. This relationship exists in both clinical and nonclinical samples, but the level specificity may vary with severity of psychopathology. Cognitive content–specificity may be more evident in more distressed samples with a wider range of disturbance than in less distressed samples with a narrower range of disturbance. In contrast, studies about the relationship between threat and danger cognitions and anxious symptoms have not consistently supported the cognitive content–specificity hypothesis. It may be that cognitive measures of anxiety, such as the CCL, are too general, and more specific cognitive measures should be developed to assess apprehensive expectation or misinterpretation of bodily symptoms. The anxious cognition–symptom relationship may be more sensitive to variations in sample characteristics, such as severity of distress. Whatever the case, it would be interesting to know why cognitive content–specificity has not been as robust in anxiety as in depression. Also, more research is needed comparing the specificity of positive versus negative cognitions. This is particularly important given the differential predictions of the cognitive and tripartite models on the role of low positive and high negative cognitions in anxiety and depression.

Psychometric studies conducted with various measures suggest that the discriminant validity of anxiety and depression measures can be improved if more specific cognitive items are included in the measures. It is likely that the inclusion of positive cognition items will also increase discriminant validity. However, we do not know whether the inclusion of cognitive items would improve the discriminant validity of anxiety and depression measures for all populations. For example, it may be that negative cognitions are more nonspecific in populations reporting mild to moderate levels of general distress without specific psychopathology, such as patients with a chronic medical illness (L. A. Clark & Watson, 1991a).

Negative anxious and depressive cognitions differentiated major depression and panic disorder. However, in two studies (Clark, Beck, & Beck, 1994; Riskind et al., 1991) measures of threat and danger cognitions (i.e., CCL) did not distinguish GAD from depression. Thus, cognitive specificity may be more evident in panic than in GAD. These results suggest that distinguishing the cognitive profile of patients with GAD from those with depressive disorders may be particularly difficult because these two disorders have a high rate of comorbidity. Clearly more research attention should be devoted to this issue in light of the diagnostic changes to GAD in DSM-IV.

Cognitive Diathesis–Stress Hypothesis

Beck's cognitive diathesis–stress hypothesis has been partially supported in recent empirical studies. Although findings vary across studies depending on the cognitive measure employed or the different types of samples drawn, most researchers have supported a significant interaction between SAS Sociotropy and negative interpersonal events. The congruent interaction of Autonomy and negative achievement events has been less encouraging, although some of the remitted depressive studies have produced more favorable results for autonomy.

A number of reasons may be proposed for why autonomy has not consistently predicted depression in the presence of negative achievement events. First, the measurement of the autonomous construct has proven to be more difficult than the measurement of sociotropy. As noted by Rude and Burnham (1993), none of the current measures of achievement vulnerability adequately assesses the construct. Revisions have been made to the SAS Autonomy scale, but it is too early to predict whether the revision will find more encouraging results than those based on the original SAS. Whether the Personal Style Inventory (PSI) developed by Clive Robins and colleagues (Robins et al., 1994) will prove to be a better measure of sociotropy and autonomy than the revised SAS also remains to be seen.

A second problem with autonomy research concerns the construct itself. Autonomy is a heterogeneous construct (Rude & Burnham, 1993) composed of concepts about achievement motivation, independence, solitude, self-criticism, interpersonal insensitivity, and discomfort over closeness. Thus, measures of autonomy will differ depending on which personality feature is emphasized. Some features of autonomy may not be related to depression, whereas other aspects are directly associated with dysphoria. Given this heterogeneity, it may be more productive for researchers to focus on more narrowly defined components of the construct, rather than to assume that autonomy is a homogeneous construct.

Finally, better research designs are required to test the cognitive diathesis–stress hypothesis. To date, most studies have employed a multiple-regression model with nonclinical student or remitted depressive samples. The problem with student·samples in the current studies is that the majority of subjects describe small changes in dysphoria in response to life stressors which, in turn, are relatively mild. Abramson, Alloy, and Metalsky (1988) have noted that cognitive diathesis–stress models, such as Beck's model, are based on sufficiency rather than necessity assumptions. That is, they recognize that many people might become depressed for reasons other than cognitive vulnerability. Also, most research on cognitive diathesis–stress has failed to adequately assess event appraisal variables which Beck argues are important in determining whether an event will be associated with a depressive response. The remitted depressive studies also have their problems. For example, it is not at all clear whether variables that lead to a relapse in depressive symptoms in remitted patients will be the same as in never depressed individuals. Thus one can question the generalizability of the findings from remitted depressive studies to never depressed samples. Haaga et al. (1991) also noted that a test of causality requires that the cognitive diathesis be measured and shown to be present *before* the depression episode. Clearly what is needed are studies, like the Temple–Wisconsin Cognitive Vulnerability to Depression Study (Alloy, Lipman, & Abramson, 1992), which follows high and low cognitively vulnerable individuals over a specified period of time and investigates their reactions to significant adverse congruent and incongruent life events. Until the next generation of cognitive vulnerability studies are completed, the empirical evidence for cognitive diathesis–stress will be at best inconclusive.

ACKNOWLEDGMENTS

Part of this research was supported by grants awarded to the first author from the University of New Brunswick Research Fund, Social Sciences and Humanities Research Council of Canada (Grant No. 410-92-0427), and Foundation for Cognitive Therapy.

REFERENCES

Abramson, L. Y., Alloy, L. B., & Metalsky, G. I. (1988). The cognitive diathesis–stress theories of depression: Toward an adequate evaluation of the theories' validities. In L. B. Alloy (Ed.), *Cognitive processes in depression* (pp. 3–30). New York: Guilford Press.

Abramson, L. Y., Metalsky, G. I., & Alloy, L. B. (1989). Hopelessness depression: A theory-based subtype of depression. *Psychological Review, 96,* 358–372.

Alloy, L. B., Lipman, A. J., & Abramson, L. Y. (1992). Attributional style as a vulnerability factor for depression: Validation by past history of mood disorders. *Cognitive Therapy and Research, 16,* 391–407.

Ambrose, B., & Rholes, W. S. (1993). Automatic cognitions and the symptoms of depression and anxiety in children and adolescents: An examination of the content specificity hypothesis. *Cognitive Therapy and Research, 17,* 153–171.

American Psychiatric Association (1994). *Diagnostic and statistical manual of mental disorders* (4th ed.). Washington, DC: Author.

Barnett, P. A., & Gotlib, I. H. (1988). *Personality and depression: New scales and a model of relationships.* Paper presented at the annual convention of the Canadian Psychological Association, Montreal, Quebec.

Beck, A. T. (1967). *Depression: Causes and treatment.* Philadelphia: University of Pennsylvania Press.

Beck, A. T. (1976). *Cognitive therapy of the emotional disorders.* New York: New American Library.

Beck, A. T. (1983). Cognitive therapy of depression: New perspectives. In P. J. Clayton & J. E. Barrett (Eds.), *Treatment of depression: Old controversies and new approaches* (pp. 265–289). New York: Raven Press.

Beck, A. T. (1987). Cognitive models of depression. *Journal of Cognitive Psychotherapy, 1*, 2–27.

Beck, A. T. (1988). *Cognitive therapy of depression: A personal reflection.* University of Aberdeen: Scottish Cultural Press.

Beck, A. T. (1991). Cognitive therapy: A 30-year retrospective. *American Psychologist, 46*, 368–375.

Beck A. T., Brown, G., Steer, R. A., Eidelson, J. I., & Riskind, J. H. (1987). Differentiating anxiety and depression: A test of the cognitive content–specificity hypothesis. *Journal of Abnormal Psychology, 96*, 179–183.

Beck, A. T., & Clark, D. A. (1988). Anxiety and depression: An information processing perspective. *Anxiety Research, 1*, 23–36.

Beck, A. T., Epstein, N., Harrison, R. P., & Emery, G. (1983). *Development of the Sociotropy–Autonomy Scale: A measure of personality factors in psychopathology.* Unpublished manuscript, Center for Cognitive Therapy, University of Pennsylvania Medical School, Philadelphia.

Beck, A. T., & Steer, R. A. (1993a). *Manual for the Beck Anxiety Inventory.* San Antonio, TX: Psychological Corporation.

Beck, A. T., & Steer, R. A. (1993b). *Manual for the Beck Hopelessness Scale.* San Antonio, TX: Psychological Corporation.

Beck, A. T., & Steer, R. A. (1993c). *Manual for the Revised Beck Depression Inventory.* San Antonio, TX: Psychological Corporation.

Blatt, S. J., & Zuroff, D. C. (1992). Interpersonal relatedness and self-definition: Two prototypes for depression. *Clinical Psychology Review, 12*, 527–562.

Burgess, E., & Haaga, D. A. F. (1994). The Positive Automatic Thoughts Questionnaire (ATQ-P) and the Automatic Thoughts Questionnaire—Revised (ATQ-RP): Equivalent measures of positive thinking. *Cognitive Therapy and Research, 18*, 15–23.

Carver, C. S., Scheier, M. F., & Weintraub, J. K. (1989). Assessing coping strategies: A theoretically based approach. *Journal of Personality and Social Psychology, 56*, 267–283.

Clark, D. A. (1986). Cognitive–affective interaction: A test of the "specificity" and "generality" hypotheses. *Cognitive Therapy and Research, 10*, 607–623.

Clark, D. A. (1988). The validity of measures of cognition: A review of the literature. *Cognitive Therapy and Research, 12*, 1–20.

Clark, D. A., & Beck, A. T. (1989). Cognitive theory and therapy of anxiety and depression. In P. C. Kendall & D. Watson (Eds.), *Anxiety and depression: Distinctive and overlapping features* (pp. 379–411). San Diego, CA: Academic Press.

Clark, D. A., & Beck, A. T. (1991). Personality factors in dysphoria: A psychometric refinement of Beck's Sociotropy–Autonomy Scale. *Journal of Psychopathology and Behavioral Assessment, 13*, 369–388.

Clark, D. A., Beck, A. T., & Beck, J. (1994). Symptom differences in major depression, dysthymia, panic disorder, and generalized anxiety disorder. *American Journal of Psychiatry, 151*, 205–209.

Clark, D. A., Beck, A. T., & Brown, G. (1989). Cognitive mediation in general psychiatric outpatients: A test of the content–specificity hypothesis. *Journal of Personality and Social Psychology, 56*, 958–964.

Clark, D. A., Beck, A. T., & Brown, G. K. (1992). Sociotropy, autonomy, and life event perceptions in dysphoric and nondysphoric individuals. *Cognitive Therapy and Research, 16*, 635–652.

Clark D. A., Beck A. T., & Stewart B. (1990). Cognitive specificity and positive–negative affectivity: Complementary or contradictory views on anxiety and depression? *Journal of Abnormal Psychology, 99*, 148–155.

Clark, D. A., Purdon, C., & Beck, A. T. (1994). *Personality and life event vulnerability to depressive symptoms: A three month prospective analogue study.* Manuscript submitted for publication.

Clark, D. A., Ross, L., Beck, A. T., & Steer, R. A. (1995). Psychometric characteristics of Revised Sociotropy and Autonomy Scales in college students. *Behaviour Research and Therapy. 33,* 325–334.

Clark, D. A., Steer, R. A., & Beck, A. T. (1994). Common and specific dimensions of self-reported anxiety and depression: Implications for the cognitive and tripartite models. *Journal of Abnormal Psychology, 103*, 645–654.

Clark, D. A., Steer, R. A., Beck, A. T., & Snow, D. (1996). Is the relationship between anxious and depressive cognitions and symptoms linear or curvilinear? *Cognitive Therapy and Research, 20*, 135–155.

Clark, D. M. (1983). On the induction of depressed mood in the laboratory: Evaluation and comparison of the Velten and musical procedures. *Advances in Behaviour Research and Therapy, 5*, 27–49.

Clark, L. A., & Watson, D. (1991a). A tripartite model of anxiety and depression: Psychometric evidence and taxonomic implications. *Journal of Abnormal Psychology, 100*, 316–336.

Clark, L. A., & Watson, D. (1991b). General affective dispositions in physical and psychological health. In C. R. Synder & D. R. Donaldson (Eds.), *Handbook of social and clinical psychology: The health perspective* (pp. 221–245). New York: Plenum Press.

Di Nardo, P. A., & Barlow, D. H. (1990). Syndrome and symptom co-occurrence in the anxiety disorders. In J. Maser & R. C. Cloninger (Eds.), *Comorbidity of mood and anxiety disorders* (pp. 205–230). Washington, DC: American Psychiatric Press.

Dobson, K. S. (1985). The relationship between anxiety and depression. *Clinical Psychology Review, 5*, 307–324.

Dobson, K. S. (1994). *Innovation in cognitive-behavioural therapy for depression.* Workshop presented to the College of New Brunswick Psychologists, Saint John, New Brunswick, Canada.

Dobson, K. S., & Block, L. (1988). Historical and philosophical bases of the cognitive behavioral therapies. In K. S. Dobson (Ed.), *Handbook of cognitive-behavioral therapies* (pp. 3–38). New York: Guilford Press.

Endler, N. S., Cox, B. J., Parker, J. D. A., & Bagby, R. M. (1992). Self-reports of depression and state-trait anxiety: Evidence for differential assessment. *Journal of Personality and Social Psychology, 63*, 832–838.

Engel, R. A., & DeRubeis, R. J. (1993). The role of cognition in depression. In K. S. Dobson & P. C. Kendall (Eds.), *Psychopathology and cognition* (pp. 83–119). San Diego, CA: Academic Press.

Feldman, L. A. (1993). Distinguishing depression and anxiety in self-report: Evidence from confirmatory factor analysis on nonclinical and clinical samples. *Journal of Consulting and Clinical Psychology, 61,* 631–638.

Frances, A., Pincus, H. A., Widiger, T. A., Davis, W. W., & First, M.B. (1990). DSM-IV: Work in progress. *American Journal of Psychiatry, 147,* 1439–1448.

Garber, J., & Hollon, S. D. (1991). What can specificity designs say about causality in psychopathology research? *Psychological Bulletin, 110,* 129–136.

Garber, J., Weiss, B., & Shanley, N. (1993). Cognitions, depressive symptoms, and development in adolescents. *Journal of Abnormal Psychology, 102*, 47–57.

Gorsuch, R. L. (1983). *Factor analysis* (2nd ed). Hillsdale, NJ: Erlbaum.

Gotlib, I. H. (1984). Depression and general psychopathology in university students. *Journal of Abnormal Psychology, 93*, 19–30.

Gotlib, I. H., & Cane, D. B. (1989). Self-Report assessment of depression and anxiety. In P. C. Kendall & D. Watson (Eds.), *Anxiety and depression: Distinctive and overlapping features* (pp. 131–169). San Diego, CA: Academic Press.

Haaga, D. A., Dyck, M. J., & Ernst, D. (1991). Empirical status of cognitive theory of depression. *Psychological Bulletin, 110*, 215–236.

Hamilton, E. W., & Abramson, L. Y. (1983). Cognitive patterns in symptomatic and major depressive disorders: A longitudinal study in a hospital setting. *Journal of Abnormal Psychology, 92*, 173–184.

Hammen, C. L., Ellicott, A., & Gitlin, M. (1989). Vulnerability to specific life events and prediction of course of disorder in unipolar depressed patients. *Canadian Journal of Behavioural Science, 21*, 377–388.

Hammen, C. L., Ellicott, A., & Gitlin, M. (1992). Stressors and sociotropy/autonomy: A longitudinal study of their relationship to the course of bipolar disorder. *Cognitive Therapy and Research, 16*, 409–418.

Hammen, C. L., Ellicott, A., Gitlin, M., & Jamison, K. R. (1989). Sociotropy/Autonomy and vulnerability to specific life events in patients with unipolar depression and bipolar disorders. *Journal of Abnormal Psychology, 98*, 154–160.

Harrell, T., Chambless, D., & Calhoun, J. (1981). Correlational relationships between self-statements and affective states. *Cognitive Therapy and Research, 5*, 159–173.

Hewitt, P. L., & Flett, G. L. (1993). Dimensions of specific perfectionism, daily stress, and depression: A test of the vulnerability hypothesis. *Journal of Abnormal Psychology, 102*, 58–65.

Hewitt, P. L., & Norton, G. R. (1993). The Beck Anxiety Inventory: A psychometric analysis. *Psychological Assessment, 5*, 408–412.

Hollon, S. D., Kendall, P. C., & Lumry, A. (1986). Specificity of depressotypic cognitions in clinical depression. *Journal of Abnormal Psychology, 95*, 52–59.

Ingram, R. E. (1989). Unique and shared cognitive factors in social anxiety and depression: Automatic thinking and self-appraisal. *Journal of Social and Clinical Psychology, 8*, 198–208.

Ingram, R. E. (1990). Depressive cognition: Models, mechanisms, and methods. In R. E. Ingram (Ed.), *Contemporary psychological approaches to depression: Theory, research, and treatment* (pp. 169–195). New York: Plenum Press.

Ingram, R. E., Kendall, P. C., Smith, T. W., Donnell, C., & Ronan, K. (1987). Cognitive specificity in emotional distress. *Journal of Personality and Social Psychology, 53*, 734–742.

Ingram, R. E., & Wisnicki, K. S. (1988). Assessment of positive automatic cognition. *Journal of Consulting and Clinical Psychology, 56*, 898–902.

Jolly, J. B., & Dykman, R. A. (1994). Using self-report data to differentiate anxious and depressive symptoms in adolescents: Cognitive content specificity and global distress? *Cognitive Therapy and Research, 18*, 25–37.

Jolly, J. B., & Kramer, T. A. (1994). The hierarchical arrangement of internalizing cognitions. *Cognitive Therapy and Research, 18*, 1–14.

Kendall, P. C., Howard, B. L., & Hays, R. C. (1989). Self-referent speech and psychopathology: The balance of positive and negative thinking. *Cognitive Therapy and Research, 13*, 583–598.

Kendall, P. C., & Ingram, R. E. (1987). The future for cognitive assessment of anxiety: Let's get specific. In L. Michelson & L. M. Ascher (Eds.), *Anxiety and stress disorders: Cognitive-behavioral assessment and treatment* (pp. 89–104). New York: Guilford Press.

LaPointe, K., & Harrell, T. (1978). Thoughts and feelings: Correlational relationships and cross-situational consistency. *Cognitive Therapy and Research, 2*, 311–322.

Laurent, J., & Stark, K. D. (1993). Testing the cognitive content–specificity hypothesis with anxious and depressed youngsters. *Journal of Abnormal Psychology, 102*, 226–237.

Martin, M. (1990). On the induction of mood. *Clinical Psychology Review, 10*, 669–697.

Metalsky, G. I., Halberstadt, L. J., & Abramson, L. Y. (1987). Vulnerability to depressive mood reactions: Toward a more powerful test of the diathesis–stress and causal mediation components of the reformulated theory of depression. *Journal of Personality and Social Psychology, 52*, 386–393.

Metalsky, G. I., & Joiner, T. E. (1992). Vulnerability to depressive symptomatology: A prospective test of the diathesis–stress and causal mediation components of the hopelessness theory of depression. *Journal of Personality and Social Psychology, 63*, 667–675.

Miller, I. W., & Norman, W. H. (1986). Persistence of depressive cognitions within a subgroup of depressed inpatients. *Cognitive Therapy and Research, 10*, 211–224.

Nietzel, M. T., & Harris, M. J. (1990). Relationship of dependency and achievement/autonomy to depression. *Clinical Psychology Review, 10*, 279–297.

Rholes, W. S., Riskind, J. H., & Neville, B. (1985). The relationship of cognitions and hopelessness to depression and anxiety. *Cognitive Therapy and Research, 3*, 36–50.

Riskind, J. H., Moore, R., Harman, B., Hohmann, A. A., Beck, A. T., & Stewart, B. (1991). The relation of generalized anxiety disorder to depression in general and dysthymic disorder in particular. In R. M. Rapee & D. H. Barlow (Eds.), *Chronic anxiety: Generalized anxiety disorder and mixed anxiety–depression* (pp. 153–171). New York: Guilford Press.

Robins, C. J. (1990). Congruence of personality and life events in depression. *Journal of Abnormal Psychology, 99*, 393–397.

Robins, C. J., & Block, P. (1988). Personal vulnerability, life events, and depressive symptoms: A test of a specific interactional model. *Journal of Personality and Social Psychology, 54*, 847–852.

Robins, C. J., Ladd, J., Welkowitz, J., Blaney, P. H., Diaz, R., & Kutcher, G. (1994). Personal Style Inventory: Preliminary validation studies of new measures of sociotropy and autonomy. *Journal of Psychopathology and Behavioral Assessment, 16*, 277–300.

Rude, S. S., & Burnham, B.L. (1993). Do interpersonal and achievement vulnerabilities interact with congruent events to predict depression? Comparisons of DEQ, SAS, DAS, and combined scales. *Cognitive Therapy and Research, 17*, 531–548.

Segal, Z. V., Shaw, B. F., & Vella, D. D. (1989). Life stress and depression: A test of the congruency hypothesis for life event content and depressive subtype. *Canadian Journal of Behavioural Science, 21*, 389–400.

Segal, Z. V., Shaw, B. F., Vella, D. D., & Katz, R. (1992). Cognitive and life stress predictors of relapse in remitted unipolar depressed patients: Test of the congruency hypothesis. *Journal of Abnormal Psychology, 101*, 26–36.

Sirota, A., & Schwartz, G. (1982). Facial muscle patterning and lateralization during elation and depression imagery. *Journal of Abnormal Psychology, 91*, 25–34.

Spitzer, R. L., Williams, J. B. W., Gibbon, M., & First, M. B. (1986). *User's guide for the Structured Clinical Interview for DSM-III-R*. Washington, DC: American Psychiatric Association Press.

Steer, R. A., Beck, A. T., Clark, D. A., & Beck, J. S. (1994). Psychometric properties of the Cognitions Checklist with psychiatric outpatients and university students. *Psychological Assessment, 6*, 67–70.

Teasdale, J., & Bancroft, J. (1977). Manipulation of thought content as a determinant of mood and corrugator electromyographic activity in depressed patients. *Journal of Abnormal Psychology, 86*, 235–241.

Teasdale, J., & Rezin, V. (1978). Effect of thought-stopping on thoughts: Mood and corrugator EMG in depressed patients. Behaviour Research and Therapy, 16, 97–102.

Thorpe, G. L., Barnes, G. S., Hunter, J. E., & Hines, D. (1983). Thoughts and feelings: Correlations in two clinical and two nonclinical samples. *Cognitive Therapy and Research, 7*, 565–574.

Vredenburg, K., Flett, G. L., & Krames, L. (1993). Analogue versus clinical depression: A critical reappraisal. *Psychological Bulletin, 113*, 327–344.

Watson, D., & Kendall, P.C. (1989). Common and differentiating features of anxiety and depression: Current findings and future directions. In P. C. Kendall & D. Watson (Eds.), *Anxiety and depression: Distinctive and overlapping features* (pp. 493–508). San Diego, CA: Academic Press.

Weissman, A. W., & Beck, A. T. (1978). *Development and validation of the Dysfunctional Attitude Scale*. Paper presented at the annual meeting of the Association for the Advancement of Behavior Therapy, Chicago.

Wickless, C., & Kirsch, I. (1988). Cognitive correlates of anger, anxiety, and sadness. *Cognitive Therapy and Research, 12*, 367–377.

Zuroff, D. C., & Mongrain, M. (1987). Dependency and self-criticism: Vulnerability factors for depressive affective states. *Journal of Abnormal Psychology, 96*, 14–22.

Chapter 5

Memory Processes in Psychotherapy

J. Mark G. Williams

Psychological theories have often been unclear about the role of unpleasant events in the etiology and maintenance of emotional disturbance. This chapter will examine the way in which memory plays a mediating role between event and psychopathology. Four aspects of memory will be distinguished: "fact memory," "behavioral memory," "event memory," and "prospective memory." Each has its own effect on emotional responses (e.g., bias in fact memory may give rise to dysfunctionl attitudes; disruption in prospective memory may give rise to intrusive thoughts). The chapter will outline how greater understanding of the processing origins of these phenomena allows researchers and therapists to work together to generate new approaches to overcome blocks in therapy.

The idea that psychotherapy has its effects by healing memories of traumatic events in the past is, of course, not new. Freud's original aim in psychoanalysis was to uncover buried traumata and it was with Breuer that he made his first breakthrough. Anna O, under hypnosis, was asked to recall the very first moment that the symptoms had appeared. She was asked to describe the event in great detail and to feel and put into words the very same feelings she had experienced at that time. Her symptoms disappeared following this "catharsis." Other patients appeared to respond equally well. Although Freud later stopped using hypnosis in favor of "free association," he continued to believe that current problems were due to past trauma, and that the memory would come to mind when he placed his hand on the client's forehead (Freud & Breuer, 1893–1895/1955).

At first, these findings were venerated to a general principle. The origins of neuroses would always be some forgotten event—an event that had been shameful, alarming, shocking, or painful. The recollection of the event had been repressed and the affect disowned. This affect had expressed itself in a neurotic symptom or, in the case of some patients (hysterics), had been converted into a physical symptom.

But as Freud treated more clients, his conviction that there was always a traumatic event waned. The general theme that emotion from the past causes problems in the present remained, but the possible causes of this past emotion was broadened. First, it was broadened to include instinctual urges or impulses that seemed too strong to resist and sought "discharge." Such impulses could arise spontaneously (endogenously) or be evoked by an event such as the sight of a person, secretly loved, but unavailable. Second, it was broadened to include events that occurred at the onset of symptoms which were not in themselves traumatic, but evoked a memory of an earlier trauma. Of all the shifts Freud made, the one that is now most famous (or infamous) is the shift he made away from the view that the majority of his patients had been seduced.

A further reason why traumatic memory was given a secondary role in analytic psychotherapy is the distinction Freud came to make between actual neurosis and psychoneurosis. Actual neuroses were reactions to "real trauma" (e. g., shell shock, injury, or endogenous sexual or aggressive urges), the potential expression of which would cause a state of inner panic and result in general fatigue, tension, dizziness, insomnia, aches, and pains. This has been variously labeled "neurasthenia," "shell shock," or "battle fatigue." Freud did not consider "actual neuroses" (especially those caused by external trauma) suitable cases for psychoanalysis. For example, he believed the nightmares of such trauma victims reflected the reality of the event and could not be subjected to dream interpretation.

The result was that psychoanalysis moved away from the idea that recovery of emotions connected with traumatic events in the past was a major factor in therapy. Although the popular image remained of the psychotherapist encouraging the client to describe his or her past until, at last, a painful episode was recalled, trauma was uncovered, and the symptoms disappeared, this is now more a feature of the Hollywood analyst than psychoanalysis as it is actually practised. When early trauma is reported, it is thought to be important in the way it reveals important features of the general atmosphere in which the client was raised at home with family or the general atmosphere at school with peers and teachers, and it raises issues about how the trauma itself has affected the person's later emotional life. This is a view common to most schools of psychotherapy (Greenberg & Safran, 1987; Segal & Blatt, 1993).

The aim of this chapter is to revisit the idea that memory plays a pivotal element in emotional disturbance, and that the healing of memory plays a central role in psychotherapy when it achieves its goal. This is partly because we now know more about the real stresses and traumas that precede psychological breakdown, including physical and sexual abuse (for a rebuttal of the argument that retrospective reports are inherently unreliable, see Brewin, Andrews, & Gotlib, 1993). However, few people would wish to suggest that there is a one-to-one correspondence between stressful events and psychological breakdown. This would be to repeat Freud's early mistake. Many people experience a great deal of trauma and do not show psychological disturbance in later life. Conversely, some people who develop emotional disturbance, as far as they or anyone else can tell, have led lives free from such unpleasant events. This is, of course, central to the cognitive model proposed by Beck throughout his writings. The power of his model is, first, that it can account for individual differences in later psychopathology, for example, by the assumptions, attitudes, and schemas acquired during childhood. Second, Beck has been able to build bridges between the interests of the clinician and the researcher. His theories inform our therapeutic practice, but they also generate testable predictions for experimental investigation. They help us to understand what might be the information processing biases that mediate vulnerability, precipitation, and maintenance of emotional disturbance. It is in this spirit of bridge building that I want to discuss the memory aspect of information processing.

THE IMPORTANCE OF MEMORY

To evaluate the importance of memory, we only have to observe what happens if we lose it. Amnesic patients find every part of their life affected; they cannot leave the house without getting lost; they cannot follow the plot of a film or keep track of a sporting event; they cannot enjoy books. They look at life through a window of a few minutes. Anything that occurred (from the film, the book, the match, or their own lives) more than those few minutes ago is lost to them.

It is from memory that we get our sense of self, a sense of being the same person through time. Our memory provides us with all the information we ever have about ourselves and how others see us. It records our social networks, our family past and present. It records what to do to fix our car when it breaks down, or where to find someone who can. It records our first day at a new school, the helpful teachers and the sarcastic ones. It records the times we fell out with our friends and the times we made up. It records that Beijing is the capital of China, and what happened in Tiananmen Square. It reminds us how to make omelettes and how to speak French. It helps plan for the future, holidays, and dental appointments, and reminds us of these arrangements when the time comes.

In order to systematize the description of what memory is, I want to divide memory into its four major systems or functions and look at each in turn. These four aspects or types of memory are *fact memory, behavioral memory, event memory,* and *prospective memory.* They define four ways in which memory can be affected by unpleasant events. First, they may affect what you "know" about yourself, your semantic self-knowledge, second, they may affect your behavioral memory, how you react to particular situations, people, activities, and places, independently of whether you consciously recall the reason why you are reacting in that way. Third, they may affect your event memory biasing recall so that positive events are harder to recall, and making memory overgeneral so that specific recording of memory is difficult and current problem solving that requires specific memory is impaired. Fourth, they may affect prospective memory, setting agendas for persons to fulfill that they may have no hope of fulfilling, but which nevertheless interrupt everyday thinking with its reminders. Let us now examine each in turn to understand exactly what can go wrong with each.

FACT MEMORY

If someone compliments another person on his or her memory, he or she often has in mind knowledge of facts and figures. This is sometimes called "semantic memory" to distinguish it from memory for specific events and episodes (episodic memory). This memory for general knowledge does not require us to recall where or when we first learned it, for its validity is not situation dependent. The fact that Paris is the capital of France or that "an object allowed to fall to the ground accelerates at 32 feet per second per second" remains true whether we first learned it through books, radio, television, or a teacher. But we use this memory system also to record knowledge about other people and ourselves: A is bossy, B is weak, C is tall, D is thin.

How, then can fact memory become distorted? It occurs because most information is partial and we create what we can out if it. There are few better illustrations of how this "embellishment of fragments" can go on than the study of rumor. Allport and Postman (1948) give an excellent account of how rumor spread in the United States during World War II. Because rumor could undermine confidence, the U.S. government was very concerned that something should be done about it. Many of the rumors were very bizarre; for example, "The Russians get most of our butter and just use it for greasing their guns"; or "The Navy has dumped three car loads of coffee into New York Harbor." The Government set up special radio programs where they would take a rumor, discuss it, and try and quash it. The problem was that listening Americans twiddled the dials on their radios. People were hearing the rumor and not the refutation, which only served to spread the rumors! So they decided to have Rumor Clinics in newspapers where a psychologist would take a rumor, refute it, and then give the psychological reasons (e.g., defense mechanism, projection, etc.) that were likely to underlie it.

However, there were problems with the Rumor Clinics too. To illustrate this, let me quote an example of a rumor that concerned the Women's Army Corps (the WACs).

Fewer items of subversive gossip have given your Rumor Clinic more dismay than the false rumors which are circulating about the WACs. Here are some examples.

"Over five hundred 'WACs' have been discharged from the service because of an illegitimate pregnancy."

"Five hundred pregnant WACs have been returned from North Africa."
"General Eisenhower says the WACs are his greatest source of trouble" [which, considering he was fighting Hitler at the time, is hardly very likely].

There is not the slightest shred of evidence to report such tales as these. The rumor about the WACs in North Africa is false for one thing because it is a mathematical impossibility [!]; the entire number of WACs stationed there is considerably less than five hundred.

This reality testing did not have an entirely convincing ring, however, especially when the next sentence said rather glumly: "The exact number is a military secret."

Separating fact from rumor and propaganda has never been easy. The trouble is that fact memory treats them all as equal. It has no basis for distinguishing one from the other. This equivalence of treatment can cause one of the biggest problems for the incubation of emotional disturbance. People who are vulnerable because of events that have happened in their lives become even more vulnerable when they turn the propaganda on themselves. Facts are mixed with self-propaganda in a very destructive way, resulting in conclusions such as "I am worthless" or "I am a failure" or "If people knew what I was really like, no one would want to know me." But why should these negative categorizations be so persistent? Often, the things about ourselves we don't like are the negative side of aspects we most value. Langer (1989) reports an experiment in which people were given some attribute and asked how much they valued it. Subjects rated highly such aspects as *consistency, serious-mindedness,* and *trust.* These same people were also asked what things they hated about themselves. Results showed that those who valued *consistency* said that they hated most *rigidity,* those who valued being *serious-minded* most hated being thought of as *grim,* those who valued their *trusting* nature wanted to be less *gullible* (Langer, 1989, p. 69).

Dysfunctional attitudes and "silent assumptions" (Beck, Rush, Shaw, & Emery, 1979) may also be characterized as "fact memory." Like a law of physics, they are learned in particular situations, yet their semantic structure gives them the appearance of timeless laws of nature. The system that records Newton's laws also records personal rules; for example, "If someone is cross with me they will never be friends with me again." This "self-knowledge" poses a problem when it is treated, like general knowledge, as a matter of fact. Precisely how many different sorts of dysfunctional schemas there are, and their interconnections, is still an open question. But there is preliminary evidence that a distinction can be made at least between dependency and achievement schemas. For example, in a prospective study Segal, Shaw, and Vella (1989) studied whether congruence between a person's schemas and type of life event was important in predicting relapse in depressed patients. They followed 46 patients who had recently recovered from depression using the Dysfunctional Attitude Scale (DAS). They were able to identify 10 ex-patients who scored high on the items reflecting dependency, and 16 ex-patients who scored high on the items reflecting self-criticism. The follow-up period lasted 6 months and people were asked to report any occurrence of life events during this period. To help them identify such events, they were given a list of 66, half of which were achievement related self-critical events and half of which were personal relationship-oriented events. If at any time during this 6 month period the Beck score of any patient exceeded 16, they were given a telephone interview to establish whether their depression was severe enough to meet the Research Diagnostic Criteria for depression. There was no significant correlation between life events and Beck scores in either the dependent or self-critical subjects while the life events were left uncategorized. Once the life events were divided into interpersonal and self-critical events a different pattern emerged, at least for the "dependent vulnerable" people. For these ex-patients there was a significant correlation between the number of interpersonal life events experienced and the level of depression ($r = .62$). These same subjects, however, were not responsive to self-critical events.

The results for the self-critical subjects remained ambiguous. For them, depression and life events continued to be uncorrelated. Neither the interpersonal negative life events nor the self-critical life events correlated with the average level of depression over the course of the study. These results partially confirmed the congruency hypothesis, but only for the dependent subjects. This is consistent, however, with the findings of specificity of cognitive therapy within the National Institute of Mental Health collaborative study of depression. Imber et al. (1990) found that cognitive therapy specifically affected a "need for approval" factor on the DAS, the only evidence for any specificity for any of the therapies within that trial.

Much of cognitive therapy aims at dealing with this fact memory aspect of psychopathology. The client and therapist spend time discovering what self-referential facts are believed and what assumptions he or she is making—how the person is categorizing him- or herself. In particular, discussion focuses on what particular events and people contributed to each assumption. The aim of this aspect of therapy is to see how these beliefs are not, in fact, laws of nature. Some therapists advocate that clients ask for further information from relatives. For example, aunts and uncles can often remember what happened to their sister/brother (the client's mother or father) in earlier years, so the client might gain a valuable alternative perspective. For example, a client may find out for the first time that his or her mother had been in the hospital for depression many times when the client was very young. Often the client will have been vaguely aware of her mother's absence for long periods, but may never have understood why, or why it was that, when her mother was home, she never seemed satisfied with her children.

Finally, the therapist in cognitive therapy encourages clients to see how many of their present reactions to people and situations are determined by these previously held "laws of nature." Gaining distance from their current reactions enables them to choose to behave in certain ways, instead of feeling that their past chooses their behavior for them; it enables them to distinguish fact from rumor.

BEHAVIORAL MEMORY

This is one of the many terms given to that aspect of memory involved in learning skills, such as car driving. This sort of "behavioral memory" or "procedural memory" is important since it does not depend on conscious awareness of having done something before. This is sometimes known as the "Claparede" phenomenon, after a neurologist at the turn of the century. Like others dealing with amnesic patients, he knew that his patients did not recognize him from one day to the next. Claparede decided to test the limits of this phenomenon by concealing a small pin in his hand. When he introduced himself to the amnesic patient he shook hands, and the patient felt the prick of the pin on the palm of the hand. The next day, the patient, of course, did not remember ever having met Claparede, but was nevertheless very reluctant to shake hands with him! The same dissociation can be found with amnesic patients' performance on a jigsaw puzzle. If given such a puzzle on consecutive days, they will not recall ever having seen it before. Despite this, they get better at it day by day. They remember, but they do not know that they remember.

An experiment illustrates how long lasting this behavioral memory is. Kolers (1976) taught people to copy sentences upside down while looking in a mirror. One year later the same people were tested again. They were given some of the sentences from 1 year ago to copy as well as some new ones. They were unable to recall or recognize which sentences they had seen before. And yet, when it came to doing the task, they were faster at performing the task using the previous year's sentences. They couldn't remember explicitly, yet their behavior showed that implicitly something was being remembered.

Brewin (1989) makes use of the same distinction in his analysis of the processes of change in psychotherapy. He distinguishes between two cognitive systems, the first for information transmission and the second for conscious experience. The relatively automatic aspect of information transmission maps closely onto the behavioral memory component while the relatively strategic aspects in his model include explicit aspects of memory (see Williams, Watts, Macleod, & Mathews, 1988, Chaps. 2 and 10). The automatic processing system is rapid, is relatively inflexible, is difficult to modify, requires minimal attention, and is activated without intention or awareness. Its function is to store the sum total of previous experiences. Its output depends on new situations matching some old situation. Under such circumstances such matching will elicit physiological responses similar to those that occurred in response to the original learning situation, but it requires no conscious deliberation. In the case of this cognitive system no account can be given by the person of the reasons why they are responding in this way.

The second cognitive system is limited by attention span and strongly influenced by a priori expectations and by simple rules and heuristics. It exists to calculate future consequences of possible actions, using knowledge of present situations. In contrast to the first cognitive system the contents of this can be verbally described.

Brewin suggests that emotional memories may be coded by both cognitive systems. In the case of the former, they will be accessed by matches between current and past situations (they are "situationally accessible"). In this case the process is not accessible to introspection although one may, on the basis of one's physical responses, infer something about what memories are stored. The example that Brewin gives of this mechanism in operation is irrational fear responses. Although spider phobics "know" that the spider will not harm them, nevertheless they react very strongly when they see a spider in front of them. The flashbacks of traumatic experiences experienced by people who have posttraumatic stress disorder are also seen as due to the activity of these sort of situationally accessible memories, as are automatic thoughts that come unbidden into the mind in depression.

In addition to these unconscious and inaccessible processes, emotional memories may also be coded by the second cognitive system. In this case they can be accessed verbally, by strategic, conscious strategies. This implies that people will be more likely to understand why they are becoming upset, for these memories are available to introspection. These conscious processes will form the basis for further metacognitive analysis: labeling and attribution, the generation of coping options, evaluation of such options, monitoring change when any action is taken, and self-reinforcement that may or may not follow. Similarly these cognitive processes are involved in the selection of coping responses (e.g., distraction, providing positive self-statements, avoidance, self-medication, relaxation, and exposure). In summary, this processing system is involved whenever particular labels, attributions, or coping options are considered.

Brewin concludes that there are two different ways in which cognitive therapy is likely to work for depression: (1) "Therapists' attempts to verbally isolate, identify, and challenge negative or dramatic thoughts may be seen as disrupting the feedback loop whereby upsetting (automatic) images and thoughts pervade consciousness, . . . re-access the situational memories, and maintain the depressed mood" (p. 388); (2) "therapists may be seen as altering the contents of verbally accessible knowledge in order to counter inappropriate stimulus classification and avoid initial accessing of nonconscious situational memories" (p. 388).

Whereas the first of these options is brought about by the patients being instructed about the links between thoughts and affect and being trained to question and argue against them, the second is achieved by the deliberate focusing on upsetting experiences and examining the evidence for different interpretations and by the systematic reality testing and relabeling of events and experiences. Brewin concludes that cognitive therapy for depression mainly "modifies access to non-conscious situational memories." Those memories may still exist unmodified, but are not accessed because either they have been overlaid with newer memories that are preferentially accessed or newer semantic categories and rules have been generated for interpreting current experience. Further discussion of Brewin's model in relation to other theories about what psychological processes underlie the changes brought about by cognitive therapy can be found in Williams (1992, pp. 249–267).

EVENT MEMORY AND
THE MNEMONIC INTERLOCK PHENOMENON

Much of our own research over the past 10 years has been examining the consequences of impairments in the retrieval system governing event memory (see Williams, 1996, for review). Increasing evidence now indicates that the sort of traumatic events which precede emotional disturbance such as depression and suicidality cause "mnemonic interlock" bringing about a nonspecific retrieval style, which then has further consequences for current problem solving.

The aim of our research on event memory was to understand how people come to react to life events and stresses in catastrophic ways. We were particularly interested in parasuicide. Although it was clear from much previous research that people who become suicidal have suffered from recent failures and losses, it was also clear that the same people had been through similar experiences before that had not precipitated a suicidal crisis. We needed to know "why now?" Likewise other people who experienced similar events were not suicidal as a result. We needed to know of our suicidal patients "why them?" Here was a case where differences in cognitive processing might well be an important mediating factor. Knowing that bad mood can often produce a negative bias in memory, we started by trying to investigate whether this might be particularly true of people who were having suicidal crises.

We used a cue word test, giving positive or negative words such as "happy," "sorry," or "clumsy" and asking people to think of any event from their past that they were reminded of by the word. We gave this test to people who had recently taken an overdose (within 2 or 3 days) and also to people from the same wards who were in the hospital for other (physical) problems. Finally, we gave the test to a matched, nonhospital control group. At first it seemed as if the overdose patients could not do the task. In response to a word, the person might say "my father'" or "going for walks with my mum" or "I'm always being clumsy." We assumed at first that we had not explained the instructions well enough. However, even after more examples had been given and they were able to say exactly what the task demanded they still found it difficult. We might have given up and moved on to another task had we not noticed the same phenomenon during cognitive therapy with a depressed suicidal client. When trying to remember times over the past year when she had succeeded in overcoming crises, she easily remembered that there *had* been such times, but couldn't recall, for a considerable time, any specific example. Could it be that this simple word cuing technique had picked up a genuine difficulty in memory?

Further studies have shown that it is a robust phenomenon, that it is not due to the drugs that patients are on or have recently taken and that it is not correlated with intelligence or education level (Williams & Broadbent, 1986; Williams & Dritschel, 1988). Further, the phenomenon is also found in depressed patients (Williams & Scott, 1988; Moore, Watts, & Williams, 1988; Puffet, Jehin-Marchot, Timsit-Berthier, & Timsit, 1991) and sufferers from posttraumatic stress disorder (McNally, Litz, Prassas, Shin, & Weathers, 1994). Finally, Robert Wahler at the University of Tennessee has found a similar phenomenon in parents who had difficulty in controlling their children, especially parents who themselves had multiple stresses in their lives. When they came to his clinics to discuss the problems they were having with their child, he would ask them to describe examples of their child's difficult behavior. The parents would say "he's awful" or "he's uncontrollable" but when asked to give specific examples, they found it difficult (Wahler & Afton, 1980).

So here is a very similar phenomenon occurring in suicidal, posttraumatic, and depressed clients and in parents who are under multiple stresses struggling to cope with their children. Two other pieces of recent research have helped us to understand what may be going on here. First, other research on parents who have poor attachments to their children find that these parents have problems with their own parents. As part of the "Adult Attachment Interview," mothers are asked about the memory of their own mothers. Interestingly, they are able to describe their mothers in general terms, but when asked to give concrete examples of each of these adjectives, find it difficult to do so.

In a second piece of related research, Kuyken and Brewin (1995) studied 58 women who met DSM-III-R criteria for major depressive disorder. Sixty-three percent of this sample reported physical and sexual abuse as children. They gave their patients the Autobiographical Memory Test[1] and found not only that the depressed people had more difficulty in being specific than the nondepressed controls, but within the depressed group, the women who had suffered sexual abuse had even more difficulty in retrieving specific episodes from their past. Furthermore, this memory impairment was particularly bad for those patients who were still having intrusive thoughts about the abuse (both physical and sexual), despite the fact that the memories themselves were not of abusive experiences. Kuyken and Brewin were also able to confirm that the difficulty in retrieving specific memories was independent of the severity of depression as measured by the Beck Depression Inventory, so it was not simply due to current depressed mood making memory more difficult or effortful.

We may therefore be on the verge of making important progress in further understanding the damage that early trauma, difficulties, and abuse can do. It is not just that it lays down traumatic memories which themselves may need addressing in later therapy, it affects memory for other events too, making people tend towards overgeneral retrieval, even overgeneral retrieval of positive events in their life. I have suggested elsewhere (Williams, 1996) that this damage is done as autobiographical memory emerges as a skill in the developing child at the age of 3 and 4. Before this time, all children are likely to speak about events in general terms (Morton, 1990; Nelson, 1991). But between the ages of 3 and 4 a number of changes take place; the child becomes more self-aware, able to attribute motives and intentions to other people (often referred to as developing a theory of mind). Psychologists studying these changes in infancy and childhood have noted that children at this stage begin to talk to their parents about particular events that have happened, rather than events in general. However, if the child is undergoing difficulty or abuse at this time the retrieval of generic memories may well persist as a defensive strategy against the recall of these particular events. Particular events evoke concrete images that bring with them sharply focused distress. General memories have their own emotional consequences, but, though painful, it is a less focused pain. An example may illustrate: It may be painful to have a general thought "I've always been a failure," but this may be preferable to remembering the particular event of your schoolteacher telling you that you had failed an important test. However, persistent use of this style of generic memory leads to mnemonic interlock in which the memory system loses its power to retrieve specific memories at will. This is because the intermediate memory descriptions that usually help in the retrieval of specific events only succeed in cuing further generic descriptions.

In cognitive therapy there is a need to refocus again on the specific events, for much of therapy involves going over events that have happened and examining possible alternative interpretations. Without being able to gain access to the specific things that happened, one cannot begin to derive alternative interpretations for the events. For example, if the ubiquitous person who passes in the street without seeing the client is encoded as one amongst a number of rejection experiences, then it is difficult to reinterpret. However, if the person is able to retrieve the specific details of the event—the busy street, the other person walking on the other side, the traffic flowing between them, the noise in the street, and so forth—then it is quite possible that he or she will be able to retrieve sufficient other cues to suggest alternative interpretations of the event.

Similarly cognitive therapy focuses on the events of each day, by emphasizing the importance of daily diaries. It is commonplace in therapy to have clients come week by week without having completed their diaries, and many therapists are inclined to interpret this as meaning that the person is undermining therapy in some way. However our research showing that depressed people find it difficult to encode specific events reminds us that for some people, completing a diary at the end of the day may be very difficult if not impossible. They simply can't remember the details of what they have been doing, and admitting that in the diary may be too much to expect. We have been too ready to interpret in a motivational way what is in fact a cognitive deficit in these people.

Evans, Williams, O'Loughlin, and Howells (1992) examined the prediction that overgeneral memory might interfere with interpersonal problem solving. They made this prediction on the basis that depressed people might try to use overgeneral memories as a "database" to generate solutions to current interpersonal problems. However, general memories are rather inadequate for this purpose. If you are feeling unhappy and you try to remember what sort of things make you happy and the only thing you come up with is a generic memory "walks with Tony," then you don't have very much specific information to help you solve your present unhappiness, especially if Tony is away at the moment. However, retrieving a specific memory ("being with Tony out for a walk when we met his friends last Tuesday and went to the pub for a drink") is likely to be more helpful in solving your current loneliness problem. Within the specific event there is "Tony," "the walk," "Tony's friends," "the pub," and "last Tuesday," each of which might activate other thoughts and memory cues that can be used in constructing possible alternative solutions to the current problem.

Evans et al. contrasted patients who had recently taken an overdose with surgical patients, matched on age, sex, and educational level. They found that the results were as predicted. Those people who had difficulty being specific in their memory also had difficulty generating effective solutions on items of the Means–Ends Problem-Solving Test (MEPS; Platt & Spivack, 1975). This was true for the group as a whole, where the correlation was .56 ($p < .01$) between effectiveness (independently rated) and specificity of memory. It was also true for the overdose patients in particular, where the correlation was .67 ($p < .02$). The authors were able to check whether the correlation might be an artifact of some people's sluggishness to respond to any task in general, by partialling out the latency of response on the memory task. If the significant correlations they found were due simply to some people being nonresponsive on all tasks, then this should also show up in slow responses to the cue words. In fact the correlation between effectiveness of problem solutions and this latency measure was low and nonsignificant, and even when latency was partialed out of the correlation between problem solving and specificity of memory, the level of correlation was unaffected.

All these results suggest that mnemonic interlock in event memory plays a critical role in contributing to depression and in preventing recovery from depression by retarding problem solving. However, we have seen that it is not just memory for the traumatic event itself which is the problem, but the effect that early negative events have on event memory in general which is responsible for much of the later problems. Similarly, it is not simply the fact that depression is associated with *memory bias*—the prepotency of negative over positive memories—which is to blame, as was once thought, but rather the *nonspecificity of memories* in general that exacerbates the problem and retards recovery. This effect of memory on the time course of depression has recently been confirmed by Brittlebank, Scott, Williams, and Ferrier (1993). They tested autobiographical memory of depressed patients on admission, along with Hamilton measures of severity of depression (Hamilton, 1967) and the DAS (Weissman & Beck, 1978). They found that neither the DAS nor Hamilton in this study predicted severity of depression at 3 and 7 months, but nonspecificity of memory (particularly in response to positive cues) did so. Out of the 22 patients in their study, they had data on 19 at the 7 month follow-up. Dividing them into specific and general using a median split on the autobiographical memory scores, they found that only 1 out of 9 patients who were overgeneral in their memories were recovered at 7 months. By contrast 8 out of 10 of the patients who had been specific in their positive memories on admission were recovered at 7 months.

PROSPECTIVE MEMORY

Finally, memory involves remembering to do things (Winograd, 1988). We must remember to keep appointments, to meet people, to pick up the children, to write to our friends, to pay that bill. Whereas the memory we have mentioned so far looks backward—it is retrospective—this memory looks forwards—it is prospective. Research shows that good retrospective memory (memory from the past) and good prospective memory (remembering to do things) are not correlated (Harris & Wilkins, 1982). Prospective memory is a memory system, the function of which is to give prompts about goals and intentions. Prospective memory is sensitive to incompleteness. Once a person has set him- or herself a goal, there will be prompts about the goal until it is satisfied (the Zeigarnik effect). However, the system can fail for a number of reasons (Reason, 1990). We see its failure in everyday life when we forget to go on an errand on the way home from work or when we forget to finish our course of antibiotics once the symptoms of the illness have subsided. The relevance for the present discussion is that a prospective memory system may set up goals that are difficult to fulfill. What will be the consequence of the activity of the normal reminder system?

If we look more closely at the research on prospective remembering we notice that when people have got to do something, thoughts about that task tend to interrupt them during the day (Ellis, 1988). If the task is at a definite time and place, and there are plenty of reminders around in your office, in your diary, and so forth, then these thought interruptions will be few. If, however, there is no fixed time (e.g., you need to phone someone at any time during the week) the responsibility for reminding falls completely on the memory system itself. Thoughts about the phone call interrupt other activities. If this does not happen, people report a general (rather uncomfortable) feeling of having something on their mind (though if you try to remember what it is you may not be successful). It is rather as if people have a goal stack retained in working memory, some goals trivial and others more important, and that working memory has a device for sampling these goals from time to time and making sure they break into ongoing activity to ensure the goals are considered.

The management of our separate goals — when we interrupt one activity (e.g., writing a letter) for another (eating supper) — is sometimes straight-forward. However, it is more difficult to prioritize between goals that are equally important or between one goal that is important but will take a great deal of effort and another goal that is less important but will take less effort. When adding up those small tasks that may be unimportant but have a deadline of 3:00 P.M. this afternoon, you can see that the "operating system" that schedules our goals and plans sometimes has to work overtime! It is adaptive for such a management system to be able to inhibit the pursuit of *some* goals so that others can proceed, however, the system needs to sample the goal stack every so often to check that there is nothing that needs pursuing. This is what causes the intrusion of thoughts related to incomplete tasks I referred to earlier.

Here is where prospective memory interacts with fact memory. The sort of facts that depressive-prone people accumulate about themselves make high-level and "difficult to obtain" goals prominent. For example, the personal law of nature, "Being happy means being liked by everyone," sets up a goal that is difficult to achieve. Thus, "someone frowning" isn't just a minor puzzling event that means "they are probably tired or concentrating hard." It means "they don't like me." This violates the goal of "being liked by everyone" and forces the conclusion "I can't be happy."

The problem is that the goal "to be liked by everyone" will sit in the goal stack alongside appointments, fixing meals, or meeting friends for lunch. Like other goals, the system will interrupt ongoing activity from time to time to check the progress of the pursuit of the goal. If depressed, the system will prioritize that goal, and since there is no very concrete solution to it (being liked by absolutely everyone may take a long time!) the interruptions — intrusive thoughts — will occur very frequently. Intrusive thoughts and ruminations are the natural consequence of an *adaptive* mechanism of mind doing its job as well as it can, to remind a person of incompleted goals (see also Greenberg & Safran, 1987, for discussion of the closely related concept of "unfinished business"). Because the system tries to prioritize these large, unfocused, incomplete goals, not only will there be repeated intrusions from them, but other smaller goals will be inhibited. That is why the adaptive mechanism is there. Yet this simply results in procrastination—the shelf that needs fixing, the letter that needs writing. Smaller things on the goal stack are inhibited (much to our continual annoyance) simply because we have, as it were, an efficient piece of software trying to make an effective scheduling of all our activities. The lack of completion of such actions then reinforces the negative view of the self that prioritized the unfocused goal in the first place.

INTERRELATIONSHIPS

Now we begin to see how all these aspects of memory may be interconnected. Damaging experiences affect behavioral or "situational" memory. Behavioral memory encodes events in a form that influences our behavioral and bodily reactions without us being able consciously to control them. Such reactions will extinguish in time, but along a different time course from that with which conscious cognitive strategies resolve. However, there is the constant danger they may be maintained or incubated, and our conscious reactions to them, if they are catastrophic, will tend to feed back into the situation that will make them incubate.

Second, damaging experiences create vulnerable attitudes and assumptions that become encoded as laws of nature in semantic memory. The assumptions translate to goals—"I must not feel pain" or "I must prevent people knowing what I'm like"—that are too global to satisfy or complete. As incomplete goals they remain in the memory system, interrupting some tasks and inhibiting others completely.

Third, damaging experiences may cause mnemonic interlock, making memory over general and unfocused. Unfocused memory itself inhibits problem solving. It reduces the number of alternatives a person can produce to resolve an interpersonal problem, and those that are produced tend to be less effective.

CONCLUSION

It now becomes clear why I said at the outset I believed the healing of memory was central to cognitive therapy. Memory is the most important thing one can know about people when attempting to listen to their problems within therapy. Not only *what* they remember but the *way* in which they remember it; not only their *conscious recollection* but their *behavioral memories* that have survived long after the initial event that precipitated them; not only their *retrospective* memory but their *prospective* memory. The research that we have done emphasizes the importance of being concrete and specific about events and not letting the smallest event go past without seeing what bigger theme it may illustrate, what uncompleted goal it may relate to. In our therapeutic practice, we need to ensure we have the range of tools with which we can deal with each of these sources of memory bias.

NOTE

1. Copies of the Autobiographical Memory Test are available from the author on request.

REFERENCES

Allport, G. W., & Postman, L. (1948). *The psychology of rumor.* New York: Holt.

Beck, A. T., Rush, A. J., Shaw, B. F., & Emery, G. (1979). *Cognitive therapy of depression.* New York: Guilford Press.

Brewin, C. R. (1989). Cognitive change processes in psychotherapy. *Psychological Review, 96,* 379–394.

Brewin C. R., Andrews, B., & Gotlib, I. H. (1993). Psychopathology and early experience: A reappraisal of retrospective reports. *Psychological Bulletin, 113,* 82–98.

Brittlebank, A. D., Scott, J., Williams, J. M. G., & Ferrier, I. N. (1993). Autobiographical memory in depression: State or trait marker? *British Journal of Psychiatry, 162,* 118–121.

Ellis, J. A. (1988). Memory for future intentions: Investigating pulses and steps. In M. M. Gruneberg, P. E. Morris, & R. N. Sykes (Eds.), *Practical aspects of memory: Current research and issues I* (pp. 371–376). Chichester, UK: Wiley.

Evans, J., Williams, J. M. G., O'Loughlin, S., & Howells, K. (1992). Autobiographical memory and problem solving strategies of parasuicide patients. *Psychological Medicine, 22,* 399–405.

Freud, S., & Breuer, J. (1955). Studies on hysteria. In *Standard edition* (Vol. 2). London: Hogarth Press. (Original work published 1893–1895)

Greenberg, L. S., & Safran, J. D. (1987). *Emotion in psychotherapy.* New York: Guilford Press.

Hamilton, M. (1967). Development of a rating scale for primary depressive illness. *Journal of Social and Clinical Psychology, 6,* 278–296.

Harris, J. E., & Wilkins, A. (1982). Remembering to do things: A theoretical framework and an illustrative experiment. *Human Learning, 1,* 123–136.

Imber, S. D., Pilkonis, P. A., Sotsky, S. M., Elkin, I., Watkins, J. T., Collins, J. F., Shea, M. T., Laber, W. R., & Glass, D. R. (1990). Mode specific effects among three treatments for depression. *Journal of Consulting and Clinical Psychology, 58,* 352–359.

Kolers, P. A. (1976). Reading a year later. *Journal of Experimental Psychology: Human Learning and Memory, 2,* 554–565.

Kuyken, W., & Brewin, C. R. (1995). Autobiographical memory functioning in depression and reports of early abuse. *Journal of Abnormal Psychology, 104,* 585–591.

Langer, E. J. (1989). *Mindfulness.* London: HarperCollins.

McNally, R. J., Litz, B. T., Prassas, A., Shin, L. M., & Weathers, F. W. (1994). Emotional priming of autobiographical memory in post-traumatic stress disorder. *Cognition and Emotion, 8,* 351–367.

Moore, R. G., Watts, F. N., & Williams, J. M. G. (1988). The specificity of personal memories in depression. *British Journal of Clinical Psychology, 27,* 275–276.

Morton, J. (1990). The development of event memory. *The Psychologist, 1,* 3–10.

Murphy, G. E., Simons, A. D., Wetzel, R. D., & Lustman, P. J. (1984). Cognitive therapy and pharmacotherapy: Singly and together in the treatment of depression. *Archives of General Psychiatry, 41,* 33–41.

Nelson, K. (1991). *Toward an explanation of the development of autobiographical memory.* Keynote address given to International Conference on Memory, Lancaster. UK.

Platt, J. J., & Spivack, G. (1975). *Manual for the means-ends-problem-solving (MEPS): A measure of interpersonal problem solving skill.* Philadelphia: Hahnemann Medical College Hospital.

Puffet, A., Jehin-Marchot, D., Timsit-Berthier, M., & Timsit, M. (1991). Autobiographical memory and major depressive states. *European Psychiatry, 6,* 141–145.

Reason, J. (1990). *Human error.* Cambridge, UK: Cambridge University Press.

Segal, Z. V., & Blatt, S. J. (Eds.). (1993). *The self in emotional distress: Cognitive and psychodynamic perspectives.* New York: Guilford Press.

Segal, Z. V., Shaw, B. F., & Vella, D. D. (1989). Life stress and depression: A test of congruency hypothesis for life event content and depressive subtype. *Canadian Journal of Behavioural Science, 21,* 389–400.

Wahler, R. J., & Afton, A. D. (1980). Attentional processes in insular and noninsular mothers: Some differences in the summary reports about child problem behaviours. *Child Behaviour Therapy, 2,* 25–41.

Weissman, A. N., & Beck, A. T. (1978). *Development and validation of the Dysfunctional Attitude Scale.* Paper presented at the annual meeting of the Association for the Advancement of Behavior Therapy, Chicago.

Williams, J. M. G. (1992). *The psychological treatment of depression: A guide to the theory and practice of cognitive behaviour therapy.* London: Routledge.

Williams, J. M. G. (1996). Depression and the specificity of autobiographical memory. In D. C. Rubin (Ed.), *Remembering our past: Studies in autobiographical memory* (pp. 244–270). Cambridge, UK: Cambridge University Press.

Williams, J. M. G., & Broadbent, K. (1986). Autobiographical memory in attempted suicide patients. *Journal of Abnormal Psychology, 95,* 144–149.

Williams, J. M. G., & Dritschel, B. H. (1988). Emotional disturbance and the specificity of autobiographical memory. *Cognition and Emotion, 2,* 221–234.

Williams, J. M. G., & Scott, J. (1988). Autobiographical memory in depression. *Psychological Medicine, 18,* 689–695.

Williams, J. M. G., Watts, F. N., Macleod, C., & Mathews, A. (1988). *Cognitive psychology and emotional disorders.* Chichester, UK: Wiley.

Winograd, E. (1988). Some observations on prospective remembering. In M. M. Gruneberg, P. E. Morris, & R. N. Sykes (Eds.), *Practical aspects of memory: Current research and issues I* (pp. 348–353). Chichester, UK: Wiley.

Chapter 6

Biology and Cognitions in Depression: Does the Mind Know What the Brain Is Doing?

Jan E. Weissenburger
A. John Rush

C ognitive and biological theories of depression have remained relatively isolated, in part because of very different theoretical orientations that pose problems for an integrative view. Similarly, very little research in depression has focused on the simultaneous evaluation of psychological and biological factors. For example, evidence has accumulated to support the presence of biological alterations in symptomatic patients with endogenous (or melancholic) depressions and psychological and social concomitants in nonendogenous (or reactive) depressions. It is important, however, to go beyond these basic categorical differences to understand how biological and psychosocial factors interact. This chapter summarizes current research that suggests potential links between psychological and biological functions in clinical depression.

Two major theoretical approaches to the understanding of depression are cognitive and biochemical. Beck's theory (1967, 1976) proposes that the state of clinical depression is characterized by the presence of a negative cognitive triad, composed of negative views of self, world, and future. Extensive work in the area has provided ample empirical confirmation of these cognitive alterations (for a review, see Haaga, Dyck, & Ernst, 1991). The well-documented negative self-characterization of depressed patients appears specific to this disorder, in both adults (Greenberg & Beck, 1989; Beck, Steer, & Epstein, 1992) and adolescents (Laurent & Stark, 1993).

In contrast to these state characteristics, the theory proposes that the etiology of depression is found in the activation of latent depressive schemas by stressors to which the individual is particularly susceptible. This so-called diathesis–stress model suggests that stressors in the interpersonal arena may precipitate depression for persons high in sociotropy; and career or materialistic setbacks are causally related to depression for persons high in autonomy. There has been some research support for the concepts of sociotropy and autonomy (Robins, Block, & Peselow, 1989; Hammen, Marks, Mayol, & deMayo, 1985; Segal, Shaw, Vella, & Katz, 1992).

Beck has suggested that the diathesis-stress model of depression applies specifically to nonendogenous (reactive) depression (Haaga et al., 1991). Confirming this theory, most research has found that nonendogenous patients report more recent stressful life events than endogenous patients (Robins, Block, & Peselow, 1990; Cornell, Milden, & Shimp, 1985; Dolan, Calloway, Fonagy, de Souza, & Wakeling, 1985). Results regarding dysfunctional attitudes are more mixed, with some studies confirming the theory (Peselow, Robins, Block, Barouche, & Fieve, 1990; Robins et al., 1990; Zimmerman, Coryell, & Pfohl, 1986) but not others (Eaves & Rush, 1984; Giles & Rush, 1982; Norman, Miller, & Dow, 1988; Zimmerman & Coryell, 1986).

A second major type of theory links clinical depression to altered neurobiology. Studies of central nervous system (CNS) metabolites suggest that the neurotransmitter systems involving norepinephrine, serotonin, acetylcholine, dopamine, and gamma-aminobutyric acid (GABA) may be altered in patients with clinical depression (Rush et al., 1991). The successful treatment of clinical depression with antidepressant medications suggests that basic neurochemical processes are involved. Changes in major neuroendocrine systems, such as the hypothalamic–pituitary–adrenal (HPA) and hypothalamic–pituitary–thyroid (HPT) axes, have also been associated with clinical depression. Several physiological and biochemical indices are abnormal in some patients with depression. The best studied of these are the dexamethasone suppression test (DST; Carroll et al., 1981), which reveals an abnormal cortisol response to dexamethasone challenge and the polysomnogram (PSG), which reveals reduced rapid-eye-movement (REM) latency (time from sleep onset to the first REM period), poor sleep continuity, reduced deep sleep, and increased REM density (see Berger & Riemann, 1993, for a review). Recent research has also utilized functional brain imaging technology to examine regional brain activity in depressed individuals (Baxter et al., 1985; Schwartz, Baxter, Mazziotta, Gerner, & Phelps, 1987).

This chapter provides a brief overview of recent findings regarding the biological and cognitive functioning of individuals with depression. Research in four areas is highlighted: (1) subtyping and classification of major depression, (2) cognitions and biology of suicide, (3) cognitions and biology relating to course of depressive illness, and (4) prediction of response to treatments.

CLASSIFICATION OF MAJOR DEPRESSION

The identification of different subtypes of major depression may lead to advances in theory and clinical treatment. Thus, the search for distinct subtypes has a long history. Several specific types have been proposed by recent diagnostic systems, including endogenous versus nonendogenous (by Research Diagnostic Criteria [RDC]; Spitzer, Endicott, & Robins, 1978), melancholic versus nonmelancholic (by the *Diagnostic and Statistical Manual of Mental Disorders*, third edition [DSM-III], third edition—revised [DSM-III-R], and fourth edition [DSM-IV]; American Psychiatric Association, 1980, 1987, 1994), endogenous versus reactive (Newcastle Scale; Carney, Reynolds, & Sheffield, 1986), and primary versus secondary (RDC) (for a review, see Rush & Weissenburger, 1994).

Research has also suggested that specific biological alterations may discriminate endogenous from nonendogenous depressions (Giles & Rush, 1982; Rush, Giles, Roffwarg, & Parker, 1982; Giles, Schlesser, et al., 1987; Rush & Weissenburger, 1994). Whereas there is general support for a biological component in endogenous (melancholic) depression (Rush et al., 1991), findings are less clear with regard to the importance of cognitive and personality factors and life stress for specific subtypes of depression.

One study (Monroe, Thase, & Simons, 1992) examined the biological marker REM latency and life stress in a group of RDC endogenous patients and found that those with precipitating stresses had normal REM latency values whereas those without such stresses had reduced REM latency. Given that the sample in this study was comprised exclusively of endogenous patients, the results suggest that even in this presumably more biologically based subgroup, life stresses contribute to some of these depressions.

In another study on REM latency, relatives of patients with reduced REM latency had more dysfunctional attitudes than relatives of patients with normal REM latency (Giles, Etzel, & Biggs, 1990). Since the relatives were asymptomatic at the time of assessment, differences in depressive state do not account for these results. However, history of depression in the relatives was found to be a significant independent correlate of the level of their dysfunctional attitudes. It is not possible to determine from this cross-sectional study whether the elevation in dysfunctional attitudes is a residual effect of the past depressive episode or a preexisting vulnerability trait. It does suggest, however, that biological and cognitive factors may independently contribute to risk of depression.

In contrast, a World Health Organization collaborative study using the DST did not find any strong symptom or psychopathological predictors of postdexamethasone cortisol levels or of DST status, beyond the well-documented effects of age and gender (Gastpar, Gilsdorf, Abou-Saleh, & Ngo-Khac, 1992). In addition, results emphasize the difficulties of measuring life stresses and the importance of using well-validated and specific instruments for this type of assessment, as there was large between-site variability in results on the stress variables.

One potential problem with research on the diathesis–stress model or other hypothesized characteristics of nonendogenous depression has been in defining a relatively homogeneous concept of this type of depression. It has often been used as a residual category for all patients who do not meet specific criteria for endogenous depression. As such, it is a mixture of potentially distinctive subtypes of depression.

With regard to this issue, a recent study by Haslam and Beck (1993) categorized outpatients with major depression based on the 21 items of the Beck Depression Inventory (BDI; Beck, Ward, Mendelson, Mock, & Erbaugh, 1961). Four distinct subtypes were identified, including a large nonspecific general type; a more severe melancholic type; a self-critical, high anxiety type; and a mild type. The latter two groups were small in comparison to the former two, accounting for only 10% and 8% of the sample, respectively. Although the results must at this time be taken as preliminary, they suggest that the term "nonendogenous" may subsume three of the four subtypes identified, with the exception being the severe melancholic type, which appears to correspond to the concept of endogenous depression.

Haslam and Beck (1993) also performed a principal components analysis on the items of the BDI to examine the structure of the variation in items. They identified four significant latent dimensions of depression which they labeled "anhedonic," "hopeless," "self-critical," and "vegetative." Results of a study by DeJong and Roy (1990) may relate to the biology of the self-critical component of depression. In this study, levels of corticotropin-releasing hormone (CRH) in the cerebrospinal fluid (CSF) of depressed patients was measured, based on previous research suggesting that hypersecretion of CRH from the paraventricular nucleus of the hypothalamus may play a role in the alterations of the HPA system found in depression (Gold et al., 1986; Nemeroff et al., 1984; Roy et al., 1987; Banki, Bissette, Arato, O'Connor, & Nemeroff, 1987). Cognitive items of self-accusation, expectation of punishment, and crying accounted for 82% of the variance in CRH levels in the sample of 17 mostly melancholic inpatients.

Two of these features (self-accusation and expectation of punishment) loaded on the self-critical component and are distinguishing features of the self-critical/anxious type of depression found by Haslam and Beck (1993). Self-accusation was associated with lower levels of CRH. When this effect was controlled, expectation of punishment was positively associated with level of CRH. These results suggest that negative view of the self (self-accusation) is associated with a lowering of CRH, whereas an independent effect is exerted in the opposite direction by the presence of cognitive aspects related to fear and anxiety (fear of punishment). Fear of punishment may arise from a negative view of how the self is perceived by others. This particular negative self-view has been theoretically related to emotions of fear and anxiety (Higgins, 1987).

In terms of related neuroanatomy, Schulkin (1994) has recently theorized that the amygdala is a major site of action in the alterations of CRH and glucocorticoids found in depression. Based on animal literature and regional cerebral blood flow studies in humans with depression using positron emission tomography (PET), he concludes that increased levels of CRH in the amygdala are related to fear and anxiety. Evidence also ties elevated levels of glucocorticoids to stress responses and lack of perceived control. Elevated glucocorticoids may thus produce anxiety, via stimulation of CRH in the amygdala. In contrast, and of relevance to the symptomatic expression of clinical depression, elevated levels of glucocorticoids *reduce* CRH levels in the paraventricular nucleus of the hypothalamus, reducing drives for food and sex. Schulkin notes that his emphasis on the role of the amygdala shifts the focus from a homeostatic mechanism (as it relates to the hypothalamic/hippocampal system and its role in regulating appetite, thirst, and sexual behavior) to the role of arousal and anticipation of negative events.

Research by Faustman, Faull, Whiteford, Borchert, and Csernansky (1990) provides more evidence for the relation between specific biochemical and symptom features in depression. In 30 depressed inpatients, cortisol level was related to "vegetative" symptoms of depression, including sleep disturbance, diurnal variation, genital symptoms, hypochondriasis, weight loss, and somatic anxiety symptoms. In contrast, CSF levels of the serotonergic metabolite 5-hydroxyindoleacetic acid (5-HIAA) were not related to these vegetative symptoms, but were related to a "cognitive" symptom cluster, which included suicidal ideation, guilt, psychic anxiety, insight, paranoia, depersonalization, work/activities, depressed mood, and psychomotor changes. Cortisol levels were also related to the cognitive symptoms, although to a lesser extent than 5-HIAA.

These results suggest that dysfunction in the HPA system and associated levels of glucocorticoids including cortisol relates highly to vegetative symptoms. This is consistent with findings relating alterations of cortisol and DST response to endogenous (melancholic) depression. RDC and DSM criteria, in particular, specify these vegetative symptoms as defining features of the endogenous subtype. Although cognitive symptoms of guilt, anxiety, paranoia, psychomotor change, and suicidal ideation also relate to levels of cortisol, they may have an additional unique association with the serotonergic system. Prior research, as discussed in the next section of this chapter, has shown a relationship between suicidality and CSF 5-HIAA.

In summary, research suggests that endogenous depression may be uniquely associated with particular biological alterations. Results are not conclusive, however, regarding the relationship of cognitive, personality, or life stress variables to depressive subtypes. Difficulties in quantifying and measuring life stress has hindered research in this area. Intriguing results suggest that self-criticality may be associated with lower levels of CRH and that symptoms of anxiety or fear may be associated with increases in this hormone. CRH levels in the amygdala may modulate glucocorticoid and paraventricular hypothalamic CRH levels, thereby influencing vegetative symptoms such as reduction in appetite and libido. There is accumulating evidence for a self-critical/anxious subtype of depression with distinct neurophysiological characteristics.

COGNITIONS AND THE BIOLOGY OF SUICIDE

Much research has examined predictors of suicidal behavior (Beck, 1986). Hopelessness has consistently been found to be related to both suicidal ideation and eventual completed suicide (Minkoff, Bergman, Beck, & Beck, 1973; Silver, Bohnert, Beck, & Marcus, 1971; Wetzel, Margulies, Davis, & Karam, 1980; Beck, Brown, Berchick, Stewart, & Steer, 1990; Beck, Steer, Kovacs, & Garrison, 1985). A cutoff score of 9 or greater on the Hopelessness Scale (HS; Beck, Weissman, Lester, & Trexler, 1974) has been suggested as a predictor of suicide in outpatients (Beck et al., 1990).

Dysfunctional attitudes have been related to suicidal ideation for inpatients (Ranieri et al., 1987) but not for outpatients (Beck, Steer, & Brown, 1993). In the latter study, the effect of dysfunctional attitudes on suicidal ideation was overshadowed by effects of hopelessness and history of a past suicide attempt. With these effects not controlled, four sets of dysfunctional attitudes were significantly related to suicidal ideation, including cognitive vulnerability, success–perfectionism, need to impress others, and disapproval–dependence.

With regard to subtypes of depression, a recent study found a higher mortality rate due to suicide among Newcastle Scale–defined nonendogenous compared to endogenous depressed patients (Buchholtz-Hansen, Wang, Kragh-Sorensen, & the Danish University Antidepressant Group, 1993). Another study focusing on a select group of severely depressed melancholic patients found that social factors appeared to be less important as suicide predictors for this group (Bradvik & Berglund, 1993).

A follow-up from the National Institute of Mental Health (NIMH) collaborative study of depression (Fawcett, 1993) found different predictors for acute (within 1 year after initial assessment) and delayed (2 to 10 years after assessment) suicides. Symptom-based predictors of suicide within 1 year of assessment included anhedonia, psychic anxiety, panic attacks, alcohol abuse, insomnia, and diminished concentration. In contrast, predictors of suicide occurring from 2 to 10 years after assessment included hopelessness, suicidal ideation, and prior suicide attempts. These results suggest that hopelessness and prior suicide attempts may predict suicide in the long run, but specific clinical symptoms may be more predictive of suicide in the short term. It is interesting that the short-term predictors of suicide include several symptoms that may be related in a general way to impulsivity, particularly anxiety, alcohol abuse, and decreased concentration. Evidence has suggested that the serotonergic system is involved in impulsivity (Linnoila et al., 1983; Coccaro et al., 1989; Gardner, Lucas, & Cowdry, 1990).

Studies that have looked at biological predictors of suicide have generally focused on the roles of corticosteroids and monoamines. Early research (Bunney & Fawcett, 1965; Bunney, Fawcett, Davis, & Gifford, 1969) found elevated levels of urinary 17-hydroxycorticosteroids in depressed patients who attempted or committed suicide. These results were replicated by others (Ostroff et al., 1982; Prasad, 1985) who also found that the elevations in corticosteroids were most pronounced in patients who used a violent method when attempting suicide. In addition, high levels of blood and plasma cortisol have also been found in suicidally depressed patients (Asberg, Schalling, Traskman-Bendz, & Wagner, 1987; Krieger, 1974).

Other evidence has pointed to the possible role of monoamines in suicidality, in particular low levels of CSF 5-HIAA, the major metabolite of serotonin (Asberg, Traskman, & Thoren, 1976; Asberg et al., 1987; Roy et al., 1986). The effect appears to be robust, occurring across diagnoses and measures of suicidality. Levels of monoamines appear to be more trait- than state-like, generally showing stability over time. Roy and colleagues (1986) have also suggested that low CSF 5-HIAA combined with high post-dexamethasone cortisol levels may predict suicide in depressed patients. A recent study has confirmed the association of low levels of 5-HIAA and high levels of 3-methoxy-4-hydroxyphenylglycol (MHPG), a norepinephrine metabolite, in violent suicide attempters (Traskman-Bendz et al., 1992).

Some investigators suggest that one of the major functions of the serotonergic system is the regulation of sleep (Griffiths, Lester, Coulter, & Williams, 1972; George, Millar, Hanley, & Kryger, 1989; Jouvet, 1984; Dugovic & Wauquier, 1987; Sommerfelt, Hauge, & Usdin, 1987). Given the suggested role for the serotonergic system in suicide, Sabo, Reynolds, Kupfer, and Berman (1991) have examined PSG measures as potential markers for suicidality. Results were consistent with the notion that suicide attempters show changes in sleep, especially in sleep onset and in the timing and intensity of REM periods.

In comparison to the research done on the serotonin system in suicidality, the dopaminergic system has received much less attention. There is evidence, however, for its potential role. Some studies have found a low level of the dopamine metabolite homovanillic acid (HVA) in CSF of depressed patients who have attempted suicide (Agren, 1980, 1983; Traskman, Asberg, Bertilsson, & Sjostrand, 1981; Montgomery & Montgomery, 1982; Roy et al., 1986). In fact, it has been suggested that a low level of HVA may be a more reliable indicator of suicidal behavior than low levels of 5-HIAA. A recent study by Pichot, Hansenne, Moreno, and Ansseau (1992) examined the relationship of postsynaptic dopamine activity to suicide attempts by administering apomorphine, a selective dopaminergic agonist, and measuring the growth hormone (GH) response. Patients with a history of suicide attempt showed a lowered GH response to apomorphine, compared to equivalently depressed patients without a history of suicide attempt. The reduced response to apomorphine challenge suggests that the patients with a history of suicide attempts have a postsynaptic dopamine receptor hyposensitivity. The time from suicide attempt to evaluation was not related to GH response, suggesting that the alteration may be stable or trait-like. No differences were found between those with violent versus nonviolent suicide attempts, although the sample size was too small to draw any firm conclusions.

Research examining the cognitive and biological correlates of suicide have suggested that there may be differences between short- and long-term predictors. Whereas hopelessness and prior attempts may predict in the longer term, short-term predictors of suicide may be related more to anxiety, panic, and impulsivity. The biological substrate for these latter characteristics may lie in the serotonergic system.

COURSE OF DEPRESSIVE ILLNESS

Evidence is mixed regarding the utility of the Dysfunctional Attitude Scale (DAS; Weissman, 1979) as a vulnerability marker for predicting onset or relapse of depression. Some studies have found the DAS to be of predictive value (Rush, Weissenburger, & Eaves, 1986; Simons, Murphy, Levine, & Wetzel, 1986) whereas others have not (Weissman & Beck, 1978; Dohr, Rush, & Bernstein, 1989; Hollon, Kendall, & Lumry, 1986). Williams, Healy, Teasdale, White, and Paykel (1990) suggested that there may be two subgroups of patients reporting high dysfunctional attitudes when depressed. One group has transient mood-related elevations, while the other has more chronic dysfunctional attitudes. The latter group would be expected to have continued depression if these attitudes were not altered. It is suggested that a combination of pharmacotherapy and psychotherapy may be indicated in cases of chronically elevated DAS scores.

This distinction may also relate to the chronicity of depressive illness itself. Individuals with so-called "characterological" chronic depression, marked by early onset and mild chronic symptoms (Akiskal, 1983), or those with episodes of major depression superimposed on chronic dysthymia (Keller, Lavori, Endicott, Coryell, & Klerman, 1983; Keller, Lavori, Lewis, & Klerman, 1983) may have chronically high dysfunctional attitudes.

A study by Frank, Kupfer, Hamer, Grochocinski, and McEachran (1992) may provide indirect support for the existence of a subgroup of patients with chronic dysfunctional attitudes who are preferentially responsive to psychotherapy. In this study, nonendogenous patients were remitted longer than endogenous patients during maintenance treatment with psychotherapy. Unfortunately, it is not known whether the nonendogenous patients who stayed well longest had more dysfunctional attitudes prior to or during acute treatment.

Several studies have examined aspects of the congruence hypothesis, which predicts that correspondence between personality type and type of life stressor is associated with onset of depression. In general, there has been support for this hypothesis (Brown, Bifulco, & Harris, 1987; Hammen, Ellicott, & Gitlin, 1989; Segal, Shaw, & Vella, 1989; Zuroff & Mongrain, 1987). Some studies have reported a greater predictive relationship for sociotropic (or dependent) patients who are susceptible to interpersonal stress (Hammen et al., 1985; Zuroff & Mongrain, 1987; Robins & Block, 1988), whereas other studies found a more powerful predictive relationship for autonomous (or self-critical) subjects who are susceptible to achievement stress (Hammen et al., 1989; Segal et al., 1992). Segal et al. (1992) suggest that these discrepancies may relate to sampling differences, with studies using student populations finding stronger congruence effects for dependent subjects experiencing interpersonal stress and patient samples showing more congruence for autonomy and achievement stress. They also suggest that there may be an interactive temporal effect, with interpersonal stress being more acute and achievement stress being more additive and insidious in its effects.

In examining biological functioning, patients with more past episodes of depression have been found to have a higher incidence of continued DST nonsuppression despite recovery (Gurguis, Meador-Woodruff, Haskett, & Greden, 1990). This result needs replication, however, because in the study cited, there were more bipolar patients in the group with continued nonsuppression. Studies have also shown that continued DST nonsuppression after clinical recovery relates to early relapse (Greden et al., 1983; Holsboer, Liebl, & Hofschuster, 1982; Targum, 1983). Pretreatment DST status has not been found to relate to number of episodes of depression (Lenox, Peyser, Rothschild, Shipley, & Weaver, 1985; Meador-Woodruff, Gurguis, Grunhaus, Haskett, & Greden, 1987). There appears to be a lag between the time of clinical recovery and the normalization of cortisol response to dexamethasone (Gerken, Maier, & Holsboer, 1985) and a number of patients continue to show abnormal DST responses despite clinical recovery (Targum, 1983; Papakostas, Fink, Lee, Irwin, & Johnson, 1981; Holsboer, Steiger, & Maier, 1983; Greden et al., 1983; Gurguis et al., 1990). In addition, DST abnormalities have been found to occur prior to clinical signs of relapse or recurrence of depression (Holsboer et al., 1983). These results suggest that although DST nonsuppression is a state characteristic associated with depression, its continued presence may indicate the potential for either incomplete recovery or early relapse.

Kupfer, Frank, McEachran, and Grochocinski (1990) have suggested that delta sleep ratio (average number of delta waves in the first non-REM period divided by the average number of delta waves in the second non-REM period) may be a correlate of early recurrence of depression. Reduced REM latency has also been suggested as a predictor of early relapse or recurrence of depression following treatment discontinuation (Giles, Jarrett, Roffwarg, & Rush, 1987; Giles, Jarrett, Biggs, Guzick, & Rush, 1989).

Course of illness has been examined in terms of both psychological and biological functioning. Unfortunately, very little has been done in the way of integrating these results. Chronic forms of depression have been related to chronically elevated DAS scores, and persistent abnormalities in the DST and PSG have been associated with early relapse/recurrence in depression.

It is not clear whether chronically depressed patients have persistent abnormalities in both cognitive and biological arenas, or if there are distinct cognitively and biologically abnormal subgroups of these patients.

PREDICTION OF TREATMENT RESPONSE

Endogenous and nonendogenous patients have been compared with respect to their response to antidepressant medication treatment (Rush et al., 1989), combined psychotherapy and medication treatment (Prusoff, Weissman, Klerman, & Rounsaville, 1980), and electroconvulsive therapy (ECT; Prudic, Devanand, Sackheim, Decina, & Kerr, 1989; Vlissides & Jenner, 1982). Results have been mixed and may have been influenced by the specific definition of endogenous (Zimmerman, Stangl, & Coryell, 1985). In general, the literature is not clear as to whether endogenous (melancholic) subtyping is useful in predicting short-term treatment outcome with antidepressant medication, especially in outpatients (Avery, Wilson, & Dunner, 1983; Paykel, Hollyman, Freeling, & Sedgwick, 1988; Georgotas et al., 1987; Coryell & Turner, 1985; Davidson, Giller, Zisook, & Overall, 1988; for a review see Rush & Weissenburger, 1994).

Results regarding the response to treatment with psychotherapy have also been inconsistent. Endogenous patients in one study did poorly when treated with interpersonal psychotherapy (IPT; Klerman, Weissman, Rounsaville, & Chevron, 1984), but responded well to a combination of IPT and amitriptyline (Prusoff et al., 1980). Nonendogenous patients in this study did best with IPT alone. In contrast, results of the NIMH collaborative study suggest that endogenous patients had a better response to IPT, whereas subtypes did not differ in their responses to cognitive-behavioral psychotherapy (CBT; Sotsky et al., 1991). Thase, Simons, Cahalane, and McGeary (1991) found a high rate of response to CBT among endogenous patients. Frank et al. (1990) found no value of endogenous subtyping for prediction of response to combination treatment with IPT and imipramine.

Studies that have focused on the factors related to antidepressant treatment response have found that short-term response may relate to early changes in specific symptoms (e.g., hostility, somatization, and anxiety; Katz et al., 1991), and higher levels of social support (Vallejo, Gasto, Catalan, Bulbena, & Menchon, 1991). Absence of life stressors during the treatment period and pretreatment DST nonsuppression have been related to long-term (6 months) response to imipramine, whereas absence of life events prior to the onset of the depressive episode was associated with a poorer long-term outcome to phenelzine (Vallejo et al., 1991).

Other evidence is mixed regarding the relevance of life events to treatment outcome. Parker, Tennant, and Blignault (1985) found that patients with preexisting life events had better response to treatment. This effect was found only for endogenous patients in another study (Monroe, Thase, Hersen, Himmelhoch, & Bellack, 1985). Life events occurring during the initial weeks of treatment have been related to poor outcome (Lloyd, Zisook, Click, & Jaffe, 1981). Other studies have not found life events to be useful predictors of either short-term response or long-term chronicity (Garvey, Schaffer, & Tuason, 1984; Hirschfeld, Klerman, Andreasen, Clayton, & Keller, 1986).

High dysfunctional attitudes have been found to predict persistence of depression in both community samples (Lewinsohn, Steinmetz, Larson, & Franklin, 1981) and inpatients (Williams et al., 1990). Similar findings have related dysfunctional attitudes to duration of hospitalization (Norman, Miller, & Keitner, 1987). In the latter study, severity and biological subtype of depression based on the DST were measured and found not to relate to results. In the study by Williams et al. (1990), dysfunctional attitudes at admission significantly related to clinical status after 6 weeks of treatment. Results were not related to severity of depression, to subtype (endogenous vs. nonendogenous), or to chronicity, defined as number of previous episodes or length of the current episode. The role of life stress was not assessed. In a follow-up at 6 months, this effect was no longer observed. This result is consistent with the suggestion that there is a difference in the prediction of relapse versus the prediction of continued depression (Keller & Shapiro, 1981; Teasdale, 1988).

In a sample of 74 outpatients treated with amitriptyline or desipramine, response to treatment at weeks 3, 7, and end of treatment (week 9 or 10) was not found to relate to pretreatment DAS scores (Rush, Gullion, Cain, & Roffwarg, 1992). In contrast, another study (Peselow et al., 1990) found that higher pretreatment DAS scores related to poorer response to both antidepressants and placebo. Interestingly, for patients with DAS scores above the median, the rate of response to drug was not significantly different than the response to placebo, suggesting that patients with high initial DAS scores may require more than pharmacotherapy alone.

Pretreatment reduced REM latency has been associated with a greater likelihood of response to amitriptyline or desipramine, with high REM latency subjects having a selectively poorer response to desipramine (Rush et al., 1989). Other studies have confirmed the association between PSG measures and response to antidepressant medication treatment (Gillin, Wyatt, Fram, & Snyder, 1978; Kupfer et al., 1981; Kupfer, Ehlers, Pollock, Nathan, & Perel, 1989; Reynolds et al., 1987; Rush et al., 1983; Shipley et al., 1985). In general, sleep continuity disturbances and reduced REM latency have been related specifically to acute medication treatment response (Kupfer et al., 1981; Rush et al., 1989).

In contrast, studies have generally not shown the effect of sleep measures on response to psychotherapy (Jarrett, Rush, Khatami, & Roffwarg, 1990; Simons & Thase, 1992; Thase & Simons, 1992). However, a recent study (Buysse et al., 1992) found that nonresponders to IPT had longer sleep latencies, lower sleep efficiency, and increased phasic REM activity when compared to responders. Responders and nonresponders also showed differences in adaptation across the two nights of sleep assessment.

In summary, response to specific treatments has not been consistently related to cognitive, personality, or life stress variables. Abnormalities in sleep continuity have been associated with a good acute response to pharmacotherapy, but their relation to response to psychotherapy is not yet certain.

SUMMARY

There has been general support for a biologically related subtype of endogenous depression that is characterized by vegetative symptoms such as sleep disturbance and loss of appetite, weight, and libido. These endogenous symptoms have been associated with reduced CRH levels in the paraventricular hypothalamus and with increased glucocorticoids. Nonendogenous depression is a residual category that may include several distinct types. One component that may be cognitively and biologically distinct is that of self-criticality/anxiety. This component may be related to chronically high levels of dysfunctional attitudes and/or alterations in specific aspects of self-esteem and interpersonal relationships. In terms of biology, alterations in serotonergic metabolism may be uniquely associated with this component of depression.

Alterations of serotonin have also been implicated in the prediction of suicide. The coexistence of altered serotonergic metabolism and elevated levels of glucocorticoids may be particularly predictive of suicidal potential. Given the serotonergic system's role in sleep and impulsivity, further work relating sleep changes and indices of central serotonergic activity to symptoms, course, treatment response, and suicide are important.

We have very little conclusive evidence about how psychological and biological factors relate to course of depressive illness, vulnerability factors, and treatment response. In general, a more protracted course and poorer response to treatment are associated with chronically poor cognitive functioning and more stable biological abnormalities. It is important to go beyond this global severity-oriented level of understanding. Longitudinal studies can provide a more idiographic approach and elucidate temporal relationships among the variables being studied.

Much research has been conducted to test the predictions of Beck's (1967, 1976) theories of depression. Results have confirmed the association of specific cognitive alterations or biases and the state of depression. Recent focus has been on the etiological implications of the theory, including the diathesis–stress model and the congruency hypothesis. Although testing these concepts is methodologically challenging, advances have been made. The role of cognitive factors, life events, and personality features in the etiology and course of depression are beginning to be elucidated. The reciprocal interaction between these factors and biological functioning is complex and not easily studied or understood. However, the few efforts made in this area have been encouraging in terms of the much richer knowledge obtained from this integrative approach. More work in this area is likely to be very informative and will shed light on the interaction between biological and psychological factors in depression.

ACKNOWLEDGMENTS

This work was supported in part by National Institute of Mental Health Center Grant No. MH-41115 to the Department of Psychiatry, University of Texas Southwestern Medical Center. We thank David Savage for secretarial support and Kenneth Z. Altshuler, MD, for administrative support.

REFERENCES

Agren, H. (1980). Symptom patterns in unipolar and bipolar depression correlating with monoamine metabolites in the cerebrospinal fluid: II. Suicide. *Psychiatry Research, 3,* 225–236.

Agren, H. (1983). Life at risk: Markers of suicidality in depression. *Psychiatric Development, 1,* 87–104.

Akiskal, M. S. (1983). Dysthymic disorder: Psychopathology of proposed chronic depressive subtypes. *American Journal of Psychiatry, 140,* 11–20.

American Psychiatric Association. (1980). *Diagnostic and statistical manual of mental disorders* (3rd ed.). Washington, DC: Author.

American Psychiatric Association. (1987). *Diagnostic and statistical manual of mental disorders* (3rd ed., rev.). Washington, DC: Author.

American Psychiatric Association (1994). *Diagnostic and statistical manual of mental disorders* (4th ed.). Washington, DC: Author.

Asberg, M., Schalling, D., Traskman-Bendz, L., & Wagner, A. (1987). Psychology of suicide, impulsivity and related phenomena. In H. Y. Meltzer (Ed.), *Psychopharmacology: The third generation of progress* (pp. 655–668). New York: Raven Press.

Asberg, M., Traskman, L., & Thoren, P. (1976). 5-HIAA in cerebrospinal fluid: A biochemical suicide predictor? *Archives of General Psychiatry, 33,* 1193–1197.

Avery, D. H., Wilson, L. G., & Dunner, D. L. (1983). Diagnostic subtypes of depression as predictors of therapeutic response. In P. J. Clayton & J. E. Barrett (Eds.), *Treatment of depression: Old controversies and new approaches* (pp. 193–205). New York: Raven Press.

Banki, C. M., Bissette, G., Arato, M., O'Connor, L., & Nemeroff, C. B. (1987). CSF corticotropin-releasing factor-like immunoreactivity in depression and schizophrenia. *American Journal of Psychiatry, 144,* 873–877.

Baxter, L. R., Phelps, M. E., Mazziotta, J. C., Schwartz, J. M., Gerner, R. H., Selin, C. E., & Sumida, R. M. (1985). Cerebral metabolic rates for glucose in mood disorders: Studies with positron emission tomography and fluorodeoxyglucose F18. *Archives of General Psychiatry, 42,* 441–447.

Beck, A. T. (1967). *Depression: Clinical, experimental, and theoretical aspects*. New York: Harper & Row.

Beck, A. T. (1976). *Cognitive therapy and the emotional disorders*. New York: International Universities Press.

Beck, A. T. (1986). Hopelessness as a predictor of eventual suicide. In J. J. Mann & M. Stanley (Eds.), *Psychobiology of suicidal behavior* (pp. 90–96). New York: Academy of Sciences.

Beck, A. T., Brown, G., Berchick, R. J., Stewart, B. L., & Steer, R. A. (1990). Relationship between hopelessness and ultimate suicide: A replication with psychiatric outpatients. *American Journal of Psychiatry, 147*, 190–195.

Beck, A. T., Steer, R. A., & Brown, G. (1993). Dysfunctional attitudes and suicidal ideation in psychiatric outpatients. *Suicide and Life-Threatening Behavior, 23*, 11–20.

Beck, A. T., Steer, R. A., & Epstein, N. (1992). Self-concept dimensions of clinically depressed and anxious outpatients. *Journal of Clinical Psychology, 48*, 423–432.

Beck, A. T., Steer, R. A., Kovacs, M., & Garrison, B. (1985). Hopelessness and eventual suicide: A 10-year prospective study of patients hospitalized with suicidal ideation. *American Journal of Psychiatry, 142*, 559–563.

Beck, A. T., Ward, C. H., Mendelson, M., Mock, J. E., & Erbaugh, J. K. (1961). An inventory for measuring depression. *Archives of General Psychiatry, 4*, 561–571.

Beck, A. T., Weissman, A. W., Lester, D., & Trexler, L. (1974). The measurement of pessimism: The Hopelessness Scale. *Journal of Consulting and Clinical Psychology, 42*, 861–865.

Berger, M., & Riemann, D. (1993). REM sleep in depression—an overview. *Journal of Sleep Research, 2*, 211–223.

Bradvik, L,. & Berglund, M. (1993). Risk factors for suicide in melancholia. *Acta Psychiatrica Scandinavica, 87*, 306–311.

Brown, G. W., Bifulco, A., & Harris, T. O. (1987). Life events, vulnerability and onset of depression: Some refinements. *British Journal of Psychiatry, 150*, 30–42.

Buchholtz-Hansen, P. E., Wang, A. G., Kragh-Sorensen, P., & the Danish University Antidepressant Group. (1993). Mortality in major affective disorder: Relationship to subtype of depression. *Acta Psychiatrica Scandinavica, 87*, 329–335.

Bunney, W. E., Jr., & Fawcett, J. A. (1965). Possibility of a biochemical test for suicidal potential. *Archives of General Psychiatry, 13*, 232–239.

Bunney, W. E., Jr., Fawcett, J. A., Davis, J. M., & Gifford, S. (1969). Further evaluation of urinary 17-hydroxycorticosteroids in suicidal patients. *Archives of General Psychiatry, 21*, 138–150.

Buysse, D. J., Kupfer, D. J., Frank, E., Monk, T. H., Ritenour, A., & Ehlers, C. L. (1992). Electroencephalographic sleep studies in depressed outpatients treated with interpersonal psychotherapy: I. Baseline studies in responders and nonresponders. *Psychiatry Research, 40*, 13–26.

Carney, M. W. P., Reynolds, E. H., & Sheffield, B. F. (1986). Prediction of outcome in depressive illness by the Newcastle Diagnosis Scale. Its relationship with the unipolar/bipolar and DSM-III systems. *British Journal of Psychiatry, 150*, 43–48.

Carroll, B. J., Feinberg, M., Greden, J. F., Tarika, J., Albala, A. A., Haskett, R. F., James, N. McI., Kronfol, Z., Lohr, N., Steiner, M., deVigne, J. P., & Young, E. (1981). A specific laboratory test for the diagnosis of melancholia. *Archives of General Psychiatry, 38*, 15–22.

Coccaro, E. F., Siever, L. J., Klar, H. M., Maurer, G., Cochrane, K., Cooper, T. B.,

Mohs, R. C., & Davis, K. L. (1989). Serotonergic studies in patients with affective and personality disorders. Correlates with suicidal and impulsive aggressive behavior. *Archives of General Psychiatry, 46*, 587–599.

Cornell, D. G., Milden, R. S., & Shimp, S. (1985). Stressful life events associated with endogenous depression. *Journal of Nervous and Mental Disease, 173*, 470–476.

Coryell, W., & Turner, R. (1985). Outcome with desipramine therapy in subtypes of nonpsychotic depression. *Journal of Affective Disorders, 9*, 149–154.

Davidson, J. R. T., Giller, E. L., Zisook, S., & Overall, J. E. (1988). An efficacy study of isocarboxazid and placebo in depression, and its relationship to depressive nosology. *Archives of General Psychiatry, 45*, 120–127.

DeJong, J. A., & Roy, A. (1990). Relationship of cognitive factors to CSF corticotropin-releasing hormone in depression. *American Journal of Psychiatry, 147*, 350–352.

Dohr, K. B., Rush, A. J., & Bernstein, I. H. (1989). Cognitive biases in depression. *Journal of Abnormal Psychology, 98*, 263–267.

Dolan, R. J., Calloway, S. P., Fonagy, P., de Souza, F. V. A., & Wakeling, A. (1985). Life events, depression, and hypothalamic–pituitary–adrenal axis function. *British Journal of Psychiatry, 147*, 429–433.

Dugovic, C., & Wauquier, A. (1987). 5-HT$_2$ receptor could be primarily involved in the regulation of slow-wave sleep in rats. *European Journal of Pharmacology, 137*, 145–146.

Eaves, G., & Rush, A.J. (1984). Cognitive patterns in symptomatic and remitted unipolar major depression. *Journal of Abnormal Psychology, 93*, 31–40.

Faustman, W. O., Faull, K. F., Whiteford, H. A., Borchert, C., & Csernansky, J. G. (1990). CSF 5-HIAA, serum cortisol, and age differentially predict vegetative and cognitive symptoms in depression. *Biological Psychiatry, 27*, 311–318.

Fawcett, J. (1993). The morbidity and mortality of clinical depression. *International Clinical Psychopharmacology, 8*, 217–220.

Frank, E., Kupfer, D. J., Hamer, T., Grochocinski, V. J., & McEachran, A. B. (1992). Maintenance treatment and psychobiologic correlates of endogenous subtypes. *Journal of Affective Disorders, 25*, 181–190.

Frank, E., Kupfer, D. J., Perel, J. M., Cornes, C., Jarrett, D. B., Mallinger, A. G., Thase, M. E., McEachran, A. B., & Grochocinski, J.J. (1990). Three year outcomes for maintenance therapies in recurrent depression. *Archives of General Psychiatry, 47*, 1093–1099.

Gardner, D. L., Lucas, P. B., & Cowdry, R. W. (1990). CSF metabolites in borderline personality disorder compared with normal controls. *Biological Psychiatry, 28*, 247–254.

Garvey, M., Schaffer, C., & Tuason, V. (1984). Comparison of pharmacological treatment response between situational and non situational depression. *British Journal of Psychiatry, 145*, 363–365.

Gastpar, M., Gilsdorf, U., Abou-Saleh, M. T., & Ngo-Khac, T. (1992). Clinical correlates of response to DST. The dexamethasone suppression test in depression: A World Health Organisation collaborative study. *Journal of Affective Disorders, 26*, 17–24.

George, C. F. P., Millar, T. W., Hanley, P. J., & Kryger, M. H. (1989). The effects of l-tryptophan on daytime sleep latency in normals: Correlation with blood levels. *Sleep, 12*, 345–353.

Georgotas, A., McCue, R. E., Cooper, T., Chang, I., Mir, P., & Welkowitz, J. (1987). Clinical predictors of response to antidepressants in elderly patients. *Biological Psychiatr, 22*, 733–740.

Gerken, A., Maier, W., & Holsboer, F. (1985). Weekly monitoring of dexamethasone suppression response in depression: Its relationship to change of body weight and psychopathology. *Psychoneuroendocrinology, 10,* 261–271.

Giles, D. E., Etzel, B. A., & Biggs, M. M. (1990). Risk factors in unipolar depression: II. Relation between proband REM latency and cognitions of relatives. *Psychiatry Research, 33,* 39–49.

Giles, D. E., Jarrett, R. B., Biggs, M. M., Guzick, D. S., & Rush, A. J. (1989). Clinical predictors of recurrence in depression. *American Journal of Psychiatry, 146,* 764–767.

Giles, D. E., Jarrett, R. B., Roffwarg, H. P., & Rush, A. J. (1987). Reduced REM latency: A predictor of recurrence in depression. *Neuropsychopharmacology, 1,* 33–39.

Giles, D. E., & Rush, A. J. (1982). Relationship of dysfunctional attitudes and dexamethasone response in endogenous and nonendogenous depression. *Biological Psychiatry, 17,* 1303–1314.

Giles, D. E., Schlesser, M. A., Rush, A. J., Orsulak, P. J., Fulton, C. L., & Roffwarg, H. P. (1987). Polysomnographic findings and dexamethasone nonsuppression in unipolar depression: A replication and extension. *Biological Psychiatry, 22,* 872–882.

Gillin, J. C., Wyatt, R. J., Fram, D., & Snyder, F. (1978). The relationship between changes in REM sleep and clinical improvement in depressed patients treated with amitriptyline. Psychopharmacology, *59,* 267–272.

Gold, P. W., Loriaux, D. L., Roy, A., Kling, M. A., Calabrese, J. R., Kellner, C. H., Nieman, L. K., Post, R. M., Pickar, D., & Gallucci, W. (1986). Responses to corticotropin-releasing hormone in the hypercortisolism of depression and Cushing's disease: Pathophysiologic and diagnostic implications. *New England Journal of Medicine, 314,* 1329–1335.

Greden, J. F., Gardener, R., King, D., Grunhaus, L., Carroll, B. J., & Kronfol, Z. (1983). Dexamethasone suppression test in antidepressant treatment of melancholia: The process of normalization and test–retest reproducibility. *Archives of General Psychiatry, 40,* 493–500.

Greenberg, M. S., & Beck, A. T. (1989). Depression versus anxiety: A test of the content–specificity hypothesis. *Journal of Abnormal Psychology, 98,* 9–13.

Griffiths, W. J., Lester, B. K., Coulter, J. D., & Williams, H. L. (1972). Tryptophan and sleep in young adults. *Psychopharmacology, 9,* 345–356.

Gurguis, G. N. M., Meador-Woodruff, J. H., Haskett, R. F., & Greden, J. F. (1990). Multiplicity of depressive episodes: Phenomenological and neuroendocrine correlates. *Biological Psychiatry, 27,* 1156–1164.

Haaga, D. A. F., Dyck, M. J., & Ernst, D. (1991). Empirical status of cognitive theory of depression. *Psychological Bulletin, 110,* 215–236.

Hammen, C., Ellicott, A., & Gitlin, M. (1989). Vulnerability to specific life events and prediction of course of disorder in unipolar depressed patients. *Canadian Journal of Behavioural Science, 21,* 377–388.

Hammen, C., Marks, T., Mayol, A., & deMayo, R. (1985). Depressive self-schemas, life stress, and vulnerability to depression. *Journal of Abnormal Psychology, 94,* 308–319.

Haslam, N., & Beck, A. T. (1993). Categorization of major depression in an outpatient sample. *Journal of Nervous and Mental Disease, 181,* 725–731.

Higgins, E. T. (1987). Self-discrepancy: A theory relating self and affect. *Psychological Review, 94,* 319–340.

Hirschfeld, R. M. A., Klerman, G., Andreasen, N., Clayton, P., & Keller, M. (1986). Psychosocial predictors of chronicity in depressed patients. *British Journal of Psychiatry, 148,* 648–654.

Hollon, S. D., Kendall, P. C., & Lumry, A. (1986). Specificity of depressotypic cognitions in clinical depression. *Journal of Abnormal Psychology, 95,* 52–59.

Holsboer, F., Liebl, R., & Hofschuster, E. (1982). Repeated dexamethasone suppression test during depressive illness: Normalization of test result compared with clinical improvement. *Journal of Affective Disorders, 4,* 93–101.

Holsboer, F., Steiger, A., & Maier, W. (1983). Four cases of reversion to abnormal dexamethasone suppression test response as indicator of clinical relapse: A preliminary report. *Biological Psychiatry, 18,* 911–916.

Jarrett, R. B., Rush, A. J., Khatami, M., & Roffwarg, H. P. (1990). Does the pretreatment polysomnogram predict response to cognitive therapy in depressed outpatients? A preliminary report. *Psychiatry Research, 33,* 285–299.

Jouvet, M. (1984). Indoleamines and sleep-inducing factors. *Experimental Brain Research, 8,* 81–94.

Katz, M. M., Koslow, S. H., Maas, J. W., Frazer, A., Kocsis, J., Secunda, S., Bowder, C. L., & Casper, R. C. (1991). Identifying the specific clinical actions of amitriptyline: Interrelationships of behaviour, affect and plasma levels in depression. *Psychological Medicine, 21,* 599–611.

Keller, M. B., Lavori, P. W., Endicott, J., Coryell, W., & Klerman, G.L. (1983). "Double depression": Two-year follow-up. *American Journal of Psychiatry, 140,* 689–694.

Keller, M. B., Lavori, P. W., Lewis, C. E., & Klerman, G. L. (1983). Predictors of relapse in major depressive disorder. *Journal of the American Medical Association, 250,* 3299–3304.

Keller, M. B., & Shapiro, R. W. (1981). Major depressive disorder: Initial results from a one-year prospective naturalistic follow-up study. *Journal of Nervous and Mental Disease, 169,* 761–768.

Klerman, G. L., Weissman, M. M., Rounsaville, B., & Chevron, E.S. (1984). *Interpersonal psychotherapy for depression.* New York: Basic Books.

Krieger, G. (1974). The plasma level of cortisol as a predictor of suicide. *Diseases of the Nervous System, 35,* 237–240.

Kupfer, D. J., Ehlers, C. L., Pollock, B. G., Nathan, R. S., & Perel, J. M. (1989). Clomipramine and EEG sleep in depression. *Psychiatry Research, 30,* 165–180.

Kupfer, D. J., Frank, E., McEachran, A. B., & Grochocinski, V. J. (1990). Delta sleep ratio: A biological correlate of early recurrence in unipolar affective disorder. *Archives of General Psychiatry, 47,* 1100–1105.

Kupfer, D. J., Spiker, D. G., Coble, P. A., Neil, J. F., Ulrich, R., & Shaw, D. H. (1981). Sleep and treatment prediction in endogenous depression. *American Journal of Psychiatry, 138,* 429–434.

Laurent, J., & Stark, K. D. (1993). Testing the cognitive content–specificity hypothesis with anxious and depressed youngsters. *Journal of Abnormal Psychology, 102,* 226–237.

Lenox, R. H., Peyser, J. M., Rothschild, B., Shipley, J., & Weaver, L. (1985). Failure to normalize the dexamethasone suppression test: Association with length of illness. *Biological Psychiatry, 20,* 329–352.

Lewinsohn, P. M., Steinmetz, J. L., Larson, D. W., & Franklin, J. (1981). Depression related cognitions: Antecedents or consequences? *Journal of Abnormal Psychology, 90,* 213–219.

Linnoila, M., Virkkunen, M., Scheinin, M., Nuutila, A., Rimon, R., & Goodwin, F. K. (1983). Low cerebrospinal fluid 5-hydroxyindoleacetic acid concentration differentiates impulsive from nonimpulsive violent behavior. *Life Science, 33,* 2609–2614.

Lloyd, C., Zisook, S., Click, M., & Jaffe, K. (1981). Life events and response to antidepressants. *Journal of Human Stress, 7,* 2–15.

Meador-Woodruff, J. H., Gurguis, G., Grunhaus, L., Haskett, R. F., & Greden, J. F. (1987). Multiple depressive episodes and plasma post-dexamethasone cortisol level. *Biological Psychiatry, 22,* 583–592.

Minkoff, K., Bergman, E., Beck, A. T., & Beck, R. (1973). Hopelessness, depression and attempted suicide. *American Journal of Psychiatry, 130,* 455–459.

Monroe, S., Thase, M., Hersen, M., Himmelhoch, J., & Bellack, A. (1985). Life events and the endogenous–nonendogenous distinction in the treatment and posttreatment course of depression. *Comprehensive Psychiatry, 26,* 175–186.

Monroe, S. M., Thase, M. E., & Simons, A.D. (1992). Social factors and the psychobiology of depression: Relations between life stress and rapid eye movement sleep latency. *Journal of Abnormal Psychology, 101,* 528–537.

Montgomery, S. A., & Montgomery, D. (1982). Pharmacological prevention of suicidal behaviour. *Journal of Affective Disorders, 4,* 291–298.

Nemeroff, C. B., Widerlov, E., Bissette, G., Walleus, H., Karlsson, I., Eklund, K., Kilts, C. D., Loosen, P. T., & Vale, W. (1984). Elevated concentrations of CSF corticotropin-releasing factor-like immunoreactivity in depressed patients. *Science, 226,* 1342–1343.

Norman, W. H., Miller, I. W., & Dow, M. G. (1988). Characteristics of depressed patients with elevated levels of dysfunctional cognitions. *Cognitive Therapy and Research, 12, 39–51.*

Norman, W. H., Miller, I. W., & Keitner, G. I. (1987). Relationship between dysfunctional cognitions and depressive subtypes. *Canadian Journal of Psychiatry, 32,* 194–198.

Ostroff, R., Giller, E., Bonese, K., Ebersole, E., Harkness, L., & Mason J. (1982). Neuroendocrine risk factors of suicidal behavior. *American Journal of Psychiatry, 139,* 1323–1325.

Papakostas, Y., Fink, M., Lee, J., Irwin, P., & Johnson, L. (1981). Neuroendocrine measures in psychiatric patients: Course and outcome with ECT. *Psychiatry Research, 4,* 55–64.

Parker, G., Tennant, C., & Blignault, I. (1985). Predicting improvement in patients with non-endogenous depression. *British Journal of Psychiatry, 146,* 132–139.

Paykel, E. S., Hollyman, J. A., Freeling, P., & Sedgwick, P. (1988). Predictors of therapeutic benefit from amitriptyline in mild depression: A general practice placebo-controlled trial. *Journal of Affective Disorders, 14,* 83–95.

Peselow, E. D., Robins, C., Block, P., Barouche, F., & Fieve, R.R. (1990). Dysfunctional attitudes in depressed patients before and after clinical treatment and in normal control subjects. *American Journal of Psychiatry, 147,* 439–444.

Pichot, W., Hansenne, M., Moreno, A. G., & Ansseau, M. (1992). Suicidal behavior and growth hormone response to apomorphine test. *Biological Psychiatry, 31,* 1213–1219.

Prasad, A. J. (1985). Neuroendocrine differences between violent and nonviolent parasuicides. *Neuropsychobiology, 13,* 157–159.

Prudic, J., Devanand, D. P., Sackheim, H. A., Decina, P., & Kerr, B. (1989). Relative response of endogenous and nonendogenous symptoms to electroconvulsive therapy. *Journal of Affective Disorders, 16,* 59–64.

Prusoff, B. A., Weissman, M. M., Klerman, G. L., & Rounsaville, B.J. (1980). Research Diagnostic Criteria subtypes of depression. *Archives of General Psychiatry, 37,* 796–801.

Ranieri, W. F., Steer, R. A., Lawrence, T. I., Rissmiller, D. J., Piper, G. E., & Beck, A. T. (1987). Relationship of depression, hopelessness, and dysfunctional attitudes to suicide ideation in psychiatric patients. *Psychological Reports, 61,* 967–975.

Reynolds, C. F., III, Kupfer, D. J., Hoch, D. D., Stack, J. A., Houck, P. A., & Berman, S. R. (1987). Sleep deprivation effects in older endogenous depressed patients. *Psychiatry Research, 21,* 95–109.

Robins, C. J., & Block, P. (1988). Personal vulnerability, life events, and depressive symptoms: A test of a specific interactional model. *Journal of Personality and Social Psychology, 54,* 847–852.

Robins, C. J., Block, P., & Peselow, E.D. (1989). Relations of sociotropic and autonomous personality characteristics to specific symptoms in depressed patients. *Journal of Abnormal Psychology, 98,* 86–88.

Robins, C. J., Block, P., & Peselow, E. D. (1990). Endogenous and non-endogenous depressions: Relations to life events, dysfunctional attitudes and event perceptions. *British Journal of Clinical Psychology, 29,* 201–207.

Roy, A., Agren, H., Pickar, D., Linnoila, M., Doran, A. R., Cutler, N. R., & Paul, S. M. (1986). Reduced CSF concentrations of homovanillic acid and homovanillic acid to 5-hydroxyindoleacetic acid ratios in depressed patients: Relationship to suicidal behavior and dexamethasone nonsuppression. *American Journal of Psychiatry, 143,* 1539–1545.

Roy, A., Pickar, D., Paul, S., Doran, A., Chrousos, G. P., & Gold, P. W. (1987). CSF corticotropin-releasing hormone in depressed patients and normal control subjects. *American Journal of Psychiatry, 144,* 641–645.

Rush, A. J., Cain, J. W., Raese, J., Stewart, R. S., Waller, D. A., & Debus, J. R. (1991). Neurobiological bases for psychiatric disorders. In R.N. Rosenberg (Ed.), *Comprehensive neurology* (pp. 555–603). New York: Raven Press.

Rush, A. J., Giles, D. E., Jarrett, R. B., Feldman-Koffler, F., Debus, J. R., Weissenburger, J., Orsulak, P. J., & Roffwarg, H.P. (1989). Reduced REM latency predicts response to tricyclic medication in depressed outpatients. *Biological Psychiatry, 26,* 61–72.

Rush, A. J., Giles, D. E., Roffwarg, H. P., & Parker, C. R., Jr. (1982). Sleep EEG and dexamethasone suppression test findings in outpatients with unipolar major depressive disorders. *Biological Psychiatry, 17,* 327–341.

Rush, A. J., Gullion, C. M., Cain, J. W., & Roffwarg, H. P. (1992). Biological and cognitive predictors of response to acute treatment in depressed outpatients. *Clinical Neuropharmacology, 15* (Suppl. 1), 576–577a.

Rush, A. J., Roffwarg, H. P., Giles, D. E., Schlesser, M. A., Fairchild, C., & Tarell, J. (1983). Psychobiological predictors of antidepressant drug response. *Pharmacopsychiatry, 16,* 192–194.

Rush, A. J., & Weissenburger, J. E. (1994). Melancholic symptom features and DSM-IV. *American Journal of Psychiatry, 151,* 489–498.

Rush, A. J., Weissenburger, J. E., & Eaves, G. (1986). Do thinking patterns predict depressive symptoms? *Cognitive Therapy and Research, 10,* 225–236.

Sabo, E., Reynolds, C. F., III, Kupfer, D. J., & Berman, S. R. (1991). Sleep, depression and suicide. *Psychiatry Research, 36,* 265–277.

Schulkin, J. (1994). Melancholic depression and the hormones of adversity: A role for the amygdala. *Current Directions in Psychological Science, 3,* 41–44.

Schwartz, J. M., Baxter, L. R., Mazziotta, J. C., Gerner, R. H., & Phelps, M. E. (1987). The differential diagnosis of depression: Relevance of positron emission tomography (PET) studies of cerebral glucose metabolism to the bipolar–unipolar dichotomy. *Journal of the American Medical Association, 258,* 1368–1374.

Segal, Z. V., Shaw, B. F., & Vella, D. D. (1989). Life stress and depression: A test of the congruency hypothesis for life event content and depressive subtype. *Canadian Journal of Behavioural Science, 21,* 389–400.

Segal, Z. V., Shaw, B. F., Vella, D. D., & Katz, R. (1992). Cognitive and life stress predictors of relapse in remitted unipolar depressed patients: Test of the congruency hypothesis. *Journal of Abnormal Psychology, 101,* 26–36.

Shipley, J. E., Kupfer, D. J., Griffin, S. J., Dealy, R. S., Coble, P. A., McEachran, A. B., Grochocinski, V. J., Ulrich, R., & Perel, J. M. (1985). Comparison of effects of desipramine and amitriptyline on EEG sleep of depressed patients. *Psychopharmacology, 85,* 14–22.

Silver, M. A., Bohnert, M., Beck, A. T., & Marcus, D. (1971). Relation of depression to attempted suicide and seriousness of intent. *Archives of General Psychiatry, 25,* 573–576.

Simons, A. D., Murphy, G. E., Levine, J. L., & Wetzel, R. D. (1986). Cognitive therapy and pharmacotherapy for depression. *Archives of General Psychiatry, 43,* 43–50.

Simons, A. D., & Thase, M. E. (1992). Biological markers, treatment outcome and one-year follow-up in endogenous depression: Electroencephalographic sleep studies and response to cognitive therapy. *Journal of Consulting and Clinical Psychology, 60,* 392–401.

Sommerfelt, L., Hauge, E. R., & Usdin, R. (1987). Similar effects on REM sleep but differential effect on slow-wave sleep of the two 5-HT uptake inhibitors ziurelidine and alaprociate in rats and cats. *Journal of Neural Transmission, 68,* 127–144.

Sotsky, S. M., Glass, D. R., Shea, M. T., Pilkonis, P. A., Collins, J. F., Elkin, I., Watkins, J. T., Imber, S. D., Leber, W. R., Moyer, J., & Oliveri, M. E. (1991). Patient predictors of response to psychotherapy and pharmacotherapy: Findings in the NIMH treatment of depression collaborative research program. *American Journal of Psychiatry, 148,* 997–1008.

Spitzer, R. L., Endicott, J., & Robins, E. (1978). Research Diagnostic Criteria: Rational and reliability. *Archives of General Psychiatry, 36,* 773–782.

Targum, S. (1983). The application of serial neuroendocrine challenge studies in the management of depressive disorder. *Biological Psychiatry, 18,* 3–19.

Teasdale, J. D. (1988). Cognitive vulnerability to persistent depression. *Cognition and Emotion, 2,* 247–274.

Thase, M. E., & Simons, A. D. (1992). The applied use of psychotherapy in the study of the psychobiology of depression. *Journal of Psychotherapy Practice and Research, 1,* 72–80.

Thase, M. E., Simons, A. D., Cahalane, J. F., & McGeary, J. (1991). Cognitive behavior therapy of endogenous depression: I. An outpatient clinical replication series. *Behavior Therapy, 22,* 457–467.

Traskman, L., Asberg, M., Bertilsson, K., & Sjostrand, L. (1981). Monoamine metabolites in CSF and suicidal behavior. *Archives of General Psychiatry, 38,* 631–636.

Traskman-Bendz, L., Alling, C., Oreland, L., Regnell, G., Vinge, E., & Ohman, R. (1992). Prediction of suicidal behavior from biologic tests. *Journal of Clinical Psychopharmacology, 12* (Suppl. 2), 21s–26s.

Vallejo, J., Gasto, C., Catalan, R., Bulbena, A., & Menchon, J. M. (1991). Predictors of antidepressant treatment outcome in melancholia: Psychosocial, clinical and biological indicators. *Journal of Affective Disorders, 21,* 151–162.

Vlissides, D. N., & Jenner, F. A. (1982). The response of endogenously and reactively depressed patients to electroconvulsive therapy. *British Journal of Psychiatry, 141,* 239–242.

Weissman, A. W. (1979). The Dysfunctional Attitude Scale: A validation study (Doctoral dissertation, University of Pennsylvania, 1979). *Dissertation Abstracts International, 40,* 1389–1390B.

Weissman, A. W., & Beck, A.T. (1978). *Development and validation of the Dysfunctional Attitude Scale: A preliminary investigation.* Paper presented at the annual meeting of the American Educational Research Association, Toronto, Canada.

Wetzel, R. D., Margulies, T., Davis, R., & Karam, E. (1980). Hopelessness, depression and suicide intent. *Journal of Clinical Psychiatry, 41,* 159–160.

Williams, J. M. G., Healy, D., Teasdale, J. D., White, W., & Paykel, E. S. (1990). Dysfunctional attitudes and vulnerability to persistent depression. *Psychological Medicine, 20,* 375–381.

Zimmerman, M., & Coryell, W. (1986). Dysfunctional attitudes in endogenous and nonendogenous depressed inpatients. *Cognitive Therapy and Research, 10,* 339–346.

Zimmerman, M., Coryell, W., & Pfohl, B. (1986). The validity of the dexamethasone suppression test as a marker for endogenous depression. *Archives of General Psychiatry, 43,* 347–355.

Zimmerman, M., Stangl, D., & Coryell, W. (1985). The Research Diagnostic Criteria for endogenous depression and the dexamethasone suppression test: A discriminant function analysis. *Psychiatry Research, 14,* 197–208.

Zuroff, D. C., & Mongrain, M. (1987). Dependency and self-criticism: Vulnerability factors for depressive affective states. *Journal of Abnormal Psychology, 96,* 14–22.

Chapter 7

Therapeutic Empathy in Cognitive-Behavioral Therapy: Does It Really Make a Difference?

David D. Burns
Arthur Auerbach

Although cognitive therapy is often perceived as a highly technical form of therapy, Beck and his colleagues (Beck, Rush, Shaw, & Emery, 1979; Beck, Wright, Newman, & Liese, 1993) have also emphasized the importance of a warm, empathic therapeutic relationship. For example, they have stated: "The efficacy of cognitive and behavioral techniques is dependent, to a large degree, on the relationship between therapist and patient. . . . The relationship requires therapist warmth, accurate empathy, and genuineness. Without these, the therapy becomes 'gimmick oriented' " (Beck et al., 1993, p. 135). In this chapter we will examine the role of therapeutic empathy in cognitive therapy and attempt to answer the following questions:

- What is therapeutic empathy? Is the cognitive view of empathy different from the traditional psychoanalytic view of empathy?
- Is there any scientific evidence that therapeutic empathy actually has a causal effect on recovery in cognitive therapy? How large is this effect?
- Are most therapists reasonably empathic? Do therapists assess their own empathy in a reasonably accurate manner? How can empathy best be evaluated by clinicians in their daily practices?
- What is the most effective way to train therapists to develop greater empathy, particularly when dealing with hostile, difficult, mistrustful patients?

WHAT IS EMPATHY? WHO CAN BEST ASSESS IT?

Since empathy is such a central concept in psychotherapy, a brief mention of the origin of the concept in general culture may be of interest (Gauss, 1973). The word "empathy" is a translation of the German word, *Einfühlung*. This concept arose in the context of the 19th century German theory of aesthetics. Philosophers were curious about how an aesthetic object could produce an emotional response in the observer. They believed that this empathic response was caused by a predisposition within the observer, who ascribed beauty or the lack of beauty to the object.

This definition of empathy was subsequently expanded to include the viewer's knowledge of the object as well as feelings, and historians and social scientists began to apply the concept to the analysis of human relationships. They theorized that sympathetic identification with another person promoted understanding of that person's point of view and motivation.

Building on this tradition, psychodynamic investigators have defined empathy in terms of the therapist's subjective experiences in response to the patient. For example, Buie (1981) states that empathy "proceeds intrapsychically in the analyst" (p. 283). In a similar vein, Basch (1983) conceptualizes empathy as an affective state within the therapist in response to the patient's appearance and behavior. Book (1988) agrees, referring to empathy as the therapist's "experiencing of the patient's . . . emotional states. . . . [Empathy is] . . . a spontaneous, intrapsychic, preconscious experience . . . within the therapist" (p. 421). Frayn (1990) agrees, claiming that "the patient's impulses stimulate corresponding fantasies in the therapist. The patient compels the therapist to experience the patient's inner world by inspiring in the therapist a feeling, thought or self-state that previously had only remained within himself." Freud (1915/1964) appeared to trigger this line of thinking when he wrote: "It is remarkable that the [unconscious] of one human being can react upon that of another . . . but . . . the fact is *incontestable*" (p. 194, italics added).

Certainly, therapists should use all available information in understanding and conceptualizing their patients, including their own subjective responses during sessions. These responses provide one source of unverbalized information about the quality and nature of the therapeutic relationship. For example, if the therapist feels frustrated during sessions with a particular patient, there is a high likelihood that the patient also feels thwarted and misunderstood. The impasse might reflect similar difficulties the patient has experienced in numerous other close relationships.

Nevertheless, from a cognitive therapy perspective, the psychodynamic view of empathy is suspect. Cognitive therapists postulate that emotional responses sometimes result more from a person's idiosyncratic perceptions than from actual, external events. Therefore, the emotional reactions of therapists to their patients will often tell us more about the therapists' perceptions, fantasies, and beliefs than the patients'. For any given patient behavior, different therapists might—and probably will—have different kinds of perceptions and feelings.

Some empirical studies suggest that therapists' formulations are frequently not systematically related to what patients are actually thinking or feeling. For example, in their study of empathy and outcome in brief dynamic therapy, Free and his collaborators (Free, Green, Grace, Chernus, & Whitman, 1985) found that therapists did not accurately estimate how their patients perceived them. The investigators reported that there "was *no significant agreement* among patients, therapists, and clinical supervisors when they used *the same scale* to rate therapist empathy for *the same sessions*. Only the patients' ratings correlated significantly with some of the outcome measures" (p. 917, italics added). In a similar vein, Squier (1990) writes: "The psychotherapy literature shows clearly that for empathy to be effective, it must be perceived and felt by the patient. Here lies a difficulty: empathy as perceived by [therapists themselves or by their] teachers, supervisors, [or] colleagues . . . has often *not* been related to that experienced by patients."

Other research on therapeutic empathy is consistent with this point of view. In their review of studies of therapeutic empathy and outcome, Orlinsky, Grawe, and Parks (1994) reported that when therapeutic empathy was assessed by patients, empathy was positively correlated with recovery in 34 of 47 studies. These correlations were positive regardless of whether the outcome was measured by patients, therapists, independent raters, or objective, psychometric tests.

In contrast, when therapists rated their own empathy, significant correlations between empathy and recovery were reported in only 4 of 15 studies. In three of these four positive reports, the outcome was assessed by therapists, raising concerns that the correlations may have been tautological. When the outcome was assessed by patients, independent raters, or objective tests, a positive correlation between the therapists' assessment of empathy and outcome was observed in only 1 of 19 studies. At the .05 level of significance, one positive correlation in 20 studies would be expected by chance alone. Taken as a whole, these findings suggest that patients may be better judges than therapists of therapeutic empathy and indicate that patients' assessments of the therapeutic alliance are far more likely to predict clinical recovery.

Certainly, a therapist's perception of the therapeutic relationship will not always be incorrect. However, therapists are not aware that their assessments of therapeutic warmth and empathy can often be very inconsistent with how their patients actually view them. To illustrate this problem, the following demonstration can be conducted during training programs. One therapist is asked to play the role of an angry patient with a borderline personality disorder. A second therapist is asked to play the role of the therapist for 1 or 2 minutes. The therapist's job is to respond to the patient in an empathic, respectful manner. The therapist is instructed to encourage the patient to open up and is cautioned not to respond in a belittling, defensive, or rejecting way.

The role play is allowed to continue for 1 or 2 minutes. The "patient" nearly always expresses anger and insists that the therapist has not been helpful and does not care or understand. Most therapists can play the role of the angry patient with considerable gusto, since nearly all of them have frequently been on the receiving end of such criticisms. After several exchanges between therapist and patient, the demonstration is stopped and the "patient" is asked to rate the therapist using the Empathy Scale (ES; Persons & Burns, 1985; Burns & Nolen-Hoeksema, 1992) which is illustrated on Table 7.1.

The ES is a 10-item questionnaire that can be used in research or in

TABLE 7.1. The Empathy Scale (Patient's Version)

Put a check (✔) in the box to the right to indicate how strongly you agree with each of the following 10 statements concerning your most recent therapy session.	0 – NOT AT ALL	1 – SOMEWHAT	2 – MODERATELY	3 – A LOT
1. I felt that I could trust my therapist during today's session.		✔		
2. My therapist felt I was worthwhile.	✔			
3. My therapist was friendly and warm toward me.		✔		
4. My therapist understood what I said during today's session.		✔		
5. My therapist was sympathetic and concerned about me.			✔	
Total score on items 1–5 →			5	
6. Sometimes my therapist did not seem to be completely genuine.		✔		
7. My therapist pretended to like me more than he or she really does.			✔	
8. My therapist did not always seem to care about me.			✔	
9. My therapist did not always understand the way I felt inside.			✔	
10. My therapist acted condescending and talked down to me.		✔		
Total score on items 6–10 →			8	

Note. Copyright 1989 by David D. Burns, MD. Revised 1991, 1992, 1994. This test was adapted from one originally developed by Jeffrey Young, PhD. Reprinted by permission.

a clinical practice. Patients rate how warm, genuine, and empathic their therapists were during the most recent therapy session. Patients record how strongly they agree with each scale item with response options ranging from "not at all" to "a lot" on a 4-point Likert scale. The first five items are written so that strong agreement indicates a good therapeutic relationship. The second five items are worded so that strong agreement indicates a poor therapeutic relationship. A total ES score can be obtained by adding the five positively worded items and subtracting the five negatively worded items. Total scores can range between -15 (the lowest possible empathy rating) and $+15$ (the highest possible rating).

The individual who plays the role of the hostile patient often gives the therapist low ratings on the ES which are similar to those in Table 7.1 These ratings indicate that the patient felt the therapist was somewhat condescending and unsupportive and did not really understand how he or she felt.

When the patient fills out the ES following the role play, the individual who played the therapist is asked to fill out the therapist's version of the ES, which is illustrated in Table 7.2. As you can see, the patient and therapist versions of the Table 7.2 contain nearly identical items but they are worded from the perspective of the patient or the therapist, respectively. For example, item 1 on the patient's version of the ES is: "I felt that I could trust my therapist during today's session." Item 1 on the therapist's version is: "My patient felt that he or she could trust me during today's session."

Once the patient and therapist have filled out the scales, their ratings can be compared. The therapist's ratings are often quite different from the patient's. Most therapists feel they've done reasonably well and rate themselves quite positively in this exercise, with responses similar to those in Table 7.2. This therapist believed he came across in a warm, trustworthy, and compassionate manner.

The participants who observe the role play can also rate the therapist. They often give the therapist low ratings similar to those of the patient. This result confirms a point made earlier—that patients may often be the best judges of their therapists' warmth, empathy, and genuineness.

The exercise can be powerful and must be conducted with great tact and sensitivity to the feelings of the individual who plays the role of the therapist. The feedback can be upsetting, especially if the therapist feels judged, vulnerable, or insecure. If conducted in supportive way, the demonstration can be quite interesting and can reveal that therapists' perceptions of how their patients feel about them are frequently inconsistent with how their patients actually view them. And even setting aside the philosophical issue of whose ratings are the more realistic, it seems clear that when discrepancies exist, the patients' ratings, but not necessarily the therapists', will predict changes in patients' self-esteem and level of depression.

TABLE 7.2. The Empathy Scale (Therapist's Version)

Put a check (✔) in the box to the right to indicate how strongly you agree with each of the following 10 statements concerning your most recent therapy session.	0 – NOT AT ALL	1 – SOMEWHAT	2 – MODERATELY	3 – A LOT
1. My felt that he or she could trust me during today's session.				✔
2. I felt this patient was worthwhile.				✔
3. I appeared friendly and warm during the session.			✔	
4. My patient felt understood during today's session.				✔
5. I appeared sympathetic and concerned about this patient.				✔
Total score on items 1–5 →				14
6. Sometimes I did not seem completely genuine.	✔			
7. I pretended to like this patient more than I really did.	✔			
8. I did not always appear to care about him or her.		✔		
9. I did not always understand how her or she felt inside.	✔			
10. Sometimes I appeared condescending and talked down to the patient.	✔			
Total score on items 6–10 →				1

Note. Copyright 1989 by David D. Burns, MD. Revised 1991, 1992, 1994. Reprinted by permission.

THE ROLE OF EMPATHY
IN COGNITIVE-BEHAVIORAL THERAPY

Although cognitive-behavioral therapy (CBT) has been shown to be an effective therapy for depression (see reviews by Dobson, 1989; Robinson, Berman, & Neimeyer, 1990), several investigators have reported that other types of psychotherapy may be equally effective (Elkin et al., 1989; Rehm, Kaslow, & Rabin 1987; Thompson, Gallagher, & Breckenridge, 1987). In addition, there appears to be a lack of specificity in the mechanism by which these different treatments work. For example, several investigators (Rehm et al., 1987; Zeiss, Lewinsohn, & Munoz, 1979) have reported that cognitive, behavioral, and interpersonal therapy had similar effects on depression as well as on cognitive, behavioral, and interpersonal target variables, even though the treatments were designed to focus only on cognitions, behaviors, or interpersonal skills, respectively. Thus, therapies that postulate very different factors in the causation and maintenance of depression and that often utilize dissimilar therapeutic interventions appear to have surprisingly similar effects in nearly all measured outcome variables.

In an attempt to explain these results, many theorists have postulated that nonspecific factors common to all forms of therapy may play a more important role in clinical improvement than the specific factors unique to each type of treatment (Bergin, 1990; Garfield, 1990). One of the most frequently cited nonspecific factors is the quality of the therapeutic relationship (Luborsky, McLellan, Woody, O'Brien, & Auerbach, 1985). The previously cited review by Orlinsky et al. (1994) supports this hypothesis. They reported that in over half of 115 studies, therapeutic empathy was significantly correlated with therapeutic outcome.

The role of empathy in CBT is somewhat controversial. Although Rogers (1957) proposed that a warm, empathic relationship is one of the necessary and sufficient conditions for personality change, Beck and his collaborators (Beck et al., 1979) have argued that a good therapeutic relationship is necessary but is not a sufficient condition for change. That is, without an adequate therapeutic relationship, technical interventions directed at modifying patients' dysfunctional attitudes and behaviors are unlikely to be effective.

Ellis (1962) has downplayed the importance of empathy, arguing that a warm therapeutic relationship is neither necessary nor sufficient. He writes: "Rogers [argues that] . . . empathic understanding . . . seems essential to therapy. . . . This contention I again must dispute . . . [and] . . . have disproved several times in my own therapeutic practice" (pp. 114–116).

Ellis (personal communication to David D. Burns, 1993) has recently suggested that therapeutic empathy may not even be desirable. He believes that empathy could actually prevent progress by addicting the client to the therapist. Thus, although a warm and supportive therapist may make the client *feel* better, this temporary mood elevation could prevent the client from doing the hard work necessary for *getting* better.

While some therapists may find themselves at odds with Ellis on this particular point, most would agree that accurate empathy does not guarantee a helpful therapeutic intervention. The therapist might empathize in a way that actually reinforces the patient's self-defeating patterns.

For example, a chronically depressed patient with narcissistic personality disorder reported difficulties at work and had been fired from numerous computer programming jobs prior to seeking therapy. He was born in Pakistan and attributed his career difficulties to racial prejudice. If his therapist buys into his point of view, this may provide emotional relief because the patient will feel vindicated and understood. However, this intervention may do little or nothing to improve the patient's inconsistent work habits or his caustic way of communicating when receiving feedback about his performance from colleagues and supervisors. By the same token, any attempt to change these dysfunctional patterns in the absence of a warm, trusting therapeutic alliance is unlikely to succeed.

RESEARCH ON EMPATHY IN CBT

In one of the few empirical tests of empathy in CBT, Persons and Burns (1985) reported that patients' perceptions of therapeutic warmth and empathy were positively and strongly correlated with the degree of improvement during individual cognitive therapy sessions. However, this was a small study involving only a single therapy session from each of 17 patients, and the effects of empathy over the course of CBT were not investigated. Furthermore, since this was a correlational analysis, it was not possible to determine whether therapeutic empathy actually caused clinical improvement.

Separating the cause and effect relationships between therapeutic empathy and clinical improvement is not straightforward. As noted above, therapists' estimates of their own empathy may be biased and often do not correlate with recovery. However, patients' perceptions of therapeutic empathy may be contaminated by the severity of depression at the time the empathy measure is obtained. Thus, patients who are severely depressed and failing to improve may be more likely to feel misunderstood and uncared about by their therapists than patients who are improving more rapidly. This type of mood-dependent bias in the patients' perceptions of therapeutic empathy could spuriously inflate the relationships between empathy and clinical recovery.

When empathy has been estimated by external observers, Orlinsky et al. (1994) reported a positive association between therapeutic empathy and clinical improvement in 19 of 43 studies. However, this does not rule out the possibility that the direction of causality is from depression severity to empathy. When patients begin to improve, they and their therapists may develop more positive feelings about each other. This could lead to an improvement in the quality of the therapeutic alliance. Thus, therapeutic empathy and clinical improvement would still be positively correlated.

It is difficult to conceptualize how this cause and effect problem could be resolved using an experimental design. Ideally one would like to assign patients randomly to therapists who were either warm and empathic or cold and judgmental. Assuming these two types of therapists were equally skillful in all other regards, then any differential outcome between the groups could be attributed to therapeutic empathy. Even if one could overcome the ethical problems in conducting an experiment of this type, training two groups of therapists who were equally skillful in all regards except empathy seems virtually impossible.

This problem presents formidable statistical challenges as well. Ordinary least squares (OLS) statistical techniques, such as correlational analysis, analysis of covariance, or multiple regression, cannot be used to estimate systems with circular causality because, no matter how large the sample, the estimates will be biased. Furthermore, the percentage of the bias may be infinite and cannot be estimated.

Given these statistical difficulties, as well as the problems of conducting a controlled experiment, other analytic strategies are needed to tease apart the cause and effect relationships between therapeutic empathy and clinical recovery. Structural equation modeling is an alternate tool that can assist the researcher in clarifying the relationships among variables that may be reciprocally and simultaneously linked. Using this strategy, Burns and Nolen-Hoeksema (1992) estimated the causal effect of therapeutic empathy on clinical improvement, while controlling for the simultaneous reciprocal causal effect of depression severity on therapeutic empathy ratings, in a group of 185 outpatients studied during the first 12 weeks of treatment with CBT. The investigators addressed the following questions:

1. Does therapeutic empathy actually lead to clinical improvement, or do patients who are improving perceive their therapists as more empathic and caring because they are feeling better?
2. How large is the effect of therapeutic empathy on recovery?
3. Does therapeutic empathy work indirectly, by facilitating patients' motivation to help themselves, which in turn leads to clinical improvement, or does therapeutic empathy have a direct effect on clinical recovery?

The investigators assigned Axis I and Axis II diagnoses at the intake evaluation using the Structured Clinical Interviews for the DSM-III Axis I (SCID-I; Spitzer & Williams, 1983) and for Axis II (SCID-II; Spitzer & Williams, 1985). Of the 185 patients in the study, 168 (90.8%) had an affective disorder (either a major depressive episode and/or dysthymic disorder), and 17 (8.2%) had an anxiety disorder or another Axis I diagnosis such as an adjustment disorder with depressed or anxious mood. In addition, 104 patients (56.2%) had one or more Axis II diagnoses. No patients in the study were schizophrenic or suffered from an organic mental disorder.

Depression severity was assessed at intake and at the 12-week evaluation using the Beck Depression Inventory (BDI; Beck, Ward, Mendelson, Mock, & Erbaugh, 1961). Therapeutic empathy was assessed at the 12-week evaluation with the ES described above (Persons & Burns, 1985; Burns & Nolen-Hoeksema, 1992).

Clinicians and researchers may be concerned that patients' scores on the ES could be biased. For example, a needy, unassertive patient may report overly positive empathy scores for fear of causing a conflict or hurting the therapist's feelings, whereas an angry or depressed patient may report overly negative empathy scores.

Burns and Nolen-Hoeksema (1992) have shown how this measurement problem can be resolved using a three-stage least squares estimation procedure (Hanushek & Jackson, 1977) to purge patients' therapeutic empathy scores of all sources of subjective bias or measurement error. Thus, the investigators were able to estimate the causal effects of "true empathy" on recovery from depression. Using a similar technique, the investigators were able to estimate the causal effects of "true depression" on patients' perceptions of therapeutic empathy.

Consistent with previous studies (see Luborsky, Crits-Christoph, Mintz, & Auerbach, 1988, and Parloff, Waskow, & Wolfe, 1978, for reviews), the patients of therapists who were the warmest and most empathic improved significantly and substantially more than the patients of the therapists with the lowest empathy ratings, when controlling for other factors. This indicates that even in a highly technical form of therapy, such as CBT, the quality of the therapeutic relationship has a substantial impact on the degree of clinical recovery.

This is the first report we are aware of that has convincingly documented the causal effects of therapeutic empathy on recovery. The magnitude of the effect was moderate to large, since each unit on the ES was associated with approximately 1.3 units on the BDI.

To understand this effect, imagine that patient A and patient B each begin therapy with a BDI score of 22, indicating moderate depression. Patient A has a warm and empathic therapist who scores + 15 on the ES. Patient B has a colder and less supportive therapist who scores only + 7 on the ES. All else being equal, patient A will improve approximately 10 BDI points more than patient B (8 ES units × 1.3) during the first 12 weeks of therapy. This is not a small degree of improvement, since an overall reduction of 15 points on the BDI will be needed to achieve a normal score. For patient A, 10 of these 15 BDI points will result from the empathy effect.

Therapeutic empathy was robustly associated with reductions in BDI scores even when homework compliance was controlled for. This suggests that therapeutic empathy has a direct effect on clinical improvement and does not operate indirectly by facilitating homework compliance. In other words, therapeutic empathy and homework compliance made *additive* and *independent* contributions to clinical improvement.

To understand the magnitude of the homework effect, imagine in the example cited above that patient A did more than 3 days per week of self-help assignments during the treatment, on the average, whereas patient B did less than 1 day per week of self-help assignments, on the average. Patient A would have a predicted 12-week BDI score 6 points lower than patient B, when controlling for all else. Because the 6 points of improvement resulting from the self-help assignments can be added to the 10 points of improvement resulting from therapeutic empathy, patient A will have a total improvement of 16 points on the BDI. Therefore, patient A's predicted 12-week BDI score will be 6, which is in the range considered normal. In contrast, patient B, lacking either the benefits of a warm therapeutic alliance or the improvement associated with the consistent completion of self-help assignments, will have a predicted 12-week BDI score of 22, indicating no improvement at all.

These findings replicate and extend previous reports (Maultsby, 1971; Burns & Nolen-Hoeksema, 1991; Persons et al., 1988) that subjects who consistently complete homework assignments between sessions improve more than subjects who do not complete them. This suggests that participation in self-help assignments may be an important ingredient of the therapeutic process in CBT.

A reciprocal causal pathway from depression severity to therapeutic empathy was also documented, but the magnitude of this effect was very small. The findings suggested that even the most extreme changes in depression severity will barely influence patients' perceptions of therapeutic empathy. This means that, all else being equal, a group of severely depressed patients and a group of happy and fully recovered patients will give their therapists nearly identical empathy scores. Thus, while the quality of the therapeutic alliance has a large impact on clinical recovery, depression appears to have only a negligible effect on patients' perceptions of therapeutic empathy. This should increase the confidence of clinicians in the usefulness of the ES and in the validity of the scores assessed with this instrument.

Patient empathy ratings were significantly and substantially lower in the patients who dropped out prematurely. Although it seems likely that a failure of therapeutic empathy contributes to premature termination, it is also possible that patients who prematurely terminate may report lower levels of therapeutic empathy because they do not have as much time to get to know their therapists.

The 20 patients (11.0% of the sample) with a diagnosis of borderline personality disorder improved significantly less than the 162 patients without this diagnosis. This result is consistent with clinical experience (Kernberg, 1975; Shapiro, 1978) and emerged even when controlling for initial severity of depression, therapeutic empathy, homework compliance, and other Axis II psychopathology. These findings indicate that the borderline patients' refractoriness to treatment is not simply the result of depression severity or difficulties forming a therapeutic alliance or adhering to the therapeutic procedures. In fact, the therapeutic empathy ratings of the borderline patients were not significantly different from the patients without this diagnosis.

CLINICAL IMPLICATIONS

If future investigators are able to replicate these findings, the results could have useful implications for clinical training as well as for treatment. Since therapist identities were used to predict patients' empathy scores, the investigators were able to identify therapists with low levels of therapeutic empathy, so that they could make corrective adjustments in their therapeutic technique. They also identified one therapist, a novice, with unusually high empathy scores. This therapist was subsequently encouraged to model empathic responses during staff training sessions. The investigators were also able to estimate precisely each therapist's effectiveness in treating depression as well as other outcome measures, such as anxiety or marital discord, so that therapists with outstanding track records, as well as those needing additional training, could be identified.

The results of this study led to significant changes in the administration and therapeutic methods at the clinic. All new patients were informed they would be required to complete the ES after every session and to return it to their therapists at the subsequent session. This procedure allowed therapists to identify and address difficulties in the therapeutic alliance immediately.

Patients were also required to complete three self-assessment tests for depression, anxiety, and relationship satisfaction, respectively, between therapy sessions so that therapists could more accurately track clinical improvement and pinpoint therapeutic logjams. This pragmatic emphasis on measurement and on gathering objective data about the patient's progress, severity of current symptoms, and perceptions about the therapist reflects the empirical spirit central to cognitive therapy. New studies will be needed to determine whether these procedures systematically improve therapeutic empathy and enhance clinical recovery.

THERAPIST RESISTANCE
TO MEASURING THERAPEUTIC EMPATHY

In informal surveys conducted during lectures and workshops to mental health professionals, the first author (D. D. B.) has discovered that very few therapists (less than 2%) require patients to fill out one or more self-assessment tests between therapy sessions. There are a number of reasons for this.

Some therapists feel that testing at every session would be time consuming or burdensome. For the most part, clinical experience has not validated these concerns. As noted above, patients complete the assessment tests on their own between therapy sessions and report the scores at the beginning of each subsequent session. The amount of therapy time required to record the scores in patients' charts and to compare them with the scores from the previous session is usually less than 1 minute.

Some patients, especially those with borderline personality disorder, resist any self-help assignment between sessions, including the self-assessment tests. An exploration of this resistance can be good grist for the therapeutic mill. In addition, to minimize this type of resistance, the self-help requirement can be negotiated with each patient as part of the intake evaluation. Patients who indicate a reluctance to participate in the self-help assignments (typically less than 1%) are not accepted for treatment, but can be referred to other therapists whose orientation is more compatible with the patients'. This procedure can result in a significant increase in patient compliance with session-by-session psychological testing as well as other self-help assignments.

Some therapists may be skeptical about the validity of self-assessment tests, fearing that patients will not answer them honestly or that the reliability of the tests will diminish over time. For the most part, clinical experience has demonstrated that these concerns are unnecessary. With the possible exception of individuals with forensic issues (such as lawsuits or disability claims), the vast majority of patients appear to answer the tests honestly and repeated administrations do not seem to bias the results.

Nevertheless, good clinical judgment must always complement the interpretation of any psychological test. For example, anxious, unassertive patients may find it difficult to express negative feelings about their therapists. Therefore, therapists need to be aware that *any* ratings other than perfect scores on the ES may point to a potential conflict that needs to be explored.

Taking this into account, a therapist might make an interpretation along these lines: "I notice your scores on the two subscales of the ES are 15 and 1. This is practically a perfect score, so I take it you felt pretty positive about our last session. However, you indicated in your response to item 10 that I sounded condescending at times. I was also concerned about this later on when I was reflecting about the session. Can you tell me a bit more about this?" This nondefensive inquiry can lead to a productive discussion that will frequently strengthen the therapeutic alliance.

Finally, some therapists are convinced that they are sensitive and *can* assess the quality of the therapeutic alliance, as well as the severity of patients' emotional distress, with reasonable accuracy. Therefore, rating scales may seem unnecessary. As noted previously, most empirical studies and role-play demonstrations do not support this notion. Unless therapists request explicit verbal or written feedback from their patients, they frequently do not accurately assess the nature of their patients' cognitions, the severity of their patients' emotions, or their patients' perceptions of the therapeutic alliance.

The use of the ES, along with the self-assessment tests for depression, anxiety, and marital discord, on a trial basis with even a few patients will usually convince the skeptical therapist that these instruments cannot only be useful but can have a revolutionary effect on one's practice, regardless of the therapist's orientation. Monitoring the session-by-session scores will make the therapist and patient alike far more accountable and accurate in the assessment of therapeutic progress or the lack of it. The awareness that the patient is stuck or that the alliance is unsatisfactory can often signal the need for a change in therapeutic strategy that will get the treatment moving forward productively again.

HOW COMMON IS EMPATHIC FAILURE?
WHAT ARE THE CONSEQUENCES?

Empathic failure in simulated role-play situations appears to be more the rule than the exception. When therapists are confronted with colleagues who play the role of difficult, critical patients, it appears that few, if any, therapists can respond in a nondefensive, empathic manner. However, it is difficult to know whether this reflects actual clinical practice because there have been very few empirical studies of how therapists respond to difficult clients in real, nonsimulated therapy sessions.

In the first Vanderbilt study of time-limited dynamic psychotherapy, Strupp (1980a) and his colleagues studied the audiotapes of therapy sessions to learn how therapists responded to difficult patients who were critical of them. They were surprised to discover that therapist defensiveness frequently contributed to failures in the therapeutic alliance. Safran and Segal (1990) quote Strupp as saying:

> [The] . . . major deterrents to the formulation of a good working alliance are not only the patients . . . maladaptive defenses but—at least equally important—the therapists. . . . In the Vanderbilt project, even highly experienced [therapists] who had undergone a personal analysis . . . tended to respond . . . with counter-hostility that took the form of coldness, distancing, and other forms of rejection. . . . In our study we failed to encounter *a single instance* in which a difficult patient's hostility and negativism were successfully confronted or resolved. (pp. 40–41, italics added)

Strupp speculated that while this might have been due to the peculiarities of the group of therapists they studied, a more likely possibility was that "therapist's negative responses to difficult patients are far more common and far more intractable than had been generally recognized" (Safran & Segal, 1990, p. 41).

Based on their analysis of data from the second Vanderbilt study, Henry, Schacht, and Strupp (1990) argued that these negative therapeutic responses may impede therapeutic progress and have a deleterious impact on patients' feelings of self-esteem. The investigators correlated therapist responses during sessions with patient outcomes in a cohort of 14 therapeutic dyads consisting of 7 good outcome and 7 poor outcome cases. Outcome was defined in terms of an improvement in the patients' levels of self-esteem and self-acceptance. The investigators reported that

> therapists in the poor outcome group were significantly more belittling and blaming and ignoring and neglecting. . . . The results indicate . . . a high degree of correspondence between patient self-blaming statements and therapist statements subtly blaming the patient ($r = -.53$). . . . Apparently, even well trained professional therapists are surprisingly vulnerable to engaging in potentially destructive interpersonal processes. . . . It seems clear that traditional training methods have not adequately prepared many therapists. (pp. 771–774)

Although the studies of Strupp and his colleagues have occurred in the context of psychodynamic therapy, it seems reasonable to assume that similar difficulties might afflict cognitive therapists as well as therapists of nearly any persuasion. There are very few empirical comparisons of the therapeutic alliance in cognitive versus other types of therapy. Raue and his colleagues (Raue, Castonguay, & Goldfried, 1993) reported significantly higher therapeutic alliance scores in individual sessions of cognitive-behavioral than in interpersonal therapy, whereas Salvio, Beutler, Wood, and Engle (1992) found no differences between cognitive therapy, Gestalt therapy, and a supportive "self-directed" therapy.

Are there any reasons to predict that training in CBT might have a positive or negative impact on a therapist's capacity for empathy? One would expect that cognitive therapy's emphasis on systematically eliciting patients' negative feelings, thoughts, and underlying beliefs during sessions should enhance therapeutic empathy.

On the other hand, empathy may sometimes pose a particular difficulty for cognitive therapists who are trained to identify the distortions in patients' dysfunctional thoughts. There is the danger that the overly zealous cognitive therapist may prematurely challenge the patient and convey the message that his or her perceptions are irrational, that is, ridiculous. This danger is particularly great when the patient is angry with the therapist. From the patient's perspective, the anger and criticism are very justified and valid. Even if the criticisms appear grossly distorted to the therapist, it is usually more effective to set one's cognitive skills temporarily on the shelf and to find the grain of truth in what the patient is saying. This requires a sudden paradigm shift that may be confusing for cognitive therapists.

Why is empathic failure so common when therapists respond to criticisms by angry patients? Empathic failure may result in part from the therapist's pride and defensiveness, as will be discussed below. But there may be other reasons as well.

Psychotherapy is still more an art than a science, and the procedures for treating depression or anxiety are not nearly as well standardized as the procedures a physician would follow when treating a urinary tract infection. Lacking a valid science of human behavior, hundreds of schools of therapy have evolved, much like competing religions, each claiming to have a handle on the truth.

Therapists must chose one or a combination of these therapeutic orientations. This choice may not be based on scientific information and is probably more often motivated by subjective values and strong personal preferences. Consequently, the therapist's faith in his or her approach is not easily shaken, in much the same way that people feel a great faith in their own religious beliefs.

Accordingly, criticism from a patient will not usually cause the therapist to do much soul searching, because there is a tendency to believe that the patient must be wrong. It is therefore not surprising therapists frequently conclude that their patients "criticism" are unreasonable and result from neurotic problems.

TECHNICAL VERSUS EMPATHIC INTERVENTIONS

The training program we will describe is based on the idea that good therapy has two basic components: technical and empathic interventions (Burns, 1989). Therapists can use technical interventions to help patients solve personal problems and modify dysfunctional thoughts, feelings, and behaviors. Empathic interventions are especially important in two situations: whenever patients express distrust or anger toward their therapists or whenever patients are upset and need to ventilate, whether or not they are in conflict with their therapists.

A therapist may have to shift back and forth between the technical and empathic modes on many occasions during any given therapy session, particularly with difficult or resistant patients. When patients are stuck or angry or expressing strong affect, therapists need to set their cognitive and behavioral techniques temporarily on the shelf and respond in on empathic manner. When patients feel relaxed and validated and trust their therapists, then technical interventions can be implemented once again.

The distinction between technical and empathic interventions is somewhat artificial, because these two modes are ideally integrated. Any cognitive or behavioral technique not embedded in the context of a trusting therapeutic relationship will probably fail.

Technical and empathic interventions require dramatically different types of therapeutic and personal aptitudes. Some therapists have excellent cognitive and behavioral skills, but appear uncomfortable in the interpersonal, empathic mode. Other therapists are good at listening and providing emotional support, but do not have highly developed cognitive or behavioral skills. The rare therapist who can seamlessly integrate the technical and empathic modes will be more flexible and effective than a therapist who is unidimensional. This integration can sometimes be quite difficult.

For example, suppose a woman has completed a 2-hour initial evaluation for severe, chronic depression and interpersonal difficulties. This evaluation reveals a definite major depressive disorder along with features of borderline personality disorder and a troubled marriage. At one of the first subsequent therapy sessions, she tells her therapist in an irate and blaming tone of voice that her depression is her husband's fault. She insists that her husband is totally self-centered, stubborn, argumentative, and unwilling to listen to her point of view. She explains that she had to fire four previous marital therapists because they were duped by her husband and wrongly and unjustly made the suggestion that they might *both* be contributing to the marital problems and that she might also need to change.

Although there is clearly some truth in what she says, most therapists will assume that it takes two to tango and that her marital difficulties result, at least in part, from her own distorted perceptions and from the self-defeating way she communicates. However, if the therapist succumbs to the temptation to help her modify her attitudes or communication style she will almost certainly react angrily and may terminate therapy prematurely once again.

In contrast, if the therapist responds in an empathic manner and listens with his or her "third ear," there is a much better chance that therapeutic bonding can occur. For example, the therapist might say, "It sounds like your relationship with your husband has been difficult, and I can imagine how frustrated and lonely and angry you must feel. Am I reading you correctly?" An alternative but equally good response might focus on her distrust of the therapist: "I gather that your previous therapists didn't do a very good job of making you feel supported or understood, and I'm concerned that I might have also sounded judgmental or unsupportive at times. Have I?"

Although there might be dozens of equally good responses a skillful therapist could make, this disarming style will avoid polarizing her, and the therapeutic alliance will in all likelihood improve. If the therapist is to have any chance of success with such a difficult patient, he or she will need to give her enough time to ventilate and develop trust. For some patients this may require as little as 20 minutes, and for others it may require several therapy sessions.

After she feels accepted and understood, then the therapist can ask her to identify several specific problems she would like to work on in the therapy. Would she like to use cognitive therapy techniques to overcome her depression? Would she like to work on improving her marriage? Would she prefer to explore the possibility of leaving her husband? Would she prefer to maintain the status quo? How hard would she be willing to work to solve these problems? Would she be willing to change herself in order to solve these problems? Would she be willing to do homework assignments every day?

This step of the therapeutic process is called "agenda setting" (Burns, 1989). Any attempt to set the agenda prematurely, when patients feel angry or emotionally overwhelmed, tends to be exceedingly unproductive. And even after the therapist and patient have bonded properly and developed a meaningful therapeutic agenda, the patient may become upset and lose trust over and over again. Whenever this occurs, the therapist must suddenly shift gears. He or she must place the cognitive and behavioral skills temporarily on the shelf and utilize the empathy skills to reestablish the patient's trust again.

Empathic responding is not easy for three reasons. First, many patients who feel angry and alienated are experts at antagonizing people. Some may subconsciously create interpersonal distance as a defense against intimacy. It may be difficult for any therapist to resist a difficult patient's subtle but forceful invitation to engage in an adversarial relationship.

Second, when patients are in great pain, therapists want to help and may propose solutions prematurely, before the therapeutic agenda has been negotiated. This may result from a therapist's subconscious fear of interpersonal conflict, especially when the patient is angry. "Helping" the angry patient can be a subtle way of establishing dominance and avoiding the patient's rage.

This is especially true when the patient's angry criticisms contain a grain of truth. Although therapists ideally think of themselves as compassionate and objective, there is a strong human tendency — in spite of psychotherapy training and personal determination — to feel unjustly accused and to respond defensively at times during sessions. Therapist defensiveness is almost as automatic and inevitable as the jerk of one's knee when tapped by the neurologist's hammer. As Strupp (1980b) has said: "The plain fact is that any therapist — indeed any human being — cannot remain immune from negative (angry) reactions to the suppressed and repressed rage regularly encountered in patients with moderate to severe difficulties" (p. 953).

DESCRIPTION OF THE EMPATHY TRAINING PROGRAM

Can therapists be trained to overcome these negative reactions and respond more empathically? We think so, but empirical studies will be needed to assess this. Much may depend on the therapist's innate aptitude and the motivation that he or she brings to the training. The capacity for empathy is partially based on the therapist's willingness to experience things as other humans experience them. This often requires a deliberate effort to adopt, temporarily, the unfamiliar mind-set of another person.

The empathy training program is based in part on the five communication techniques listed in Table 7.3. There are three listening skills and two self-expression skills. A great many therapeutic logjams can be rapidly resolved using these techniques, as long as they are implemented tactfully and respectfully.

Although all of the techniques appear to be quite straightforward, novices and experienced practitioners alike will discover that they can be surprisingly difficult to apply when therapists are under attack from difficult clients. These methods can usually be mastered after several months of persistent practice with colleagues. The reward for this effort is frequently a significant improvement in therapeutic warmth and effectiveness.

The Disarming Technique

The first of the three listening skills is called the disarming technique: You find truth in what the angry patient is saying, even if the patient's statements seem entirely unfair or illogical. This is nearly always difficult, because from the therapist's perspective it may appear that the patient's criticisms are not valid.

The disarming technique is based on a concept known as the law of opposites (Burns, 1989). Burns (1989) has emphasized that if you defend

TABLE 7.3. The Five Secrets of Effective Communication

Listening skills

1. *The disarming technique:* You find truth in what the patient is saying, even if it seems totally distorted and unreasonable.

2. *Empathy:* You put yourself in the patient's shoes and try to see the world through his or her eyes.
   - *Thought empathy:* You paraphrase the patient's words.
   - *Feeling empathy:* You acknowledge how the patient is probably feeling.

3. *Inquiry:* You ask gentle, probing questions to learn more about what the patient is thinking and feeling.

Self-expression skills

4. *"I feel" statements:* You use "I feel" statements (such as "I'm feeling a bit on the defensive") in order to maintain credibility and genuineness when attacked. Avoid "you" statements (such as "you seem to have a problem with anger").

5. *Stroking:* You find something genuinely positive to say and convey an attitude of respect, even though the interaction may feel adversarial or tense.

Note. Copyright 1989 by David D. Burns, MD. Revised 1991, 1992, 1993. Reprinted by permission.

yourself from a criticism that is *entirely* untrue and unfair, you will often validate the criticism in the patient's mind. If, in contrast, you find the grain of truth in the criticism, you will often put the lie to it. This is a paradox.

This concept is anti-intuitive and may initially be difficult to comprehend. An example may make it more understandable. The most common complaint from patients is that the therapist has not been helpful and does not understand or care. This complaint may be expressed many different ways by many different patients, but this is usually the essence of the criticism.

Many therapists will feel the urge to defend themselves, and some may respond along these lines: "I want you to know that I *do* care about you and I *can* understand how you are suffering. Even though you may feel stuck just now, I believe that we have been making progress and that I *can* help you." This statement may be well intentioned and may sound supportive. Given a sufficiently warm and respectful tone of voice, it might even be appreciated by some patients, but this is not a likely result.

According to the law of opposites, any defense will validate the criticism. Is this the case here?

The therapist, in essence, is saying, "I am right and you are wrong." This is a subtle put-down that will probably not sound very understanding or compassionate from the patient's perspective. The therapist has not explored the patient's feelings of anger or mistrust but is talking about him- or herself. The implication is, "I am okay, and you are mistaken since you do not agree with me." This sounds self-serving and confirms the patient's criticisms.

How could the therapist use the disarming technique to respond more effectively? First, we need to ask if there is some truth in the patient's criticisms. The patient says that the therapist has not been helpful and does not care or understand. The patient is right in the sense that he or she has *not* recently been helped, even if the interventions seemed quite reasonable, since the patient is quite depressed. An examination of the patients' scores on the depression, anxiety, and relationship satisfaction tests will confirm that the patient is in tremendous pain. The therapy may have been helpful previously, and may be helpful later on, but at this moment the patient is clearly stuck.

We can also say that the therapist has probably *not* conveyed an understanding of the patient's inner feelings, since the patient feels angry and misunderstood. An empathic relationship, by definition, is one in which the patient feels understood and accepted.

Finally, the patient's insistence that the therapist does not care is right on target. The therapist may have been trying incredibly hard to be helpful, both during and between sessions. There may have been a number of stressful emergency calls on weekends or in the middle of the night. In spite of these efforts, the therapist has probably been repeatedly rebuffed and has not have heard many expressions of gratitude or appreciation—only complaints and demands.

How has this therapist been feeling about the patient? Warm and caring? It's not very likely! Many therapists would understandably feel frustrated, burned out, or resentful. On some level, the patient and therapist are both vividly aware of this negative dynamic, and the patient is verbalizing what they both know to be true.

This example is not unusual. On some level, patients' criticisms nearly always contain a considerable amount of truth, even when the criticisms are expressed in an exaggerated manner.

The therapist could acknowledge the validity of the patient's criticism by saying, "You know, what you're saying is important, and I agree with you. I can see from your depression and anxiety scores that you've been extremely upset in the past several weeks. I've also noticed some tension in our relationship, and I'm concerned that recently I haven't done a good job of helping you or understanding how you feel. I can imagine you may be feeling quite discouraged and angry with me. Am I reading you right? I'd like to hear more about how you feel."

The paradox is that by respectfully acknowledging a certain degree of therapeutic failure, the therapist increases the likelihood of success because the therapist and patient end up on the same team. If the therapist can find the truth in the patient's criticisms, the antagonism and mistrust will frequently diminish.

The patient may feel the same way about many people, and not just the therapist. Probably *none* of them will ever admit to any validity in what the patient says. When the therapist responds nondefensively and expresses genuine curiosity about how the patient feels, this will come as an unexpected surprise to the patient. This may be the *first* time that anyone has listened or acknowledged that the patient's negative perceptions have some value.

Many therapists fear that any attempt to agree with an angry borderline patient with a strong sense of entitlement will make the therapist appear weak. These therapists may resist the disarming technique, thinking it will simply open the door for more sadistic attack. Clinical experience indicates that just the opposite occurs. The escalation of the patient's attack nearly always results from the therapist's subtle defensiveness. The loud banging occurs because the patient rightly senses that the door is tightly closed. Because the patient desperately wants to be understood, the accusations become louder and more extreme. In contrast, when the therapist genuinely acknowledges the validity in the patient's criticisms, the intensity of the interaction is usually reduced.

There are several caveats. First, the therapist must be genuine and compassionate and must communicate a sense of respect for the patient. If the therapist disarms the patient with a tone of voice that sounds condescending, sarcastic, or manipulative, the method will backfire.

Second, the therapist must comprehend that the patients' criticisms really may contain significant truth, no matter how illogical or unreasonable they sound. This is a stumbling block for many therapists. Wile (1984) has emphasized how therapeutic training may contribute to this unfortunate tendency to discredit what patients say:

> Certain interpretations commonly made in psychoanalysis and psychodynamic therapy are accusatory. Therapists appear to make them not because they are hostile or insensitive, but because of the dictates of their theory. Clients are seen as gratifying infantile impulse, being defensive, having developmental defects, or resisting therapy. . . . Even therapists who reject the psychoanalytic model may nevertheless view clients as dependent, narcissistic, manipulative, . . . and refusing to face the responsibilities of adulthood. Therapists who conceptualize people in these ways may have a hard time making interpretations that do not communicate at least some element of this pejorative view. (p. 353)

Of course, most human beings (including therapists as well as patients!) do at times behave in a dependent, narcissistic, or manipulative manner. These deficiencies often precipitate the need for treatment in the first place. It is clearly important to deal with these difficulties, but this requires careful attention to timing along with infinite tact. When the patient is angry and the therapist is under attack, it is unwise to draw attention to the patient's deficiencies. This can be dealt with far more effectively when the patient feels relaxed and validated by the therapist. Even then, the therapist must use a tone of voice and language that conveys objectivity and support, rather than accusations.

At times disarming may not be indicated or helpful. Suppose that a female patient angrily wrongly accuses a male therapist of having a sexual attraction to her. An effective and ethical response might be, "I want to reassure you that I am here to help you, and not to have a personal or sexual relationship, which would be exceedingly abusive and unethical. Nevertheless, I realize that I must have said or done something that sounded unprofessional or hurtful. You seem to be saying that it is difficult for you to trust in me. Can you tell me more about this? I feel badly that I have upset you, and I'm extremely grateful that you're telling me how you feel." Notice that even though the therapist reassures the patient that the specific content of the criticism is not correct, he still disarms her lack of trust.

Thought and Feeling Empathy

The two types of empathy are called thought empathy and feeling empathy. Thought empathy is defined as repeating the patient's words so that the patient knows the therapist listened and received the message. The therapist can simply say, "It sounds like you're saying that . . . " (or another similar phrase) and then repeat the patient's words as exactly as possible. After paraphrasing the patient's words, the therapist can acknowledge what the patient is likely to be feeling, given what the patient said. This latter step is called feeling empathy.

Suppose a patient says, "I've been coming to see you for 18 months and I feel more depressed today than I've ever felt in my entire life." Using thought and feeling empathy, the therapist could say, "You say that you've been coming to sessions for 18 months and yet you feel more depressed today than ever. I can imagine you must be feeling frustrated and discouraged and maybe even angry with me. Are you?"

There are several benefits of thought and feeling empathy. The discipline of repeating the patient's statement verbatim forces the therapist to process the message correctly and gives the therapist a few moments to think about what to say next. Many therapists become so nervous and distracted by their own negative thoughts when confronted with angry patients that they lose track of the content of what the patient said. Then the therapist's subsequent response will reveal that he or she did not hear what the patient said. This irritates the patient and tensions escalate. In contrast, when therapists paraphrase accurately and acknowledge how the patient feels, the patient is often relieved because it is clear that the therapist is tuned in.

Feeling empathy can be difficult if the therapist does not identify with the patient's emotional reactions. Sometimes therapists can translate a patient's feelings into experiences that are more familiar.

For example, suppose a patient describes anger attacks in traffic when commuting to work, and the therapist rarely or never reacts this way. The patient's anger results from highly competitive, personalized cognitions such as, "He thinks he can get away with cutting in front of me. I'll show him a thing or two!" If the therapist points out that these cognitions are irrational and dysfunctional, it may intensify the anger. Many patients will defend their perceptions and feelings if they feel misunderstood. Rather, the therapist's empathic effort should consist of silently remembering anger that he or she has experienced in some other situation and acknowledging that people can, indeed, be aggressive and irritating.

Accurate empathy can also guide the therapist's choice of technical interventions. For example, there is a pronounced tendency for people to want to hold on to their anger. This is because anger frequently creates feelings of power and moral superiority. Noting these reactions from personal experience, the therapist may chose a motivational technique such as the Cost–Benefit Analysis (Burns, 1980, 1989) before attempting to challenge the angry patient's distorted cognitions. After listing the advantages and disadvantages of feeling angry, the patient may conclude that the advantages are greater. Then the therapist can point out that the anger does not seem to be a problem and ask whether there are other problems that patient may prefer to work on during the session. This intervention may paradoxically intensify the patient's desire to work on the anger.

Thought and feeling empathy seem straightforward but can be challenging because of a difficulty called "anger phobia" or "conflict phobia" (Burns, 1989). Some therapists feel threatened by conflict and may subtly avoid acknowledging or exploring the patient's anger. This phenomenon can be quite striking.

During a recent demonstration at a psychotherapy training center, the director of training volunteered for a role-play demonstration on how to empathize with an angry patient with borderline personality disorder. He was instructed to respond as empathically as possible, using the three listening techniques described above. He was advised that the patient would probably be furious and was strongly encouraged to acknowledge any angry feelings the patient might express.

Another staff member volunteered to play the role of the patient. She made a scathing attack, using four-letter words liberally. She called him a phony and criticized his lack of understanding.

When she finished, there was a long silence, and you could hear a pin drop as he struggled desperately to think of an adequate response. Finally, in a patronizing tone of voice he said, "You must be a *very lonely* person!"

In this exercise, the patient is allowed only one attack on the therapist, and the therapist is only allowed one response. Then the therapist's response is critiqued by the "patient" and by the colleagues who observed the demonstration.

The group pointed out that he had carefully avoided any acknowledgment of her anger, even though he was specifically instructed to do so. Instead of finding some truth in what she said, he had subtly blamed her for the therapeutic impasse by labeling her as "a lonely" (and therefore inadequate) person.

When therapists observe colleagues making such obvious mistakes during training sessions, they are surprised and convinced they would not make similar errors. Nevertheless, when they take their turns in the role of the therapist, they frequently make similar mistakes. Persistent practice, with numerous role reversals, is usually needed before therapists can relax and empathize effectively.

Inquiry

When therapists use the thought and feeling empathy techniques, it can be helpful to add an open-ended question at the end. For example, the therapist can say, "Am I reading you right?" or "Can you tell me a bit more about this?" This technique, inquiry, is the third listening skill. Therapists use gentle, probing questions to invite patients to share their thoughts and feelings. The idea is to encourage patients to open up and discuss their most negative feelings and perceptions. Inquiry also allows patients to validate or correct the therapist's perceptions of how they are thinking and feeling.

"I Feel" Statements

The first self-expression skill involves the use of "I feel" statements. Therapists can sometimes express their own feelings in an "I'm feeling x" format, where x refers to an emotion word such as "concerned," "frustrated," etc. An "I feel" statement is quite different from a "you statement." An "I feel" statement would be, "I'm feeling a bit frustrated." In contrast, a "you statement" would be, "*You're* being stubborn" or "*You're* making me angry." "You statements" sound accusational and will cause the other person to become defensive.

The use of "I feel" statements in therapy is controversial. Many therapists with a psychoanalytic orientation do not believe it is appropriate to express personal feelings during sessions. They often respond to a patient's criticisms with silence or may simply reflect what the patient is saying. The idea is that the therapist is not a real person but a blank screen who reflects other significant figures in the patient's life. The more the therapist reveals of him- or herself, the more this transference reaction is contaminated by what the therapist is really like.

Nevertheless, there are circumstances when the expression of feelings by therapists can be important. Several guidelines can help therapists decide whether the expression of feelings will be ethical or hurtful. The first rule is that the expression of feelings by a therapist should be done with respect for the patient, using tactful language rather than street language which sounds crude or offensive.

The second rule is that the purpose of the "I feel" statement should be to help the patient rather than to help the therapist. If the therapist were to confess to feelings of hopelessness or inadequacy in a dispirited tone of voice, this would be demoralizing to the patient.

The third rule is that the therapists should express their feelings with an attitude of self-esteem, and not in a self-demeaning or guilty manner. When in doubt, a consultation with a colleague can be quite helpful.

As noted previously, it is natural for therapists to feel frustrated or defensive from time to time during sessions. Many therapists are afraid to acknowledge these feelings, thinking it would be unprofessional. The therapist may feel ashamed or fear losing face in the eyes of the patient. The therapist may be thinking: "This patient is getting to me. I *shouldn't* feel upset. I *should* be more objective. What's wrong with me? I *must* appear confident and maintain control."

The therapist who censors him- or herself in this manner may rely on stock expressions picked up during training, such as "tell me more" or "have you had this difficulty in other relationships as well?" These responses will sound patronizing and usually irritate the patient. An assertive patient may become even more critical and point out that the therapist sounds phony and defensive.

How could the therapist respond under these circumstances? What would you say if a patient said this to you and you actually were feeling brittle and defensive?

You could disarm the patient and use an "I feel" statement along these lines: "You know, I *am* feeling a bit defensive and I realize that I sounded phony just now. I realize there's some truth in your criticisms, and I apologize for being so off track."

By admitting that he or she feels defensive, the therapist no longer appears phony. Therapeutic humility and respect for the patient frequently have a positive effect because the therapist creates a level playing field and the patient is no longer in a "one down" position. This will frequently increase the therapist's stature in the eyes of the patient.

As a caveat, this type of response, like all the techniques described, will fail if the therapist does not genuinely agree with the patient or if the patient sees the therapist's statement as a ploy. Even given the same words, the slightest change in a therapist's attitude or tone of voice can make a dramatic difference in how the therapist is perceived and experienced by the patient. Substantial training is frequently required before therapists can apply any of these techniques in a natural and effective manner.

Stroking

The second self-expression skill is called stroking. Stroking simply means that therapists should express respect for patients, even in the heat of battle. Many people have difficulties integrating anger with liking or respect and naturally expect that any conflict will inevitably end in punishment or rejection. If the therapist reassures the patient that the frank discussion of the patient's anger and distrust will enhance the relationship, this will make it easier for the patient to open up.

Stroking can be conveyed verbally or nonverbally. Sometimes a therapist's relaxed demeanor, warmth, and genuine interest in what the patient is saying naturally conveys an attitude of respect. It is always a pleasure to encounter the rare therapist with the natural gift of a compassionate interpersonal style.

Stroking sometimes needs to be explicitly spelled out with a statement like: "I can see you are feeling quite angry and misunderstood right now. I know it might be awkward to talk this out. Nevertheless, I believe we will end up with a much better sense of understanding and mutual respect. With that in mind, can you tell me more about how you've been thinking and feeling?" This statement reassures the patient that the therapist will not reject the patient or lose respect for the patient—no matter what the patient says—and that the therapist does not expect to be rejected, either. This message can soften the interaction and increase feelings of trust.

These five technique have been presented separately to facilitate learning. There is no simple formula for how to apply them, and the skillful therapist will integrate them in a wide variety of ways, depending on the needs of the situation. They can be viewed as the five keys on a musical instrument, and an infinite variety of melodies are possible. Although the mastery of these techniques requires considerable training and determination, the reward will usually be more profound, compassionate, and effective therapeutic style.

CONCLUSION

Nineteenth-century aesthetic philosophers emphasized the importance of intuition and subjective responses in understanding another person. This concept of empathy was subsequently incorporated into psychoanalytic therapy by Freud and has been accepted by nearly all psychodynamic theorists.

Although a therapist's subjective responses can sometimes enhance his or her understanding of the patient, there are two reasons to question this view of empathy. First, a therapist's emotional reactions can sometimes be quite idiosyncratic and may not always reflect what the patient is actually thinking and feeling. Second, empirical studies indicate that therapists' and patients' assessments of the therapeutic alliance are frequently not correlated and that only patients' perceptions of therapists' empathy are reliably associated with clinical improvement.

Although positive correlations between therapeutic empathy and clinical recovery have been reported by many previous investigators, the causal relationships between these variables remain controversial. A nearly insurmountable technical problem plaguing all previous researchers has been the "chicken versus the egg" question: Does therapeutic empathy actually lead to recovery, or do patients who recover feel more positively about their therapists? Ordinary least squares statistical techniques cannot be used to resolve this problem because of the possibility of reciprocal causality.

Recent studies which utilize structural equation modeling have indicated, for the first time, that the causal effects of therapeutic empathy on recovery appear to be large, even in a highly technical form of therapy such as CBT. In contrast, depression does not appreciably affect patients' perceptions of the therapeutic alliance. These findings indicate that therapeutic empathy is a two-edged sword. A warm and trusting therapeutic relationship can significantly enhance treatment and speed recovery, but an unsatisfactory therapeutic alliance may have a negative impact on a patient's self-esteem and delay recovery.

The session-by-session assessment of empathy can help therapists evaluate the quality of the therapeutic alliance and pinpoint therapeutic logjams more rapidly. Session-by-session testing can also help therapists assess the severity of other symptoms such as depression, anxiety, and satisfaction in intimate relationships so that clinical progress—or the lack of it—can be monitored more accurately.

Although some therapists resist these procedures, clinical experience indicates they are accepted by most patients and can be surprisingly helpful, in much the same way the use of a thermometer helps a physician monitor the course of the patient's fever. This emphasis on systematic measurement reflects the collaborative and empirical spirit that is so central to the cognitive model of therapy. Although most therapists see themselves as relatively objective and compassionate, they often respond to hostile, critical patients in a defensive, controlling, or subtly distancing manner. Empathy training can make therapists more aware of these reactions.

The training program is based on the idea that good therapy consists of technical and empathic interventions. Empathic interventions are needed whenever patients feel angry or distrustful toward the therapist or when they feel demoralized and overwhelmed with emotion. These technical and empathic interventions are based on significantly different paradigms and require different personal aptitudes. Many therapists seem stuck in one or the other mode and have difficulty integrating them.

Five listening and self-expression techniques can help therapists improve their interpersonal skills. Learning to implement these methods requires systematic training and persistent effort over a period of many months. The incorporation of these methods into training programs for cognitive behavioral therapists may provide novice and advanced practitioners with a broader range of interventions and a more compassionate and creative way of helping difficult patients. Further studies will be needed to determine whether these techniques, along with the session-by-session assessment procedures, can significantly increase therapeutic empathy and effectiveness.

REFERENCES

Basch, M. F. (1983). Empathic understanding: A review of the concept and some theoretical considerations. *Journal of the American Psychoanalytic Association, 31,* 101–126.

Beck, A. T., Rush, A. J., Shaw, B. F., & Emery, G. (1979). *Cognitive therapy of depression.* New York: Guilford Press.

Beck, A. T., Ward, C. H., Mendelson, M., Mock, J., & Erbaugh, J. (1961). An inventory for measuring depression. *Archives of General Psychiatry, 4,* 561–571.

Beck, A. T., Wright, F. D., Newman, C. F., & Liese, B. S. (1993). *Cognitive therapy of substance abuse.* New York: Guilford Press.

Bergin, A. (1990). *Common and specific factors in psychotherapy.* Paper presented at the annual meeting of the Society for the Exploration of Psychotherapy Integration, Philadelphia.

Book, H. E. (1988). Empathy: Misconceptions and misuses in psychotherapy. *American Journal of Psychiatry, 145*(4), 420–424.

Buie, D. H. (1981). Empathy: Its nature and limitations. *Journal of the American Psychoanalytic Association, 29,* 281–307.

Burns, D. D. (1980). *Feeling good: The new mood therapy.* New York: William Morrow. (Paperback edition published 1981 by New American Library)

Burns, D. D. (1989). *The feeling good handbook.* New York: William Morrow.

Burns, D. D., & Nolen-Hoeksema, S. (1991). Coping styles, homework assignments and the effectiveness of cognitive-behavioral therapy. *Journal of Consulting and Clinical Psychology, 59*(2), 305–311.

Burns, D. D., & Nolen-Hoeksema, S. (1992). Therapeutic empathy and recovery from depression in cognitive-behavioral therapy: A structural equation model. *Journal of Consulting and Clinical Psychology, 59*(2), 305–311.

Dobson, K. S. (1989). A meta-analysis of the efficacy of cognitive therapy for depression. *Journal of Consulting and Clinical Psychology, 57*(3), 414–419.

Elkin, I., Shea, T., Watkins, J. T., Imber, S. D., Sotsky, S. M., Collins, J. F., Glass, D. R., Pilkonis, P. A., Leber, W. R., Docherty, J. P., Fiester, S. J., & Parloff, M. B. (1989). National Institute of Mental Health treatment of depression collaborative research program: General effectiveness of treatments. *Archives of General Psychiatry, 46,* 971–982.

Ellis, A. (1962). *Reason and emotion in psychotherapy.* Secaucus, NJ: Citadel Press.

Frayn, D. H. (1990). Intersubjective processes in psychotherapy. *Canadian Journal of Psychiatry, 35,* 434–438.

Free, N. K., Green, B. L., Grace, M. D., Chernus, L. A., & Whitman, R. M. (1985). Empathy and outcome in brief, focal dynamic therapy. *American Journal of Psychiatry, 142,* 917–921.

Freud, S. (1964). The unconscious. In *Standard edition* (Vol. 14). London: Hogarth Press. (Original work published 1915)

Garfield, S. L. (1990). *Common and specific factors in psychotherapy: Association.* Paper presented at the annual meeting of the Society for the Exploration of Psychotherapy Integration, Philadelphia.

Gauss, C. E. (1973). Empathy. In P. P. Wiener (Ed.), *Dictionary of the history of ideas* (Vol. II, p. 85). New York: Scribner's.

Hanushek, E. A., & Jackson, J. E. (1977). *Statistical methods for social scientists.* Orlando, FL: Academic Press.

Henry, W. P., Schacht, T. E., & Strupp, H. (1990). Patient and therapist introject, interpersonal process, and differential outcome. *Journal of Consulting and Clinical Psychology, 58*(6), 768–774.

Kernberg, O. S. (1975). Transference and counter-transference in the treatment of borderline patients. *Journal of the National Association of Private Practice Psychiatric Hospitals, 7,* 14–24.

Luborsky, L., Crits-Christoph, P. Mintz, J., & Auerbach, A. (1988). *Who will benefit from psychotherapy? Predicting therapeutic outcomes.* New York: Basic Books.

Luborsky, L., McLellan, T., Woody, G., O'Brien, C., & Auerbach, A. (1985). Therapist success and its determinants. *Archives of General Psychiatry, 37,* 471–481.

Maultsby, M. C. (1971). Systematic, written homework in psychotherapy. *Psychotherapy: Theory, Research, and Practice, 8*(3), 195–198.

Orlinsky, D. E., Grawe, K., & Parks, B. K.. (1994). Process and outcome in psychotherapy—noch einmal. In A. E. Bergin & S. L. Garfield (Eds.), *Handbook of psychotherapy and behavior change* (4th ed., pp. 270–376). New York: Wiley.

Parloff, M. B., Waskow, I. E., & Wolfe, B. E. (1978). Research on therapist variables in relation to process and outcome. In S. L. Garfield & A. E. Bergin (Eds.), *Handbook of psychotherapy and behavior change* (2nd ed.) New York: Wiley.

Persons, J. B., & Burns, D. D. (1985). Mechanism of action of cognitive therapy: Relative contribution of technical and interpersonal intervention. *Cognitive Therapy and Research, 9*(5), 539–551.

Persons, J. B., Burns, D. D., & Perloff, J. M. (1988). Predictors of dropout and outcome for cognitive therapy for depression in a private practice setting. *Cognitive Therapy and Research, 12*(6), 557–575.

Raue, P., Castonguay, L., & Goldfried, M. (1993). The working alliance: A comparison of two therapies. *Psychotherapy Research, 3,* 197–207.

Rehm, L. P., Kaslow, N. J., & Rabin, A. S. (1987). Cognitive and behavioral targets in a self-control therapy program for depression. *Journal of Consulting and Clinical Psychology, 55*(1), 60–67.

Robinson, L. A., Berman, J. S., & Neimeyer, R. A. (1990). Psychotherapy for the treatment of depression: A comprehensive review of controlled outcome research. *Psychological Bulletin, 108,* 30–49.

Rogers, C. R. (1957). The necessary and sufficient conditions of therapeutic personality change. *Journal of Consulting Psychology, 21,* 95–103.

Safran, D. S., & Segal, Z. V. (1990). *Interpersonal process in cognitive therapy.* New York: Basic Books.

Salvio, M., Beutler, L., Wood, J., & Engle, D. (1992). The strength of the therapeutic alliance in three treatments for depression. *Psychotherapy Research, 2*(1), 31–36.

Shapiro, E. R. (1978). The psychodynamics and developmental psychology of the borderline patient: A review of the literature. *American Journal of Psychiatry, 135,* 1305–1315.

Spitzer, R. L., & Williams, J. B. (1983). *Structured Clinical Interview for DSM-III.* New York: Biometrics Research Department, New York State Psychiatric Institute.

Spitzer, R. L., & Williams, J. B., (1985). *Structured Clinical Interview for DSM-III— Personality Disorders (SCID-II).* New York: Biometrics Research Department, New York State Psychiatric Institute.

Squier, R. W. (1990). A model of empathic understanding and adherence to treatment regimens in practitioner–patient relationships. *Social Science and Medicine, 30*(3), 325–339.

Strupp, H. H. (1980a). Success and failure in time-limited psychotherapy. *Archives of General Psychiatry, 37,* 595–603.

Strupp, H. H. (1980b). Success and failure in time-limited psychotherapy: A systematic comparison of two cases—Comparison 4. *Archives of General Psychiatry, 37,* 947–954.

Thompson, L. W., Gallagher, D., & Breckenridge, J. S. (1987). Comparative effectiveness of psychotherapies for depressed elders. *Journal of Consulting and Clinical Psychology, 55*(3), 385–390.

Wile, D. B. (1984). Kohut, Kernberg, and accusatory interpretations. *Psychotherapy, 21,* 353–364.

Zeiss, A., Lewinsohn, P., & Munoz, R. (1979). Nonspecific improvement effects in depression using interpersonal skills training, pleasant activities schedules or cognitive training. *Journal of Consulting and Clinical Psychology, 47,* 427–439.

Chapter 8

Cognitive Therapy of Personality Disorders

Judith S. Beck

C ognitive therapy, as Aaron T. Beck, M.D., first conceived it, was primarily a short-term, problem-focused form of psychotherapy for the treatment of depression, although Beck also noted its application to anxiety (Beck, 1964, 1967). Since the 1960s, Beck and his colleagues worldwide have expanded cognitive therapy both conceptually and clinically. One notable expansion has been to the area of personality disorders (Beck, Freeman, & Associates, 1990). While many cognitive and cognitive-behavioral theorists have written about a cognitive approach to personality disorders (e.g., Linehan, 1993; Liotti, 1992; Safran & McMain, 1992), this chapter focuses on the theory and approach derived directly from Beck's work.

There has been little controlled research on the efficacy of cognitive therapy for personality disorders. Most of the research conducted to date has consisted of uncontrolled clinical reports, single-case design studies, and studies of the effects of personality disorders on treatment outcome. In general these studies indicate that cognitive therapy is a promising approach (Pretzer & Beck, 1996). Turkat and Maisto (1985) reviewed a number of single-case experimental design studies using individualized conceptualizations with specific treatment plans. In general, they found that the implementation of these individualized treatment plans was more effective than treatment that matched interventions to symptoms. Beck et al. (1990) conclude that "standard" cognitive therapy, utilized for straightforward cases of depression and anxiety, is often ineffective for personality disorder cases and that research is essential to test whether a more comprehensive approach, such as that outlined in the 1990 book by Beck and his colleagues, is efficacious for this difficult population.

Personality disorder patients, according to the fourth edition of the *Diagnostic and Statistical Manual of Mental Disorders* (DSM-IV; American Psychiatric Association, 1994), are characterized by "an enduring pattern of inner experience and behavior that deviates markedly from the expectations of the individual's culture, is pervasive and inflexible, has an onset in adolescence or early adulthood, is stable over time, and leads to distress or impairment" (p. 630). The pervasiveness, early onset, rigidity, chronicity, and enduring dysfunctionality help separate Axis II personality disorders from the usually more acute, episodic Axis I disorders. The inflexibility, dysfunctionality, and compulsive use of certain behavioral strategies distinguish the personality disorder patient from patients who also display "enduring patterns of perceiving, relating to, and thinking about the environment and oneself that are exhibited in a wide range of social and personal contexts" (American Psychiatric Association, 1994, p. 630) but whose personality traits are relatively more flexible and who can vary their behavior more adaptively, according to the situation.

Beck became interested in Axis II disorders when he recognized that a significant number of patients who had recovered from a major depression still experienced reduced but enduring or intermittent distress and continued to demonstrate faulty thinking and maladaptive behavior patterns (Beck, in press). Simultaneously, he began to explore the connection between evolutionary theory and psychiatric disorders. Mankind, he noted, has developed behavioral strategies to promote the primary evolutionary goals of survival and reproduction. The inflexible, maladaptive, compulsive use of these strategies in the current environment is one of the most salient characteristics of personality disorder patients.

DYSFUNCTIONAL STRATEGIES

Evolutionarily derived patterns of functioning include such behaviors or strategies as competitiveness, dependence, avoidance, resistance, suspiciousness, dramatics, control, aggression, isolation, and self-aggrandizement. Beck (in press) notes that the strategies "represent each individual's unique solutions to the problems of reconciling internal pressures for survival and bonding and external obstacles, threats and demands."

The healthy individual in our technologically advanced society flexibly employs many, if not all, of these strategies in adaptive ways, in specific circumstances. It is functional, for example, for an individual to be suspicious, vigilant, and on guard in a crime-ridden part of town. An individual whose task it is to persuade a group to adopt a certain viewpoint may need to be somewhat dramatic or theatrical. In a championship match it is to the individual's advantage to be highly competitive.

The personality disorder patient may display these same behaviors but tends consistently to overutilize a small set of strategies in an inflexible, compulsive way, when doing so is often distinctively disadvantageous. Unlike the individual with a healthier personality, he or she lacks the ability to assess particular situations realistically and select from a wide spectrum of strategies. For example, a paranoid patient may react quite suspiciously in interactions with people even when objective data and his own experience indicate they are most likely trustworthy. A histrionic patient may act in a highly unsuitable, dramatic fashion in a serious situation such as a formal job interview. A narcissistic patient may act in a self-aggrandizing, competitive manner when assigned to an egalitarian team at work.

Beck notes that not all individuals with a significantly skewed distribution of genetically influenced traits or strategies experience significant distress. Some seek an environment that accommodates their characteristic strategies. A dependent, help-seeking individual may select friends and mates who are strong, decisive caretakers. A suspicious, overly guarded individual may choose to live alone, in a rather anonymous fashion, and seek a job that requires little interaction with others. A compulsive, perfection-driven individual may create an environment that is highly structured and ordered. Note, too, that some individuals with inflexible strategies may not experience much subjective distress themselves but may inflict distress on others. Individuals who consistently act in a superior, entitled, demanding way often have disturbed relationships, for example, as do those who are manipulative, exploitive, and aggressive.

SCHEMAS AND BELIEF SYSTEMS

Early in their developmental period, children seek to make sense of themselves and their world. They develop schemas, or cognitive structures, to organize the massive amount of data they are constantly receiving. Schemas are the means by which they understand what they are experiencing and decide how to proceed. Beck drew on the works of Bartlett, Piaget, and Kelly in his elaborated conception of schemas (Weishaar, 1993).

The content of some schemas is often idiosyncratic for a given person. A schema relevant to policemen will elicit a positive response in one child, for example, or an anxious, contemptuous, or neutral reaction in others. Schemas "provide the instructions to guide the focus, direction, and qualities of daily life and special contingencies" (Beck et al., 1990, p. 4).

Schemas have various characteristics. At any given time a schema might be highly activated or completely dormant or somewhere in between. A schema can be relatively narrow or broad, rigid or modifiable, prominent or relatively quiescent. When highly activated, a schema influences how the individual is processing information. The hypervalence of one schema may inhibit the activation of contrary schemas that are more adaptive to the specific situation (Beck, 1967).

An avoidant patient, for example, may have a prepotent schema of threat or danger activated even when she is with nonjudgmental coworkers who are actively making supportive comments to her. A passive–aggressive patient with a schema relevant to vulnerability may inaccurately perceive his supervisor as trying to control him when the supervisor is actually trying to help.

According to Beck et al. (1990), there are in addition to cognitive schemas, affective, motivational, action (or instrumental), and control schemas. The avoidant patient who is describing his project to his coworkers has an activation of his cognitive schema (threat), his affective schema (anxiety), his motivational schema (desire to avoid), and his action schema (mobilization to deal with threat by fleeing).

Young (1990) elaborates on the characteristics and functioning of "early maladaptive schemas," or "extremely stable and enduring themes that develop during childhood and are elaborated upon throughout an individual's lifetime . . . [which are] templates for the processing of later experience" (p. 9). He notes that these schemas are accepted as a priori truths, self-perpetuating, difficult to change, significantly dysfunctional, activated by environmental events, and associated with high levels of affect. He describes three processes of schemas: schema maintenance (the individual processes information in such a way as to reinforce the schema), schema avoidance (the individual avoids thinking about situations that might trigger a schema, avoids negative feelings associated with a schema, or behaviorally avoids situations that might trigger a schema), and schema compensation (the individual consistently acts in a way opposite to what might be expected from their schemas).

Beck (1967) terms the content of cognitive schemas as "beliefs," which represent individuals' understanding of themselves, their world, and others. The healthy personality has stable, adaptive, relativistic basic or core beliefs ("I am a reasonably competent person; my world has some danger but is predominantly a safe enough place for me; other people may be beneficent, neutral, or malevolent toward me"). Personality disorder patients, in contrast, have extreme, negative, global, rigid beliefs ("I am incompetent; my world is out of my control; other people are untrustworthy"). When their schemas are activated, they apply these beliefs to situations that do not warrant such a negative view. They act and react as if their perceptions are accurate, despite sometimes strong evidence to the contrary. They develop a perceptual bias that interferes with reasonable and adaptive information processing.

One individual, for example, when presented with an intellectually challenging assignment at which he usually excels suddenly feels terrified because his beliefs "I am inadequate" and "Others will judge and criticize me" have been activated. Another person with a strongly activated belief such as "Others always take advantage of me" feels quite angry in this same situation. Thus individuals' schemas influence how they process information and which beliefs will guide their reactions. The personality disorder patient often selectively attends to, distorts, stores, and retrieves information in a dysfunctional way.

The rigidity and inflexibility of the personality disorder patient's beliefs and strategies can be understood by a lack of accommodation to new environmental input in a meaningful and useful manner. A histronic patient, for example, may fail to notice that she is often more appreciated when she interacts with others in a subtle, low-key way. An antisocial patient may believe others did not exploit him because they didn't have a clear opportunity to do so. A paranoid patient may recognize that another person did not treat her badly on a number of occasions but account for the lack of mistreatment to a hidden motive. People who have relatively healthier personalities are able to assimilate incoming information in a more appropriate way, adjust their schemas to match the reality of their worlds more accurately, and develop a wider range of behavior patterns that are relatively more adaptive and functional.

Beck (in press) proposes that core beliefs about the self are of central importance in conceptualizing personality disorder patients. He describes these negative beliefs as falling into two categories: those beliefs associated with helplessness (e.g., "I am helpless," "I am powerless," "I am inadequate," "I am not good enough [in achievement]," "I am weak," "I am vulnerable," "I am trapped") and those associated with unlovability (e.g., "I am unlovable," "I am unworthy," "I am defective," "I am undesirable," "I am not good enough [to be loved by others]"). These core beliefs are quite painful to patients and they develop strategies to help them cope with or prevent the activation of these distressing ideas.

These strategies are often expressed as rules (e.g., "I must not let others take advantage of me"), attitudes (e.g., "It would be terrible if others saw me as weak"), and conditional assumptions (e.g., "If others take advantage of me, then it means I'm a thoroughly weak person"). Patients may not articulate their core beliefs and assumptions until therapy when their therapist probes to uncover the underlying meaning of their current perceptions across situations. For the most part, dysfunctional beliefs are not difficult to identify and therapists build their conceptualizations based on patients' characteristic perceptions of, meanings attributed to, and reactions in a variety of problematic situations.

Each personality disorder has a specific set of beliefs and accompanying behavioral pattern (Beck et al., 1990). Dependent personality disorder patients, for example, believe that they are incompetent and unable to cope. Therefore, they tend to have overdeveloped strategies of relying on others and avoiding important decisions and challenges, but they are underdeveloped in autonomy and decisiveness. Avoidant personality disorder patients believe they are unlovable and vulnerable. They tend to avoid intimacy, criticism, and negative emotion and are thus underdeveloped in openness, assertion, and emotional tolerance. Obsessive–compulsive personality disorder patients believe that they are vulnerable to their world's falling apart and therefore overemphasize rules, responsibility, and control and are deficient in spontaneity, lightness, and flexibility. Borderline personality disorder patients share a number of extremely rigid, negative beliefs with other personality disorders (Layden, Newman, Freeman, & Morse, 1993) ("I am defective," "I am vulnerable," "I am out of control," "I can't cope," "I will be abandoned") leading to more extreme patterns of behavior.

Patients who suffer from an Axis I disorder without a comorbid Axis II disorder may also demonstrate extreme, negative beliefs. Depressed patients, for example, may view themselves as total failures or as completely unlovable. Patients with an anxiety disorder may believe "I am vulnerable." These beliefs, however, become activated only during the acute episode and become latent once the Axis I disorder remits, when their relatively more positive core beliefs once again predominate. Axis II patients, in contrast, describe themselves as "always feeling this way" about themselves, others, and their world, though the degree of belief may intensify during a concomitant Axis I episode. The development of such beliefs, according to Beck (in press), is partly genetically influenced but also significantly affected by childhood events.

DEVELOPMENT EXPERIENCE

Core beliefs originate as individuals develop and start to make sense of themselves, their personal world, and other people. Most healthy children are able to incorporate both positive and negative events and adopt a balanced, stable view of themselves and others. Personality disorder patients, on the other hand, usually had either subtly or dramatically traumatic childhoods, during which they began, accurately or inaccurately, to view themselves in a distinctively negative way. Some trauma is blatant: sexual, physical, verbal abuse. Other trauma is less acute but agonizingly chronic: highly critical parents, demeaning siblings or peers, overly harsh teachers or caretakers. Since not all children who experience early trauma develop personality disorders, however, Beck (in press) proposes that some individuals may be genetically predisposed to develop a more extreme personality disorder or may have lacked supportive figures who would have helped to buffer the childhood traumas.

As children begin to develop a negative core belief, based on their experiences, they begin to process information in a distorted way. They interpret negative events as broad, global confirmation for their negative core beliefs. Positive events are either unnoticed, and therefore unprocessed, or distorted so that the core belief is not undermined (J. S. Beck, 1995). For example, a child who believes he is inadequate may not recognize his increasing mastery of skills or challenges or may discount them ("Anyone can do this," "This [task] might not be hard for me, but most other things are"). The process of readily incorporating negatively perceived data and omitting or discounting positive data solidifies dysfunctional schemas in the individual's formative period. The specific beliefs and strategies that the child develops are, again, idiosyncratic to the individual.

One child with an alcoholic parent, for example, may view himself as unprotected, vulnerable, and helpless when the parent rages at the family during bouts of drinking, and these beliefs about himself may become more generalized and global. He may begin to believe "I am vulnerable" or "I am helpless" in a range of situations in which these judgments are wholly or at least partially invalid. Depending on certain biases in his genetic make-up, the child may develop strategies of overcontrol, and overresponsibility and may become overly rule-driven in order to cope in an environment he experiences as chaotic. Another child might become quite avoidant, blame himself for his parent's dysfunctional behavior, start to believe that he is defective, and distance himself from other people who he fears will also find him lacking. A third child with a relatively healthier sense of self may accurately perceive that she is not in acute danger and that it is her parent, rather than she herself, who has problems. This third child, who perhaps has better insight due to a better "genetic shuffle," develops a healthier personality without a skewed set of overdeveloped and underdeveloped strategies. Thus it is that children develop their own characteristic ways of perceiving and relating to their world.

REACTIONS TO CURRENT SITUATIONS

Personality disorder patients often have strong emotional reactions to current situations. Their underlying beliefs influence their perceptions and interpretations. These perceptions are often distorted, yet are accepted as true, and, in turn, influence patients' emotional, physiological, and behavioral reactions. Thus a narcissistic patient who believes "If people don't treat me in a special way, they are being unfair or unreasonable" may have automatic thoughts such as "How dare they treat me like this" and may become quite angry and belligerent when he is forced to wait for an appointment or denied a request. An obsessive–compulsive patient may become very upset if others create even minor disorder because of her belief, "Terrible things can happen if everything is not done in just the right way." Automatic thoughts such as "What if the work isn't good enough? What if it isn't finished in time? What if the project doesn't get approved?" in a work situation may lead to anxiety and to her spending an inordinate amount of time on relatively unimportant tasks.

In order to facilitate the modification of these dysfunctional reactions, it is important to conceptualize for patients the relationship between the activation of their core beliefs in specific current situations and their automatic thoughts, emotional response, and behavior. Figure 8.1 presents a Cognitive Conceptualization Diagram for Kim, a personality disorder patient described later in this chapter. Filling in this diagram with patients (based on data they present) helps them understand how their childhood experiences have led to the development of their dysfunctional beliefs and assumptions and maladaptive behavior patterns (J. S. Beck, 1995).

Pt's initials: ___K.___   **Therapist's name:** ___Judith Beck, PhD___

Pt's diagnosis: Axis I: _Panic disorder in remission_ **Axis II:** _Avoidant Personality Disorder_

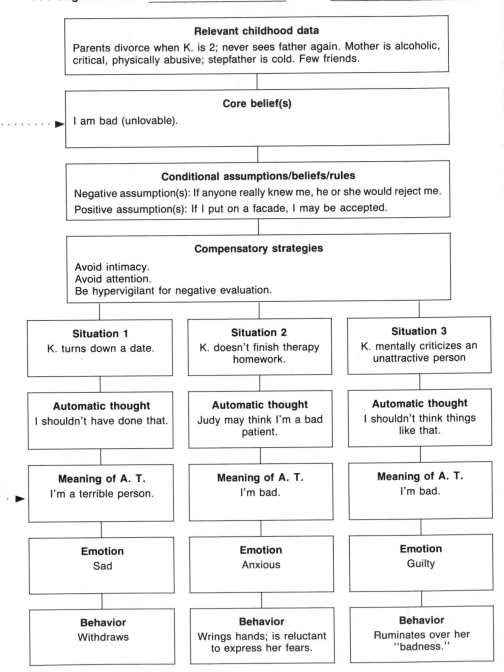

FIGURE 8.1. Cognitive Conceptualization Diagram. Copyright 1996 by Judith S. Beck, PhD. Reprinted by permission.

TREATMENT OF PERSONALITY DISORDER PATIENTS

The treatment of this difficult population shares some commonalties with cognitive therapy for Axis I depression and anxiety disorders. The therapist emphasizes collaboratively setting goals, solving problems, modifying dysfunctional thoughts and beliefs, changing dysfunctional behavior, and preventing relapse through teaching patients to be their own therapists. Treatment usually focuses first on the more acute Axis I diagnosis, if one is present. Collaborative empiricism and guided discovery are emphasized, though more persuasive techniques are often used in order to modify strongly held beliefs.

Several notable differences do exist, however, between Axis I and Axis II treatment. Perhaps of paramount importance is the establishment and maintenance of a sound therapeutic alliance (essential for all patients but often challenging for patients who characteristically exhibit disturbed relationships within and outside of therapy). Also, there is a much stronger focus on modifying core beliefs and assumptions, in addition to recognizing and responding to automatic thoughts. This additional emphasis requires a focus not only on the here and now (as therapists and patients analyze patients' distressed reactions to current situations both within and outside of therapy sessions) but also on the developmental origins of dysfunctional beliefs, through both "rational" and "emotional" or experiential methods. Modification of Axis II–related beliefs requires consistent work over a considerable period of time and treatment may continue for 9 months to 2 years or even longer for severely disordered patients. (See Beck et al., 1990, and Fleming & Pretzer, 1990, for additional guidelines in treating personality disorders.)

Case Example

Kim (see Figure 8.1) was an avoidant personality disorder patient in her mid-20s. She originally sought treatment for panic disorder and after 12 sessions this Axis I disorder fully remitted. However, she chose to remain in therapy to ameliorate some of her long-standing problems in relationships and work.

Kim had few friends and was not intimate with those she did have. She was hypersensitive to criticism from other people and consistently misread neutral or even slightly positive reactions from other people as negative. She was inhibited in social situations and tried to avoid drawing attention to herself. She avoided challenges at work even though she was competent and talented. Kim behaved in this dysfunctional manner in large part because of her strong core belief that she was bad and unlovable. She was certain that if people really got to know her, they would reject her because they would find out just how bad she really was. Although she appeared to others to be an attractive, well-groomed, articulate, intelligent, accomplished person, she believed almost completely that she was actually the opposite. She occasionally had images of "contaminating" innocent people with her badness by just being in their presence.

How did Kim develop such a distorted self-view? Kim's parents divorced when she was quite young and her mother continuously attributed the divorce to Kim's birth. Her mother was alcoholic, highly critical, and physically abusive. She may have had a borderline personality disorder herself. Her mother remarried when Kim was 10 and she and Kim's stepfather subsequently had two children whom they blatantly favored over Kim. Kim's stepfather was volatile and alcoholic and he, too, was quite verbally critical of Kim.

At a very early age Kim developed the idea that she must be bad and unlovable for her mother (and later her stepfather) to treat her so badly. She believed this negative idea so strongly that once she started school and was exposed to others, she began to withdraw from her classmates, neighborhood children, and most adults. She describes herself as having been a physically unattractive child who wore her hair in her face so that people couldn't really see her or get to know her. Her inhibition and withdrawal contributed to Kim's having few friends as she grew up. Her interpretation of lack of friends was that other children could see that she was bad and unlovable and therefore did not make overtures to her. Of course, a more likely explanation is that Kim did not present herself as a desirable or attractive person because her beliefs that she was bad and unlovable were so intense.

In addition to frequent physical abuse from her mother, Kim experienced many small traumas from her family on a daily basis. For example, whenever she received good grades her mother would say to her, "Don't think you're so smart. The teacher probably gave you good marks because you're well-behaved or you're quiet." When Kim won a statewide math competition, her mother characteristically remarked, "I hope you don't think too highly of yourself here. The judges probably gave you that award because they felt sorry for you." Kim's core belief, "I'm bad and unlovable," became stronger with each passing year. Although she did have occasional positive experiences (some teachers and a cousin treated her warmly), she did not interpret these events in a positive way. Instead, she discounted them, believing, "They only like me because they don't really know me well enough."

Kim's college years away from home were relatively better. With the diminishing influence of her family, she began to realize, to a limited degree at least, that other people did find her appealing. However, she once again interpreted this positive experience in a distorted way. "The reason they like me is because I put on a facade. If they really knew me, they would reject me."

Kim's personality disorder treatment had two major focuses. The first involved helping her solve problems, adaptively respond to her distorted thinking in current situations, learn new skills, and change her behavior. Second, toward the middle and end of therapy, her therapist strongly emphasized both testing Kim's assumption that if anyone really knew her she would be rejected and modifying her core belief of being bad and unlovable.

Kim will be used as an example to illustrate the following principles of treatment:

Establishing and Maintaining a Therapeutic Alliance

As mentioned above, the personality disorder patient brings the same negative assumptions about relationships outside of therapy to the therapy session itself. While this is an impediment in eliciting the full cooperation and trust of the patient, these problems within the session also provide an opportunity to conceptualize the patient's difficulties in relationships, to test the patient's assumptions about the therapist, and to learn new, more functional ways of relating to other people.

Kim, for example, was initially anxious in therapy because she assumed, "If my therapist really knew me, she would reject me." This assumption resulted in numerous automatic thoughts Kim had during the therapy session itself that interfered with her ability to relate important data to the therapist. She felt certain that if she revealed her problems (and especially her troubled history with her mother) the therapist would evaluate her negatively, verbally criticize her, and terminate the therapeutic relationship. Kim continually believed that she was on the brink of rejection.

Kim's anxiety within the therapy session allowed the therapist to conceptualize Kim's difficulties on the spot. First the therapist attempted to elicit Kim's automatic thoughts in the session. Fearful of the therapist's reaction, Kim replied that she couldn't relate what was going through her mind. The therapist did not push her to identify her cognitions but instead elicited her fears about revealing her thoughts. Kim was able to relate that she feared negative evaluation and rejection by the therapist. The therapist then helped her test that thought by examining supporting and disconfirmatory evidence, based on Kim's experience in prior therapy sessions. Through Socratic questioning, Kim realized that it was unlikely the therapist would judge her harshly and eject her from therapy.

After several sessions in which the therapist helped Kim realistically evaluate her fears of rejection, Kim's anxiety reduced and she was able to be more open. In small steps over several more sessions, Kim revealed her mother's abusiveness toward her when she was a child. The therapist anticipated that Kim might misread her reaction to these revelations and so encouraged Kim to question her directly. Kim's therapist then provided her honest reaction: She felt sad for Kim that she had undergone such trauma, she was sorry Kim had suffered, she was pleased that Kim had trusted her enough to confide in her, and she was also pleased because such information was vital for the therapist to be able to conceptualize Kim's present difficulties and plan her treatment. After several such interventions in which Kim discovered her fears about her therapist to be groundless, she was able to generalize what she had learned to other relationships. Over time Kim became less fearful of rejection by others, more willing to risk intimacy, and more successful in establishing and maintaining good, productive relationships.

Thus, establishing the therapeutic relationship poses both a challenge to therapists (when patients bring dysfunctional assumptions to therapy) and an opportunity for therapists to gain a "window" into the patients' reactions to other people. And monitoring their own emotional responses to patients' behavior also provides therapists with a window into how others may in turn be reacting to the patient.

Patients provide a variety of different challenges in therapy according to their dysfunctional beliefs and strategies. The narcissistic patient who has a belief "If others don't treat me in a special way, it means I'm nothing" may demand extra time with a therapist. The dependent patient who believes "If I rely on myself, I'll fail" may avoid tackling problems she can solve on her own. The passive–aggressive patient who believes "If I do what others want me to, it means they're controlling me" may fail to do homework assignments suggested by the therapist. The obsessive–compulsive personality disorder patient who believes "If my therapist doesn't understand me perfectly, I won't get helped" may insist on relating numerous unnecessary details. The histrionic patient who believes "If I'm not entertaining to my therapist, she won't like me or pay enough attention to me" may regale the therapist with amusing stories instead of focusing on her problems. Identifying and modifying these dysfunctional beliefs within the therapy relationship enables the patient to learn additional strategies to relate to others.

Modifying Underlying Assumptions and Beliefs

In general the therapist initially focuses on the patient's distressing automatic thoughts in specific current situations and teaches the patient how to identify thoughts and images and systematically evaluate them. Automatic thoughts are usually less rigid and global than beliefs and thus more easily modifiable. For example, Kim had little difficulty in evaluating and adaptively responding to her automatic thought, "It's terrible that I didn't pay my utilities bill." Modifying her global core belief "I'm a bad person," however, took months of sustained work with many types of interventions, as described below.

The use of a Cognitive Conceptualization Diagram (Figure 8.1) can aid the therapist in formulating a case and identifying the patient's core beliefs, underlying assumptions, compensatory strategies, and reactions to current situations (J. S. Beck, 1995). The therapist can fill in the diagram itself with a patient or verbally review its contents (without presenting the diagram) in several parts over several sessions. It is important for patients to understand their cognitive profile and how their core beliefs shape their interpretations of reality. By reviewing examples of their faulty information processing, the therapist shows patients how their negative core beliefs have become strengthened over time while positive, more realistic beliefs never developed or became attenuated. These explanations help patients comprehend why their beliefs can "feel" so true and yet be untrue or mostly untrue.

Having educated patients about their core beliefs, the therapist helps them identify advantages and disadvantages of modifying them. Through Socratic questioning the therapist fortifies each advantage and undermines each disadvantage. ("An advantage to seeing myself as an okay person is that I'll be more likely to initiate new relationships, improve the relationships I already have, speak my mind, be more interesting to people, have more fun, not feel like I'm always on the brink of rejection, not have to guard everything I say and do." "A disadvantage is that I'll feel anxious about questioning my sense of self but the anxiety will be time-limited, I'll most likely be able to tolerate it, and there may be a big payoff in seeing myself less negatively, more realistically.")

Initial interventions aimed at modifying core beliefs of personality disorder patients are present focused. A Core Belief Worksheet (Figure 8.2) allows the patient to recognize when she is processing information in a distorted way and thereby reinforcing a negative core belief. It aids the patient in reframing her negative interpretations and in attending to positive data that she might otherwise fail to recognize or discount. The worksheet also helps therapist and patient monitor over time the progress made toward attenuating the negative core belief and strengthening a new, more realistic belief (J. S. Beck, 1995).

Therapists must be creative to devise interventions that demonstrate the invalidity of patients' core beliefs. Extreme contrasts helped Kim carefully analyze how she differed from someone she considered to have even more of a negative quality than she herself had. Through Socratic questioning, for example, Kim compared herself to a public figure whom she viewed as a truly bad person and she recognized that she shared few attributes with him. A cognitive continuum, in which she ranked acts of "badness," helped her realize that she was not 100% bad for inadvertently misleading a coworker but rather only 1% bad. Her therapist helped her begin to judge her own and others' behavior by creating "yardsticks" of reasonable, borderline, and unreasonable behavior. Through guided questioning, Kim was able to provide examples of clearly unreasonable, mean-spirited responses to a man's request for a date and to judge that she herself had declined the date in a reasonable manner. This realization undermined her belief that she was bad for not accepting an invitation from a man she didn't like. Through evaluating others' behavior via a "yardstick," she began to recognize when they were acting unreasonably toward her. She stopped labeling herself as "bad," for example, when she resisted her housemate's unreasonable demands.

Behavioral experiments helped Kim test her assumptions. She believed that a friend would reject her if she proposed they see a movie different from

Name: Kim

Old core belief: I'm bad

How much do you believe the old core belief right now?	(0–100) __70%__
***What's the most you've believed it this week?**	(0–100) __95%__
***What's the least you have believed it this week?**	(0–100) __70%__

New belief: ____I'm okay_____

How much do you believe the new belief right now?	(0–100) __50%__

Evidence that contradicts old core belief and supports new belief	Evidence that supports old core belief with reframe
Jean asked me to have lunch with her.	I didn't want to go to the movies with my housemate *but* that doesn't mean I'm bad; it means I'm a normal person with reasonable preferences.
I took time to show (the new secretary) around the office.	I complained to Judy during therapy *but* she didn't consider it complaining and I'm supposed to bring up problems.
I called my sister and offered to help her move.	
(Boyfriend) invited me to a family wedding.	I told Norman that I was too busy to talk to him *but* he was really bugging me. I told him nicely, and okay people are appropriately assertive with others.

*Should situations related to an increase or decrease in the strength of the belief be topics for the agenda?

FIGURE 8.2. Core Belief Worksheet. Copyright 1996 by Judith S. Beck, PhD. Reprinted by permission.

his initial suggestion and that her boss would view her as critical and "uppity" if she made a constructive suggestion for improvement. After discussing and role-playing these situations, Kim approached her friend and her boss and discovered that they responded positively. "Acting as if" Kim believed a new, more functional belief (before she actually did) helped her modify her core belief and practice more functional behavior. Kim's therapist had her imagine in detail what she would do at a particular social gathering if she truly believed that she was an "okay" person whom others would like. Even though Kim did not yet hold this new belief strongly, she was nevertheless able to imagine herself acting more functionally and then actually did so at a party. Such behavioral change in many situations fortified the new, more adaptive belief. And as the new belief grew stronger, Kim found herself more and more easily able to "act as if."

The interventions described above are all present oriented. Personality disorder patients also benefit from a reexamination of the validity of their core belief from a developmental perspective. Kim and her therapist conducted a historical review (see Young, 1990) in which they examined her life in chunks of years (actually by school periods). Kim first recalled evidence that seemed to support her negative core belief for each time period. Then through Socratic questioning she identified evidence that contradicted the core belief and fortified the new, more functional belief. Next the therapist helped Kim to reframe each piece of negative data in a more adaptive way. Finally, Kim summarized this time period, more realistically assessing the validity of the core belief.

"Emotional" level interventions may be necessary for patients who develop an intellectual realization that their core beliefs are not valid but still "feel" them to be true. During rational/emotional role plays, Kim portrayed her "emotional" side that held a core belief strongly while her therapist played the "intellectual side" that recognized the core belief to be false or mostly false. Her therapist urged Kim to argue as strongly as she could so all of her "emotional" reasons could be voiced aloud. The therapist countered each emotional reason with a more realistic viewpoint, based on data Kim had provided in previous sessions. When Kim exhausted all her "emotional" reasons, they switched parts. Now the therapist expressed the same emotional reasons and Kim provided the more reasonable interpretations, having just heard these rational counters in the previous role play. Later in therapy Kim was encouraged to play both roles with the therapist intervening only when she was unable to produce an appropriate rational response.

Exercise

A final intervention for patients who still "feel" their core beliefs to be true even though they intellectually understand them to be invalid involves restructuring the meaning of earlier memories (J. S. Beck, 1995; Edwards, 1989). Kim's therapist had her vividly reexperience in imagination early traumas that contributed to the origination or maintenance of her core belief. When Kim related an intense activation of her core belief and intense emotion her therapist interviewed Kim's "younger self." The therapist helped Kim reinterpret the experience, by suggesting that another person or her "older self" enter the image immediately following the trauma and help the younger Kim understand an alternative explanation for what had just transpired. During several therapy sessions Kim vividly recalled her mother's physical abuse for imagined or minor infractions. Through her therapist's suggestions, she was able to imagine her older self comforting her younger self, explaining that the 5-year-old Kim was not bad but rather that her mother had serious problems of her own and so treated Kim badly. By eliciting and then responding to the younger Kim's doubts about the validity of such an interpretation, the younger Kim (actually the "emotional" part of Kim's mind) was able to change the meaning of these experiences.

CONCLUSION

Thus the treatment of personality disorder patients shares many commonalities with the treatment of the Axis I patient, especially the initial emphasis on solving here-and-now problems, learning to identify and modify dysfunctional thoughts in current situations, and behavioral change. A solid formulation of the case is critical in identifying the core beliefs, assumptions, and compensatory strategies in order for patients and therapist to understand the patients' reactions to current situations. A strong emphasis on modifying patients' assumptions and beliefs is necessary for patients to see themselves and others in a more realistic way, leading to more functional behavior, decreased reliance on just one or a few compensatory strategies, and greater ability to reach their goals.

When Aaron T. Beck conceived of cognitive therapy as a treatment for depression, he had little notion of its wide applicability to the range of Axis I disorders, much less characterological disorders. His elaboration of schemas, his application of evolutionary theory to individuals' current functioning, his notions of information processing, and his development of specific cognitive profiles for each of the personality disorders led to the development and refinement of an effective treatment for Axis II patients. This major accomplishment is, of course, but one of the extraordinary contributions Beck has made to the fields of psychiatry and psychotherapy.

REFERENCES

American Psychiatric Association. (1994). *Diagnostic and statistical manual of mental disorders* (4th ed.). Washington, DC: Author.

Beck, A. T. (1964). Thinking and depression: 2. Theory and therapy. *Archives of General Psychiatry, 10,* 561–571.

Beck, A. T. (1967). *Depression: Clinical, experimental, and theoretical aspects.* New York: Harper & Row.

Beck, A. T. (in press). Cognitive aspects of personality disorders and their relation to syndromal disorders: A psychoevolutionary approach. In C. R. Cloninger (Ed.), *Personality and psychopathology.* Washington, DC: American Psychiatric Press.

Beck, A. T., Freeman, A., & Associates. (1990). *Cognitive therapy of personality disorders.* New York: Guilford Press.

Beck, J. S. (1995). *Cognitive therapy: Basics and beyond.* New York: Guilford Press.

Edwards, D. J. A. (1989). Cognitive restructuring through guided imagery: Lessons from Gestalt therapy. In A. Freeman, K. M. Simon, L. E. Beutler, & H. Arkowitz (Eds.), *Comprehensive handbook of cognitive therapy* (pp. 283–297). New York: Plenum.

Fleming, B., & Pretzer, J. (1990). Cognitive-behavioral approaches to personality disorders. In M. Hersen, R. Eisler, & P. Miller (Eds.), *Progress in behavior modification* (Vol. 25, pp. 119–151). Newbury Park, CA: Sage.

Layden, M., Newman, C., Freeman, A., & Morse, S. (1993). *Cognitive therapy of borderline personality disorder.* Boston: Allyn & Bacon.

Linehan, M. M. (1993). *Cognitive-behavioral treatment of borderline personality disorder.* New York: Guilford Press.

Liotti, G. (1992). Egocentrism and the cognitive psychotherapy of personality disorders. *Journal of Cognitive Psychotherapy: An International Quarterly, 6,* 43–58.

Pretzer, J. L., & Beck, A. T. (1996). A cognitive theory of personality disorders. In J. F. Clarkin & M. F. Lenzenweger (Eds.), *Major theories of personality disorder.* New York: Guilford Press.

Safran, J., & McMain, S. (1992). A cognitive-interpersonal approach to the treatment of personality disorders. *Journal of Cognitive Psychotherapy: An International Quarterly, 6,* 59–68.

Turkat, I. D., & Maisto, S. A. (1985). Personality disorders: Application of the experimental method to the formulation and modification of personality disorders. In D. H. Barlow (Ed.), *Clinical handbook of psychological disorders: A step-by-step treatment manual* (pp. 503–570). New York: Guilford Press.

Weishaar, M. E. (1993). *Aaron T. Beck: Key figures in counseling and psychotherapy.* Thousand Oaks, CA: Sage.

Young, J. (1990). *Cognitive therapy for personality disorders: A schema-focused approach.* Sarasota, FL: Professional Resource Exchange.

Chapter 9

Schema-Focused Therapy

Lata K. McGinn
Jeffrey E. Young

R ecent trends in cognitive therapy, such as a growing interest in examining the core structures and processes that facilitate or inhibit personal growth and change (Mahoney, 1993), have led to the development of new paradigms for treating patients with character pathology. As
cognitive therapists began to move from treating Axis I disorders like depression to more chronic, characterological problems,[1] some limitations of
Beck's early model of cognitive therapy, developed for acute states of depression (Beck, Rush, Shaw, & Emery, 1979) became apparent. Influenced by
the constructivist movement (Mahoney, 1993), Young (1994a) has proposed
an integrative model called *schema-focused therapy,* designed to extend Beck's
original model of cognitive therapy and to specifically address the needs
of patients with long-standing characterological disorders.

The chapter elucidates both the theoretical postulates and practical applications of schema-focused therapy. However, the historical antecedents
to schema-focused therapy, principally Beck's earlier model of cognitive therapy and the work of the constructivists, will first be elaborated to illustrate
their influence on the development of the schema-focused model.

HISTORICAL ROOTS OF SCHEMA-FOCUSED THERAPY

Beck's Cognitive Therapy

Beck's cognitive therapy traditionally focuses on distorted patterns of thinking. In order to understand why patients experience distressing emotional
states or engage in dysfunctional behaviors, the cognitive therapist tries to
understand how they interpret events in their lives. If the therapist can help
patients to change these interpretations, which take the form of distorted
thoughts and images, then the accompanying maladaptive emotional states
and behaviors will usually improve as well.

Cognitive therapy developed as a movement away from both the theoretical and practical limitations of classical psychoanalysis and the restrictive nature of radical behaviorism (Dobson, 1988). By the 1970s a number of distinct cognitive therapies had evolved, including those of Beck (1976) and Ellis (1962). Beck's cognitive therapy stemmed directly from his efforts to test Freud's theory that at the core of depression is anger turned on the self. Through examining the thoughts and dreams of depressed patients, Beck repeatedly observed feelings of defeat, along with a consistent bias toward negativity, rather than themes of internalized anger as would have been predicted by Freud's theory. On the basis of studies like these, Beck concluded that depression was characterized by a consistent bias toward negative interpretations of the self, the environment, and the future. This eventually developed into his more general cognitive theory of emotional disorders which stated that shifts in information processing are central to psychopathology. Emotions were explained as the result of ongoing cognitive appraisals—negative emotions and the distorted appraisals from which they resulted became the focus of the cognitive model.

In further contrast to the psychoanalytic model, which assumes we are driven by unconscious motives and impulses, and to the behavioral tradition, which assumes we are governed by external contingencies, Beck proposed that dysfunctional thoughts, which could readily be brought into conscious awareness, are responsible for a great deal of emotional dysfunction.

While Beck did not dispute the central psychoanalytic claim of unconscious determinants of behavior, he challenged the notion of active repression. According to Beck, core assumptions about the self and the world, formed in early childhood, remain unconscious because of the same normal, nonpathological mechanisms by which other habits of thinking and behaving become automatic.

This led Beck to very different therapeutic procedures from psychoanalysis. He trained patients to increase awareness of their ongoing "stream of consciousness," exposing the rigid, automatic thoughts that preceded their characteristic emotional responses. Beck then taught patients procedures for utilizing reason to combat these dysfunctional "automatic thoughts." He advocated active dialogue with patients, rather than passive listening, through which he trained patients to develop empirical, reality-based arguments to combat distortions in their thinking.

By training patients to process information in a more accurate and reasonable fashion, patients learned to gain distance from their depressive feelings and their symptoms gradually improved. Because the therapist and patient work together as a team, systematically testing the validity of the patient's thoughts and beliefs, the working style of cognitive therapy was called "collaborative empiricism." From the beginning, cognitive therapy was present-oriented, time limited, structured, and educative. The therapist was active, directive, and problem focused.

Through Beck's emphasis on scientific outcome studies to test its efficacy, cognitive therapy became one of the most widely researched psychotherapies. Most of the early research conducted on depressed outpatients demonstrated that cognitive therapy is as effective as pharmacotherapy in reducing acute symptomatology, and there is promising evidence that it may be superior to pharmacotherapy and nonbehavioral psychotherapies in preventing relapse (Dobson, 1989). Growing evidence indicates that cognitive therapy is also effective for anxiety and other disorders, but questions of process and outcome are still being actively researched (Beckham & Watkins, 1989; Robins & Hayes, 1993).

The clinical impact of the cognitive movement has been enormous. However, the hope of a single, integrated paradigm has not been realized. Instead a multitude of theoretical and practical formulations that all claim to be cognitive therapy have been developed. By 1990, more than 20 different types of cognitive therapy had been identified (Haaga & Davison, 1991).

The Constructivist Movement

As cognitive therapists began to focus on personality disorders and other chronic disorders, many of the limitations of Beck's original model as applied to this subgroup of patients became apparent. Young (1994a) proposed that, for patients to succeed with Beck's original model, several conditions had to be met: that patients have ready access to their feelings and thoughts, that patients have identifiable life problems to focus on, that they are motivated and able to do homework assignments, that they can engage in a collaborative relationship with the therapist, and that their cognitions are flexible enough to be modified using established cognitive behavioral procedures. Unfortunately, patients with personality disorders often violate these conditions, and, to the extent that patients cannot meet these conditions, Young suggested that Beck's earlier model would fail unless the approach was significantly altered to address these limitations.

Several developments in psychology also challenged many of the core assumptions and intervention strategies of mainstream cognitive therapy (Mahoney, 1993). These included new research findings on the nature of emotions; the incorporation of experiential techniques into clinical practice; the study of unconscious processes in cognitive psychology; an increasing focus on self-organizing and self-protective processes in life span and personality development; and the acknowledgment of social, biological, and embodiment processes in therapy. As a result of these recent developments, the constructivist movement in the cognitive sciences was born.

Constructivists reject a "correspondence theory" of truth, the idea that thoughts and beliefs should bear a direct correspondence to external reality, as well as the corollary assumption that beliefs that fail to correspond to objective reality are dysfunctional. Instead, they hold that the viability of any given construction is a function of its consequences for the individual who adopts it. Human systems are characterized by self-organizing dynamics and evolve in such a way as to protect their internal coherence. Human cognition is seen as proactive and anticipatory rather than passive and determined. As a consequence, constructivist therapists tend to target changes in broader systems of personal constructs, rather than disputing circumscribed thought units (Neimeyer, 1993). Because these belief systems and personal accounts are seen as having enduring continuity over time, developmental dimensions of the patient's psychopathology are emphasized, with particular attention given to primary attachment relationships.

The goal of constructivist therapies is creative rather than corrective and interventions are likely to be elaborative, reflective, and intensely personal rather than persuasive, analytic, or technically instructive. There is a focus on the personal meanings that form the subtext of the patients' statements, so metaphor and idiosyncratic imagery are used extensively. Emotions are viewed as informative, in that they reflect the nature of the patients' attempts to construct meaning out of their experiences. Likewise, resistance is seen as a form of self-protection at points in therapy when the therapist threatens the patients' core ordering processes.

DEVELOPMENT OF SCHEMA-FOCUSED THERAPY

Characterological Problems: Why Modification of Cognitive Therapy Is Necessary

The schema-focused approach was formulated specifically to address the needs of patients with long-standing characterological disorders. According to Young (1994a), patients with characterological problems have several unique psychological characteristics that distinguish them from straightforward Axis I cases and make them unsuitable candidates for standard cognitive therapy alone.

Diffuse Presentation

Patients with characterological problems often do not have readily identifiable problems that can become the focus of treatment. These patients often present with vague, ill-defined complaints without specific triggers, yet exhibit significant disturbance in personal adjustment over time. Because no specific target problems can be identified, standard techniques used in cognitive therapy require modification.

Interpersonal Problems

In traditional cognitive therapy, patients are expected to engage in a collaborative relationship with the therapist within a few sessions. This often presents a formidable challenge for these patients, who typically have long-standing dysfunctional interpersonal relationships. In fact, interpersonal difficulties are emphasized in the DSM-IV definitions of personality disorders (American Psychiatric Association, 1994) and are often the core problem for many of these patients. Some patients often find it difficult to engage in a therapeutic relationship while others may become overly reliant on their therapist. If these interpersonal difficulties are viewed as a barrier to the real tasks of therapy, then the core problem is often missed. Unfortunately, the early model of cognitive therapy does not offer sufficient guidelines for addressing problems within the therapeutic relationship.

Rigidity

In traditional cognitive therapy, patients are taught to observe distortions in their thinking and, with reasonable practice and rehearsal, are expected to challenge and modify their cognitive and behavioral patterns. Patients are assumed to have a certain flexibility that enables them to modify their thoughts and behaviors through empirical analysis, logical discourse, experimentation, gradual steps, and practice.

However, since one of the hallmarks of personality disorders is the presence of rigid, inflexible traits, standard cognitive therapy techniques alone often meet with limited or no success with these patients. Patients with personality disorders typically display entrenched patterns of thinking and behaving that may not yield to months of therapeutic work. Even patients who are able to acknowledge their maladaptive thoughts or actions still maintain a sense of hopelessness about ever changing their core feelings, behaviors, and beliefs.

Avoidance

In traditional cognitive therapy, patients are presumed to have relatively free access to their thoughts and feelings. However, since patients with characterological problems chronically block or avoid painful feelings (affective avoidance; see Young, 1994a) and thoughts (cognitive avoidance), standard techniques utilized in cognitive therapy are often unsuccessful in gaining access to their thoughts and feelings. Young hypothesized that this chronic avoidance develops as a result of aversive conditioning—anxiety and depression become conditioned to memories and cognitions, leading to avoidance.

Although patients with uncomplicated Axis I disorders also exhibit avoidance (e.g., patients with panic disorder who avoid looking at their catastrophic thoughts or avoid going to places where they fear an attack will occur), they have relatively free access to their thoughts and feelings. That is, with sufficient training these patients are generally able to access their automatic thoughts and thus challenge and modify their thoughts and behaviors.

Differences between Schema-Focused Therapy and Cognitive Therapy

Schema-focused therapy integrates cognitive, behavioral, experiential, and interpersonal techniques, utilizing the concept of a "schema" as the unifying element. It adapts techniques used in traditional cognitive therapy but goes beyond the short-term approach by combining interpersonal and experiential techniques within a cognitive-behavioral framework.

Compared to traditional cognitive therapy, the schema-focused model involves greater use of the therapeutic relationship as a vehicle for change and more extensive discussion of early life experiences and childhood origins of problems. There is also more emphasis on affective experience (e.g., imagery, role-playing), and, as a result, the level of affect is much higher in schema-focused sessions. The schema-focused approach relies less on guided discovery and instead advocates more active confrontation of cognitive and behavioral patterns. And finally, because patients with personality disorders exhibit far more resistance to change than patients with uncomplicated Axis I conditions, the course of treatment is often longer in schema-focused therapy.

SCHEMA-FOCUSED MODEL: THEORETICAL FRAMEWORK

The schema-focused model is not intended as a comprehensive theory of psychopathology but rather as a working theory to integrate and guide the clinical interventions with patients who present with character disorders. Four main constructs are proposed: early maladaptive schemas, schema domains, schema processes, and schema modes. Some of these constructs represent an extension of the short-term cognitive model proposed by Beck and his colleagues (1979), while others represent new constructs based on our growing work within this model.

Early Maladaptive Schemas

Central to Young's model of therapy (1994a) is the concept of schemas. Schemas have been previously defined as "organized elements of past reactions and experience that form a relatively cohesive and persistent body of knowledge capable of guiding subsequent perception and appraisals." (Segal, 1988, p. 147). In fact, the importance of schemas was noted by Beck (1967) in some of his earliest work on depression where he noted that "a schema is a (cognitive) structure for screening, coding, and evaluating the stimuli that impinge on the organism. . . . On the basis of the matrix of schemas, the individual is able to orient himself in relation to time and space and to categorize and interpret experiences in a meaningful way" (p. 283).

Rather than present a competing theory of schemas, Young (1994a) proposes a subset of schemas called the "early maladaptive schema." In contrast to short-term cognitive therapy which focuses primarily on two levels of cognitive phenomena—automatic thoughts and underlying assumptions—the schema-focused approach proposes a primary emphasis on this deepest level of cognition, the early maladaptive schema (the term "schemas" will be used to refer to "early maladaptive schemas" in the present chapter).

The schema-focused model defines schemas as broad, pervasive themes regarding oneself and one's relationship with others, developed during childhood and elaborated throughout one's lifetime, which are dysfunctional to a significant degree (Young, 1994a). For example, children who receive no nurturance, empathy, or protection from their parents may develop the Emotional Deprivation schema. As adults, such individuals may hold exaggerated beliefs that they are not being cared for and understood by others, may feel lonely and empty, and may behave by becoming overly reliant on others.

Several defining characteristics of schemas are noted. Schemas are essentially implicit, unconditional themes held by individuals. They are perceived to be irrefutable and are taken for granted. Schemas serve as a template to process later experiences and, as a result, become elaborated throughout life and define an individual's behaviors, thoughts, feelings, and relationships with other people. In contrast to underlying assumptions, schemas are usually unconditional and, therefore, far more rigid.

Schemas develop as the result of ongoing, dysfunctional experiences with parents, siblings, and peers during childhood and develop as children attempt to make sense of their experiences and to avoid further pain. Essentially, schemas are usually valid representations of the noxious experiences during childhood.

However, schemas eventually become elaborated over time into deeply entrenched patterns of distorted thinking and dysfunctional behaviors. They become self-perpetuating and, therefore, are extremely resistant to change. Because schemas develop early in life, they become comfortable and familiar and are often central to people's self-concept and their conception of an environment. Even when presented with evidence that refutes the schema, individuals persistently distort information to maintain the validity of the schema. For example, an adult with the Defectiveness schema may continue to feel flawed and defective despite being told repeatedly that she is lovable. The threat of schematic change is too disruptive to the core cognitive organization and hence a variety of cognitive and behavioral maneuvers (schema processes, outlined below) reinforce the schema.

Schemas are usually activated throughout life by events in the environment relevant to the particular schema. For example, an individual's Abandonment schema may be triggered if his wife goes out of town to attend a business meeting. When triggered, schemas generate high levels of affect in the individual and lead directly or indirectly to a variety of psychological problems such as depression or panic; feelings of loneliness or destructive relationships; inadequate work performance; addictions like alcohol, drugs, or overeating; or psychosomatic disorders like ulcers or insomnia.

By definition, schemas are significantly dysfunctional. They interfere with one's ability to satisfy basic needs for stability and connection, autonomy, desirability, and self-expression, and with one's ability to accept reasonable limits and boundaries in relationships with others.

Schema Domains and Developmental Origins

Young has developed 18 schemas and has outlined specific cognitive, behavioral, experiential, and interpersonal strategies for each one (Bricker, Young, & Flanagan, 1993; Young, 1994a). Each of the schemas is grouped within five domains or broad categories, and each of the five domains is believed to interfere with a core need in childhood. This listing is tentative and constantly open to modification and elaboration based on our growing work within this model. Recent studies generally confirm the factor structure of the Young Schema Questionnaire (2nd edition), a self-report questionnaire derived through clinical experience and designed to assess the early maladaptive schemas (Schmidt, 1994; Schmidt, Joiner, Young, & Telch, 1995; Young & Brown, 1994).

In the following section, we will provide a description of each schema domain. A list of the 18 schemas is presented in the Appendix.

Disconnection and Rejection

Patients with these schemas expect that their need for security, safety, stability, nurturance, empathy, sharing of feelings, acceptance, and respect will not be met in a constant or predictable manner. Schemas in this domain (Abandonment/Instability, Mistrust/Abuse, Emotional Deprivation, Defectiveness/Shame, and Social Isolation/Alienation) typically result from early experiences of a detached, cold, rejecting, withholding, lonely, explosive, unpredictable, or abusive family environment.

Impaired Autonomy and Performance

Essentially, patients with these schemas (Dependence/Incompetence, Vulnerability to Danger [Random Events], Enmeshment/Undeveloped Self, and Failure) have certain expectations about themselves and the environment that interfere with their perceived ability to separate, survive, function independently, or perform successfully. The typical family origin is enmeshed, undermining of the child's confidence, or overprotective, or there is a failure to reinforce the child for performing competently outside the family.

Impaired Limits

Schemas within this domain (Entitlement/Grandiosity, Insufficient Self-Control/Self-Discipline) pertain to deficiency in internal limits, responsibility to others, or long-term goal orientation. These schemas lead to difficulty respecting the rights of others, cooperating with others, making commitments, or setting and meeting realistic personal goals. Patients with these schemas typically have families characterized by permissiveness, indulgence, lack of direction, or a sense of superiority, rather than appropriate confrontation, discipline, and limits in relation to taking responsibility, cooperating in a reciprocal manner, and setting goals. In some cases, the child may not have been pushed to tolerate normal levels of discomfort or may not have been given adequate supervision, direction, or guidance.

Other-Directedness

Within this domain, there is an excessive focus on the desires, feelings, and responses of others, at the expense of one's own needs, in order to gain love and approval, maintain one's sense of connection, avoid retaliation, or alleviate the pain of others. Patients with these schemas (Subjugation, Self-Sacrifice, Approval-Seeking/Recognition-Seeking) usually suppress and lack awareness regarding their own anger and natural inclinations. Typical family origin for these patients is based on conditional acceptance, where children must suppress important aspect of themselves in order to gain love, attention, and approval. In many such families, the parents' emotional needs and desires, or social acceptance and status, are valued more than the unique needs and feelings of each child.

Overvigilance and Inhibition

Schemas within this domain include Negativity/Vulnerability to Error (Controllable Events), Overcontrol/Emotional Inhibition, Unrelenting Standards/Hypercriticalness, and Punitiveness. Within this domain, there is an excessive emphasis on controlling one's spontaneous feelings, impulses, and choices in order to avoid making mistakes *or* on meeting rigid, internalized rules and expectations about performance and ethical behavior, often at the expense of happiness, self-expression, relaxation, close relationships, or health. Typical family origin is grim (and sometimes punitive): performance, duty, perfectionism, and following rules and avoiding mistakes predominate over pleasure, joy, and relaxation. There is usually an undercurrent of pessimism and worry that things could fall apart if one fails to be vigilant and careful at all times.

Schema Processes

As stated earlier, when the threat of schematic change is too disruptive to the core cognitive organization of the self, the individual engages in a variety of cognitive and behavioral maneuvers or schema processes to maintain the validity of the schema. Three schema processes are proposed: maintenance, avoidance, and compensation. These processes (which were adaptive in childhood and which overlap with the psychoanalytic concepts of resistance and defense mechanisms) later become maladaptive styles of coping used by the individual that are activated by and, in turn, reinforce the schemas.

Schema Maintenance

Schema maintenance refers to cognitive distortions and maladaptive behavior patterns that directly reinforce or perpetuate a schema (e.g., exaggerating information that confirms the schema, engaging in behaviors that are consistent with the schema). For example, an individual with the Defectiveness schema may tolerate critical friends because she perceives herself as defective.

Schema Avoidance

Schema avoidance refers to the cognitive, behavioral, or emotional strategies by which the individual attempts to avoid triggering a schema and the related intense affect (e.g., distracting oneself from thinking about schema-related issues or avoiding situations likely to trigger the schema). For example, a patient with the Failure schema may avoid working on his project because he believes that it will be poorly evaluated. By doing so, he makes it likely that he will obtain a negative evaluation, thus further reinforcing the schema (self-fulfilling prophecy).

Schema Compensation

Schema compensation refers to behaviors or cognitions that overcompensate for a schema; they appear to be the opposite of what one would expect from a knowledge of their early schemas. Schema compensations represent early functional attempts by the child to redress and cope with the pain of early mistreatment by parents, siblings, or peers. However, when extended into adulthood, schema compensations often become too extreme to be functional in a healthier environment and thus overshoot the mark. Overcompensations ultimately backfire and serve to maintain the schema. For example, an individual with the Emotional Deprivation schema who demands excessive amounts of attention may, in fact, alienate others and ultimately feel even more deprived.

Schema Modes

Although several schemas may underlie an individual's behaviors, thoughts, feelings, and relationships with other people, all the schemas may not be active at the same time. In fact, some schemas may be triggered while others remain dormant. A schema mode represents a group of schemas that are *currently active* for a particular individual. Young defines a schema mode as "a facet of the self, involving a natural grouping of schemas and schema processes, that has not been fully integrated with other facets" (Young & Flanagan, in press). As an individual shifts into another schema mode, a different group of schemas, previously dormant, now become active.

Severe characterological patients, such as patients with borderline personality disorder, abruptly flip from one mode to another, primarily in response to environmental circumstances or life events. These schema modes or facets of the self are more or less cut off from each other and patients may display different cognitions, behaviors, and emotions in each mode.

For example, patients with a narcissistic personality disorder may often flip between three modes, the Self-Aggrandizer, the Lonely Child, and the Detached Self-Soother. Many narcissists spend a majority of their time in the Self-Aggrandizer mode, which comprises the Entitlement, Approval-Seeking, Unrelenting Standards, and Mistrust schemas. Narcissists in this mode act superior, status-oriented, entitled, and critical of others, showing little empathy. They may flip to the Lonely Child mode (comprising the schemas of Defectiveness, Emotional Deprivation, and Subjugation) if they are cut off from sources of approval and validation, for example, when they receive negative feedback or criticism. In this mode, these individuals acutely experience the loss of special status and feel devalued. Finally, to escape the pain of being average and devalued, narcissists either flip back into the Self-Aggrandizer or, failing attempts to regain approval and validation, they switch into the third mode, the Detached Self-Soother. This mode is a form of schema avoidance: its purpose is to distract or numb themselves to the pain of the Emotional Deprivation and Defectiveness schemas. Self-soothing can take many forms, including drug and alcohol abuse, compulsive sexual activity, stimulation seeking (e.g., high-stakes gambling or investing), overeating, fantasies of grandiosity, and workaholism.

Patients with a borderline personality disorder may switch between four modes: the Detached Protector, Angry Child, Abandoned Child, and Punitive Parent. The Detached Protector is the default mode for most of these patients and serves to detach them from people and from experiencing emotions. Patients with borderline personality disorder usually experience a sense of depersonalization, emptiness, or boredom and may appear excessively obedient or compliant. Substance abuse, bingeing, self-mutilation, and psychosomatic complaints are characteristic of this mode. Such patients may flip to the Abandoned Child mode when they feel overwhelmed by threats of harm or abandonment. They characteristically experience intense depression, hopelessness, fear, worthlessness, unlovability, victimization, and intense neediness while in this mode. As a result, they may engage in frantic efforts to avoid abandonment and may even attempt suicide. A shift to the Punitive Parent mode occurs when patients with borderline personality disorder believe that they may have done something wrong, for example, having some "inappropriate" feelings, such as anger. They begin to experience self-hatred and self-directed anger and tend to punish themselves harshly for making mistakes. For example, they may deny themselves pleasures, may become self-critical, and, in severe cases, may even cut or mutilate themselves.

The Detached Protector and Abandoned Child modes create tremendous anger in patients with borderline personality disorder because they involve the suppression of intense needs and feelings. When the anger builds up and can no longer be contained, often due to an event perceived as the last straw, these individuals flip to the Angry Child mode. In this mode, their previously pent-up emotions become unleashed, and they often become enraged, demanding, devaluing, manipulative, controlling, and abusive. These individuals now also become focused on getting their needs met but do so in destructive ways. For example, they become impulsive, make suicide attempts, engage in promiscuity, etc.

Since schema modes are more or less cut off from each other, and because characterological patients display different cognitions, behaviors, and emotions in each mode, the therapist must utilize different treatment strategies in response to each mode. The therapeutic goal is to eliminate unhealthy modes, while developing, nurturing, and integrating healthy modes.

PRACTICAL APPLICATIONS OF SCHEMA-FOCUSED THERAPY

Schema-focused treatment is divided into two phases: assessment and change. The assessment phase focuses on the identification and activation of the particular schemas that are most relevant for each patient while the change phase attempts to modify the relevant schemas by altering the distorted views of self and others.

Assessment

The assessment phase is roughly divided into four stages. (1) *Schema identification*: During this stage, relevant schemas are identified via clinical analysis of the presenting problem and life review; inventories such as the Young Schema Questionnaire (2nd edition), the Multimodal Life History Inventory, Thought Records, diaries, mood log, the Young Parenting Inventory (YPI), the Young Compensation Inventory (YCI), and the Young-Rygh Avoidance Inventory; as well as by observing patterns in the therapy relationship. (2) *Schema activation*: In this stage, identified schemas and affect are triggered through imagery, dialogues, and role plays to confirm the role of the schemas and to overcome affective avoidance. (3) *Schema conceptualization*: In preparation for the change phase, the therapist develops an overall conceptualization of relevant schemas and a treatment plan. (4) *Schema education*: In the final stage, the conceptualization of the problem in schema terms and treatment plan are discussed with the patient.

Schema Identification

Lifelong patterns are initially identified during the clinical interview so that the patient's presenting problems may be conceptualized within the context of the schemas. Supporting information is then derived from other sources, including the Young Schema Questionnaire (2nd edition; Young & Brown, 1994), a 205-item self-report inventory that consists of self-statements related to each schema; the Multimodal Life History Inventory (Lazarus & Lazarus, 1991), a record of important historical events in the patient's life that permits the clinician to generate hypotheses about schema origins; the YPI (Young, 1994b), which taps the origins of schemas by asking patients to rate their mother and father separately on many statements regarding their childhood (e.g., "criticized me a lot"); the YCI (Young, 1994c), which taps the degree and type of schema compensation; and the Young-Rygh Avoidance Inventory (Young & Rygh, 1994), which measures the degree and type of schema avoidance. The Schema Diary, a mood log given to patients to document thoughts, feelings, and behaviors during periods of stress or anxiety (Young, 1994d), also provides important information about underlying schemas.

Once specific schemas are identified, the clinician must explore how patients characteristically maintain, avoid, and compensate for the schemas. For example, a patient identified as having the Defectiveness schema may enter into an intimate relationship with someone overly critical and thereby continue to feel even more defective. Identifying these schema processes helps the clinician determine how schemas are perpetuated by the patient and also provides further confirmation for the primacy of certain schemas over others.

Finally, schema modes are also identified during this stage. Clinicians must not only distinguish the different modes, they must be alert to situational triggers or life that activate each mode and note the different cognitions, emotions, and behaviors displayed by patients in each schema mode.

Schema Activation

Once schema identification is complete, the therapist now focuses on activating the primary schemas during the assessment sessions. One of the most valuable components of this phase involves the use of experiential techniques, such as asking a patient to imagine an early childhood scene that comes to mind, to trigger affect associated with the identified schemas.

The goal of schema activation is twofold. First, activating schemas during assessment confirms the primacy of the identified schemas. That is, schemas that elicit (or are associated with) high levels of affect during schema activation sessions may be considered primary while those that do not elicit significant affect may be considered secondary for the patient.

Schema activation is also used to overcome schema avoidance; however, this process is not intended to modify the schemas but merely to facilitate schema modification during the change phase. Activating schemas enables patients, particularly those who exhibit schema avoidance, to tolerate painful feelings without escaping so that the change phase may proceed effectively. As we mentioned earlier, characterological patients exhibit tremendous affective and cognitive avoidance. As long as they continue to avoid thoughts and memories that cause painful emotions, therapy cannot proceed effectively because the therapist and patient do not have access to vital information that is out of awareness. Experiential techniques, such as imagery, are employed to facilitate patients' ability to experience painful emotions that are triggered by their schemas, and thus recall the events and cognitions associated with the affect. In essence, the role of the therapist in this phase is to help patients tolerate low levels of schema-related affect and then to gradually intensify the experience until patients are able to tolerate the full imagery exercise without retreating from the image. This process ultimately enables patients to gain access to previously avoided thoughts and emotions and facilitates modification of the underlying schemas during the change phase.

Schema Conceptualization

Before the change phase can begin, the material obtained during the assessment phase is integrated into an overall map of the patient's problems using the Schema Conceptualization Form (Young, 1992). It may require several sessions to get to this point, depending on the duration and complexity of the issues involved and how wounded, self-protective, compensated, or avoidant the patient is. The conceptualization is always tailored to the individual patient, in that the patterning of schemas and the particular way in which they interact is different for everyone. Two patients with the core schema of Defectiveness may present very different clinical pictures. As well as being different in age, intelligence, ethnicity, and so on, some patients with the Defectiveness schema may come across as flamboyant, self-absorbed, and eager to talk about superficial aspects of themselves, whereas others might be very guarded and threatened by any personal questions, however gently posed.

Schema Education

Finally, before change is initiated, it is essential to explain the nature of their schemas to patients in order to develop a shared understanding of their problems and core issues. This also allows the patient and therapist to agree on a conceptualization of the problem and treatment in the context of the schema model. To further consolidate their understanding of schemas, we recommend that patients read *Reinventing Your Life* (Young & Klosko, 1994), a self-help book based on the schema-focused approach. We also routinely supply new patients with *A Client's Guide to Schema-Focused Therapy* (Bricker & Young, 1994). This six-page booklet explains the schema-focused approach and provides illustrative examples of how each schema operates.

The Change Phase

As stated earlier, the schema-focused model is an integrative approach to the treatment of patients with characterological disorders that incorporates experiential and interpersonal techniques within a cognitive-behavioral framework. Since many of the cognitive and behavioral strategies are similar to the ones used in standard cognitive therapy, we will merely summarize these techniques. Schema-focused techniques unique to this model will be presented in more detail.

Throughout the change phase, the basic stance of the therapist toward the patient is that of "empathic confrontation." This involves consistently empathizing with the underlying schemas while confronting the patient with the need to change his or her dysfunctional thoughts, feelings, and behaviors. The therapist should strive to balance empathy with confrontation or reality-testing continuously throughout this phase.

Cognitive Techniques

The overall aim of cognitive techniques is to alter the distorted view of self and others that stems from the schema by presenting contrary objective evidence to refute it. Cognitive exercises are intended to improve the way patients habitually process information, so that they are able to maintain gains made in therapy.

Cognitive exercises include the "life review," where patients are asked to provide evidence from their lives that supports and contradicts the schema. The goal of the life review is to (1) help patients appreciate how their schemas distort their perceptions and feelings, thereby rigidly maintaining the schema and to (2) begin the process of distancing from, rather than identifying with, the schemas.

Schema Flashcards (Young, 1996) are also used in this phase so that patients may continue the distancing process outside therapy. Flashcards are essentially index cards developed jointly by the therapist and patient that incorporate the most powerful evidence and counterarguments against the schemas. Patients are encouraged to carry these flashcards with them wherever they go and are required to read them repeatedly, especially when a schema is triggered (i.e., when they have a "schema attack"). The constant repetition of rational responses and the acknowledgment of evidence contradictory to the schema at the time of its activation help patients to gain distance from the schema and the related feeling and to identify more with the newer, healthier, and more objective voice.

Experiential Techniques

Experiential techniques have been increasingly incorporated into cognitive therapy in recent years (e.g., see Daldrup, Beutler, Engle, & Greenberg, 1988; Safran & Segal, 1990) and are used to bring the patients' emotions in sync with cognitive changes. These techniques appear to be among the most useful of all strategies in schema-focused therapy and are believed to change the underlying schemas in a fundamental way that is often more powerful than with cognitive techniques alone. Experiential techniques enable the patient to experience affective arousal associated with the schema, which, in turn, facilitates modification of the underlying schema. Among the two most commonly used techniques are imagery exercises and schema dialogues.

Imagery Techniques. Imagery techniques are among the most dramatic approaches to changing schemas. Instead of merely recalling and tolerating the pain and discomfort in the image as required in the assessment phase, patients are now encouraged to modify the image. For example, a patient with the Emotional Deprivation schema may be encouraged to confront a depriving parent in the safety of the image.

Patients are asked to visualize the scene as vividly as possible. To facilitate this, the therapist may ask patients to describe details of the situation such as how they looked at that age; how the parents, siblings, or peers appeared; what the scene looked like; time of day; and so forth. During the imagery procedure, particular attention is also paid to accessing feelings and thoughts relevant to the visualized scene.

Patients are encouraged to stay with their feelings and ultimately respond to the image with the healthy, newer part of themselves. For example, during the image, a patient with the Defectiveness schema may be encouraged to express to a critical father how he made her feel and to get angry at him for mistreating her. This work allows patients to continue distancing from their schemas by helping them change their perception of their childhood. For example, confronting a critical father in imagery may enable a patient to recognize the parent's role in forming her Defectiveness schema, instead of attributing the criticism to herself.

Schema Dialogue. In a schema dialogue, patients learn to reject the feelings elicited by the schema and strengthen the healthy aspects of themselves. They are encouraged to confront the schema by providing contradictory evidence to refute it. Just as the life review enables patients to experience cognitive distance from the schema, the schema dialogue allows patients to experience emotional freedom and self-efficacy while increasing their emotional distance from the schema.

With this technique, patients are asked to go back and forth between two chairs. In one chair, they role play the "voice" of the schema (i.e., thoughts consistent with their schema). Patients usually do this with ease because their schema-driven thoughts form the core of their self-concept. In the other chair, patients are encouraged to respond to the "voice" of the schema from the "healthy side." Because patients experience more difficulty refuting the schema, the clinician can "coach" them by pointing out contradictory evidence from his or her knowledge of the patients' lives and by encouraging them to focus on how living with the schema makes them feel.

In addition to providing distance from the schema, the schema dialogue also enables patients to appreciate that it is the voice of the schema maintaining their negative feelings and, therefore, these feelings are not inherently valid. With sufficient practice, patients gradually learn to assume the role of the healthy voice and contradict the voice of the schema. When they get to this stage, their ability to ventilate feelings and to reject the schema provides them with a sense of liberation from this habitual way of thinking and facilitates a newer, healthier way of thinking and feeling.

Interpersonal Techniques

Since many characterological patients have difficulty establishing a therapeutic relationship, and since interpersonal problems are often the core issue for these patients, the therapeutic relationship is often a potent vehicle for schema modification.

Limited Reparenting. One aspect of the therapist's role is construed as "limited reparenting," where the therapist attempts to provide a therapeutic relationship that counteracts the schemas. The patient's schemas and schema domains guide the therapist in deciding what aspects of the reparenting process might be especially important. Limited reparenting is most valuable for patients with schemas in the Disconnection and Rejection domain, particularly for those who experienced extreme criticism, abuse, instability, deprivation, or rejection as children. For example, if a patient's parents were extremely critical, the therapist attempts to be as accepting as possible and to praise the patient directly and frequently. If the patient's parents were withholding, the therapist endeavors to be as nurturing as possible. Of course, the therapist only offers an approximation of the missed emotional experience, while maintaining the ethical and professional boundaries of the relationship. No attempt is made by the therapist to reenact being the parent, nor to regress the patient to a child-like state of dependency.

Schemas Triggered within the Therapy Relationship. Since many of the patients' schematic issues (e.g., Emotional Deprivation, Subjugation, Dependence, and Defectiveness) arise in relation to the therapist, the patient's thoughts and feelings about the therapist also become relevant in identifying, triggering, and modifying schemas.

Unlike traditional psychoanalytic therapy, the schema-focused therapist works collaboratively and directly with patients to identify schemas when they arise during sessions. When a schema is believed to be activated in relation to the therapist, the therapist gives patients the opportunity to test the validity of their schemas. This may involve self-disclosure on the therapist's part to correct patients' distortions. Often the therapist offers direct feedback that contradicts the patients' schema-driven beliefs and expectations, and provides patients with the opportunity to express highly charged feelings directly in the session. Through repeated empathic confrontation, patients are taught to understand the role of the schemas in maintaining their thoughts and expectations and to challenge and modify them as they arise during sessions.

Interpersonal Relationships. Schemas are also maintained by the patient's current interpersonal environment, including friends and partners. Patients are gradually made aware of the role of their schemas in maintaining interpersonal relationships. Patterns observed within the therapeutic relationship may also be applied to interpersonal relationships outside the therapeutic environment.

When possible, friends or spouses may be invited to sessions to help patients assess the validity of their schemas and to modify their dysfunctional relationships. During these sessions, the therapist confronts patients' schema-driven thoughts and expectations and helps them to draw accurate inferences about others. Such sessions also enable patients to communicate their previously unexpressed thoughts and feelings in a safe environment The results of such meetings can often be dramatic, particularly when participants can see how their schemas interact to produce conflict and disappointment.

Behavioral Techniques

Behavioral techniques are utilized in schema-focused therapy to modify self-defeating patterns of behavioral avoidance, maintenance, and compensation that have been perpetuating the patients' schemas. Although cognitive exercises weaken the schema, thoughts related to the schema may still be triggered in specific situations, causing patients to continue behaving in ways that reinforce the schema. Therefore, behavioral exercises are used in conjunction with cognitive exercises to further challenge thoughts and behaviors in specific situations. Schema-focused therapy incorporates, when appropriate, many well-established behavioral and operant techniques, such as social skills, assertiveness training, systematic exposure, and behavioral programming, to change behaviors that reinforce the schema.

Performing New Behaviors. Sometimes, an exposure hierarchy is constructed jointly by the therapist and patient to enable patients to challenge their thoughts systematically and to perform new behaviors that contradict the schema. Before *in vivo* exposure takes place, patients are imaginally exposed to each step in the hierarchy during the therapy session. This process reduces their anxiety and increases the likelihood of success outside therapy, because these new behaviors, not currently in their repertoire, will be primed in the image. Once patients successfully complete each step on the hierarchy through imaginal exposure, they are required to perform it outside the session (*in vivo* exposure).

If patients perform the exercise successfully outside the session, they are reinforced during the next session and are then guided through the next, more difficult exercise on the hierarchy. If patients are unsuccessful, the situation is discussed at length to pinpoint exactly how or where it failed. Often flashcards are useful to help patients fight schemas while making behavioral changes. Once the source of the failure is identified, the same exercise is rehearsed again during the session before the patient attempts to do it outside therapy.

Behavioral Pattern Breaking. In addition to exercises that focus on adding new behaviors to their repertoire, patients are also encouraged to stop behaving in ways that reinforce the schema. For example, since patients with the Defectiveness schema often perceive well-intentioned suggestions as harsh criticism (schema maintenance), they may be helped to distinguish helpful suggestions from excessive derogatory criticism. Once they are able to make this distinction, they are taught to confront partners who are inappropriately critical and to terminate the relationship if the partners do not change. They may also be taught to respond more appropriately to friends who offered helpful feedback instead of becoming depressed or defensive.

CLINICAL AND EMPIRICAL VALIDATION
OF SCHEMA-FOCUSED THERAPY

In our clinical experience, Young's schema-focused model has been successfully applied to patients with a range of DSM-IV disorders including prevention of relapse in depression and anxiety disorders (Young, Beck, & Weinberger, 1993); avoidant, dependent, compulsive, passive–aggressive, histrionic, borderline, and narcissistic personality disorders; substance abuse during the recovery phase; and those with a history of eating disorders, chronic pain, or childhood abuse (McGinn, Young, & Sanderson, 1995). However, controlled clinical outcome trials comparing the relative efficacy of schema-focused therapy versus standard cognitive therapy for the treatment of these disorders have yet to be conducted.

Future investigations may compare treatment outcome for Axis I patients with and without a personality disorder on both short-term cognitive therapy and schema-focused therapy. Specifically, patients presenting with a principal Axis I disorder with and without a comorbid personality disorder may be treated with either short-term cognitive therapy alone or cognitive therapy plus schema-focused therapy. This type of design would determine if adding a schema-focused component maintains gains, prevents relapse, and so on, over cognitive therapy alone. Additionally, patients with a principal Axis II disorder may be treated with either traditional cognitive therapy or schema-focused therapy. This would enable us to determine if schema-focused therapy is superior to short-term cognitive therapy for these patients as proposed.

CONCLUSION

Schema-focused therapy is a promising new integrative model of treatment for a wide range of lifelong patterns. Schema-focused therapy adapts techniques used in traditional cognitive therapy but goes beyond the short-term approach by combining interpersonal and experiential techniques within a cognitive-behavioral framework, utilizing the concept of the early maladaptive schema as the unifying element.

APPENDIX: EARLY MALADAPTIVE SCHEMAS[2]

Domain I. Disconnection and Rejection

1. Abandonment/Instability

The perceived instability or unreliability of those available for support and connection. This schema includes the sense that significant others will not be able to continue providing emotional support, connection, strength, or practical protection because they are emotionally unstable and unpredictable (e.g., angry outbursts), unreliable, or erratically present; because they will die imminently; or because they will abandon the patient in favor of someone better.

2. Mistrust/Abuse

The expectation that others will hurt, abuse, humiliate, cheat, lie, manipulate, or take advantage. This schema usually involves the perception that the harm is intentional or the result of unjustified and extreme negligence. May include the sense that one always ends up being cheated relative to others or "gets the short end of the stick."

3. Emotional Deprivation

The expectation that one's desire for a normal degree of emotional support will not be adequately met by others. The three major forms of deprivation are (a) deprivation of nurturance: absence of attention, affection, warmth, or companionship; (b) deprivation of empathy: absence of understanding, listening, self-disclosure, or mutual sharing of feelings from others; (c) deprivation of protection: absence of strength, direction, or guidance from others.

4. Defectiveness/Shame

The feeling that one is defective, bad, unwanted, inferior, or invalid in important respects; or that one would be unlovable to significant others if exposed. May involve hypersensitivity to criticism, rejection, and blame; self-consciousness, comparisons, and insecurity around others; or a sense of shame regarding one's perceived flaws. These flaws may be private (e.g., selfishness, angry impulses, unacceptable sexual desires) or public (e.g., undesirable physical appearance, social awkwardness).

5. Social Isolation/Alienation

The feeling that one is isolated from the rest of the world, different from other people, and/or not part of any group or community.

Domain II: Impaired Autonomy and Performance

6. Dependence/Incompetence

The belief that one is unable to handle one's everyday responsibilities in a competent manner, without considerable help from others (e.g., take care of oneself, solve daily problems, exercise good judgment, tackle new tasks, make good decisions). Often presents as helplessness.

7. Vulnerability to Danger (Random Events)

Exaggerated fear that "random" catastrophe could strike at any time and that one will be unable to prevent it. Fears focus on one or more of the following: (a) medical (e.g., heart attack, AIDS), (b) emotional (e.g., go crazy), (c) natural/phobic (e.g., elevators, crime, airplanes, earthquakes).

8. Enmeshment/Undeveloped Self

Excessive emotional involvement and closeness with one or more significant others (often parents), at the expense of full individuation or normal social development. Often involves the belief that at least one of the enmeshed individuals cannot survive or be happy without the constant support of the other. May also include feelings of being smothered by, or fused with, others *or* insufficient individual identity. Often experienced as a feeling of emptiness and floundering, having no direction, or, in extreme cases, questioning one's existence.

9. Failure

The belief that one has failed, will inevitably fail, or is fundamentally inadequate relative to one's peers in areas of achievement (career, sports, etc.). Often involves beliefs that one is stupid, inept, untalented, ignorant, lower in status, less successful than others, and the like.

Domain III: Impaired Limits

10. Entitlement/Grandiosity

The belief that one is superior to other people; entitled to special rights and privileges, or not bound by the rules of reciprocity that guide normal social interaction. Often involves insistence that one should be able to do or have whatever one wants, regardless of what is realistic, what others consider reasonable, or the cost to others; *or* an exaggerated focus on superiority (e.g., being among the most successful, famous, wealthy) in order to achieve power or control (not primarily for attention or approval). Sometimes includes excessive competitiveness toward, or domination of, others — asserting one's power, forcing one's point of view, or controlling the behavior of others in line with one's own desires — without empathy or concern for others' needs or feelings.

11. Insufficient Self-Control/Self-Discipline

Pervasive difficulty or refusal to exercise sufficient self-control and frustration tolerance to achieve one's personal goals,) or to restrain the excessive expression of one's emotions and impulses. In its milder form, patient presents with an exaggerated emphasis on discomfort-avoidance — avoiding pain, conflict, confrontation, responsibility, or overexertion — at the expense of personal fulfillment, commitment, or integrity.

Domain IV: Other-Directedness

12. Subjugation

An excessive surrendering of control to others because one feels coerced — usually to avoid anger, retaliation, or abandonment. The two major forms of subjugation are (a) subjugation of needs: suppression of one's preferences, decisions, and desires; and (b) subjugation of emotions: suppression of emotional expression, especially anger. This schema usually involves the perception that one's own desires, opinions, and feelings are not valid or important to others. Frequently presents as excessive compliance, combined with hypersensitivity to feeling trapped. Generally leads to a buildup of anger, manifested in maladaptive symptoms (e.g., passive–aggressive behavior, uncontrolled outbursts of temper, psychosomatic symptoms, withdrawal of affection, "acting out," substance abuse).

13. Self-Sacrifice

Excessive focus on voluntarily meeting the needs of others in daily situations, at the expense of one's own gratification. The most common reasons are to prevent causing pain to others, to avoid guilt from feeling selfish, or to maintain the connection with others perceived as needy. Often results from an acute sensitivity to the pain of others. Sometimes leads to a sense that one's own needs are not being adequately met and to resentment of those who are taken care of (overlaps with concept of codependency).

14. Approval-Seeking/Recognition-Seeking

An excessive emphasis on gaining approval, recognition, or attention from other people or fitting in, at the expense of developing a secure and true sense of self. One's sense of esteem is dependent primarily on the reactions of others rather than on one's own natural inclinations. Sometimes includes an overemphasis on status, appearance, social acceptance, money, or achievement as means of gaining approval, admiration, or attention (not primarily for power or control). Frequently results in major life decisions that are unauthentic or unsatisfying, or in hypersensitivity to rejection.

Domain V: Overvigilance and Inhibition

15. Negativity/Vulnerability to Error (Controllable Events)

A pervasive, lifelong focus on the negative aspects of life (pain, death, loss, disappointment, conflict, guilt, resentment, unsolved problems, potential mistakes, betrayal, things that could go wrong, etc.) while minimizing or neglecting the positive or optimistic aspects *or* an exaggerated expectation—in a wide range of work, financial, or interpersonal situations that are typically viewed as "controllable"—that things will go seriously wrong, or that aspects of one's life that seem to be going well will fall apart at any time. Usually involves an inordinate fear of making mistakes that might lead to financial collapse, loss, humiliation, being trapped in a bad situation, or loss of control. Because potential negative outcomes are exaggerated, these patients are frequently characterized by chronic worry, vigilance, pessimism, complaining, or indecision.

16. Overcontrol/Emotional Inhibition

The excessive inhibition of spontaneous action, feeling, or communication—usually to create a sense of security and predictability or to avoid making mistakes, disapproval by others, catastrophe and chaos, or losing control of one's impulses. The most common areas of excessive control involve (a) inhibition of anger and aggression; (b) compulsive order and planning; (c) inhibition of positive impulses (e.g., joy, sexual excitement, play); (d) excessive attention to routine or rituals; (e) difficulty expressing vulnerability or communicating freely about one's feelings, needs, and so forth; or (f) excessive emphasis on rationality while disregarding emotional needs. Often the overcontrol is extended to others in the patient's environment.

17. Unrelenting Standards/Hypercriticalness

The underlying belief that one must strive to meet very high internalized standards of behavior and performance, usually to avoid criticism. Typically results in feelings of pressure or difficulty slowing down and in hypercriticalness toward oneself and others. Must involve significant impairment in pleasure, relaxation, health, self-esteem, sense of accomplishment, or satisfying relationships. Unrelenting standards typically present as (a) perfectionism, inordinate attention to detail, or an underestimate of how good one's own performance is relative to the norm; (b) rigid rules and "shoulds" in many areas of life, including unrealistically high moral, ethical, cultural, or religious precepts; or (c) preoccupation with time and efficiency, so that more can be accomplished.

18. Punitiveness

The belief that people should be harshly punished for making mistakes. Involves the tendency to be angry, intolerant, punitive, and impatient with those people (including oneself) who do not meet one's expectations or standards. Usually includes difficulty forgiving mistakes in oneself or others, because of a reluctance to consider extenuating circumstances, allow for human imperfection, or empathize with feelings.

NOTES

1. The terms "characterological problems," "character pathology," and "personality disorders" will be used interchangeably in the present chapter.

2. Developed by Jeffrey E. Young, PhD. Copyright 1996 by Jeffrey E. Young. Unauthorized reproduction without written consent of the author is prohibited. For more information, write to: Cognitive Therapy Center of New York, 8 East 80th Street, PH, New York, NY 10021.

REFERENCES

American Psychiatric Association. (1994). *Diagnostic and statistical manual of mental disorders* (4th ed.). Washington, DC: Author.

Beck, A. T. (1967). *Depression: Clinical, experimental and theoretical aspects.* New York: Harper & Row.

Beck, A. T. (1976). *Cognitive therapy and the emotional disorders.* New York: International Universities Press.

Beck, A. T., Emery, G., & Greenberg, R. L. (1985). *Anxiety disorders and phobias: A cognitive perspective.* New York: Basic Books.

Beck, A. T., Rush, A. J., Shaw, B. F., & Emery, G. (1979). *Cognitive therapy of depression.* New York: Guilford Press.

Beckham, E. E., & Watkins, J. T. (1989). Process and outcome in cognitive therapy. In A. Freeman, K. Simon, L. Beutler, & H. Arkowitz (Eds.), *Comprehensive handbook of cognitive therapy* (pp. 61–81). New York: Plenum Press.

Bricker, D. C., & Young, J. E. (1994). *A client's guide to schema-focused therapy.* In J. E. Young, *Cognitive therapy for personality disorders: A schema-focused approach* (Rev. ed., pp. 79–90). Sarasota, FL: Professional Resource Press.

Bricker, D. C., Young, J. E., & Flanagan, C. M. (1993). Schema-focused cognitive therapy: A comprehensive framework for characterological problems. In K. T. Kuehlwein & H. Rosen (Eds.), *Cognitive therapies in action* (pp. 88–125). San Francisco: Jossey-Bass.

Daldrup, R. J., Beutler, L. E., Engle, D., & Greenberg, L. S. (1988). *Focused expressive psychotherapy: Freeing the overcontrolled patient.* New York: Guilford Press.

Dobson, K. S. (Ed.). (1988). *Handbook of cognitive-behavioral therapies.* New York: Guilford Press.

Dobson. K. S. (1989). A meta-analysis of the efficacy of cognitive therapy for depression. *Journal of Consulting and Clinical Psychology, 57,* 414–419.

Ellis, A. (1962). *Reason and emotion in psychotherapy.* New York: Lyle Stuart.

Haaga, D. A., & Davison, G. C. (1991). Disappearing differences do not always reflect healthy integration: An analysis of cognitive therapy and rational-emotive therapy. *Journal of Psychotherapy Integration, 1,* 287–303.

Lazarus, A. A., & Lazarus, C. N. (1991). *Multimodal life history inventory* (2nd ed.). Champaign, IL: Research Press.

Mahoney, M. J. (1993). Introduction to special section: Theoretical developments in the cognitive psychotherapies. *Journal of Consulting and Clinical Psychology, 2,* 187–193.

McGinn, L. K., Young, J. E., & Sanderson, W. C. (1995). When and how to do longer-term therapy without feeling guilty. *Cognitive and Behavioral Practice, 2*(1), 187–212.

Neimeyer, R. A. (1993). An appraisal of constructivist psychotherapies. *Journal of Consulting and Clinical Psychology, 2,* 221–234.

Robins, C. J., & Hayes, A. M. (1993). An appraisal of cognitive therapy. *Journal of Consulting and Clinical Psychology, 2,* 205–214.

Safran, J. D., & Segal, Z. V. (1990). *Interpersonal processes in cognitive therapy.* New York: Basic Books.

Schmidt, N. B. (1994). The Schema Questionnaire and the Schema Avoidance Questionnaire. *Behavior Therapist, 17*(4), 90–92.

Schmidt, N. B., Joiner, T. E., Young, J. E., & Telch, M. J. (1995). The Schema Questionnaire: Investigation of psychometric properties and the hierarchical structure of a measure of maladaptive schemas. *Cognitive Therapy and Research, 19*(3), 295–321.

Segal, Z. V. (1988). Appraisal of the self-schema construct in cognitive models of depression. *Psychological Bulletin, 103*(2), 147–162.

Young, J. E. (1992). *Schema Conceptualization Form.* (Available from the Cognitive Therapy Center of New York, 3 East 80th Street, PH, New York, NY 10021)

Young, J. E. (1994a). *Cognitive therapy for personality disorders: A schema-focused approach* (Rev. ed.). Sarasota, FL: Professional Resource Press.

Young, J. E. (1994b). *Young Parenting Inventory.* (Available from the Cognitive Therapy Center of New York, 3 East 80th Street, PH, New York, NY 10021).

Young, J. E. (1994c). *Young Compensation Inventory.* (Available from the Cognitive Therapy Center of New York, 3 East 80th Street, PH, New York, NY 10021)

Young, J. E. (1994d). *Schema Diary.* (Available from the Cognitive Therapy Center of New York, 3 East 80th Street, PH, New York, NY 10021)

Young, J. E. (1996). *Schema Flashcard.* (Available from the Cognitive Therapy Center of New York, 3 East 80th Street, PH, New York, NY 10021)

Young, J. E., Beck, A. T., & Weinberger, A. (1993). Depression. In D. H. Barlow (Ed.), *Clinical handbook of psychological disorders* (2nd ed., pp. 240–277). New York: Guilford Press.

Young, J. E., & Brown, G. (1994). *Young schema questionnaire* (2nd ed.). In J. E. Young, *Cognitive therapy for personality disorders: A schema-focused approach* (Rev. ed., pp. 63–76). Sarasota, FL: Professional Resource Press.

Young, J. E., & Flanagan, C. (in press). Schema-focused therapy for narcissistic patients. In E. Ronningstam (Ed.), *Disorders of narcissism—Theoretical, empirical, and clinical implications*. Washington, DC: American Psychiatric Press.

Young, J. E., & Klosko, J. (1994). *Reinventing your life*. New York: Plume.

Young, J. E., & Rygh, J. (1994). *Young–Rygh Avoidance Inventory*. (Available from the Cognitive Therapy Center of New York, 3 East 80th Street, PH, New York, NY 10021)

Chapter 10

Inpatient Cognitive Therapy

Jesse H. Wright

The application of cognitive therapy principles to the treatment of inpatients is taking place at a critical juncture in the history of hospital psychiatry. Length of stay in most North American hospitals has fallen dramatically, and the patients that qualify for hospitalization under strict utilization review programs are usually quite ill. A typical patient may have been admitted because of a suicide attempt or a psychotic episode complicated by comorbid disorders such as characterological disturbance, substance abuse, or significant medical problems. Severe disruption of social relationships and occupational functioning also is common.

Inpatient therapists now frequently have to accomplish a great deal in a very short time. They must reduce symptoms substantially and rehabilitate social and occupational functioning so that the patient can be discharged to outpatient care. All of this must be done at an acceptable cost. In some cases, these conditions have led to abandoning attempts to form a treatment milieu (Kleepsies, 1986). However, cognitive therapy models have emerged as a method of providing substantive psychosocial interventions in an era of "managed care." As will be detailed later in this chapter, cognitive therapy has many attributes that make it highly suitable for use in short-term inpatient treatment.

Cognitively oriented inpatient programs were initially developed in academic centers when research on inpatient cognitive therapy was begun. An inpatient cognitive therapy treatment center was established in 1980 at the Norton Psychiatric Clinic of the University of Louisville, and the first report on treating inpatients with cognitive therapy came from the University of Western Ontario in the same year (Shaw, 1980). Subsequently, Miller, Bishop, Norman, and Keitner (1985) began to use cognitive therapy as an adjunct to standard inpatient treatment at Brown University, and Bowers (1990) implemented a similar program at the University of Iowa. In the United Kingdom, Scott and coworkers (Barker, Scott, & Eccleston, 1987; Scott, 1988; Scott, 1992; Scott, Byers, & Turkington, 1993) have contributed a series of papers on treating depression in a cognitively oriented hospital milieu. Inpatient cognitive therapy units also have been developed in for-profit hospitals (Fidaleo & Creech, 1989), long-term rehabilitation centers, and community-based facilities (Perris et al., 1987).

These inpatient programs have diverse goals, structures, and methods of implementing cognitive therapy, but they all share a common link to the work of Aaron T. Beck. The fundamental concepts of cognitive therapy outlined by Beck in the early 1960s (Beck, 1963, 1964), and refined during the next three decades, form the backbone for inpatient cognitive therapy. Beck's personal interest in many of these inpatient units has played a significant role in their development. He has visited inpatient programs on a regular basis, served as a consultant, stimulated ideas for research, convened discussion groups on hospital psychiatry, and made major contributions to the first treatment manual for inpatient cognitive therapy (Wright, Thase, Beck, & Ludgate, 1993).

This chapter details the general features of a cognitive milieu and describes several different types of cognitive therapy units that have wide applicability. Modifications of therapy techniques for inpatients are briefly outlined. After reviewing research on cognitive therapy in hospital settings, the chapter concludes with consideration of prospects for future growth of inpatient cognitive therapy.

THE COGNITIVE MILIEU

The term "cognitive milieu" is used to describe inpatient programs that have three main features: (1) psychosocial treatment interventions are based predominantly on the theoretical constructs and methods of cognitive therapy, (2) the broad therapeutic milieu is considered in planning and implementing treatment, and (3) cognitive therapy is joined together with biological psychiatry and other approaches in an integrated treatment delivery model (Wright & Davis, 1993). No inpatient programs have relied upon cognitive therapy as the sole treatment modality, but many units have evolved to the point where cognitive therapy acts as the primary organizing theory for psychotherapy (Wright, Thase, & Beck, 1992). An exclusionary emphasis on cognitive therapy would be unwise for several reasons, such as the potential for biasing against other effective treatments (e.g., pharmacotherapy or systems approaches to family therapy) and downplaying of valuable contributions from previous models of hospital psychiatry (Wright & Davis, 1993).

Wright and Davis (1993) have identified nine general features of inpatient cognitive therapy programs: (1) treatment is based on specific cognitive theories; (2) the collaborative nature of cognitive therapy stimulates good working relationships between patients, members of the treatment team, and families; (3) the structured format of cognitive therapy helps organize the unit in a productive manner; (4) the problem-oriented, short-term nature of cognitive therapy is especially useful for hospitalized patients who are attempting to improve as quickly as possible and resume occupational and social functioning; (5) the proven effectiveness of cognitive therapy provides patients with hope for significant improvement during a hospital stay; (6) cognitive therapy is integrated with biological psychiatry in clinical practice; (7) psychoeducational methods are used extensively; (8) relapse prevention is a major focus of treatment; and (9) significant contributions from earlier models of inpatient therapy, including the therapeutic community, are adapted for use in the treatment milieu. An example of the latter feature of cognitive therapy units is the reformulation of group therapies, unit—community meetings, and unit governance procedures—hallmarks of the therapeutic community—to be consistent with the cognitive approach to treatment (Wright, Thase, Beck, & Ludgate, 1993; Bowers, 1989). Cognitive milieus did not appear *de novo*. They owe much to individuals such as Maxwell Jones (1953), Jerrold Maxmen (Maxmen, Tucker, & Lebow, 1974), and others who developed earlier methods for hospital psychiatry.

The defining features of inpatient cognitive therapy described above set this form of therapy apart from other contemporary models of inpatient treatment including rational eclecticism (Moline, 1976) and "pure" biological psychiatry. In the next section of the chapter, specific forms of inpatient cognitive therapy are defined and illustrated.

MODELS FOR INPATIENT COGNITIVE THERAPY

A number of different forms of hospital-based cognitive therapy have developed in response to local needs, resources, and constraints. Cognitive therapy units have ranged from closed-staff, university affiliated programs, in which all the primary therapists have received intensive training in cognitive therapy, to open-staff, for-profit hospitals, in which cognitive therapy is delivered by nurses and other staff members or consultants who are hired to perform cognitive therapy as an adjunct to the existing treatment system. Four common types of cognitive therapy units have been described previously (Wright, et al.,1993). Features of these inpatient cognitive therapy models (*primary therapist, "add-on," staff,* and *comprehensive*) and an additional method of treatment (the *flexible* model) are summarized in Table 10.1.

The *primary therapist* model was originally constructed to introduce cognitive therapy to academic units in which outcome research was being conducted. Emphasis is placed on training primary therapists to perform individual cognitive therapy at a high level of competence. Some effort may be expended on educating staff members so they can assist with cognitive therapy homework assignments or psychcoeducational procedures, but the weight of responsibility for psychotherapy is clearly placed upon primary therapists such as psychiatrists, psychologists, and social workers. In con-

TABLE 10.1. Models for Inpatient Cognitive Therapy

	Primary therapist	"Add-on"	Staff	Comprehensive	Flexible
Intensive training	Psychiatrist; primary therapists	Adjunctive therapist(s)	Support staff	All therapists; support staff	Most therapists; support staff
Minimal training	Support staff	Psychiatrists; support staff	Psychiatrists	None	Some therapists
Physician role	Cognitive therapist; pharmacotherapist	Referral source; pharmacotherapist	Referral source; pharmacotherapist	Cognitive therapist; pharmacotherapist	Cognitive therapist; pharmacotherapist
Nurse role	Cognitive orientation	Traditional	Cognitive therapist	Cognitive therapist	Variable
Group and family therapy	Variable	Variable	Variable	Cognitive therapist	Cognitive therapist
Activities therapy	Cognitive orientation	Traditional	Cognitive orientation	Cognitive therapist	Cognitive therapist

trast, the *staff* model shifts responsibility for cognitive therapy toward nurses, aides, and adjunctive therapists (occupational, recreational, and expressive therapists). These units have been formed at for-profit and open-staff hospitals where psychiatrists admit the patient and agree to allow the staff to implement the psychotherapy program. The doctor retains responsibility for the diagnostic evaluation and pharmacotherapy. Usually a medical director or other program director who has received training in cognitive therapy devotes considerable time to educating and supervising staff members in the application of cognitive therapy methods. Although a cohesive milieu can be developed with the staff model, there is considerable potential for conflict between the treatment goals and methods of the admitting physician and staff members.

The *add-on* model has been used widely in a number of different settings. This type of inpatient treatment is less complicated, more rapidly employed, and less costly than any of the other systems described here. However, cognitive therapy may be utilized only to a limited extent in the overall treatment program. When this approach is used, a cognitive therapy module is added to the treatment milieu without attempting to make significant changes in the other ongoing therapeutic programs. This model has been used for research studies where cognitive therapy is compared to other interventions that are added to "treatment as usual" (Miller, Norman, & Keitner, 1989). The add-on model also has been adapted by clinical programs that wish to initiate cognitive therapy without the effort and expense of training large groups of primary therapists or staff and refitting the entire milieu. In this case, an experienced cognitive therapist is recruited to perform individual cognitive therapy with selected patients or to conduct cognitive group therapy. Some education of staff members is usually necessary so they will be oriented to cognitive therapy principles, but staff members do not have a prominent role in implementing cognitive therapy.

The *comprehensive* model is the most fully developed form of inpatient cognitive therapy. This treatment system combines the best features of the primary therapist and staff models. The comprehensive approach to inpatient cognitive therapy involves extensive training of both primary therapists and staff members, so that all members of the multidisciplinary team can join together in constructing a treatment milieu based on the concepts and methods of cognitive therapy. All of the venues for treatment (e.g., individual, group, recreational, occupational, family, nursing interventions, unit–community meetings, etc.) employ cognitive therapy, and treatment planning is used to integrate the activities of the team.

Primary therapist and staff model units can evolve to a comprehensive approach as their programs mature. However, many roadblocks can be encountered in attempting to implement a comprehensive cognitive therapy program. Staff turnover and fluctuations of the patient population often are significant problems. The ideal environment for the development of a comprehensive cognitive therapy milieu would include: (1) a closed-staff or limited-staff physician system in which all psychiatrists are knowledgeable and supportive of cognitive therapy, (2) availability of many other primary therapists and adjunctive therapists who are experienced in cognitive therapy or who are interested in learning this approach, (3) strong and consistent administrative support for a cognitive therapy program and, (4) ability to select the unit patient population for suitability for cognitive therapy. These ideal conditions are rarely if ever met. Thus, most current units have not been able to fully implement a comprehensive milieu.

The *flexible* model is especially useful when many of the elements of a comprehensive milieu have been developed, but the patient population on the unit varies significantly from day to day. Psychiatric units in general hospitals or small free-standing hospitals may not have the luxury of screening out organic or floridly psychotic patients from their units. At some times the patient population of the unit may be comprised primarily of individuals with affective disorders who can benefit from an intense cognitive therapy program. However, with a short length of stay and rapid patient turnover, the ward environment may quickly change to the point where heavy demands are placed on staff for medical interventions, limit setting, or even restraint. Although cognitive therapy methods have been developed for psychotic patients, this type of therapy (in its standard form) is not really-suitable for acute, severe psychosis or patients with significant organicity. Instead, a reality-oriented, truncated approach that has been termed "supportive cognitive therapy" is recommended (Casey & Grant, 1993).

When the flexible model is applied, group therapies and treatment plans for individual patients are adjusted daily to account for the types of patients on the unit and to most effectively use the resources of the hospital. This form of inpatient cognitive therapy requires a well-trained and dedicated staff that can perform a full range of treatment interventions while maintaining the core functions of a cognitively oriented treatment milieu.

ADAPTATIONS OF COGNITIVE THERAPY FOR HOSPITALIZED PATIENTS

The cognitive therapy approach to inpatients uses all of the procedures (e.g., collaborative empiricism, agenda setting, behavioral interventions, and eliciting and testing automatic thoughts) that are widely employed in the treatment of outpatients. However, inpatients usually have more severe symptoms such as profound hopelessness, intense suicidal ideation, marked psychomotor retardation, unrelenting panic, or psychosis. Also, hospitalized patients are more likely to have had major stressful life events or marked disruption in interpersonal relationships. Therapy techniques must be modified to account for these differences (Thase & Wright, 1991).

A full description of methods for individual, group, and family therapy with inpatients is not possible here. The reader is referred to recent accounts of therapy procedures for hospitalized patients (Bowers,1989; Davis & Casey, 1990, Ludgate, Wright, Bowers, & Camp, 1993; Freeman, Schrodt, Gilson, & Ludgate, 1993; Miller, Keitner, Epstein, Bishop, & Ryan, 1993; Wright & Beck, 1993) for detailed guidelines on this form of treatment. In addition, specific approaches have been developed for inpatients with eating disorders (Bowers, 1993), substance abuse (Barrett & Meyer, 1993), chronic depression (Scott, 1992; Scott et al., 1993), schizophrenia (Perris, 1989; Scott et al., 1993), and personality disorders (Scott et al., 1993). Also, specialty programs have been initiated for treatment of adolescents (Schrodt & Wright, 1987; Schrodt, 1993) and geriatric patients (Casey & Grant, 1993). Several of the general modifications of therapy procedures for inpatients are outlined here.

The most obvious adaptation of cognitive therapy for hospital use is the involvement of a multidisciplinary team. This change in therapy conditions can offer distinct advantages. The therapy program can continue throughout the day and can be reinforced by large numbers of individuals in the milieu. There also can be disadvantages, especially if communication problems or conflicts exist among team members. In the hospital environment, the individual cognitive therapist needs to extend his or her work beyond the boundaries of the usual therapy dyad to include involvement with other team members. This effort can be time consuming and frustrating, but if the team works well together, results can be gratifying. Some of the positive aspects of the milieu approach include the ability to assign homework that can be carried out under supervision, the opportunity for multiple psychoeducational programs that teach the basics of cognitive therapy, use of the hospital setting to recognize "hot cognitions," and utilization of ancillary therapists (e.g., occupational therapy, pastoral counseling, and art therapy) who may reach some patients not readily accessible with standard cognitive therapy.

Individual therapy with hospitalized patients typically employs more structure and more of a behavioral emphasis, especially early in treatment, than usually is the case in treatment of outpatients (Thase & Wright, 1991). Intensive work on identifying and modifying cognitions may be overwhelming to patients who are profoundly depressed and are having difficulties with concentration. Usually therapy begins with the development of a collaborative relationship, generation of a problem list, activity scheduling and recording, and socialization to the cognitive model (Ludgate et al., 1993). It is also important to address hopelessness early in the therapy. Frequently it is possible to identify a few key cognitive distortions (e.g., "There's no future"; "I'm a complete failure"; "Everyone would be better off if I were dead") that can be modified with cognitive therapy techniques and thereby reduce the risk of suicide. One of the most useful techniques with inpatients is to write out a list of reasons to live. With the majority of depressed inpatients, this procedure usually can be performed on the first day of hospitalization.

As the hospitalization proceeds, inpatients learn to recognize automatic thoughts and cognitive distortions and to use procedures such as the Daily Record of Dysfunctional Thoughts (Beck, Rush, Shaw, & Emery, 1979) to modify distorted thinking. Considerable effort is usually directed at helping the patient acquire problem-solving skills and improved coping strategies through behavioral procedures, psychoeducational sessions, and cognitive interventions. Therapeutic work on schemas may be delayed to the latter part of hospitalization, or even for the outpatient or partial hospitalization phase of treatment. However, some patients are able to benefit from schema-level interventions early in treatment (Wright, 1992). One of the more important components of inpatient therapy is a focus on relapse prevention during the middle and late phases of the hospital stay. An attempt is made to identify triggers in the home or work environment that may lead to a return of symptoms. The therapist then uses procedures such as role play or cognitive behavioral rehearsal to help the patient learn strategies for managing potentially stressful situations. Cognitive and behavioral methods of enhancing compliance with pharmacotherapy are also emphasized (Rush, 1988; Wright & Schrodt, 1989).

Many inpatient programs utilize group therapies as a primary mode of treatment. Several different formats for inpatient group cognitive therapy have been described (Freeman et al., 1993). Most cognitive therapy units have an open-ended group. Because of the rapid turnover of patients, most open-ended groups have a different composition at each session. Nevertheless, there usually is enough stability in the milieu to provide a nucleus of carryover patients for each group. Generally, inpatient core groups follow Yalom's (1983) suggestion that each meeting should be self-contained (Freeman et al., 1993). A variety of techniques are used to ensure that group therapy will be valuable to patients, even if the individual is only able to attend a single session. However, most patients attend four or more meetings of the group.

Freeman et al. (1993) have recommended methods for making each group therapy session a "therapy within a therapy." They suggest placing an emphasis on the psychoeducational aspects of treatment so that patients are provided with tools they can use elsewhere during their hospital stay and during the outpatient phase of therapy. Thus, group therapists may be somewhat more didactic in inpatient settings than they would be in longer-term outpatient work. Agenda setting is another important component of inpatient group cognitive therapy. An attempt is made to elicit meaningful agenda items from each patient and then to focus the group on topics of broad relevance. The group retains a "here and now," problem oriented focus and is especially directed toward achieving cognitive and behavioral changes that will prepare one for discharge. It has been noted that turnover of patients can provide an advantage for inpatient group cognitive therapy because it keeps individuals focused on the primary task of resuming a level of functioning that is compatible with leaving the hospital (Freeman et al., 1993).

Core groups have a flexible agenda based on the unique issues and concerns of the patients in the group. Two other forms of inpatient group cognitive therapy use a more structured approach. The *rotating theme* group concept was developed by Bowers (1989) in an attempt to counter the problems of the instability of inpatient group composition. A series of themes, such as reactions to hospitalization, setting and reaching goals, or building self-esteem, is used to organize the group. Topics are posted in advance, and staff members help patients prepare for the group. The therapist develops psychoeducational materials relevant to each theme, but also asks patients to suggest agenda items related to the chosen theme for the session.

Methods for *programmed* groups are derived from the work of Covi and coworkers (Covi, Roth, & Lipman, 1982; Covi & Lipman, 1987) who demonstrated the effectiveness of a curriculum-based group therapy with outpatients. Specific learning goals and methods are established for each group, and the sessions are arranged in a developmental sequence. For example, session 1 might be directed at understanding the cognitive model for depression and anxiety, while later sessions are devoted to recognizing cognitive errors or mastering cognitive-behavioral rehearsal techniques (Freeman et al., 1993). When this form of group cognitive therapy is used in a hospital setting, each session is designed so that attendance at previous meetings is not a prerequisite for understanding material that is presented. However, patients will obviously gain more if they are able to go through the entire sequence of sessions and build their cognitive therapy skills in multiple areas.

A number of other different types of group therapy are used in cognitive therapy units, including unit community meetings, focused groups for patients who have significant problems with reality testing, family groups to provide education and support, homework groups to review assignments from individual or group therapy, psychoeducational groups about medication or stress management, occupational therapy groups, and transition or relapse prevention groups. In a cognitively oriented milieu, patients usually are involved in multiple interlocking group therapies designed to maximize the application of cognitive therapy methodology during the short time available for inpatient treatment.

COMPUTER-ASSISTED THERAPY FOR INPATIENTS

Another form of treatment, computer-assisted cognitive therapy, has been recently introduced to the inpatient milieu. Bowers, Stuart, MacFarlane, and Gorman (1993) studied the usefulness of the computer program "Overcoming Depression" (Colby & Colby, 1990) in hospitalized depressed patients and found that computerized therapy was inferior to therapist-administered cognitive therapy. However, it should be noted that the Colby and Colby program requires the patient to type responses on a keyboard and is tutorial in nature. The computer "mirrors" the patient's responses and is programmed toward responding toward "key" words (Bowers et al., 1993). Although the program introduces the concept that dysfunctional thoughts are involved with depression, it does not duplicate the usual elements of therapist-administered cognitive therapy (such as behavioral homework assignments).

Bowers et al. (1993) did not study the possibility that a computer program could augment standard inpatient cognitive therapy. It would seem unlikely that a computer could take the place of a human therapist for a severely depressed inpatient, but computer-assisted interventions might be helpful in socializing the patient to treatment, giving instructions on the basic principles of cognitive therapy, providing opportunities to practice cognitive behavioral procedures, and reinforcing the self-help component of therapy.

A new form of computer-assisted therapy that uses multimedia technology may be more "user friendly" for inpatients with significant levels of symptomatic distress. "Cognitive Therapy: A Multimedia Learning Program" (Wright, Salmon, Wright, & Beck, 1995a, 1995b) is now being studied in hospitalized patients at the University of Louisville. This computer program uses full-screen video to involve the patient in real-life situations that show cognitive therapy at work. Familiarity with keyboards or computers is not required. The patient moves through a series of highly interactive exercises by using a touch screen or a mouse. The basic features of cognitive therapy—the cognitive-behavioral model, recognizing and changing automatic thoughts, using behavioral procedures, and modifying schemas—are covered, and homework assignments are completed in a companion workbook.

The place of computer-assisted cognitive therapy in hospital-based treatment is still unknown. Empirical studies are clearly needed. However, the continued pressure to reduce length of stay and still achieve a favorable outcome may stimulate efforts to use computer technologies with inpatients.

PARTIAL HOSPITALIZATION PROGRAMS

All five of the models for inpatient psychiatry described here also can be used for partial hospitalization programs. The more highly developed forms such as the comprehensive and flexible models may actually be easier to implement in partial hospital settings because the numbers of staff members and primary therapists are usually much smaller than in a traditional full-service inpatient unit. Thus, the training and supervision of therapists may require fewer resources, and the consistency of approach may be easier to maintain. Also, because the acuity of symptoms can be less extreme in day hospital patients, this group of individuals may be able to concentrate more effectively on the work of therapy.

Group cognitive therapy is often the backbone of cognitively oriented partial hospitalization programs. The day hospital program at the Norton Psychiatric Clinic at the University of Louisville relies heavily on group therapy methods. On most days there are two to three group sessions utilizing the open-ended and rotating theme formats for group cognitive therapy. Patients also have individual sessions (approximately three per week) and participate in computer-assisted cognitive therapy (Wright, Salmon, Wright, & Beck, 1995a, 1995b).

The adaptations of cognitive therapy for inpatients described earlier in this chapter also apply to the day hospital. However, because the symptoms often are less severe, the patient may be able to engage in more demanding therapy exercises. For example, homework assignments may be made for more *in vivo* exposure to anxiety-provoking situations or the therapist may focus more intensively on modifying underlying schemas. Partial hospital programs are usually geared toward increasing functional capacity to allow full return to social and occupational roles. Thus, the therapy is usually directed at learning how to use cognitive-behavioral principles to improve social skills, increase self-esteem, and effectively manage real-life problems.

The push to rapidly move patients out of intensive inpatient units to day hospitals has been a recent phenomenon in the United States, and the efficacy of this type of treatment is still unclear. Outcome research has not yet been reported on cognitively oriented partial hospitalization programs. It is expected that the "managed care" environment will encourage further growth of partial hospital programs, and that many inpatient cognitive therapy units will be associated with day hospitals that use cognitive-behavioral treatment methods. Thus, the definition of the "cognitive milieu" will need to be expanded to include the continuum between the inpatient and partial hospitalization components of treatment. Also, studies of inpatient cognitive therapy will need to include day treatment programs as part of the therapy package being evaluated.

OUTCOME RESEARCH

Controlled investigations of cognitive therapy for inpatients have been limited so far to studies of the effect of adding individual cognitive therapy to other forms of treatment used in medical model or eclectic milieus. No comparisons of treatment efficacy in a full cognitive milieu versus "standard" psychiatry hospital care have been done. However, available evidence indicates that cognitive therapy can have an additive effect, even when a full range of other treatments is employed.

Several open trials of cognitive therapy with inpatients have suggested that this form of therapy can be associated with substantial reductions in symptoms of depression. Shaw (1980) treated 10 medication-free patients with cognitive therapy three times a week for a mean length of stay of 8.1 weeks. The mean Beck Depression Inventory (BDI) scores in this group of patients fell from 29.8 before treatment to 15.6 at discharge. Thase, Bowler, and Hardin (1991) also examined the effect of cognitive therapy without medication. In their first study, 16 depressed inpatients who received daily cognitive therapy (mean number of sessions = 12.8) were found to have a decrease in mean Hamilton Rating Scale for Depression (HRSD) scores from 21.7 to 7.7. Although 13 of 16 patients (18%) met criteria for treatment response at discharge, three out of four subjects who did not receive follow-up outpatient cognitive therapy relapsed. In contrast, relapse was observed in just 1 of 7 (14%) patients who received outpatient cognitive therapy after hospitalization. Thase's group (Thase, 1994) also reported an outcome of a larger group of 30 depressed inpatients who were noted to have a 70% response rate (HRSD < 10) to inpatient cognitive therapy.

Additional evidence for the usefulness of inpatient cognitive therapy has come from open trials of cognitive therapy in patients who also received antidepressant medication (Wright, 1986; Barker et al., 1987; Scott, 1992; Simoneau, Konen, & Gabris, 1992). Wright (1986) found that 42 depressed inpatients who were randomly assigned to three different doses of nortriptyline (50, 100, and 150 mg per day, respectively) responded well to combined cognitive therapy. Although it was predicted that patients who had nortriptyline plasma levels in the therapeutic range would have a superior response, plasma levels were not significantly associated with outcome. In another study, Barker et al. (1987) noted that 8 inpatients with refractory chronic depression improved after 12 weeks of cognitive therapy but still had some evidence of residual depression at the conclusion of therapy (mean posttreatment HRSD = 13.1). Scott (1992) also observed that 16 patients with chronic depression who were treated with a more intensive cognitive therapy protocol (three sessions per week) had a reduction in mean HRSD scores from 24.5 to 10.6 after inpatient treatment.

Another open trial examined the effects of group cognitive therapy on depressed inpatients (Simoneau et al., 1992). Although the treatment program was not described in detail, it appears that multiple group therapies were utilized. Unfortunately, data were not provided on duration of hospitalization or the frequency and format of treatment modalities. Mean HRSD scores fell from 22.2 before treatment to 8.7 at discharge. Further, mean HRSD scores remained stable after 1 year (9.0) and 2 years (8.5) of follow-up.

Three controlled trials of inpatient cognitive therapy have been reported to date. DeJong, Treiber, and Henrich (1986) completed the first controlled study of inpatient cognitive therapy. Although subjects were treated with cognitive therapy without medication, the design did not allow for adequate comparisons of experimental groups. Thirty patients with chronic depression were treated with individual inpatient cognitive therapy, inpatient cognitive restructuring, or outpatient supportive psychotherapy. Individuals who received the intensive inpatient cognitive therapy had the greatest reduction in BDI scores after a maximum of 6 weeks of treatment. However, the two inpatient treatment groups had similar HRSD scores at the time of discharge. Six out of 10 patients who received cognitive therapy were classified as treatment responders, whereas only 1 out of 10 of the outpatient control group members met criteria for treatment response. The similar forms of treatment used for the two inpatient samples and the inclusion of an outpatient control group confounded interpretation of results from this study.

Miller and coworkers (Miller et al., 1985; Miller, Norman, Keitner, Bishop, & Dow, 1989; Miller, Norman, & Keitner, 1989; Miller, Norman, & Keitner, 1990) have studied inpatient cognitive therapy in an "add-on" model milieu at a large university-affiliated psychiatric hospital. Their first report described an open pilot study of 6 inpatients with chronic depression who responded well to cognitive therapy plus medication (Miller et al., 1985). In a later controlled trial, Miller, Norman, Keitner, Bishop, and Dow (1989) randomly assigned 47 inpatients to standard inpatient therapy (treatment "as usual" including medication of the doctor's choice), standard therapy plus cognitive therapy, or standard therapy plus social skills training. No significant differences in treatment outcome were observed at the end of hospitalization (about 3 to 4 weeks); however, after the outpatient continuation phase of treatment (17 to 18 sessions) patients in the psychotherapy groups had lower BDI scores (Miller, Norman, & Keitner, 1989). These differences reached statistical significance for the group who received social skills training.

Patients treated with cognitive therapy by Miller et al. had a nonsignificant trend ($p = .06$) for superior outcome. At the end of treatment, patients who received cognitive therapy had a significantly higher response rate (HRSD < 7) than those who were treated with standard hospital therapy. Sixty-four percent of the cognitive therapy group responded to treatment (using HRSD criteria), while only 24% of the subjects assigned standard therapy were judged to be treatment responders. The response rate for the patients who received social skills training was midway (43%) between the other two groups. After 12 months of follow-up, there were no differences between the three groups in respect to HRSD and BDI scores, but patients treated with either form of psychotherapy (pooled together in the statistical analysis) had a significantly higher rate of recovery (68%) than those who received standard hospital treatment (33%). A subsequent analysis of data from this investigation revealed that individuals who had high levels of cognitive dysfunction exhibited considerably more improvement in HRSD and BDI scores and were more likely to be recovered (57%) after cognitive therapy than those with lower levels of cognitive dysfunction (18%) (Miller, Norman, & Keitner, 1990).

In another study, Bowers (1990) randomly assigned 30 inpatients to nortriptyline alone, nortriptyline plus cognitive therapy, or nortriptyline plus relaxation training. Patients in all three groups also received other therapies that were provided on the unit. At the end of hospitalization (average length of stay = 29.4 days) all three treatment groups were improved, but patients who received combined psychotherapy and pharmacotherapy had significantly lower BDI scores and were more likely to have reached BDI criteria for recovery (BDI < 7). Although there were no differences in mean HRSD scores at the end of treatment between the three groups, patients who received cognitive therapy had a significantly higher rate of recovery based on Hamilton scale criteria (HRSD < 7).

FUTURE PROSPECTS FOR INPATIENT COGNITIVE THERAPY RESEARCH

The overall results of research on inpatient cognitive therapy suggest that this approach can be an effective treatment for severely depressed hospitalized patients. However, there are many limitations to the research that has been completed and significant barriers will impede future investigations. The most obvious concerns in this area of research are the paucity of controlled investigations, the small number of subjects in most studies, and difficulties in controlling the impact of other treatments in the hospital milieu. Bowers (1990) and Miller, Norman, Keitner, Bishop, and Don (1989) have made the most concerted efforts to use a controlled research design. However, they were unable to document or study the influences of multiple variables that may affect outcome with inpatients (e.g., stressful events, family structure and support, therapeutic relationships with physicians and other professionals, treatment with group therapy and other psychotherapies commonly used with inpatients, medical illnesses, Axis II disorders). Both the Bower and Miller et al. studies had only 10 to 12 patients in each treatment condition.

Another difficulty with inpatient research is a general reluctance to treat hospitalized patients with psychotherapy alone. The standard expectation for inpatient care is to provide relief of symptoms as soon as possible through pharmacotherapy. However, Shaw (1980) and Thase and coworkers (1991) have demonstrated that cognitive therapy can relieve depression even if used without pharmacotherapy. Although their work would appear to set the stage for controlled trials of cognitive therapy alone versus pharmacotherapy and combined treatment, the current economic environment in the United States is placing severe constraints upon inpatient research. With vigorous utilization review and a shortened length of stay, randomized assignment of inpatients to psychotherapy alone for 3 to 4 weeks may not be possible. Alternate designs that utilize a longitudinal treatment program, including a brief hospital stay of 1 to 2 weeks followed by a continuation of intensive cognitive therapy on an outpatient basis and a subsequent maintenance phase of therapy, may be preferable. Also, controlled studies of longer forms of inpatient treatment may be feasible in countries with different systems for financing health care.

One of the advantages of inpatient cognitive therapy is that the model can be readily adapted for use in multiple therapies such as group treatment, occupational therapy, and nursing interventions. However, this advantage becomes a disadvantage with most research designs. It is quite difficult to limit cognitive therapy to one patient group only and to ensure that other patients in the same hospital are not influenced at all by this treatment approach. An ideal research design would include randomized assignment of patients to a comprehensive cognitive therapy milieu as compared to another treatment milieu where cognitive therapy methods are not used in any form. This design would give valuable information on how a full cognitive therapy program compares to other treatments. However, studies such as this would be extremely difficult to implement and would require significant commitments from a regional or national health care system.

It is likely that research on inpatient cognitive therapy will proceed on a smaller scale than randomized comparisons of entire treatment milieus. Further studies could refine comparisons of cognitive therapy with pharmacotherapy and other treatments and could examine components or forms of therapy. Examples could include studies of the costs and benefits of group versus individual cognitive therapy, the optimum timing or "dosing" of cognitive therapy sessions, and the impact of psychoeducational groups on acquisition of cognitive therapy skills. Other areas for potential investigation could include inpatient cognitive therapy for special patient populations (e.g., eating disorders, adolescents, chronic pain, characterological disorders), the interaction between cognitive therapy and pharmacotherapy, cognitive therapy models for partial hospitalization, and the effect of cognitive therapy on relapse prevention. Hopefully a continued investigative effort will help clarify the role that cognitive therapy should play in the psychiatric hospital.

SUMMARY

Cognitive therapy has emerged as a significant influence on the changing scene of inpatient psychiatry. As the length of stay has diminished and pressure has increased for rapid symptom resolution, the need for effective, brief psychotherapies has been heightened. Cognitive therapy methods have been successfully adapted for use with hospitalized patients in individual, group, and family therapy formats. Treatment procedures are usually carried out in multiple settings in the milieu so that basic concepts can be reinforced and the patient has the opportunity to operationalize cognitive therapy skills *in vivo*. Some inpatient programs use cognitive therapy as a specialty track or as an "add-on" to an eclectic treatment model, while other units utilize cognitive therapy as the primary method for psychosocial interventions and as an organizing theory for the milieu.

Research on inpatient cognitive therapy has been limited to trials of the effectiveness of individual or group therapy added to the other forms of treatment utilized with inpatients. Taken together, the results of these studies suggest that treatment with cognitive therapy can be associated with substantial reduction in symptoms of depression. However, there have been few controlled studies, and it has been difficult to separate cognitive therapy effects from the host of other treatment influences operative in hospital settings. Additional research on hospital applications of cognitive therapy is clearly needed, but it will be difficult to carry out definitive studies. It is anticipated that the short-term, pragmatic, and problem-oriented features of cognitive therapy will promote further growth of this method of inpatient treatment.

REFERENCES

Barker, W. A., Scott, J., & Eccleston, D. (1987). The Newcastle chronic depression study: Results of a treatment regime. *International Clinical Psychopharmacology, 2,* 261–272.

Barrett, C. L., & Meyer, R. G. (1993). Cognitive therapy of alcoholism. In J. H. Wright, M. E. Thase, A. T. Beck, & J. W. Ludgate (Eds.), *Cognitive therapy with inpatients: Developing a cognitive milieu* (pp. 313–336). New York: Guilford Press.

Beck, A. T. (1963). Thinking and depression. *Archives of General Psychiatry, 9,* 324–333.

Beck, A. T. (1964). Thinking and depression, 2: Theory and therapy. *Archives of General Psychiatry, 10,* 561–571.

Beck, A. T., Rush, A. J., Shaw, B. F., & Emery, G. (1979). *Cognitive therapy of depression.* New York: Guilford Press.

Bowers, W. A. (1989). Cognitive therapy with inpatients. In A. Freeman, K. M. Simon, L. E. Beutler, & H. Arkowitz (Eds.), *Comprehensive handbook of cognitive therapy* (pp. 583–596). New York: Plenum Press.

Bowers, W. A. (1990). Treatment of depressed inpatients: Cognitive therapy plus medication, relaxation plus medication, and medication alone. *British Journal of Psychiatry, 156,* 73–78.

Bowers, W. A. (1993). Cognitive therapy for eating disorders. In J. H. Wright, M. E. Thase, A. T. Beck, & J. W. Ludgate (Eds.), *Cognitive therapy with inpatients: Developing a cognitive milieu* (pp. 337–356) New York: Guilford Press.

Bowers, W. A., Stuart, S., MacFarlane, M. A., & Gorman, L. (1993). Use of computer-administered cognitive-behavior therapy with depressed inpatients. *Depression, 1,* 294–299.

Casey, D. A., & Grant, R. W. (1993). Cognitive therapy with depressed elderly patients. In J. H. Wright, M. E. Thase, A. T. Beck, & J. W. Ludgate (Eds.), *Cognitive therapy with inpatients: Developing a cognitive milieu* (pp. 295–314). New York: Guilford Press.

Colby, K. M., & Colby, P. M. (1990). *Overcoming depression* [Computer software]. Malibu, CA: Malibu Artificial Intelligence Works.

Covi, L., & Lipman, R. (1987). Cognitive behavioral group psychotherapy combined with imipramine in major depression. *Psychopharmacology Bulletin, 23,* 173–176.

Covi, L., Roth, D., & Lipman, R. S. (1982). Cognitive group psychotherapy of depression: The close-ended group. *American Journal of Psychotherapy, 36*(4), 459–469.

Davis, M. H., & Casey, D. A. (1990). Utilizing cognitive therapy on the short-term psychiatric inpatient unit. *General Hospital Psychiatry, 12,* 170–176.

DeJong, R., Treiber, R., & Henrich, G. (1986). Effectiveness of two psychological treatments for inpatients with severe and chronic depressions. *Cognitive Therapy and Research, 10*(6), 645–663.

Fidaleo, R. A., & Creech, R. (1989). *Cognitive therapy on an affective disorders unit: First 15 months evaluation.* Paper presented at World Congress of Cognitive Therapy, Oxford, England.

Freeman, A., Schrodt, G., Jr., Gilson, M., & Ludgate, J. W. (1993). Group cognitive therapy with inpatients. In J. H. Wright, M. E. Thase, A. T. Beck, & J. W. Ludgate (Eds.), *Cognitive therapy with inpatients: Developing a cognitive milieu* (pp. 121–153). New York: Guilford Press.

Jones, M. (1953). *The therapeutic community: A new treatment method in psychiatry.* New York: Basic Books.

Kleespies, P. M. (1986). Hospital milieu treatment and optimal length of stay. *Hospital and Community Psychiatry, 37,* 509–510.

Ludgate, J. W., Wright, J. H., Bowers, W. A., & Camp, G. F. (1993). Individual cognitive therapy with inpatients. In J. H. Wright, M. E. Thase, A. T. Beck, & J. W. Ludgate (Eds.), *Cognitive therapy with inpatients: Developing a cognitive milieu* (pp. 91–120). New York: Guilford Press.

Maxmen, J. S., Tucker, G. J., & Lebow, M. (1974). *Rational hospital psychiatry.* New York: Brunner/Mazel.

Miller, I. W., Bishop, S. B., Norman, W. H., & Keitner, G. I. (1985). Cognitive-behavioral therapy and pharmacotherapy with chronic, drug-refractory depressed inpatients: A note of optimism. *Behavioral Psychotherapy, 13,* 320–327.

Miller, I. W., Keitner, G. I., Epstein, N. B., Bishop, D. S., & Ryan, C. E. (1993). Inpatient family treatment: General principles. In J. H. Wright, M. E. Thase, A. T. Beck & J. W. Ludgate (Eds.), *Cognitive therapy with inpatients* (pp. 154–175). New York: Guilford Press.

Miller, I. W., Norman, W. H., & Keitner, G. I. (1989). Cognitive-behavioral treatment of depressed inpatients: Six- and twelve-month follow-up. *American Journal of Psychiatry, 146,* 1274–1279.

Miller, I. W., Norman, W. H., & Keitner, G. I. (1990). Treatment response of high cognitive dysfunction depressed inpatients. *Comprehensive Psychiatry, 30,* 62–71.

Miller, I. W., Norman, W. H., Keitner, G. I., Bishop, S. T., & Dow, M. G. (1989). Cognitive behavioral treatment of depressed inpatients. *Behavior Therapy, 20,* 25–47.

Moline, R. A. (1976). Hospital psychiatry in transition: From the therapeutic community toward a rational eclecticism. *Archives of General Psychiatry, 33,* 1234–1238.

Perris, C. (1989). *Cognitive therapy with schizophrenic patients.* New York: Guilford Press.

Perris, C., Rodhe, K., Palm, A., Abelson, M., Hellgren, S., Livja, C., & Soderman, H. (1987). Fully integrated in- and outpatient services in a psychiatric sector: Implementation of a new mode for the care of psychiatric patients favoring continuity of care. In A. Freeman & V. Greenwood (Eds.), *Cognitive therapy: Applications in psychiatric and medical settings* (pp. 117–131). New York: Human Sciences Press.

Rush, A. J. (1988). Cognitive approaches to adherence. In A. J. Frances & R. E. Hales (Eds.), *American Psychiatric Press review of psychiatry* (Vol. 7, pp. 627–642). Washington, DC: American Psychiatric Press.

Schrodt, G. R. (1993). Adolescent inpatient treatment. In J. H. Wright, M. E. Thase, A. T. Beck, & J. W. Ludgate (Eds.), *Cognitive therapy with inpatients: Developing a cognitive milieu* (pp. 273–294). New York: Guilford Press.

Schrodt, G. R., & Wright, J. H. (1987). Inpatient treatment of adolescents. In A. Freeman & V. B. Greenwood (Eds.), *Cognitive therapy: Applications in psychiatric medical settings* (pp. 69–82). New York: Human Sciences Press.

Scott, J. (1988). Cognitive therapy with depressed inpatients. In W. Dryden & P. Trower (Eds.), *Developments in cognitive psychotherapy* (pp. 177–189). London: Sage Publications.

Scott, J. (1992). Chronic depression: Can cognitive therapy succeed when other treatments fail? *Behavioral Psychotherapy, 20,* 25–36.

Scott, J., Byers, S., & Turkington, D. (1993). The chronic patient. In J. H. Wright, M. E. Thase, A. T. Beck, & J. W. Ludgate (Eds.), *Cognitive therapy with inpatients: Developing a cognitive milieu* (pp. 357–392). New York: Guilford Press.

Shaw, B. F. (1980). *Predictors of successful outcome in cognitive therapy: A pilot study.* Paper presented at the First World Congress on Behavioral Therapy, Jerusalem, Israel.

Simoneau, J. F., Konen, A., & Gabris, G. (1992). *Combined cognitive group therapy for depressed inpatients: A specialized therapeutic programme.* Paper presented at the World Congress of Cognitive Therapy, Toronto, Canada.

Thase, M. E. (1994). Cognitive behavior therapy of severe unipolar depression. In L. Grunhaus & J. F. Greden (Eds.), *Severe depressive disorders* (pp. 269–296). Washington, DC: American Psychiatric Press.

Thase, M. E., Bowler, K., & Hardin, T. (1991). Cognitive behavior therapy of endogenous depression: Part 2. Preliminary findings in 16 unmedicated inpatients. *Behavior Therapy, 22,* 469–477.

Thase, M. E., & Wright, J. H. (1991). Cognitive behavior therapy manual for depressed inpatients: A treatment protocol outline. *Behavior Therapy, 22,* 579–595.

Wright, J. H. (1986). Nortriptyline effects on cognition in depression. *Dissertation Abstracts International, 47*(6B), 2667.

Wright, J. H. (1992). Combined cognitive therapy and pharmacotherapy of depression. In A. Freeman & F. M. Dattilio (Eds.), *Comprehensive casebook of cognitive therapy* (pp. 285–292). New York: Plenum Press.

Wright, J. H., & Beck, A. T. (1993). Family cognitive therapy with inpatients. In J. H. Wright, M. E. Thase, A. T. Beck, & J. W. Ludgate (Eds.), *Cognitive therapy with inpatients* (pp. 176–192). New York: Guilford Press.

Wright, J. H. & Davis, M. H. (1993). Hospital psychiatry in transition. In J. H. Wright, M. E. Thase, A. T. Beck, & J. W. Ludgate (Eds.), *Cognitive therapy with inpatients: Developing a cognitive milieu* (pp. 35–60). New York: Guilford Press.

Wright, J. H., Salmon, P., Wright, A. S., & Beck, A. T. (1995a). *Cognitive therapy: A multimedia learning program* [Computer software]. Louisville, KY: MindStreet.

Wright, J. H., Salmon, P., Wright, A. S., and Beck, A. T. (1995b). *Cognitive therapy: A multimedia learning program.* Paper presented at the annual meeting of the American Psychiatric Association, Miami Beach, FL.

Wright, J. H., & Schrodt, G. R. (1989). Combined cognitive therapy and pharmacotherapy. In A. Freeman, K. M. Simon, L. E. Beutler, & H. Arkowitz (Eds.), *Comprehensive handbook of cognitive therapy* (pp. 267–282). New York: Plenum Press.

Wright, J. H., Thase, M. E., & Beck, A. T. (1992). *Inpatient cognitive therapy: Structures, processes, and procedures.* Paper presented at the World Congress of Cognitive Therapy, Toronto, Canada.

Wright, J. H., Thase, M. E., Beck, A. T., & Ludgate, J. W. (Eds.). (1993). *Cognitive therapy with inpatients: Developing a cognitive milieu.* New York: Guilford Press.

Wright, J. H., Thase, M. E., Ludgate, J. W., & Beck, A. T. (1993). The cognitive milieu: Structure and process. In J. H. Wright, M. E. Thase, A. T. Beck, & J. W. Ludgate (Eds.), *Cognitive therapy with inpatients: Developing a cognitive milieu* (pp. 61–90). New York: Guilford Press.

Yalom, I. D. (1983). *Inpatient group psychotherapy.* New York: Basic Books.

Chapter 11

Cognitive Risk Factors in Suicide

Marjorie E. Weishaar

Cognitive therapy research, most notably the work of Aaron T. Beck and his associates, has contributed considerably to our understanding of the clinical risk factors in suicide. Beck's suicide research was a natural outgrowth of his research on unipolar depression and, thus, benefited from his use of clinical samples and the conceptual model generated from his findings on depression.

The model posits that during psychological distress a person's thinking becomes more rigid and biased, judgments become absolute, and the individual's core beliefs about the self, one's personal world, and the future become fixed. Errors in logic, called cognitive distortions, negatively skew perceptions and inferences, and lead to faulty conclusions.

The notion of a cognitive vulnerability to depression rests on the schema concept. Schemas are cognitive structures that hold core beliefs. These beliefs are usually out of a person's awareness until triggered by a life event, at which time they emerge accompanied by strong emotion. In depression, these core beliefs and assumptions reflect themes of loss, deprivation, defeat, and worthlessness. Beck's definition of the cognitive triad—the negative view of the self as a failure, the world as harsh and overwhelming, and the future as hopeless—encapsulates the themes apparent in depressogenic beliefs. Thus, in depression, these beliefs are negative, maladaptive, and idiosyncratic, as are those accompanying personality disorders.

For many, cognitive flexibility returns and negative thinking decreases as depression remits. For others, negative beliefs and assumptions, particularly those established early in life, persist and lead to more chronic depressions and, in some cases, incipient suicidality.

In order to investigate risk factors in suicide, cognitive therapy research used the classification of suicidal behaviors developed by the National Institute of Mental Health (NIMH) task force on suicide prevention (Beck et al., 1973). Cognitive therapy research developed scales to assess suicide ideation and intent and conducted prospective studies with clinical samples. The finding that hopelessness is a key psychological variable in suicide paved the way for the identification of additional cognitive variables and the construction of models to describe and explain the paths to suicide.

ASSESSMENT SCALES

As part of the task force of the National Institute of Mental Health Center for Studies of Suicide Prevention, Beck helped to establish a tripartite classification system to describe suicidal behaviors: suicide ideation, suicide attempt, and completed suicide (Beck et al., 1973). These categories are further subdivided by suicide intent, lethality of attempt, and method of suicide or attempt. Such distinctions aid in investigating differences among groups and reinforce the finding that intent cannot always be inferred by the lethality of an attempt. While some (Goldney, 1981) have found an association between intent and the lethality of an attempt, Beck, Beck, and Kovacs (1975) found that intent and lethality are positively correlated only when the person has an accurate conception of the lethality of his of her chosen method of suicide.

In addition, cognitive therapy research has yielded assessment scales to investigate the nature of suicide. These scales were originally intended for prospective studies, but have clinical utility as well. Beck's use of prospective studies was a major contribution to suicide research, for their longitudinal dimension allowed for the identification of risk factors not due to chance or hindsight bias. The cognitive therapy scales developed are the Beck Depression Inventory (BDI; Beck & Steer, 1987), the Dysfunctional Attitude Scale (DAS; Weissman & Beck, 1978), the Scale for Suicide Ideation (SSI; Beck, Kovacs, & Weissman, 1979), the Suicide Intent Scale (SIS; Beck, Schuyler, & Herman, 1974), the Beck Hopelessness Scale (BHS; Beck, Weissman, Lester, & Trexler, 1974), and the Beck Self-Concept Test (BST; Beck, Steer, Epstein, & Brown, 1990). These scales have been used to identify cognitive risk factors in suicide. Thus, in addition to demographic, proximate, and clinical risk factors, we may consider cognitive precursors to suicide as well.

Beck Depression Inventory

The BDI (Beck & Steer, 1987) is a 21-item, self-report questionnaire that asks respondents to rate, on a 4-point scale, their depressive symptoms over the past week. Among the symptoms assessed are vegetative signs of depression as well as feelings of failure, guilt, and pessimism, and suicidal wishes. Beck and Steer (1987) present the psychometric properties of the BDI.

The BDI has been found to correlate with suicide intent when a broad, heterogeneous sample, such as a general clinic population, is studied. When a homogeneous group, specifically a highly depressed population of suicide ideators, is studied, the BHS (Beck, Weissman, et al., 1974) and the BST (Beck, Steer, et al., 1990) are better indicators of intent.

Dysfunctional Attitude Scale

The DAS (Weissman & Beck, 1978) is a 100-item scale designed to measure the assumptions and beliefs underlying clinical depression. In addition to identifying beliefs that might interact with life stress to produce clinical symptoms (Beck & Weishaar, 1989), the total score is presumed to reflect the overall severity of negative dysfunctional attitudes. The DAS was originally developed to measure specific beliefs and assumptions, but has been used as a general measure of cognitive vulnerability to depression (Shaw & Segal, 1988). Dysfunctional attitudes have been correlated with suicidal ideation in a number of studies (Bonner & Rich, 1987, 1988a; Ellis & Ratliff, 1986; Ranieri et al., 1987).

Scale for Suicide Ideation

The SSI (Beck, Kovacs, & Weissman, 1979; Beck & Steer, 1991) assesses the degree to which someone is presently thinking of suicide. The SSI is a 19-item scale administered in a structured clinical interview, with ratings made on a 3-point scale. It evaluates the intensity of specific attitudes, plans, and behaviors concerning suicide such as the frequency and duration of suicidal thoughts, subjective feelings of control, the relative strengths of the wish to live and the wish to die, deterrents, and the availability of method. Studies of the reliability and validity of the SSI support its usefulness (Beck, Kovacs, & Weissman, 1979). A self-report version of the SSI has been developed (Beck, Steer, & Ranieri, 1988) as has a modified version (Miller, Norman, Bishop, & Dow, 1986).

Suicide Intent Scale

The SIS is a 15-item questionnaire administered in a clinical interview to individuals who have attempted suicide. It assesses the severity of the individual's psychological intent to die at the time of the attempt by investigating relevant aspects of the attempter's behavior before, during, and after the attempt. Items include the degree of isolation and likelihood of being discovered, final acts, conception of lethality and medical rescuability, attitudes toward living and dying, and purpose of the attempt.

The SIS has been consistently validated as a measure of the seriousness of intent to die (Beck, Kovacs, & Weissman, 1975; Beck & Lester, 1976; Beck, Morris, & Beck, 1974; Beck, Schuyler, & Herman, 1974; Minkoff, Bergman, Beck, & Beck, 1973; Silver, Bohnert, Beck, & Marcus, 1971). The Precautions subscale of the SIS was found to be the only predictor, compared to the BDI and the BHS, of eventual suicide among alcoholics (Beck, Steer, & Trexler, 1989; Beck & Steer, 1989). Alcoholic suicide attempters who eventually killed themselves took more precautions against discovery at the time of their index attempt than did those who did not die.

Beck Hopelessness Scale

The BHS (Beck, Weissman, et al., 1974) is a 20-item, true–false, self-report questionnaire. It assesses the level of pessimism or negative view of the future held by the respondent. The psychometric properties of the BHS are presented by Beck, Kovacs, and Weissman (1975). A version of the BHS has been developed for use with children (Hopelessness Scale for Children; Kazdin, Rodgers, & Colbus, 1986). In additon, a rating scale based on clinical interview, the Clinician's Hopelessness Scale (CHS), has been developed (Beck, Weissman, et al., 1974). It appears comparable to the BHS in terms of sensitivity, but lower in specificity for both inpatient and outpatient samples (Beck, Brown, & Steer, 1989). The BHS itself has a high false positive rate (Beck, Brown, Berchick, Stewart, & Steer, 1990) which is reduced by adding the BST to the research protocol. For clinical use, the BHS is the most sensitive indicator of suicide risk; in research, the combination is recommended.

Beck Self-Concept Test

The BST (Beck, Steer, et al., 1990) asks respondents to rate themselves, using a 5-point scale, on each of 25 personal characteristics. A total score reflects overall self-concept. The BST has been found to be of greater specificity than the BHS, but also to decrease the number of true positives.

A number of researchers have identified cognitive characteristics of suicidal individuals beyond Beck's establishment of hopelessness and low self-concept as risk factors. These cognitive differences between suicidal and nonsuicidal people persist even with degree of pathology or level of depression controlled. The cognitive factors in suicide that have been examined are hopelessness, low self-concept, cognitive rigidity, dysfunctional assumptions, attributional style, poor interpersonal problem-solving skills, the view of suicide as a "desirable" solution, and deficient reasons for living. Some of these factors have stronger support than others and, thus, make varying contributions to models of suicidality.

HOPELESSNESS

Hopelessness, or a negative view of the future, is the cognitive feature most consistently related to suicide ideation, intent, and completion in adult (Beck, Brown, et al., 1990; Beck, Steer, Kovacs, & Garrison, 1985; Fawcett et al., 1987; Goldney, 1981; Wetzel, 1976) and child (Asarnow & Guthrie, 1989; Carlson & Cantwell, 1982; Kazdin, French, Unis, Esveldt-Dawson, & Sherrick, 1983) clinical populations. In terms of *suicide ideation,* Beck, Kovacs, and Weissman (1975) found hopelessness to be a better indicator of current suicide ideation among suicide attempters than depression. Also,

Nekanda-Trepka, Bishop, and Blackburn (1983) found an association between hopelessness and increased suicidal wishes among psychiatric outpatients.

Hopelessness has been found to be more strongly related to *suicide intent* than is depression per se among clinical samples of suicide ideators (Beck, Kovacs, & Weissman, 1975; Bedrosian & Beck, 1979; Wetzel, Margulies, Davis, & Karam, 1980) and suicide attempters (Dyer & Kreitman, 1984; Goldney, 1981; Wetzel, 1976). In a study of depressed and nondepressed (schizophrenic) patients, those who had high levels of hopelessness, even in the absense of depression, had high levels of suicide intent (Minkoff et al., 1973). Beck, Kovacs, and Weissman (1975) report that hopelessness mediates the relationship between depression and suicidal intent among suicide attempters.

Among drug abusers, hopelessness has been found more strongly associated with suicide intent than is depression (Emery, Steer, & Beck, 1981) or drug use per se (Weissman, Beck, & Kovacs, 1979). However, the role of hopelessness in the relationship between alcoholism and suicide attempts is less clear. Although it was thought to play a mediating role (Beck, Weissman, & Kovacs, 1976), it has not been found predictive of eventual suicide in alcoholic suicide attempters (Beck, Steer, & Trexler, 1989). In this sample, only the Precautions subscale of the SIS, compared to the BDI and the BHS, predicted suicide over a 5- to 10-year period.

Prospective studies have found hopelessness to be predictive of eventual suicide in adults (Beck et al., 1985; Beck, Brown, et al., 1990; Drake & Cotton, 1986; Fawcett et al., 1987). Fawcett et al. (1987) identified hopelessness, loss of pleasure or interest, and mood fluctuations as variables discriminating those who committed suicide from those who didn't. Longitudinal studies by Beck and his associates found that a score of 9 or more on the BHS predicted suicide over a 10-year period for both patients hospitalized with suicide ideation (Beck et al., 1985; Beck, Brown, & Steer, 1989) and psychiatric outpatients (Beck et al., 1990). In the sample of outpatients, the BHS yielded a high percentage of false positives (59%), so hopelessness is more accurately conceptualized as a risk factor than as a predictor of suicide. Nevertheless, in clinical decision making, such overinclusiveness is preferable to missing some true positives.

Hopelessness may be conceptualized as a relatively stable schema incorporating negative expectations. During psychiatric distress, such as a depressive episode, hopelessness increases, posing an acute risk to suicide. For most, hopelessness decreases as the depression remits. Yet, high hopelessness in one episode is predictive of high hopelessness in subsequent episodes (Beck, 1988; Beck, Brown, et al., 1990). For other individuals, hopelessness is more chronic and suicide becomes a more constant threat (Beck, 1987). Thus, hopelessness can be conceived as both an acute and chronic risk factor in suicide.

Among adolescents and in nonclinical samples, the relationship of hopelessness to suicide ideation and intent is less clear. While a number of researchers have found that hopelessness increases with severity of suicidal ideation in child and adolescent psychiatric patients (Asarnow & Guthrie, 1989; Brent, Kolko, Goldstein, Allan, & Brown, 1989; Carlson & Cantwell, 1982; Kazdin et al., 1983; Rich, Kirkpatrick-Smith, Bonner, & Jans, 1992; Spirito, Williams, Stark, & Hart, 1988), others have found that this relationship drops to a nonsignificant level when depression is partialed out (Asarnow, Carlson, & Guthrie, 1987).

Gender differences may be important in adolescents, for Cole (1989) found that, after controlling for depression, hopelessness had a modest correlation with suicidal behavior for girls, but not for boys.

In contrast, Rotheram-Borus and Trautman (1988, p. 703) argue that "hopelessness is not a meaningful predictor of suicide intent for girls and young women." They found that, among minority adolescent girls, hopelessness did not differentiate suicide attempters from psychiatrically disturbed nonattempters. In this study, although depression and hopelessness were highly correlated, neither predicted suicide intent. Similar findings were achieved by Dyer and Kreitman (1984) among females 15 to 34 years old.

So different are the findings on adolescents that most youthful suicide attempters do not even have high intent (Brent, 1987; Hawton, Osborn, O'Grady, & Cole, 1982). When suicide intent is present, however, it is an indication of the need for hospitalization (Brent & Kolko, 1990).

Results are similarly equivocal in nonclinical samples. Cole (1989) and Rudd (1990) both found depression to be more related to suicide ideation and self-reported behavior than was hopelessness in adolescent groups. Rich et al. (1992) found that both depression and hopelessness, along with substance abuse and few reasons for living, were predictive of suicidal ideation in high school students.

In a college sample of suicide ideators, Clum and his associates (Clum, Patsiokas, & Luscomb, 1979; Schotte & Clum, 1982) found that depression was the best predictor of suicide intent at low levels of suicide ideation. Hopelessness was the best predictor of suicide intent at high levels of suicide ideation. So, the relationship between hopelessness and intent in nonclinical, adolescent samples may be different at differing levels of suicide ideation.

SELF-CONCEPT

Self-concept has been identified in adults as an indicator of suicide risk independent of hopelessness (Beck, Steer et al., 1990b; Beck & Stewart, 1989; Wetzel & Reich, 1989). Among children as well, negative expectations of oneself as well as negative views of the future are related to depression and to suicide intent (Kazdin et al., 1983). In terms of the cognitive model of depression, negative self-concept or low self-esteem represents one component of the cognitive triad: the negative view of the self. Hopelessness, the negative view of the future, is another component of the triad.

COGNITIVE DISTORTIONS AND DYSFUNCTIONAL ASSUMPTIONS

Cognitive Distortions

Some evidence indicates that particular cognitive distortions are associated with suicidal ideation. For example, Prezant and Neimeyer (1988) found, among moderately depressed persons, that once the level of depression was controlled for selective abstraction and overgeneralization emerged as predictors of suicide ideation. Selective abstraction is a perceptual error by which an individual attends to only a portion of relevant information. Overgeneralization is an error of inference in which a person abstracts a general rule from a single event and applies it to both related and unrelated events. Prezant and Neimeyer conclude that the combination of cognitive distortions and depressive symptomotology is a superior predictor of suicidality over self-reported level of depression alone.

Cognitive Rigidity

In addition to selective abstraction and overgeneralization, the cognitive distortion of dichotomous or all-or-nothing thinking has been found characteristic of suicidal persons (Neuringer, 1961, 1967, 1968; Neuringer & Lettieri, 1971). Dichotomous thinking is viewed as a form of cognitive rigidity and has been incorporated into that category in more recent research on problem solving. It is discussed below.

Dysfunctional Assumptions

Some studies have endeavored to ascertain whether particular dysfunctional assumptions lead to suicidal thinking. Ellis and Ratliff (1986) compared suicide attempters to equally depressed nonsuicidal patients using a battery of cognitive measures. They found that the suicidal patients scored higher than the nonsuicidal patients in terms of irrational beliefs, hopelessness, and depressogenic attitudes. Bonner and Rich (1987) found dysfunctional assumptions to play an important role in predicting suicide ideation in college students. Lastly, Ranieri et al. (1987) found overall severity of dysfunctional assumptions to be positively correlated with suicidal ideation in psychiatric inpatients, even after hopelessness and depression were controlled for. In addition, perfectionistic attitudes toward the self and sensitivity to social criticism accounted for independent variance in suicide ideation.

Additional work by Beck, Steer, and Brown (1993) with psychiatric outpatients attempted to determine whether specific sets of dysfunctional attitudes distinguished suicide ideators from nonideators, and whether certain dysfunctional attitudes were asssociated with the severity of suicidal ideation. In this sample, the overall severity of dysfunctional attitudes as well as four sets of specific attitudes—feeling vulnerable to becoming depressed, accepting other people's expectations, feeling that it is important to impress others, and being sensitive to the opinions of others—were positively associated with being a suicide ideator. However, these attitudes did not discriminate ideators from nonideators when age, sex, a clinical diagnosis of a primary mood or panic disorder, comorbidity, presence of a personality disorder, history of past suicide attempt, BDI score, BHS score, and BST score were controlled for. History of past suicide attempt and hopelessness were the two most important variables for identifying suicide ideators. Hopelessness superimposed on dysfunctional attitudes may increase one's wish to die.

In addition to the work of Ranieri et al. (1987), Hewitt, Flett, and Turnbull-Donovan (1992) found a type of perfectionism associated with suicidal threat or impulses, as measured by the Minnesota Multiphasic Personality Inventory (MMPI). The authors examined three types of perfectionism—expectations of self (self-oriented), expectations of others (other-oriented), and expectations that others hold for the person (socially prescribed perfectionism)—and their possible relationships to suicide ideation in psychiatric inpatients. Only socially prescribed perfectionism predicted variance in suicide ideation scores that was not accounted for by depression or hopelessness. This finding indicates that the tendency to perceive others as holding unrealistic expectations for oneself is associated with suicide ideation. This may relate to the third aspect of Beck's cognitive triad: that the world holds exorbitant demands for the individual.

ATTRIBUTIONAL STYLE

Attributional style has been investigated in suicide research because of its demonstrated relationship to depression (Abramson, Metalsky, & Alloy, 1989). According to the model, depressed individuals are more likely than nondepressed persons to attribute causality of negative events to internal, stable, and global factors. Positive events would be attributued to external, unstable, and specific causes. There is evidence that life events precipitate many suicide attempts, particularly among adolescents (Spirito, Overholser, & Stark, 1989), alcoholics (Heikkinen, Aro, & Lonnqvist, 1993), and those with personality disorders (Lester, Beck, & Steer, 1989). Thus, the study of attributional style may illuminate the manner in which suicidal persons evaluate events.

The findings on the role of attributional style in suicide are mixed.

Rotheram-Borus, Trautman, Dopkins, and Shrout (1990) found, in a study of suicide-attempting and non-suicide-attempting female minority adolescents, that the adolescent suicide attempters did not fit the pattern observed in depressed adults. Rather, the adolescent attempters perceived positive events as due to one's own intiative, stable across time, and global. Adolescent attempters reported significantly fewer dysfunctional attributions in positive situations than did the psychiatrically disturbed nonattempters.

Spirito, Overholser, and Hart (1991) also compared adolescent suicide attempters with a sample of psychiatrically hospitalized adolescents. Differences in attributional style by diagnostic groups were not found. However, adolescent patients on welfare were more likely than those not on welfare to attribute negative events to global causes and positive events to specific causes. The authors conclude that the consistent lack of relationships between attributional style and suicide attempts indicates that a specific attributional style does not exist among adolescent attempters.

Results more consistent with the pattern in depressed adults were obtained by Priester and Clum (1992), who studied the relationship of attributional style to depression, hopelessness, and suicide ideation in college students. A failing grade on an exam was the negative event imposed on students who had pre- and postexam measures taken on all three criteria. It was found that the negative–stable attributional style was related to all criteria: A tendency to attribute exam failue to stable causes was associated with higher levels of depression, hopelessness, and suicidal ideation. Those who attributed positive events (i.e., good grades) to internal causes were less likely to feel depressed, hopeless, or suicidal. It was the interaction between a poor exam score and the negative–stable attributional style that was key. Poor performance alone did not relate to suicidal ideation.

PROBLEM-SOLVING DEFICITS

Much of the recent research on cognitive risk factors in suicide has focused on the poor problem-solving skills of suicide ideators and attempters. Problem-solving deficits have been found to be characteristic of suicidal children (Asarnow et al., 1987; Orbach, Rosenheim, & Hary, 1987), adolescents (Curry, Miller, Waugh, & Anderson, 1992; Levenson & Neuringer, 1971; Rotheram-Borus et al., 1990), and adults (Linehan, Camper, Chiles, Strosahl, & Shearin, 1987; Schotte & Clum, 1987), and these difficulties become more profound as problems increase in interpersonal content (McLeavey, Daly, Murray, O'Riodan, & Taylor, 1987).

Suicidal children, adolescents, and adults have limited abilities to find solutions to impersonal tasks, for they have difficulty producing new ideas, identifying solutions (Orbach et al., 1987; Patsiokas, Clum, & Luscomb, 1979), and deliberating alternatives (Cohen-Sandler & Berman, 1982; Levenson, 1974). Suicidal adolescents were found to persist with ineffective solutions even when a more effective strategy was offered to them (Levenson & Neuringer, 1971). Such stereotyped responsivity and cognitive rigidity help explain how repeated suicide attempts get established as a behavioral outcome.

Interpersonal problem solving has greater clinical relevance to the study of suicide for several reasons. First, suicide attempters report greater difficulty with interpersonal problems than do suicide ideators, nonsuicidal psychiatric patients, and general population controls (Linehan, Chiles, Egan, Devine, & Laffaw, 1986). Second, there is evidence that suicide ideators (Mraz & Runco, 1994) and attempters (Rotheram-Borus et al., 1990) perceive more numerous problems but generate fewer solutions than do patient and non-patient controls. Third, suicide attempters, compared to nonsuicidal patients and normal controls, are less likely to engage in interpersonal problem solving when it is called for. In one of the few studies of the coping strategies of suicidal children, Asarnow et al. (1987) found them less likely than nonsuicidal children to use instrumental problem solving in the face of stressful life events.

Lack of active problem solving has also been noted in adult suicide attempters as compared to suicide ideators and nonsuicidal medical patients (Linehan et al., 1987). The suicide attempters waited for problems to resolve or found someone else to solve the problems. This finding, however, is contradicted by the findings of Orbach, Bar-Joseph, and Dror (1990) who compared the problem-solving styles of adult suicide ideators, suicide attempters, and nonsuicidal psychiatric patients. Both the suicide attempters and the nonsuicidal patients generated more active solutions than did the suicide ideators. The clinical implication is that active problem solving needs to be channeled in a positive direction.

Avoidance, or lack of engagement in problem solving, has also been noted in adolescent suicide attempters. Rotheram-Borus et al. (1990) found that suicide-attempting, female, minority adolescents were more likely to use wishful thinking under stress than were normal controls. Spirito et al. (1989) found that suicidal adolescents used social withdrawal more frequently than did psychiatric and normal controls. It appears that, like the control groups, the suicidal adolescents used a variety of coping strategies, but at some point they gave up and withdrew from others.

The above studies of "coping style" address whether or not suicidal individuals attempt to solve problems, not how well they do. Some people cope by avoiding; others cope by trying to solve their problems. Schotte and Clum (1987) argue that, among other deficits, suicidal patients lack an appropriate orientation toward problem solving. They have trouble engaging in problem solving and have difficulty accepting problems as a normal part of life.

Coping style has been systematically investigated by Josepho and Plutchik (1994). They define it as "the methods people use to handle particular classes of emotional conflicts" (p. 50). They compared the coping styles of hospitalized suicide attempters with those of nonsuicidal patients. Suppression, the avoidance of the person or problem that one believes created the situation, had the strongest positive relationship to suicidality. It amplifies suicide risk. Conversely, replacement, the effort to improve stressful situations or limitations in oneself, had the strongest negative association with suicide risk. Increased use of suppression and decreased use of replacement were asssociated with increased risk of suicidal behavior.

Once suicidal individuals engage in interpersonal problem solving, the same deficits accompanying impersonal problem solving emerge, but are magnified (McLeavey et al., 1987). McLeavey et al. (1987) found that, compared to nonsuicidal psychiatric patients and nonpatient controls, suicide attempters were less able to orient themselves to a goal and conceptualize a means of moving toward it. They were less able to generate alternatives, anticipate consequences of various solutions, and deal with actual problems in their own lives.

Schotte and Clum (1987) similarly found that hospitalized suicide ideators were able to generate fewer than half as many potential solutions to interpersonal problems selected from their own lives as were depressed control subjects. In addition, suicide ideators tended to focus on the potential negative consequences of implementing any solutions. This "yes, but . . . " reaction to potential solutions may be an important characteristic of suicidal thinking (Priester & Clum, 1993b).

Orbach et al. (1990) compared the problem-solving styles of adult suicide ideators, suicide attempters, and nonsuicidal psychiatric patients. The solutions offered by the suicidal patients to interpersonal dilemmas showed less versatility, less relevance, more avoidance, more negative affect, and less reference to the future than did the solutions of nonsuicidal patients. Orbach and his associates (Orbach et al., 1987) similarly found that suicidal children were less able than medically ill and normal children to generate alternatives to life-and-death dilemmas in stories. Moreover, they were the only group to show an interaction between such cognitive rigidity and an attraction to death.

The research literature on problem solving has recently encompassed the notion of *perceived,* rather than actual, problem-solving ability (Bonner & Rich, 1988b; Dixon, Heppner, & Anderson, 1991; Rudd, Rajab, & Dahm, 1994). Bonner and Rich (1988b) and Dixon et al. (1991) found that both life stress and self-appraised problem-solving skills predicted hopelessness and suicide ideation in college students. However, Priester and Clum (1993a) found that college students who rated their problem-solving lower at time 1 were more vulnerable to the stress of a low grade and showed higher levels of depression and hopelessness, but *not* suicidal ideation, at time 2 than students with higher self-appraisal. Rudd et al. (1994) also found problem-solving appraisal more predictive of hopelessness than suicide ideation in a clinical sample.

Problem-solving self-appraisal is more a measure of self-efficacy than of problem-solving ability (Bonner & Rich, 1988b). Indeed, a person's confidence in his or her ability to solve problems may be quite different from actual performance, particularly among depressed persons. The construct needs to be clarified: Is it a measure of self-efficacy or of outcome expectations? In addition, it is not clear whether problem-solving ability, self-appraisal, or some combination is most important in predicting hopelessness. It could also be argued that hopelessness causes low problem-solving appraisal (Bonner & Rich, 1988b). Thus, the theoretical and clincal significances of the observed relationship among problem-solving skills, problem-solving appraisal, and hopelessness need to be established.

SUICIDE AS A "DESIRABLE" SOLUTION

In *Cognitive Therapy of Depression* (Beck, Rush, Shaw, & Emery, 1979), Beck observes that suicidal individuals have a unique cognitive deficit in solving interpersonal problems: When their usual strategies fail, they become paralyzed and view suicide as a way out. He describes the attraction to suicide in these cases as an "opiate."

Suicidal persons may have difficulty tolerating the anxiety of problem solving. Suicidal children, for example, have been found less able than non-suicidal children to generate self-comforting statements in the face of stresful life events (Asarnow et al., 1987).

Linehan et al. (1987) report that the level of expectancy that suicide can solve one's problems predicts higher suicide intent. In addition, Strosahl, Chiles, and Linehan (1992) found, among parasuicides with high intent to die, a positive relationship between survival/coping beliefs and suicide intent. As intent increases, the person becomes more focused on the problem-solving effects of suicide.

Orbach et al. (1987) found evidence of the view of suicide as a desirable solution among children. In comparing suicidal children, medically ill children, and normal children, they found that the interaction between the inability to generate solutions to life-and-death dilemmas in stories and an attraction to death was unique to suicidal children. There was no such interaction for either the chronically ill or normal children, who may not have been adept at problem solving, but weren't attracted to suicide.

Thus, suicide may appear as a solution when a person is unable to shift to a new strategy, is incapable of tolerating the anxiety of problem solving, or has faulty assumptions about suicide's effectiveness to solve problems.

REASONS FOR LIVING

In contrast to hopelessness is the notion of adaptive beliefs or positive expectations that may serve to keep people alive or buffer them from life events.

The role of positive attitudes in preventing suicide has been explored by a number of researchers, most notably Linehan and her colleagues (Linehan, Goodstein, Nielson, & Chiles, 1983; Strosahl et al., 1992; Strosahl, Linehan, & Chiles, 1983). They take the point of view that suicidal people lack positive expectations rather than, or in addition to, having negative ones. The Reasons for Living Inventory (RFLI; Linehan et al., 1983a) was devised to assess the influence of adaptive or coping beliefs on suicidal behavior. Additionally, BHS is a global measure of pessimism; it is not suicide specific. The RFLI, in contrast, identifies suicide-specific beliefs. As one becomes increasingly suicidal, cognitions may shift from generalized hopelessness to appraisals of suicide as a solution. For these reasons, the RFLI has been used to study suicidal cognitions. Indeed, a study of inpatients and normal controls found RFLI scores to be inversely related to suicide ideation and previous suicide attempts (Linehan et al., 1983). Suicidal individuals were significantly less likely to endorse reasons to live. Recent life stress and pathology in general did not identify those who had few reasons to live.

Six sets of reasons for living distinguished nonsuicidal individuals from suicidal ones: (1) survival and coping beliefs, (2) responsibility to family, (3) child-centered concerns, (4) fear of suicide, (5) fear of social disapproval, and (6) moral objections to suicide. Survival and Coping Beliefs include such items as "I have future plans I am looking forward to carrying out" and "I believe I can learn to adjust or cope with my problems." Linehan et al. (1983) describe this set of beliefs as combining beliefs that are the converse of some beliefs on the BHS with beliefs of self-efficacy and beliefs supporting the value of life. Survival and Coping Beliefs is the subset of the RFLI that has received the most attention, as will be discussed below.

Using a sample of college students, Westefeld, Cardin, and Deaton (1992) developed the College Student Reasons for Living Inventory (CSRFLI). Factor analysis yielded six factors, five of which are the same identified by Linehan et al. (1983) with the addition of "friends" to the factor Responsibility to Family and Friends. Among college students, the Child-Related Concern was, understandably, not present. Instead, the factor College and Future-Related Concerns was unique to this group.

Research has investigated the role of coping beliefs in suicidal ideation, intent, and behavior. Specifically, attention has been devoted to establishing whether the BHS and the RFLI measure different constructs (Dyck, 1991; Strosahl et al., 1983) and how hopelessness and reasons for living differentially influence suicidal ideation and behavior at various levels of intent (Strosahl et al., 1992) and in different populations (Cole, 1989; Connell & Meyer, 1991; Rich et al., 1992). In several studies, Linehan and her associates (Linehan et al., 1983; Strosahl et al., 1992; Strosahl et al., 1983) established the Survival and Coping Beliefs subscale of the RFLI as a useful predictor of suicide intent. Strosahl et al. (1983) demonstrated that Survival and Coping Beliefs could discriminate among levels of suicide intent even among patients with significant levels of hopelessness. A further study of hospitalized parasuicides (Strosahl et al., 1992) identified Survival and Coping Beliefs, hopelessness, and depression as the most important predictors of suicide intent. Survival and Coping Beliefs emerged as the single best predictor of suicide intent for parasuicides. Hopelessness achieved a significant predictor effect only when analyzed apart from Survival and Coping Beliefs, but even then not among repeat parasuicides.

The findings on both repeat parasuicides and a subsample of high-intent parasuicides in this study support the idea that suicide as a solution becomes fixed in a self-limiting response repertoire. Lester, Beck, and Narrett (1978) found that suicide intent increases with successive attempts, and among these high-intent parasuicidal patients there was a positive association between Survival and Coping Beliefs and intent. Theoretically, this could reflect the focus on suicide as a solution, however maladaptive. It could also indicate that as one becomes more suicidal, cognitions shift from general hopelessness to suicide-specific beliefs. Moreover, the presence of a set of suicidal expectancies may establish a "readiness to respond" (Strosahl et al., 1992, p. 371) to negative life events, making what appears to be impulsive acts actually based in a highly specific belief system.

Social Desirability, Hopelessness, and Coping

One of the debates to emerge from the identification of cognitive risk factors in suicide revolves around the concept of social desirability or the tendency to attribute socially desirable qualities to oneself and reject socially undesirable values.

Linehan and her associates (Linehan & Nielson, 1981, 1983; Strosahl, Linehan, & Chiles, 1984) found that the BHS negatively correlated with the Edwards Social Desirability Scale (ESD; Edwards, 1970) and, therefore, questioned the predictive validity of the BHS. It was argued that people might not fully divulge the extent of their hopelessness, suicidal ideation, and past suicidal behavior and thus bias results.

In fact, social desirability was found to play a greater role in the responses of the general population than among psychiatric patients (Strosahl et al., 1984). Cole (1988), in a study of college students, also found that social desirability influenced the relationship between hopelessness and parasuicide only among those who were not seeking psychological treatment. For students seeking treatment, hopelessness was related to parasuicide even controlling for depression and social desirability. Cole's study concluded that both the nature of the sample and the manner in which social desirability is operationalized affect the results.

In studies of nonclinical groups, social desirability has come to be defined as a reflection of good social and psychological adjustment (Strosahl et al., 1984; Connell & Meyer, 1991). This has led to some confusion over what the construct measures: Is it an attempt to portray oneself in the most favorable light or is it a self-report measure of general capability? While the theoretical meaning of social desirability remains unclear, the clinical implication is that one should interpret self-reports of hopelessness with the possibility of social desirability in mind.

Finally, Holden, Mendonca, and Serin (1989) examined the relationships among suicide, hopelessness, and a two-factor model of social desirability. One factor of social desirability contained items reflecting focused and realistic thinking, social integration, self-confidence, and hardiness. The other factor contained items relating to considerateness, social sensitivity, and tolerance. The authors define hopelessness as pessimistic cognitions about the future and negative social desirability as a low sense of self-efficacy and coping. In two studies of clinical and nonclinical groups, Holden et al. (1989) found that both hopelessness and a component of social desirability representing a general sense of capability are important for the prediction of suicidal behavior. There is an interaction in which this general sense of capability moderates the relationship between hopelessness and suicidality. Lack of self-efficacy and pessimistic expectations are both associated with suicide, but self-capability reduces the link between hopelessness and suicide. Thus, it is argued that different sets of cognitions are relevant for understanding suicide.

MODELS OF SUICIDAL BEHAVIOR

Models that integrate cognitive risk factors for suicide have been proposed and tested in various samples. These models are based primarily of the stress–vulnerability format in which life stressors imposed on a set of cognitive risk factors result in suicidal behavior. Thus, the risk factors pose a vulnerability to suicide that becomes apparent under adverse conditions.

Bonner and Rich constructed (Bonner & Rich, 1987) and tested (Rich & Bonner, 1987) a model based on a college student sample in which cognitive distortions, social–emotional alienation, and deficient reasons for living predispose an individual to suicide ideation. Once suicide ideation is elicited, the person is at risk for increased alienation, depression, and stress. At this point, hopelessness can develop which can lead to overt suicidal behavior. A linear combination of social–emotional alienation, cognitive distortions, deficient adaptive resources, hopelessness, and life stress was found to account for both past suicidal behavior (Bonner & Rich, 1987) and current suicidal ideation (Rich & Bonner, 1987). A further test of the interaction of the variables (Bonner & Rich, 1988a) concluded that any or all of the factors may increase the risk for suicide ideation; they are independent risk factors.

Clum and his colleagues (Clum et al., 1979; Schotte & Clum, 1982) developed models that focus on the relationship between problem-solving deficits and hopelessness. They proposed that the combination of life stress and poor problem-solving ability leads to hopelessness which, in turn, discourages the person from trying to solve problems (Clum et al., 1979). A test of this model with suicidal patients, however, found no relationship between hopelessness and levels of interpersonal problem-solving skill (Schotte & Clum, 1987). This finding supports the hypothesis that they are independent risk factor in suicide.

The relationships among problem-solving skills, depression, and suicide have been examined in longitudinal work. Schotte, Cools, and Payvar (1990) followed the course of hospitalized suicide ideators and found that problem-solving ability was not a trait, but fluctuated with levels of depression, state anxiety, hopelessness, and suicide intent. This suggests that problem-solving deficits are concomitant to, rather than the cause of, depression, hopelessness, and suicide intent.

Schotte et al. (1990) called into question the notion that problem-solving deficits are antecedents of depression, hopelessness, and suicidal behavior. So, Priester and Clum (1993b) assessed the role of problem-solving deficits prior to a stressor in the eventual development of these criteria. The results generally support the hypothesis that problem-solving deficits alone and in interaction with levels of stress predict depression, hopelessness, and suicide ideation, but not all aspects of problem solving were important in predicting all criteria. The pattern of predictive relationships was most similar for hopelessness and suicide ideation, but different for symptoms of depression. Specifically, individuals who could think of only negative consequences for their identified solutions became hopeless and suicidal when stressed by a life event. This attitude of rejecting solutions prevents them from implementing solutions. It was not, however, related to depression. Subjects who became depressed and hopeless were those less able to generate relevant solutions to problems.

There are several implications of these findings: (1) The finding that different problem-solving variables were predicitve of hopelessness, suicide ideation, and depression suggests that it is important to measure all aspects of problem solving, for specific deficits may lead to specific dysfunctions; (2) the finding that, if profound enough, problem-solving deficits alone can lead to suicide ideation suggests that they are more trait-like than state-like for this sample; and (3) the tendency to focus on negative consequences was associated with both hopelessness and suicide ideation. This same variable did not covary with mood in the Schotte et al. (1990) study. So, it may be a good measure of enduring problem-solving deficits.

Beck's research (Beck, 1987; Lester et al., 1989) on suicide ideation and repeat attempters also provides information on the state- or trait-like aspects of problem-solving deficits. The suicide ideators in this study were depressed patients hospitalized for suicide ideation. When depressed, they were also hopeless and had negative self-concepts and problem-solving deficits. These features resolved when the depression remitted. For them, problem-solving deficits were state dependent.

In contrast, the suicide attempters were characterized by personality disorders, alcoholism, and antisocial behavior. Their hopelessness and low self-concepts were chronic and reinforced by society. This group displayed cognitive rigidity, impulsivity, and poor problem-solving deficits that persisted between suicidal episodes (Lester et al., 1989) and were trait-like. At the time of suicidal crises, both groups had low self-concepts, elevated levels of hopelessness, and poor interpersonal problem-solving skills, but from different "causes."

CLINICAL PRESENTATION OF SUICIDAL CLIENTS

The cognitive factors investigated help form a clinical picture of suicidal clients. Persons at high risk for suicide display high levels of hopelessness with each depressive episode or, especially in the case of clients with personality disorders, whenever a life event precipitates an interpersonal crisis. Selective abstraction would allow the individual to see only part of the picture, overgeneralization would lead to faulty and broad conclusions, and dichotomous thinking would lead to extreme emotions and behavior. Incidentally, one can easily imagine the influence alcohol would have on this cognitive processing. Such cognitive distortions serve to maintain the person's depressogenic or dysfunctional assumptions by screening out other, relevant information. The inability to generate alternative perspectives or solutions to problems leads the client to a mental impasse. Suicide, particularly if it has been previously attempted, appears as a way out of this gridlock, and becomes a stereotyped response. Suicide ideation that is frequent or continuous, over which the individual feels little control, and that provides some solace is indication of high risk.

In assessing for suicide risk, it is necessary to ascertain how the client has previously responded to stressful life events. What types of self-control strategies or coping skills has the client employed? These might include distraction from persistent suicide ideation, disputing suicidal ideas, utilizing social supports, engaging in alternative behaviors, and taking a problem-solving stance. Someone at risk of suicide might feel incapable of or hostile towards problem solving and avoid it altogether. Instead, the client might demonstate an attraction to death as a way of solving problems.

Finally, the cognitive rigidity apparent in suicidal clients may be accompanied by difficulty tolerating the process of problem solving. Certainly, a challenge to the therapist is to engage the patient in this process and create some disequilibrium in a fixed set of beliefs while encouraging and teaching the patient to withhold judgment until an alternative solution can safely be chosen.

CONCLUSION

Cognitive characteristics of suicidal individuals may be conceptualized as both acute and chronic risk factors in the development of suicidal behavior.

There is strong support for the independent roles of hopelessness, problem-solving deficits, and few reasons for living in the paths to suicide. The relationships among these cognitive features may vary by level of suicide ideation and intent, with other factors, such as stressful life events, posing a more proximate risk.

Identification of cognitive factors in suicide can lead to therapeutic interventions to reduce suicide risk. For example, both cognitive therapy (Rush, Beck, Kovacs, Weissenburger, & Hollon, 1982) and problem-solving training (Lerner & Clum, 1990; Salkovskis, Atha, & Storer, 1990) have been found to reduce hopelessness and, in one study (Salkovskis et al., 1990), suicide ideation and short-term frequency of attempts. In addition, the importance of coping beliefs in ameliorating suicide risk has been noted. Such a finding lends further support to interventions that reduce cognitive distortions and bolster more adaptive ways of thinking. Therapeutic strategies aimed at increasing cognitive flexibility, toleration of anxiety in interpersonal conflicts, and suspension of judgment until a solution has been tested would, presumably, reduce the use of suicide as a response to seemingly intolerable situations.

REFERENCES

Abramson, L. Y., Metalsky, G. I., & Alloy, L. B. (1989). Hopelessness depression: A theory-based subtype of depression. *Psychological Review, 96*(2), 358–372.

Asarnow, J. R., Carlson, G. A., & Guthrie, D. (1987). Coping strategies, self-perceptions, hopelessness, and perceived family environments in depressed and suicidal children. *Journal of Consulting and Clinical Psychology, 55,* 361–366.

Asarnow, J. R., & Guthrie, D. (1989). Suicidal behavior, depression, and hopelessness in child psychiatric inpatients: A replication and extension. *Journal of Clinical Child Psychology, 18,* 129–136.

Beck, A. T. (1987, November). *Cognitive approaches to hopelessness and suicide.* Paper presented at the annual meeting of the Association for Advancement of Behavior Therapy, Boston.

Beck, A. T. (1988). *Stability of hopelessness scale scores over repeated admissions.* Unpublished manuscript, Center for Cognitive Therapy, Philadelphia.

Beck, A. T., Beck, R. W., & Kovacs, M. (1975). Classification of suicidal behaviors: I. Quantifying intent and medical lethality. *American Journal of Psychiatry, 132,* 285–287.

Beck, A. T., Brown, G., Berchick, R. J., Stewart, B. L., & Steer, R. A. (1990). Relationship between hopelessness and ultimate suicide: A replication with psychiatric outpatients. *American Journal of Psychiatry, 147*(2), 190–195.

Beck, A. T., Brown, G., & Steer, R. A. (1989). Prediction of eventual suicide in psychiatric inpatients by clinical ratings of hopelessness. *Journal of Consulting and Clinical Psychology, 57*(2), 309–310.

Beck, A. T., Davis, J. H., Frederick, C. J., Perlin, S., Pokorny, A. D., Schulman, R. E., Seiden, R. H., & Wittlin, B. J. (1973) Classification and nomenclature. In H. C. P. Resnik & B. C. Hathorne (Eds.), *Suicide prevention in the seventies* (DHEW Publication No. HSM 72-9054, pp. 7–12). Washington, DC: U.S. Government Printing Office.

Beck, A. T., Kovacs, M., & Weissman, A. (1975). Hopelessness and suicidal behavior: An overview. *Journal of the American Medical Association, 234*(11), 1146–1149.

Beck, A. T., Kovacs, M., & Weissman, A. (1979). Assessment of suicidal intention: The Scale for Suicide Ideation. *Journal of Consulting and Clinical Psychology, 47*(2), 343–352.

Beck, A. T., & Lester, D. (1976). Components of suicidal intent in completed and attempted suicides. *Journal of Psychology, 92,* 35–38.

Beck, A. T., Rush, A. J., Shaw, B. F., & Emery, G. (1979). *Cognitive therapy of depression.* New York: Guilford Press.

Beck, A. T., Schuyler, D., & Herman, I. (1974). Development of suicidal intent scales. In A. T. Beck, H. C. P. Resnik, & D. Lettieri (Eds.), *The prediction of suicide* (pp. 45–56). Bowie, MD: Charles Press.

Beck, A. T., & Steer, R. A. (1987). *Manual for the revised Beck Depression Inventory.* San Antonio, TX: Psychological Corporation.

Beck, A. T., & Steer, R. A. (1989). Clinical predictors of eventual suicide: A 5- to 10-year prospective study of suicide attempters. *Journal of Affective Disorders, 17,* 203–209.

Beck, A. T., & Steer, R. A. (1991). *Manual for the Beck Scale for Suicide Ideation.* San Antonio, TX: Psychological Corporation.

Beck, A. T., Steer, R. A., & Brown, G. (1993). Dysfunctional attitudes and suicidal ideation in psychiatric outpatients. *Suicide and Life-Threatening Behavior, 23*(1), 11–20.

Beck, A. T., Steer, R. A., Epstein, N., & Brown, G. (1990b). The Beck Self-Concept Test. *Psychological Assessment: A Journal of Consulting and Clinical Psychology, 2*(2), 191–197.

Beck, A. T., Steer, R. A., Kovacs, M., & Garrison, B. (1985). Hopelessness and eventual suicide: A ten-year prospective study of patients hospitalized with suicidal ideation. *American Journal of Psychiatry, 142*(5), 559–563.

Beck, A. T., Steer, R. A., & Ranieri, W. F. (1988). Scale for Suicide Ideation: Psychometric properties of a self-report version. *Journal of Clinical Psychology, 44*(4), 499–505.

Beck, A. T., Steer, R. A., & Trexler, L. D. (1989). Alcohol abuse and eventual suicide: A five to ten year prospective study of alcohol abusing suicide attempters. *Journal of Studies on Alcohol, 50*(3), 202–209.

Beck, A. T., & Stewart, B. (1989). *The self-concept as a risk factor in patients who kill themselves.* Uunpublished manuscript, Center for Cognitive Therapy, Philadelphia.

Beck, A. T., & Weishaar, M. (1989). Cognitive therapy. In A. Freeman, K. M. Simon, L. E. Beutler, & H. Arkowitz (Eds.), *Comprehensive handbook of cognitive therapy* (pp. 21–36), New York: Plenum Press.

Beck, A. T., Weissman, A., & Kovacs, M. (1976). Alcoholism, hopelessness and suicidal behavior. *Journal of Studies on Alcohol, 37*(1), 66–77.

Beck, A. T., Weissman, A., Lester, D., & Trexler, L. (1974). The measurement of pessimism: The Hopelessness Scale. *Journal of Consulting and Clinical Psychology, 42,* 861–865.

Beck, R. W., Morris, J. B., & Beck, A. T. (1974). Cross-validation of the Suicide Intent Scale. *Psychological Reports, 34,* 445–446.

Bedrosian, R. C., & Beck, A. T. (1979). Cognitive aspects of suicidal behavior. *Suicide and Life-Threatening Behavior, 9*(2), 87–96.

Bonner, R. L., & Rich, A. R. (1987). Toward a predictive model of suicidal ideation and behvaior: Some preliminary data in college students. *Suicide and Life-Threatening Behavior, 17,* 50–63.

Bonner, R. L., & Rich, A. R. (1988a). A prospective investigation of suicidal ideation in college students: A test of a model. *Suicide and Life-Threatening Behavior, 18*(3), 245–258.

Bonner, R. L., & Rich, A. (1988b). Negative life stress, social problem-solving, self-appraisal, and hopelessness: Implications for suicide research. *Cognitive Therapy and Research, 12*(6), 549–556.

Brent, D. A. (1987). Correlates of medical lethality of suicide attempts in children and adolescents. *Journal of the American Academy of Child Psychiatry, 26,* 87–89.

Brent, D. A., & Kolko, D. J. (1990). The assessment and treatment of children and adolescents at risk for suicide. In S. J. Blumenthal & D. J. Kupfer (Eds.), *Suicide over the life cycle: Risk factors, assessment and treatment of suicidal patients* (pp. 253–302). Washington, DC: American Psychiatric Press.

Brent, D., Kolko, D., Goldstein, C., Allan, M., & Brown, R. (1989, October). *Cognitive distortion, familial stress, and suicidality in adolescent inpatients.* Poster presented at the annual meeting of the American Academy of Child and Adolescent Psychiatry, New York.

Carlson, G. A., & Cantwell, D. P. (1982). Suicidal behavior and depression in children and adolescents. *Journal of the American Academy of Child Psychiatry, 21,* 361–368.

Clum, G. A., Patsiokas, A. T., & Luscomb, R. L. (1979). Empirically based comprehensive treatment program for parasuicide. *Journal of Consulting and Clinical Psychology, 47,* 937–945.

Cohen-Sandler, R., & Berman, A. L. (1982). *Training suicidal children to problem-solve in nonsuicidal ways.* Paper presented at the annual meeting of the American Association of Suicidology, New York.

Cole, D. A. (1988). Hopelessness, social desirability, depression, and parasuicide in two college student samples. *Journal of Consulting and Clinical Psychology, 56*(1), 131–136.

Cole, D. A. (1989). Psychopathology of adolescent suicide: Hopelessness, coping beliefs, and depression. *Journal of Abnormal Psychology, 98*(3), 248–255.

Connell, D. K., & Meyer, R. G. (1991). The Reasons for Living Inventory and a college population: Adolescent suicidal behaviors, beliefs, and coping skills. *Journal of Clinical Psychology, 47*(4), 485–489.

Curry, J. F., Miller, Y., Waugh, S., & Anderson, W. B. (1992). Coping responses in depressed, socially maladjusted, and suicidal adolescents. *Psychological Reports, 71,* 80–82.

Dixon, W. A., Heppner, P. P., & Anderson, W. (1991). Problem-solving appraisal, stress, hopelessness, and suicide ideation in a college population. *Journal of Counseling Psychology, 38,* 51–56.

Drake, R. E., & Cotton, P. G. (1986). Depression, hopelessness, and suicide in chronic schizophrenia. *British Journal of Psychiatry, 148,* 554–559.

Dyck, M. J. (1991). Positive and negative attitudes mediating suicide ideation. *Suicide and Life-Threatening Behvaior, 21*(4), 360–373.

Dyer, J. A. T., & Kreitman, N. (1984). Hopelessness, depression and suicidal intent in parasuicide. *British Journal of Psychiatry, 144,* 127–133.

Edwards, A. (1970). *The measurement of personality traits by scales and inventories.* New York: Holt, Rinehart & Winston.

Ellis, T. E., & Ratliff, K. G. (1986). Cognitive characteristics of suicidal and nonsuicidal psychiatric patients. *Cognitive Therapy and Research, 10*, 625–634.

Emery, G. D., Steer, R. A., & Beck, A. T. (1981). Depression, hopelessness and suicidal intent among heroin addicts. *International Journal of the Addictions, 16*(3), 425–429.

Fawcett, J., Schefter, W., Clark, D., Hedeker, D., Gibbons, R., & Coryell, W. (1987). Clinical predictors of suicide in patients with major affective disorder: A controlled prospective study. *American Journal of Psychiatry, 144*, 35–40.

Goldney, R. D. (1981). Attempted suicide in young women: Correlates of lethality. *British Journal of Psychiatry, 139*, 382–390.

Hawton, K., Osborn, M., O'Grady, J., & Cole, D. (1982). Classification of adolescents who take overdoses. *British Journal of Psychiatry, 140*, 124–131.

Heikkinen, M., Aro, H., & Lonnqvist, J. (1993). Life events and social support in suicide. *Suicide and Life-Threatening Behavior, 23*(4), 343–358.

Hewitt, P. L., Flett, G. L., & Turnbull-Donovan, W. (1992). Perfectionism and suicide potential. *British Journal of Clinical Psychology, 31*, 181–190.

Holden, R. R., Mendoca, J. D., & Serin, R. C. (1989). Suicide, hopelessness, and social desirability: A test of an interactive model. *Journal of Consulting and Clinical Psychology, 57*(4), 500–504.

Josepho, S. A., & Plutchik, R. (1994). Stress, coping and suicide risk in psychiatric inpatients. *Suicide and Life-Threatening Behavior, 24*(1), 48–57.

Kazdin, A. E., French, N. H., Unis, A. S., Esveldt-Dawson, K., & Sherrick, R. B. (1983). Hopelessness, depression, and suicidal intent among psychiatrically disturbed inpatient children. *Journal of Consulting and Clinical Psychology, 51*, 504–510.

Kazdin, A. E., Rodgers, A., & Colbus, D. (1986). The Hopelessness Scale for Children: Psychometric characteristics and concurrent validity. *Journal of Consulting and Clinical Psychology, 54*, 241–245.

Kovacs, M., Beck, A. T., & Weissman, A. (1975). Hopelessness: An indicator of suicidal risk. *Suicide and Life-Threatening Behavior, 5*(2), 98–103.

Lerner, M. S., & Clum, G. A. (1990). Treatment of suicide ideators: A problem-solving approach. *Behavior Therapy, 21*, 403–411.

Lester, D., Beck, A. T., & Narrett, S. (1978). Suicidal intent in successive suicidal actions. *Psychological Reports, 43*, 110.

Lester, D., Beck, A. T., & Steer, R. A. (1989). Attempted suicide in those with personality disorders. *European Archives of Psychiatry and Neurological Sciences, 239*, 109–112.

Levenson, M. (1974). Cognitive characteristics of suicide risk. In C. Neuringer (Ed.), *Psychological assessment of suicide risk* (pp. 150–163). Springfield, IL: Charles C. Thomas.

Levenson, M., & Neuringer, C. (1971). Problem-solving behavior in suicidal adolescents. *Journal of Consulting and Clinical Psychology, 37*, 433–436.

Linehan, M. M., Camper, P., Chiles, J., Strosahl, K., & Shearin, E. (1987). Interpersonal problem-solving and parasuicide. *Cognitive Therapy and Research, 11*, 1–12.

Linehan, M. M., Chiles, J. A., Egan, K. J., Devine, R. H., & Laffaw, J. A. (1986). Presenting problems of parasuicides versus suicide ideators and nonsuicidal psychiatric patients. *Journal of Consulting and Clinical Psychology, 54*, 880–881.

Linehan, M. M., Goodstein, J. L., Nielson, S. L., & Chiles, J. A. (1983). Reasons for staying alive when you are thinking of killing yourself: The Reasons for Living Inventory. *Journal of Consulting and Clinical Psychology, 51*, 276–286.

Linehan, M., & Nielson, S. (1981). Assessment of suicide ideation and parasuicide: Hopelessness and social desirability. *Journal of Consulting and Clinical Psychology, 49,* 773–775.

Linehan, M., & Nielson, S. (1983). Social desirability: Its relevance to the measurement of hopelessness and suicidal behavior. *Journal of Consulting and Clinical Psychology, 51,* 141–143.

McLeavey, B. C., Daly, R. J., Murray, C. M., O'Riodan, J., & Taylor, M. (1987). Interpersonal problem-solving deficits in self- poisoning patients. *Suicide and Life-Threatening Behavior, 17,* 33–49.

Miller, I. W., Norman, W. H., Bishop, S., & Dow, M. G. (1986). The modified Scale for Suicidal Ideation: Reliability and validity. *Journal of Consulting and Clinical Psychology, 54,* 724–725.

Minkoff, K., Bergman, E., Beck, A. T., & Beck, R. (1973). Hopelessness, depression, and attempted suicide. *American Journal of Psychiatry, 130*(4), 455–459.

Mraz, W., & Runco, M. A. (1994). Suicide ideation and creative problem-solving. *Suicide and Life-Threatening Behavior, 24*(1), 38–47.

Nekanda Trepka, C. J. S., Bishop, S., & Blackburn, I. M. (1983). Hopelessness and depression. *British Journal of Clinical Psychology, 22,* 49–60.

Neuringer, C. (1961). Dichotomous evaluations in suicidal individuals. *Journal of Consulting Psychology, 25,* 445–449.

Neuringer, C. (1967). The cognitive organization of meaning in suicidal individuals. *Journal of General Psychology, 76,* 91–100.

Neuringer, C. (1968). Divergencies between attitudes towards life and death among suicidal, psychosomatic, and normal hospitalized patients. *Journal of Consulting and Clinical Psychology, 32,* 59–63.

Neuringer, C., & Lettieri, D. J. (1971). Cognition, attitude, and affect in suicidal individuals. *Suicide and Life-Threatening Behavior, 1,* 106–124.

Orbach, I., Bar-Joseph, H., & Dror, N. (1990). Styles of problem solving in suicidal individuals. *Suicide and Life-Threatening Behavior, 20*(1), 56–64.

Orbach, I., Rosenheim, E., & Hary, E. (1987). Some aspects of cognitive functioning in suicidal children. *Journal of the American Academy of Child and Adolescent Psychiatry, 25*(2), 181–185.

Patsiokas, A. T., Clum, G. A., & Luscomb, R. L. (1979). Cognitive characteristics of suicide attempters. *Journal of Consulting and Clinical Psychology, 47,* 478–484.

Prezant, D. W., & Neimeyer, R. A. (1988). Cognitive predictors of depression and suicide ideation. *Suicide and Life-Threatening Behavior, 18*(3), 259–264.

Priester, M. J., & Clum, G. A. (1992). Attributional style as a diathesis in predicting depression, hopelessness, and suicide ideation in college students. *Journal of Psychopathology and Behavioral Assessment, 14*(2), 111–122.

Priester, M. J., & Clum, G. A. (1993a). Perceived problem-solving ability as a predictor of depression, hopelessness and suicidal ideation in a college population. *Journal of Counseling Psychology, 40*(1), 79–85.

Priester, M. J., & Clum, G. A. (1993b). The problem-solving diathesis in depression, hopelessness and suicide ideation: A longitudinal analysis. *Journal of Psychopathology and Behavioral Assessment, 15*(3), 239–254.

Ranieri, W. F., Steer, R. A., Lavrence, T. I., Rissmiller, D. J., Piper, G. E., & Beck, A. T. (1987). Relationship of depression, hopelessness, and dysfunctional attitudes to suicide ideation in psychiatric patients. *Psychological Reports, 61,* 967–975.

Rich, A. R., & Bonner, R. L. (1987). Concurrent validity of a stress vulnerability model of suicidal ideation and behavior: A follow-up study. *Suicide and Life-Threatening Behavior, 17*(4), 265–270.

Rich, A. R., Kirkpatrick-Smith, J., Bonner, R. L., & Jans, F. (1992). Gender differences in psychosocial correlates of suicidal ideation among adolescents. *Suicide and Life-Threatening Behavior, 22*(3), 364–373.

Rotheram-Borus, M. J., & Trautman, P. D. (1988). Hopelessness, depression, and suicidal intent among adolescent suicide attempters. *Journal of the American Academy of Child and Adolescent Psychiatry, 27,* 700–704.

Rotheram-Borus, M. J., Trautman, P. D., Dopkins, S. C., & Shrout, P. E. (1990). Cognitive style and pleasant activities among female adolescent suicide attempters. *Journal of Consulting and Clinical Psychology, 58*(5), 554–561.

Rudd, M. D. (1990). An integrative model of suicidal ideation. *Suicide and Life-Threatening Behavior, 20*(1), 16–30.

Rudd, M. D., Rajab, M. H., & Dahm, P. F. (1994). Problem-solving appraisal in suicide ideators and attempters. *American Journal of Orthopsychiatry, 64*(1), 136–149.

Rush, A. J., Beck, A. T., Kovacs, M., Weissenburger, J., & Hollon, S. (1982). Comparison of the differential effects of cognitive therapy and pharmacotherapy on hopelessness and self-concept. *American Journal of Psychiatry, 139,* 862–866.

Salkovskis, P. M., Atha, C., & Storer, D. (1990). Cognitive-behavioural problem solving in the treatment of patients who repeatedly attempt suicide: A controlled trial. *British Journal of Psychiatry, 157,* 871–876.

Schotte, D. E., & Clum, G. A. (1982). Suicide ideation in a college population: A test of a model. *Journal of Consulting and Clinical Psychology, 50,* 690–696.

Schotte, D. E., & Clum, G. A. (1987). Problem-solving skills in suicidal psychiatric patients. *Journal of Consulting and Clinical Psychology, 55,* 49–54.

Schotte, D. E., Cools, J., & Payvar, S. (1990). Problem solving deficits in suicidal patients: Trait vulnerability or state phenomenon? *Journal of Consulting and Clinical Psychology, 58*(5), 562–564.

Shaw, B. F., & Segal, Z. V. (1988). Introduction to cognitive theory and therapy. In A. J. Frances & R. E. Hales (Eds.), *Review of Psychiatry* (Vol. 7, pp. 538–553). Washington, DC: American Psychiatric Press.

Silver, M. A., Bohnert, M., Beck, A. T., & Marcus, D. (1971). Relation of depression of attempted suicide and seriousness of intent. *Archives of General Psychiatry, 25,* 573–576.

Spirito, A., Overholser, J., & Hart, K. (1991). Cognitive characteristics of adolescent suicide attempters. *Journal of the American Academy of Child and Adolescent Psychiatry, 30*(4), 604–608.

Spirito, A., Overholser, J., & Stark, L. J. (1989). Common problems and coping strategies II: Findings with adolescent suicide attempters. *Journal of Abnormal Child Psychology, 17*(2), 213–221.

Spirito, A., Williams, C., Stark, L. J., & Hart, K. (1988). The Hopelessness Scale for Children: Psychometric properties and clinical utility with normal and emotionally disturbed adolescents. *Journal of Abnormal Child Psychology, 16,* 445–458.

Strosahl, K., Chiles, J. A., & Linehan, M. (1992). Prediction of suicide intent in hospitalized parasuicides: Reasons for living, hopelessness, and depression. *Comprehensive Psychiatry, 33*(6), 366–373.

Strosahl, K., Linehan, M., & Chiles, J. (1983, August). *Predictors of suicide intent in psychiatric patients: Reasons for living, hopelessness, and depression.* Paper presented at the annual convention of the American Psychological Association, Anaheim, CA.

Strosahl, K. D., Linehan, M. M., & Chiles, J. A. (1984). Will the real social desirability please stand up? Hopelessness, depression, social desirability, and the prediction of suicidal behavior. *Journal of Consulting and Clincal Psychology, 52*(3), 449–457.

Weissman, A. N., & Beck, A. T. (1978, November). *Development and validation of the Dysfunctional Attitude Scale: A preliminary invesitgation.* Paper presented at the meeting of the Association for Advancement of Behavior Therapy, Chicago.

Weissman, A., Beck, A. T., & Kovacs, M. (1979). Drug abuse, hopelessness, and suicidal behavior. *International Journal of the Addictions, 14,* 451–464.

Westefeld, J. S., Cardin, D., & Deaton, W. L. (1992). Development of the College Student Reasons for Living Inventory. *Suicide and Life-Threatening Behavior, 22*(4), 442–452.

Wetzel, R. D. (1976). Hopelessness, depression and suicide intent. *Archives of General Psychiatry, 33,* 1069–1073.

Wetzel, R. D., Margulies, T., Davis, R., & Karam, E. (1980). Hopelessness, depression, and suicide intent. *Journal of Clinical Psychology, 41,* 159–160.

Wetzel, R. D., & Reich, T. (1989). The cognitive triad and suicide intent in depressed inpatients. *Psychological Reports, 65,* 1027–1032.

Chapter 12

Cognitive Vulnerability to Depression

Ivy-Marie Blackburn

Through the centuries, theoretical, clinical, and research studies in depression have sought possible factors that may predispose some individuals to develop a depressive illness. Biological, psychological, and sociological factors have been implicated, although these classes of predisposing or vulnerability factors are not necessarily independent and most researchers now accept that vulnerability is likely to be multifactorial.

That there should be vulnerability factors in depression has compelling and empirical validity. Research evidence supporting the view of a biological predisposition derives primarily from family genetic studies (McGuffin & Katz, 1986), indicating that depression appears to have a hereditary component, while Brown and Harris (1978), in their influential sociological study of women in Camberwell, described several environmental factors that appear to render people vulnerable to a depressive reaction in the face of adversity. Psychological investigations have tended to focus primarily on internal personality factors. The concept of a depressive personality has a long history dating back to at least the time of Kraepelin (1921), who described the "depressive temperament" as innate and persistent and sometimes erupting into the full melancholic syndrome. Other authors have since implicated personality traits such as introversion and neuroticism (Murray & Blackburn, 1974) and obsessional traits (Kendell & DiScipio, 1970).

Cognitive theories of depression have revived interest in research in psychological vulnerability to depression by postulating certain basic attitudes or cognitive styles as depressogenic or as predisposing to depression. This diathesis–stress model first described by Beck (1967) and further expanded by Kovacs and Beck (1978) describes latent attitudes that can be triggered by certain key situations or events and that then become hyperactive and applied to increasingly more inappropriate stimuli. This hypothesis has received little empirical backing, with most studies finding evidence for a state-dependent cognitive style instead of a stable personality trait (Persons & Miranda, 1992). Other cognitive theories, such as the reformulated learned helplessness theory (Abramson, Seligman, & Teasdale, 1978), have similarly looked for stable cognitive patterns in attributional style as predisposing to depression, with inconsistent results. Costello (1992) attributes the poor results in this area to methodological problems rather than to the invalidity of a concept of cognitive vulnerability. For example, the disappointing results obtained in the use of the Dysfunctional Attitude Scale (DAS; Weissman & Beck, 1978) may be due, according to Costello, to the use of "incontrovertible concepts"—that is, the association of negative self-schemas with depression. Hence most studies indicate that dysfunctional attitudes "wax and wane with the clinical state" and appear "to refute the hypothesis that they are stable traits" (Persons & Miranda, 1992, p. 487).

Teasdale (1988) has proposed an alternative to Beck's vulnerability theory that he calls the "differential activation hypothesis." This "suggests that it is the patterns of information processing that occur once a person is at least mildly depressed that are crucial in determining whether an initial depressed state will escalate to the level of major depression" (Teasdale, 1988, p. 256). This hypothesis assumes rightly that mild, transient depression is a common phenomenon, but only some people develop severe and/or chronic depression. Several empirical studies are quoted by Teasdale in support of his hypothesis. For example, interpretations of experience in global negative terms while in mild depressed mood and elevated scores on the DAS have been found to be predictive of severe depression. The level of these patterns of negative cognitive processing once the individual is depressed also predicts the persistence of depression. The particular style of information processing implicated by Teasdale—that is, global negative self-evaluations—is probably related to high levels of neuroticism (Martin, 1985).

Recent studies in cognitive vulnerability to depression have focused on personality traits that are deemed to be more stable than depressogenic assumptions. Beck (1983, 1987) described two personality constructs, sociotropy and autonomy, that can act as vulnerability markers in that they sensitize individuals to certain types of events. A sociotropic individual is described as socially dependent—that is, he or she is highly invested in positive interchange with others, valuing above all acceptance, intimacy, support, and guidance. On the other hand, an autonomous individual is described as invested in independent functioning, mobility, freedom, choice, and achievement, valuing above all the integrity of his or her own domain. These concepts resemble the concepts of dependency and self-criticism described by other authors from a psychodynamic view as involved in depression (Blatt, Quinlan, Cherron, McDonald, & Zuroff, 1982). A scale has been developed, the Sociotropy–Autonomy Scale (SAS; Beck, Epstein, & Harrison, 1983) consisting of 60 items, rated on 5-point scales, from which three factors have been extracted as relating to sociotropy (Disapproval, Attachment, and Pleasing Others) and three factors as relating to autonomy (Individualistic Achievement, Freedom from Control, and Preference for Solitude).

Beck (1983) hypothesized that excessive sociotropy or autonomy would predispose to depression in response to particular events; determine the pattern of symptoms, nonendogenous symptoms being associated with sociotropy and endogenous symptoms with autonomy, and they would influence response to particular forms of treatment. A large number of studies have been published to date investigating the validity and reliability of the SAS and testing some of the predictions described above (see Clark & Beck, 1991, for a review). In general, the construct validity of the sociotropy subscale has been well supported but there are less consistent findings for the autonomy subscale. The Edinburgh University Cognitive Therapy Research Group has used the SAS as part of a test battery in a large treatment and follow-up study investigating the prophylactic effect of cognitive therapy in recurrent depression. This study is just completed and some results relating to sociotropy and autonomy will be reported below.

Another aspect of cognitive vulnerability to depression has been described as a general pessimistic style of thinking. This negativity has sometimes been defined as a distortion of reality, or as a bias, which is not necessarily a distorted view of the world, but a negative bias in situations where reality is not evident. An influential paper by Alloy and Abramson (1979), with the catchy subtitle "Sadder But Wiser?," discussed a study of perception of control in undergraduates described as depressed (Beck Depression Inventory [BDI] score $\geq$ 9) and nondepressed (BDI score $\leq$ 8). They found that, contrary to expectation, depressed subjects were more accurate than nondepressed subjects in contingency computer tasks with no control over outcome. The nondepressed subjects exhibited an optimistic bias which led to errors of judgment in their degree of control. The depressed subjects showed excessive realism and appeared to be dysfunctional only insofar as they did not exhibit the normal self-serving bias that has been found in many studies (Ackerman & Derubeis, 1991). In this chapter, I also report briefly on a study comparing judgment of control in depressed subjects and normal controls.

The four studies described below were carried out by my research group as part of an ongoing program investigating various aspects of cognitive vulnerability to depression. The first three studies relate to sociotropy and autonomy while the fourth study is a partial repliction of Alloy and Abramson (1979).

SOCIOTROPY AND AUTONOMY IN DEPRESSION

Study 1: Sociotropy, Autonomy, and Personal Memories

The SAS allows us to define subgroups of depressed individuals on the basis of groups of attitudes that may render them vulnerable to particular kinds of events, perhaps through the mediation of particular types of cognitive bias. Moore and Blackburn (1993) described a study of depressed patients aimed to test the hypothesis that particular kinds of negative bias would be related to sociotropy and autonomy. We used autobiographical memory as the experimental task instead of self-rated questionnaires which may have some overlap with the independent questionnaire measure of personality — that is, the SAS. As this study was fully described in Moore and Blackburn (1993), only a brief account will be given here.

Twenty unipolar depressed inpatients and outpatients took part in the study, 6 males and 14 females with a mean age of 37 years ($SD = 12$). The mean Hamilton Rating Scale for depression (HRSD, 17 items; Hamilton, 1960) score was 19.6 ($SD = 4.9$) and the mean BDI (13-item version; Beck & Beck, 1972) score was 19.2 ($SD = 6.5$). Sixteen prompts were independently validated by three judges to elicit four positive and four negative sociotropy-related memories and four positive and four negative autonomy-related memories. The dependent measure was the latency of recall for a specific memory elicited by the prompt. The 16 prompts were presented in a balanced design and subjects rated on a scale of 1 (much sadder) to 7 (much happier) how the event had made them feel.

The specific hypotheses of the study were:

1. Sociotropy will be related with faster recall of sociotropic and negative events.
2. Autonomy will be related with faster recall of autonomous negative events.
3. Speed of recall of positive memories relative to negative memories will be positively related to level of depression.

The results indicated that the ratio of the latency for memory of negative sociotropic events was significantly and negatively correlated with level of sociotropy ($r = -.47$, $n = 19$, $p < .05$, one-tailed), that is, the higher the level of sociotropy of the individual, the quicker the speed of memory for sociotropic negative events relative to speed of memory in general. The relationship of autonomy with relative speed of memory for negative autonomous events was not significant. Speed of recall for positive memories relative to negative memories increased with level of depression (as predicated in hypothesis 3), the correlation with HRSD being significant ($r = .44$, $n = 20$, $p < .05$, one-tailed), but the correlation with the BDI not reaching significance $r = .34$).

Importantly, none of the correlations of sociotropy and autonomy with level of depression were significant, indicating that sociotropy and autonomy were more trait-like than state-like. Moreover, when the association of sociotropy with depression was partialed out, the correlation of sociotropy with the speed of recall of negative sociotropic memories remained significant (partialing out BDI, $r = -.43$, $n = 18$; partialing out HRSD, $r = -.50$, $n = 19$, $p < .05$, one-tailed). There did not seem to be a recency effect, as the correlation between sociotropy and speed of recall for negative sociotropic events remained significant when recency of events was partialed out ($r = -.47, n = 19, p < .05$, one-tailed). A specific effect was also shown by the significant difference between the correlation of sociotropy with relative speed of recall for negative sociotropic events and sociotropy with relative speed of recall for negative autonomous events.

This study, although based on small numbers, is important for two reasons: It is based on a patient sample and it is the first study to show the effect of sociotropy on cognitive functions, in this instance recall of negative sociotropic events. The primacy of negative memories relative to positive memories in depression is well established (Blaney, 1986). This study indicates a specificity effect for type of negative memories, at least in the case of sociotropy. The hypothesis relating to autonomy was not supported. Clark and Beck (1991) indicate that the construct validity of the autonomy subscale can be increased by deletion of 10 of the original items and the addition of 24 new items.

The next two studies were conducted in a large group of patients recruited to take part in a 3-year outcome and follow-up study to investigate the prophylactic effect of cognitive therapy relative to antidepressant medication.

Study 2: The Relationship of Sociotropy and Autonomy to Symptoms, Cognition, and Personality in Depressed Patients

In this study (Moore & Blackburn, 1994), we looked at the relationship of sociotropy and autonomy with depression and anxiety, as well as with well-established personality features (neuroticism and extraversion, Eysenck Personality Questionnaire; Eysenck & Eysenck, 1975), with negative content of thought (Automatic Thoughts Questionnaire [ATQ]; Hollon & Kendall, 1980), and with specific dysfunctional attitudes (DAS, Weissman & Beck, 1978).

Although it now seems clear that sociotropy, in particular, is associated with depressive symptoms (Nietzel & Harris, 1990), it has not been established that any such association is specific to depression rather than reflecting general psychological distress. One aim of this study was to examine the specificity of the relationship of sociotropy and autonomy with depression as compared with anxiety. A second aim was to clarify the relationship between sociotropy and autonomy and neuroticism and extraversion. As mentioned in the introduction, neuroticism has been associated with vulnerability to depression and Gilbert and Reynolds (1990) reported a relationship between sociotropy and neuroticism but not extraversion, while autonomy was not related to either personality dimension. Thirdly, it might be predicted that, as potential vulnerability factors, higher levels of sociotropy and autonomy would be related to higher levels of conscious negative automatic thoughts and with higher levels of dysfunctional attitudes. In particular, it would be expected that sociotropy and autonomy would be differentially related to the dependency-related and achievement-related clusters derived from the DAS (Imber et al., 1990).

One hundred eighteen depressed in- and outpatients satisfying Research Diagnostic Criteria (Spitzer, Endicott, & Robins, 1978) for primary major depression and suffering from at least a second episode of depression took part in the study. There were 72 outpatients, 46 inpatients, 61% of the sample was female, and the mean age was 40 years (SD = 13),

Internal Reliability

Cronbach's alpha indicated that both scales of the SAS were highly internally consistent (alpha = .87, n = 118 in both instances). For comparison, the correlation of sociotropy and autonomy was .23, n = 118, $p <$ .05. Table 12.1 shows the various correlations that were calculated.

Specificity of Relationship with Depression

As Table 12.1 shows, sociotropy correlated significantly with both measures of severity of depression and with severity of anxiety, while autonomy correlated significantly only with the observer rating scale of depression (the HRSD). Specificity was tested by partial correlations. For sociotropy scores the correlation with the BDI (Beck, Ward, Mendelson, Mock, & Erbaugh, 1961) remained significant when state scores on the State–Trait Anxiety Inventory (STAI-S; Spielberger, Gorsuch, & Lushener, 1970) were partialed out (r = .36, n = 118, $p <$ .0001). However, the correlation of STAI-S with sociotropy was no longer significant when BDI scores were controlled for (r = .03). On the other hand, the correlation with HRSD was no longer

TABLE 12.1. Correlations of Sociotropy and Autonomy with Measures of Severity, Cognition, and Personality

	Sociotropy	Autonomy
Severity		
BDI	.44**	.14
HRSD	.22*	.21*
STAI-S	.26**	.06
Negative thoughts		
ATQ	.45**	.18
Attitudes		
DAS	.38**	.05
Social approval (DAS)	.59***	.10
Perfectionism (DAS)	.26**	.19*
Personality		
Neuroticism	.22*	.13
Extraversion	− .03	− .20*

$*p < .05; **p < .01; ***p < .001.$

significant when STAI-S scores were partialed out ($r = .17$), whereas the correlation of sociotropy and STAI-S remained significant when HRSD scores were partialed out ($r = .22, n = 118, p < .05$). However, the relationship of autonomy with HRSD remained significant when anxiety level was partialed out ($r = .21, n = 118, p < .05$). Thus some degree of specificity for the relationship of sociotropy with depression was demonstrated as far as self-rated depression is concerned. The HRSD is known to be heavily weighted on anxiety symptoms (Cleary & Guy, 1977) and it is perhaps not surprising that the relationship of sociotropy and HRSD was no longer significant when anxiety was controlled for. On the other hand, specificity for autonomy and level of depression was only shown for the HRSD and not the BDI. The HRSD and the BDI are known to tap different aspects of depression, the two scales correlating only moderately (Prusoff, Klerman, & Paykel, 1972).

Relationship with Neuroticism and Extraversion

The pattern of correlations indicates that higher levels of sociotropy were significantly associated with higher levels of neuroticism, while higher levels of autonomy were associated with lower levels of extraversion. Since neuroticism has often been described as a vulnerability factor in depression (Martin, 1985), this finding, which is in accord with Gilbert and Reynolds (1990), adds support to the view of sociotropy as a vulnerability factor in depression. The mild but significant relationship between autonomy and introversion has face validity but was not found by Gilbert and Reynolds (1990).

Relationship with Cognitive Variables Implicated in Depression

Sociotropy was highly significantly correlated with frequency of negative automatic thoughts (the ATQ) and with level of dysfunctional attitudes (the DAS), but autonomy was not. The relationship with specific factors of the DAS indicated, as would be expected, that sociotropy was highly significantly correlated with social approval but sociotropy was also, unexpectedly, significantly associated with perfectionism, although less so. Specificity was demonstrated by the significant difference between the two correlations ($t = 4.79, n = 118, p < .0001$). Autonomy was significantly correlated with perfectionism but not with social approval, again the difference between the two correlations being highly significant ($t = 3.57, n = 118, p < .001$).

In summary, in this large study of depressed patients satisfying criteria for primary major unipolar depression, the following findings were obtained:

1. Both the sociotropy and autonomy subscales proved to be highly internally reliable.
2. Sociotropy was moderately but significantly associated with level

of depression and of anxiety. The association with self-rated depression was not mediated by anxiety whereas the association with observer-rated depression was.

3. Neuroticism was associated with sociotropy and introversion with autonomy.
4. Negative content of thought and depressive attitudes were related to higher levels of sociotropy but not of autonomy.
5. Sociotropy was more highly related to need for social approval than to perfectionism and autonomy was more highly related to perfectionism than to need for social approval.

In conclusion, sociotropy appears to be a vulnerability marker for depression but the autonomy subscale, although reliable, appears to have less conceptual validity.

The next study investigated the stability over time of the concepts of sociotropy and autonomy. As pointed out in the introduction, several putative vulnerability factors, for example dysfunctional attitudes as measured by the DAS, have proved elusive when measured in a longitudinal design, pre- and posttreatment.

Study 3: The Stability of Sociotropy and Autonomy over the Course of Treatment

As part of the study described above, patients were tested on two occasions: time 1 (at entry into the study, after screening for diagnosis and history) and time 2 (at the end of 16 weeks of treatment). Treatment consisted either of cognitive therapy or of antidepressants alone, or of the combination of these two treatments, after randomized allocation.

If the SAS behaves as a personality measure indicating particular vulnerabilities to depression, it would be expected to show some degree of stability over time—that is, no significant change should occur with the remission of symptoms. Both sociotropy and autonomy were stable over time as indicated by correlations (sociotropy, $r = .77, n = 90, p < .001$; autonomy, $r = .72, n = 90, p < .001$).

The magnitude of changes was calculated by paired t tests as shown in Table 12.2. The highly significant changes in depression were not reflected in changes in sociotropy and autonomy which remained remarkably stable over time. However, these comparisons may be misleading as, at time 2, not all patients were fully recovered, as indicated by the high mean BDI and HRSD scores. We therefore set the more stringent test of comparing the scores of patients who had fully recovered to a significant degree, that is, with HRSD scores of eight or less. As can be seen in Table 12.2, the mean sociotropy score dropped by nearly 7 points ($p < .01$), while autonomy remained static. When treatment responders were divided into two groups, those who were treated with medication alone ($n = 24$) and those

TABLE 12.2. Mean Scores (and Standard Deviations) on the SAS, BDI, and HRSD at Time 1 (Baseline) and Time 2 (16 Weeks Later)

	Time 1	Time 2	n
		All subjects	
BDI	27.1 (9.3)	16.6 (13.4)	8.2 (94) $p < .001$
HRSD	21.0 (4.2)	10.2 (7.4)	14.4 (100) $p < .001$
Sociotropy	77.9 (17.1)	75.7 (19.3)	1.7 (89) $p < .10$
Autonomy	69.2 (16.0)	69.6 (16.9)	0.3 (89) n.s.
		Only subjects with time 2 HRSD < 8	
Sociotropy	76.0 (14.7)	69.3 (17.7)	3.3 (41) $p < .01$
Autonomy	67.8 (14.6)	67.6 (16.5)	0.1 (41) n.s.

who received cognitive therapy alone, or in combination with medication ($N = 18$), a two-way analysis of variance of sociotropy scores, with time and treatment as factors, indicated a significant time effect, as already shown in the paired t test, but no treatment effect and no time × treatment interaction. A similar analysis of autonomy scores indicated no significant time, treatment, or interaction effect.

It is noteworthy, however, that although sociotropy scores decreased significantly with remission of symptoms, the mean score remained high relative to normative scores (our own data for 30 nondepressed controls [Blackburn, Roxborough, Muir, Glabus, & Blackwood, 1990; Roxborough, 1991] mean HRSD score = 1.5 [SD 1.7]; mean sociotropy score = 57.2 [SD = 15.8]). These means are significantly different ($t = 3.05$, $df = 70$, $p < .01$).

In summary, the correlations of scores over time in treated patients indicated that the relative levels of sociotropy and autonomy remain consistent over time. Further evidence for stability of both characteristics was obtained for the group as a whole. However, for patients who do respond to treatment, sociotropy, but not autonomy, decreases significantly. Nonetheless, there is some indication that the level of sociotropy in remitted depressed patients remains higher than normal. This finding is not dissimilar to that found in neuroticism, as indicated by several studies (e.g., Murray & Blackburn, 1974).

The last study is different in that it employs an experimental design to test, in depressed patients, the dysfunctional realism hypothesis in judgments of control where, in fact, no control exists.

NEGATIVE BIAS OR DEPRESSIVE REALISM

Study 4: "Sadder But Wiser"

As indicated in the introduction, another aspect of cognitive vulnerability to depression may be how inferences are drawn about degree of control in uncertain situations. From an evolutionary point of view, a helpful style of thinking may require a degree of unrealistic optimism, which would combat helplessness and hopelessness and hence dysfunctional depression. Alloy and Abramson's study (1979) appeared to indicate that realism, in a laboratory computer task involving judgments of contingency, was characteristic of depressed mood.

In this study (Mountford, 1992), we tested 20 depressed patients and 20 nondepressed controls matched as far as possible for demographic characteristics. There were 10 males and 10 females in each group. The depressed group had a mean age of 35.5 years (SD = 11.0) and a mean IQ of 103.6 (SD = 9.3). The mean age of the control group was 36.9 years (SD = 12.1 and their mean IQ was 104.1 (SD = 10.2). The depressed subjects all satisfied criteria for primary major unipolar depression The judgement of control task was similar to that used by Alloy and Abramson (1979), consisting of the relationship between an outcome, the appearance of a star on the computer screen, and a response, pressing (active response) or not pressing (nonactive) a button.

Subjects were asked to guess the amount of control they were able to exert over the appearance or nonappearance of the star on the computer screen. Each subject carried out four different conditions of the task in a balanced order:

1. 70% control (active or inactive response)
2. 30% control (active or inactive response)
3. 0% control with 70% frequency of star appearance (high reinforcement)
4. 0% control with 30% frequency of star appearance (low reinforcement)

Subjects were fully briefed and started the experiment after they had had a chance to practice and fully understood the task. A summary of the results and the implications that can be derived from them will be given here. Two hypotheses were made from Alloy and Abramson's (1979) experiments 1 and 2. A third hypothesis was made, deriving from the depressive realism proposition:

1. In the *contingent conditions* (70% and 30% control), there will be no differences between groups regardless of response type (active and nonactive), both depressed and nondepressed groups judging the degree of contingency accurately. There will also be no difference between males and females both within and across groups.

2. In the *noncontingent conditions* (0% control) there will be no difference between groups in the low level of reinforcement (30% star appearance); but in the high level of reinforcement (70% star appearance), the nondepressed group will overestimate their degree of control and the depressed group will be accurate. Response type (active and nonactive) will

not be a significant factor. Nondepressed females, relative to other groups, will overestimate degree of control in the high level of reinforcement conditions.

3. Nondepressed subjects, as a group, will view their general performance overoptimistically as being above average, while depressed subjects, as a group, will view their performance realistically, as average.

The results relating to hypotheses 1 and 2 are shown in Figures 12.1 and 12.2. Two four-way mixed analyses of variance were carried out. To test hypothesis 1 (Figure 12.1), the factors were mood (depressed or nondepressed) × sex (male and female) × response type (active or nonactive) × level of control which is a repeated factor (70% or 30%). To test hypothesis 2 (Figure 13.2), the factors were mood × sex × response type × level of reinforcement, which is repeated (70% or 30% appearance of star).

Figure 12.1 indicates, as was predicted, that both groups behave remarkably similarly in the 70% degree of control: They are relatively accurate in the active response condition but they underestimate their control in the inactive response condition. The two groups also respond similarly in the 30% control, active response condition (both groups overestimating their control), but in the 30% control, inactive response condition, *the nondepressed are relatively accurate while the depressed underestimate control.*

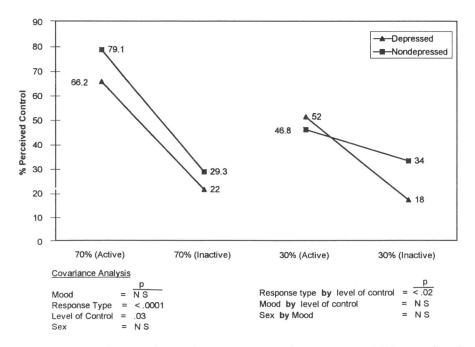

FIGURE 12.1. Judgment of control in contingent conditions (70% or 30% control) and active or inactive response type.

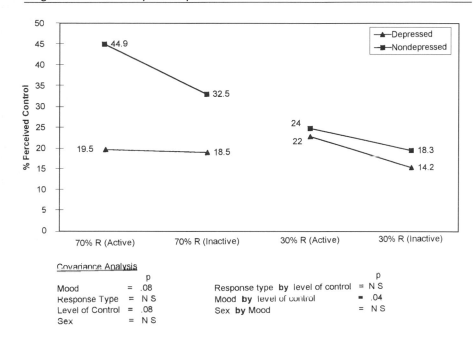

FIGURE 12.2. Judgment of control in noncontingent conditions (0% control), two levels of reinforcement (R), and active or inactive response type.

The analysis of variance indicates that hypothesis 1 was only partly supported: There was no group (Mood) difference and no sex or sex × mood difference, but response type (Active or Inactive) was a highly significant factor ($F = 23.7$, $df = 1,32$, $p < .0001$), and level of control was also significant ($F = 5.8$, $df = 1,32$, $p < .03$). There was a significant interaction between response type and level of control ($F = 6.2$, $df = 1,32$, $p < .02$). Thus, the depressed and nondepressed groups did not differ significantly, but level of control and response type did affect judgment.

Figure 12.2 indicates that in the noncontingent condition (0% control), the results obtained with dysphoric students (Alloy & Abramson, 1979) were replicated. With high frequency of star appearance (70% reinforcement), both groups overestimate their level of control but the nondepressed overestimate far more in both the active and nonactive response type. The difference between groups is less obvious in the low reinforcement (30%) condition.

The multiple analysis of variance shows that group (Mood) showed a trend towards significance ($F = 3.3$, $df = 1,32$, $p < .08$) as did level of reinforcement ($F = 3.3$, $df = 1,32$, $p < .08$). However, as predicted, there was a significant interaction between mood and level of reinforcement ($F = 4.3$, $df = 1,32$, $p < .04$), indicating that the nondepressed subjects overestimated degree of control relative to depressed subjects in the high reinforcement condition. Also, as predicted, response type (active or nonactive) was not a significant factor. However, contrary to prediction, sex and sex × mood were not significant, indicating that, unlike the nondepressed undergraduate females, nondepressed females in this experiment did not overestimate their degree of control in the high reinforcement condition.

In hypothesis 3, we predicted that the nondepressed would overestimate their performance as a group and the depressed would not. At the end of the experiment, all subjects were asked to rate their performance relative to the other people who took part in the experiment on a scale of 1 to 3, where 1 = above average, 2 = average, and 3 = below average. The nondepressed, as a group, were realistic, rating their performance as average (mean = 2.0, SD = 0.64) and the depressed, as a group, rated their performance as below average (mean = 2.7, SD = 0.47). Thus, in their self-evaluation, the depressed patients showed an unrealistic negative bias, in that the large majority rated themselves as performing at a lower level than other group members, and the nondepressed were realistic. This does not support the hypothesis of depressive realism.

In summary, essentially the phenomenon of "depressive realism," as found in the original Alloy and Abramson (1979) study, was supported as far as judgment of control was concerned, when there was in fact 0% control, but a highly reinforcing condition. When self-evaluation was concerned, the more typical overly negative bias was found in the depressed group, while the nondepressed were realistic. Thus, depressive realism may be applicable to only some situations, namely evaluation of control, while depressive negative bias is applicable to self-evaluation. It could therefore be argued, if the findings of a laboratory experiment could be extended to apply to more general day-to-day functioning, that the characteristics of depressive thinking involve considering oneself as relatively helpless and, furthermore, considering oneself as performing less well than others.

GENERAL CONCLUSION

In these four studies, I have given an overview of work carried out by a group of colleagues whom I acknowledge at the end of the chapter. It is my opinion that research in cognitive vulnerability to depression is only in its infancy and that promising trends are now in place. These include the role of basic personality dimensions such as sociotropy and autonomy and the role of particular cognitive styles in specific situations.

Sociotropy has, to date, been shown to be a more reliable vulnerability factor than autonomy. The revision of the SAS (Clark & Beck, 1991) may help in increasing the construct validity of the scale or it may be possible that the need for autonomy does not, in reality, play a large part in depression. The interpersonal context of depression, as discussed by several authors (e.g., Klerman, Rounsaville, Chevron, & Weissman, 1984, Safran & Segal,

1990), is congruent with the finding that high levels of sociotropy can be a real vulnerability factor.

Depressive realism in judgments of control and depressive negative bias in evaluations of performance are but two aspects of information processing that may be important. Other authors have implicated other aspects—for example, a ruminative response style (Nolen-Hoeksema, Morrow, & Fredrickson, 1993); dimensions of perfectionism (Hewitt & Flett, 1993) that may be related to autonomy, as indicated in study 2; and overgeneral recall, especially for positive autobiographical memories (Brittlebank, Scott, Williams, & Ferrier, 1993).

The search for psychological vulnerability factors does not preclude the role of other classes of vulnerability factors. These are likely to interact to produce the final common pathway of depression. For example, Harris, Brown, and Bifulco (1990) and Brown, Bifulco, and Andrews (1990) have shown how psychological variables, such as helplessness and low self-esteem, interact with life events to produce depression. Biological vulnerability factors are certainly also implicated, although they have been difficult to establish. Family genetic studies (McGuffin & Katz, 1986) and, more tentatively, genetic marker studies, attest to a substantial heritability factor in depression. However, the interplay of environmental, psychological, and heritability factors is complex and not yet clarified.

ACKNOWLEDGMENTS

I am grateful for the collaboration of Richard Moore, now at the MRC Applied Psychology Unit in Cambridge; Louise Mountford, now at the Royal Edinburgh Hospital; Hilary Roxborough, now at the Department of Psychiatry, Manchester; and Angela Wilson and Michelle Hipwell, Royal Edinburgh Hospital.

REFERENCES

Abramson, L. T., Seligman, M. E. P., & Teasdsale, J. D. (1978). Learned helplessness in humans: Critique and reformulations. *Journal of Abnormal Psychology, 87,* 49–74.

Alloy, L. B., & Abramson, L. Y. (1979). Judgement of contingency in depresssed and non-depressed college students: Sadder but wiser? *Journal of Experimental Psychology: General, 108,* 441–485.

Beck, A. T. (1967). *Depression: Clinical, experimental and theoretical aspects.* New York: Harper & Row.

Beck, A. T. (1983). Cognitive therapy of depression: New perspectives. In P. J. Clayton & J. E. Barrett (Eds.), *Treatment of depression: Old controversies and new approaches.* New York: Raven Press.

Beck, A. T. (1987). Cognitive model of depression. *Journal of Cognitive Psychotherapy, 1,* 2–27.

Beck, A. T., & Beck, R. W. (1972). Screening depressed patients in family practice: A rapid technique. *Postgraduate Medicine, 52,* 81–85.

Beck, A. T., Epstein, N.., & Harrison, R. (1983). Cognitions, attitudes and personality dimensions in depression. *British Journal of Cognitive Psychotherapy, 1,* 1–16.

Beck, A. T., Ward, C. H., Mendelson, M., Mock, J., & Erbaugh, J. (1961). An inventory for measuring depression. *Archives of General Psychiatry, 4,* 561–571.

Blackburn, I. M., Roxborough, H. M., Muir, W. J., Glabus, M., & Blackwood, D. H. R. (1990). Perceptual and physiological dysfunction in depression. *Psychological Medicine, 20,* 95–103.

Blaney, P. H. (1986). Affect and memory: A review. *Psychological Bulletin, 99,* 229–246.

Blatt, S. J., Quinlan, D. M., Chevron, E. S., McDonald, C., & Zuroff, D. (1982). Dependency and self-criticism: Psychological dimensions of depression. *Journal of Consulting and Clinical Psychology, 50,* 113–124.

Brittlebank, A. D., Scott, J., Williams, J. M. G., & Ferrier, I. N., (1993). Autobiographical memory in depression: State or trait marker? *British Journal of Psychiatry, 162,* 118–121.

Brown, G., Bifulco, A., & Andrews, B. (1990). Self-esteem and depression. III. Etiological issues. *Social Psychiatry and Psychiatric Epidemiology, 25,* 235–243.

Brown, G., & Harris, T. (1978). *The social origins of depression.* London: Tavistock.

Clark, D. A., & Beck, A. T. (1991). Personality factors in dysphoria: A psychometric refinement of Beck's Sociotropy–Autonomy Scale. *Journal of Psychopathology and Behavioral Assessment, 13,* 369–388.

Cleary, P., & Guy, W. (1977). Factor analysis of the Hamilton Depression Scale. *Drugs in Experimental and Clinical Research, 1,* 115–120.

Costello, C. G. (1992). Conceptual problems in current research on cognitive vulnerability to psychopathology. *Cognitive Therapy and Research, 16,* 379–390.

Eysenck, H. J., & Eysenck, S. B. G. (1975). *Manual of the Eysenck Personality Questionnaire.* London: Hodder and Stoughton.

Gilbert, P., & Reynolds, S. (1990). The relationship between the Eysenck Personality Questionnaire and Beck's concepts of sociotropy and autonomy. *British Journal of Clinical Psychology, 29,* 319–325.

Hamilton, M. (1960). A rating scale for depression. *Journal of Neurology, Neurosurgery and Psychiatry, 23,* 56–62.

Harris, T., Brown, G., & Bifulco, A. (1990). Depression and situational helplessness/Mastery in a sample selected to study childhood parental loss. *Journal of Affective Disorders, 20,* 27–41.

Hewitt, P. L., & Flett, G. L. (1993). Dimensions of perfectionism, daily stress and depression: A test of the specific vulnerability hypothesis. *Journal of Abnormal Psychology, 102,* 58–65.

Hollon, S. D., & Kendall, P. C. (1980). Cognitive self-statements in depression: Development of an Automatic Thoughts Questionnaire. *Cognitive Therapy and Research, 4,* 383–395.

Imber, S. D., Pilkonis, P. A., Sotsky, S. M., Elkin, I., Watkins, J. T., Collings, J. F., Shea, M. T., Leber, W. R., & Glass, D. R. (1990). 'Mode'-specific effects among three treatments for depression. *Journal of Consulting and Clinical Psychology, 58,* 352–359.

Kendell, R. E., & DiScipio, W. J. (1970). Obsessional symptoms and obsessional personality traits in patients with depressive illnesses. *Psychological Medicine, 1,* 65–72.

Klerman, G. L., Rounsaville, B., Chevron, E., & Weissman, M. (1984). *Interpersonal psychotherapy of depression.* New York: Basic Books.

Kovacs, M., & Beck, A. T. (1978). Maladaptive cognitive structures in depression. *American Journal of Psychiatry, 135, 525–535.*

Kraepelin, E. (1921). *Manic depressive insanity and paranoia* (R. M. Barclay, Trans.) Edinburgh, Scotland: E & S Livingstone.

McGuffinn, N. P., & Katz, R. (1986). Nature, nurture and affective disorder. In J. F. W. Deakin (Ed.), *Biology of depression.* London: Royal College of Psychiatrists, Gaskell.

Martin, M. (1985). Neuroticism as cognitive predisposition to depression: A cognitive mechanism. *Personality and Individual Differences, 6, 353–365.*

Moore, R. G., & Blackburn, I. M. (1993). Sociotropy, autonomy and personal memories in depression. *British Journal of Clinical Psychology, 32, 460–462.*

Moore, R. G., & Blackburn, I. M. (1994). The relationship of sociotropy and autonomy to symptoms, cognition and personality in depressed patients. *Journal of Affective Disorders, 32, 239–245.*

Mountford, L. A. (1992). *An investigation of "depressive realism."* Unpublished thesis, University of Edinburgh, Edinburgh, Scotland.

Murray, I. G., & Blackburn, I. M. (1974). Personality differences in patients with depressive illness and anxiety neurosis. *Acta Psychiatrica Scandinavica, 50, 183–191.*

Nietzel, M. T., & Harris, M. J. (1990). Relationship of dependency and achievement/autonomy to depression. *Clinical Psychology Review, 10, 279–297.*

Nolen-Hoeksema, S., Morrow, J., & Fredrickson, B. L. (1993). Response styles and the duration of episodes of depressed mood. *Journal of Aboral Psychology, 102, 20–28.*

Persons, J. B., & Miranda, J. (1992). Cognitive theories of vulnerability to depression: Reconciling negative evidence. *Cognitive Therapy and Research, 16, 485–502.*

Prusoff, B. A., Klerman, G. L., & Paykel, E. S. (1972). Concordance between clinical assessments and patients' self-report of depression. *Archives of General Psychiatry, 26, 546–552.*

Roxborough, H. M. (1991). *Psychological and cognitive dysfunction in depression.* Unpublished doctoral dissertation, University of Edinburgh, Edinburgh, Scotland.

Safran, J. D., & Segal, J. D. (1990). *Interpersonal process in cognitive therapy.* New York: Basic Books.

Spielberger, C. D., Gorsuch, R. L., & Lushene, R. E. (1970). *Manual for State–Trait Anxiety Inventory.* Palo Alto, CA: Consulting Psychologists Press.

Spitzer, R. L., Endicott, J., & Robins, E. (1978). Research diagnostic criteria: Rationale and reliability. *Archives of General Psychiatry, 35, 773–782.*

Teasdale, J. D. (1988). Cognitive vulnerability to persistent depression. *Cognition and Emotion, 2, 247–274.*

Weissman, A., & Beck, A. T. (1978). *Development and validation of the Dysfunctional Attitude Scale.* Paper presented at the 12th annual meeting of the Association for Advancement of Behavior Therapy, Chicago.

Chapter 13

Developing Cognitive Therapist Competency: Teaching and Supervision Models

Christine A. Padesky

C ognitive therapy was one of the first therapies to provide detailed specifications for treatment stages, structure, and methods. The seminal text on the therapy, *Cognitive Therapy of Depression* (Beck, Rush, Shaw, & Emery, 1979), was originally written as a therapist training manual to standardize treatment interventions. Clear specificity in treatment methods allowed researchers to evaluate how closely therapists adhered to treatment protocols and whether different elements of these protocols correlated with positive treatment outcome.

While treatment outcome is generally used to measure the efficacy of therapy models, it can also be used as a measure of therapist competency. Several studies suggest that therapists obtain better treatment outcome for depression if they adhere closely to the structure of cognitive therapy (Shaw, 1988) and follow the standardized procedures of the therapy (Thase, 1994). Therefore, two possible criteria for therapist competency are knowledge of and adherence to treatment protocols.

While these studies have not been duplicated for all the various problems treated with cognitive therapy, the development of specific cognitive therapy protocols for specific disorders assumes that protocol adherence is linked to therapy outcome. Therefore, programs teaching therapists to conduct cognitive therapy usually teach cognitive conceptualizations for particular problems as well as specific procedures to be administered according to the principles and structure specified in cognitive therapy treatment protocols.

Therapist adherence to general cognitive therapy principles is often measured by ratings on the Cognitive Therapy Scale (CTS; Young & Beck, 1980) which was devised to measure therapist competency in applying cognitive therapy. The CTS seems to be a reliable and valid measure of therapist competency (Dobson, Shaw, & Vallis, 1985; Hollon et al., 1981; Vallis, Shaw,

& Dobson, 1986; Young, Shaw, Beck, & Budenz, 1981) with intraclass reliability coefficients ranging from .54 to .96 (Beckham & Watkins, 1989). Instructors and therapists wishing to rate therapists' cognitive therapy skills can use the CTS to rate an audiotape or videotape of a therapy session on general therapy skills (e.g., collaboration, interpersonal rapport, pacing of the session) and on specific cognitive therapy skills (e.g., focus on key cognitions, strategies for change, quality of homework assigned).

TEACHING COGNITIVE THERAPY TO THERAPISTS

Competency as a cognitive therapist requires knowledge of cognitive therapy theory and the ability to apply this theory in a structured fashion. To do so, therapists must be able to formulate a useful case conceptualization and skillfully apply empirically based clinical methods within a collaborative therapeutic relationship. Programs that teach cognitive therapy must therefore teach therapists conceptualization skills, interpersonal processes necessary to the formation and maintenance of a collaborative therapeutic relationship, a range of clinical procedures, and treatment protocols that specify how and when to use particular procedures for particular problems.

Content Required for Therapist Competency

Teaching cognitive therapy in the final decade of this century is more complex than it was in the late 1970s when a single treatment model existed for a single disorder, depression. Today there are specific cognitive therapy conceptualizations and treatment protocols for most syndromes described in the fourth edition of the *Diagnostic and Statistical Manual of Mental Disorders* (American Psychiatric Association, 1994). Further, positive treatment outcomes obtained in empirical studies contribute to the expectation that cognitive therapists should be able to treat multiproblem clients in brief format therapy. This complex task requires therapists to form rapid conceptualizations and be knowledgeable and skilled in the treatment of varied and interrelated problems. A brief history of the content taught in cognitive therapy training programs will illustrate this evolution and explosion in the knowledge base required to achieve "competency" as a cognitive therapist.

The Evolution of the Cognitive Therapy Knowledge Base

When Beck introduced cognitive therapy for depression in the 1970s, other therapies for depression were highlighting affect, biology, interpersonal relationships, and sometimes behavior. Beck proposed cognition and behavior as primary focal points for therapeutic intervention. Therapists wishing to learn this new therapy read *Cognitive Therapy of Depression* (Beck et al.,

1979) as the new template for depression treatment. To achieve competency, one learned Beck's cognitive model for understanding depression (Beck, 1967) and mastered the techniques described in the treatment manual (Beck et al., 1979).

The primary therapist skills taught in this latter book were methods for changing behavior, identifying cognitions, and teaching clients to test out negative thoughts and beliefs. Since affect was already predominant in this clinical population, only cursory discussion was given to the importance of cultivating affect in therapy. Therapists were taught to do therapy in a relatively new way. Each session was structured with a clear agenda, problem focus, and development of homework assignments to encourage client learning, observation, and experimentation between therapy sessions. Within sessions, there was a new concept of "collaborative empiricism" (Beck et al., 1979, p. 6) in which the therapist employed "Socratic questions" to guide client learning and reevaluation of negative depressogenic beliefs.

As cognitive therapy's efficacy for treating depression was established (Rush, Beck, Kovacs, & Hollon, 1977; Shaw, 1977; Blackburn, Bishop, Glen, Whalley, & Christie, 1981; Murphy, Simons, Wetzel, & Lustman, 1984; Beck, Hollon, Young, Bedrosian, & Budenz, 1985), the therapy became increasingly popular among therapists and researchers around the world. Paradigms evolved that applied its principles to an ever expanding array of problems including anxiety disorders, eating disorders, and relationship difficulties. With each new application, new conceptual models were developed and empirically tested. In addition, new content requirements for therapist competency were added.

By the mid-1980s, cognitive therapy was a treatment of choice for anxiety disorders. Beck and others developed cognitive conceptualizations for anxiety disorders (cf. Beck, Emery, & Greenberg, 1985; Butler & Matthews, 1983; Clark, 1986; Salkovskis, 1985) . Cognitive therapists wishing to attain competency now needed to learn conceptual models for both depression and anxiety. In addition, while still structured and grounded in collaborative empiricism, the anxiety treatments required new skills for therapists.

Anxious cognitions often occurred as images so therapists learned methods for assessing and cognitively restructuring images. In contrast with depression treatment, affect was not omnipresent in sessions. Therapists needed to learn methods for inducing affect in session because "cognitive therapy cannot be done in the absence of affect" (Beck, 1990). Unlike depression, which was successfully treated by similar cognitive therapy methods regardless of type, anxiety disorders responded differentially to treatment. Therefore, cognitive therapists learned specific conceptualizations and treatment protocols for each anxiety disorder.

In addition to cognitive therapy for anxiety disorders, research-based treatment paradigms emerged for many other problems in the 1980s. Cognitive conceptualizations and treatment paradigms were developed for problems as diverse as eating disorders (Garner & Bemis, 1982; Fairburn, 1985), substance abuse (Beck, Wright, Newman, & Liese, 1993), relationship problems (Beck, 1988; Baucom & Epstein, 1990; Dattilio & Padesky, 1990), and schizophrenia (Perris, 1988; Kingdon & Turkington, 1994).

In the late 1980s cognitive therapists began discussing applications of cognitive therapy principles to the treatment of personality disorders (Padesky, 1988; Pretzer & Fleming, 1989). By 1990 these ideas were collected in a text that outlined specific treatment emphases and strategies for each of the personality disorders (Beck et al., 1990). Cognitive therapy of personality disorders requires therapists to develop individualized case conceptualizations that include deeper schematic beliefs as well as the automatic thoughts and underlying assumptions that are the primary focus of depression and anxiety treatment. Conceptualizations of clients with personality disorders also include a greater emphasis on early developmental history and client interactions with environmental factors (especially familial and social) which influence schema development and maintenance.

Cognitive therapists treating personality disorders also emphasize the therapist–client relationship more than is required in the treatment of depression and anxiety. This is because the schemas central to personality disorder treatment often emerge most clearly within the therapy relationship. Schema change is central in the treatment of personality disorders. While therapists help clients with personality disorders evaluate and change maladaptive automatic thoughts and underlying assumptions, Beck and his colleagues proposed that the key to personality disorder treatment was changing maladaptive schemas (Beck et al., 1990). Thus, the required cognitive therapy knowledge base expanded to include methods designed to weaken maladaptive schemas and construct new ones. These skills include use of continuum methods, psychodrama, historical tests of schemas, and core belief data logs (Padesky, 1994a).

State-of-the-Art Content Requirements for Therapist Competency

As the previous summary illustrates, the content to be mastered by cognitive therapists has grown enormously over the past 20 years. As always, cognitive therapy continues to evolve as clinical practice is teamed with research data. Each specific clinical application includes interventions to be learned and mastered. Once the basics are learned, a competent cognitive therapist develops an artful ability to conceptualize interlocking problems, make intervention choices, and solve problems in an efficient and effective manner to facilitate client learning and change. These ideals are challenging to achieve.

Clinical Processes Required for Therapist Competency

Bridging the various domains of clinical application are the necessity for a positive therapy relationship and therapist ability to follow basic principles of cognitive therapy process: collaboration, guided discovery, and structure. These principles have remained the same throughout cognitive therapy's evolution, although cognitive therapists specify them more clearly over time.

Therapy Relationship Factors

Beck's initial treatment manual (Beck et al., 1979) dedicated a chapter to the necessity for a positive therapeutic relationship including such nonspecific treatment factors as warmth, accurate empathy, genuineness, trust, and rapport. In addition, this book briefly discussed transference and countertransference issues in therapy, acknowledging their importance in cognitive therapy and the direct manner with which cognitive therapists address them. Thus, from the beginning, competent cognitive therapists were expected to be able to form and maintain positive therapeutic relationships.

Some later texts devote considerable discussion to interpersonal processes in cognitive therapy, especially important in therapy with clients with personality disorders (cf. Beck et al., 1990; Safran & Segal, 1990; Wright & Davis, 1994). Strategies for using a positive client–therapist relationship to promote change and using conflict in the therapy relationship to foster client learning are central to cognitive therapy (Newman, 1994; Padesky with Greenberger, 1995; Rane & Goldfried, 1994; Safran & Muran, 1995).

To promote schema change in personality disorders, cognitive therapists use the therapy relationship as a laboratory for testing core beliefs. For example, a client who mistrusts others is encouraged to risk trusting the therapist in small ways. Therapist and client examine affective, cognitive, behavioral, and relationship consequences of these experiments. To fully participate in this type of relationship "laboratory," a cognitive therapist needs good self-awareness in addition to relationship skills.

Cognitive Therapy Process

The fundamental therapy processes in cognitive therapy are collaboration, guided discovery, and structure. Collaboration means therapist and client work together as a team jointly choosing therapy goals, constructing a meaningful conceptualization of problems, and developing plans for change. A collaborative relationship requires both therapist and client to be active and interactive within the therapy relationship. Each seek and receive feedback from the other; questions back and forth are encouraged. Collaboration in cognitive therapy requires the client also to be active outside the session as an observer, reporter of experiences, and experimenter. Therapists who are not willing to participate in a highly interactive therapy relationship are poor candidates for cognitive therapy training.

Guided discovery is the primary learning process in cognitive therapy. Therapists guide discovery both verbally through questioning and experientially by helping clients devise experiments conducted in and outside of therapy sessions. Guided discovery is the engine that drives client learning in cognitive therapy. Encouragement of active client observation and examination of thoughts, emotions, behaviors, interpersonal patterns, and physiological responses is fundamental to guided discovery. Therapists with an understanding of scientific method and an enthusiasm for helping others learn for themselves are ideally suited to guide client discovery.

Finally, cognitive therapy is structured. Within sessions, cognitive therapists collaboratively set agendas with clients, clearly define goals, provide frequent summaries, and help construct specific, structured learning assignments. Across sessions, skills are taught in a stepwise fashion, clients are encouraged to keep therapy notes and records, and treatment protocols are followed as closely as ideal for a particular client's treatment.

The degree and form this structure takes can be quite different depending upon the client and the problems addressed. For example, cognitive therapy of panic disorder follows a highly structured treatment protocol over a brief number of sessions. Alternatively, cognitive therapy for posttraumatic stress disorder with a rape victim with concurrent borderline personality disorder would require more flexibility in structure, collaborating with the client to determine the types and degrees of session structure that can be therapeutically tolerated week to week. Therefore, the ideal cognitive therapist is capable of being highly structured in therapy, comfortable tracking a number tasks within a session, and yet sensitive to adapting therapy structure to individual clients in order to maximize collaboration and a positive therapeutic relationship.

In the following section a variety of teaching methods are described that foster the development of therapist competency in content, relationship factors, and cognitive therapy process. It is ideal if training and supervision programs model mastery of content, positive relationships (between instructor and student), collaboration, guided discovery, and structure.

Teaching Processes

From the earliest years of cognitive therapy training, Beck preferred teaching methods that modeled the therapy and provided therapists with learning experiences to guide their discovery. His workshops and presentations include frequent use of Socratic dialogue to help participants discover theoretical principles. In addition, Beck employs experiential exercises to encourage students to gather data regarding their own thoughts, emotions, and physiological responses, linking these personal experiences to the topics of discussion. In these ways, from the beginning, cognitive therapy has been taught using principles of collaboration, guided discovery, conceptualization, and structure.

Collaboration

Collaboration between instructor and student is central in the teaching and learning of cognitive therapy. Students are encouraged to play an active role in learning by (1) questioning the instructor, (2) participating in exercises designed to teach key therapy principles, and (3) thoughtfully answering instructor questions by drawing on clinical experiences and self-observation. Cognitive therapy instructors collaborate with students by (1) openly discussing the teaching agenda, (2) encouraging student input regarding topics and learning processes, (3) asking questions to guide student discovery, and (4) inviting student feedback on clinical demonstrations and theoretical principles.

Cognitive therapy instructors foster supportive, investigative teams. In large learning groups, these teams can be small groups of two to six members that learn via role plays and discussion, followed by instructor feedback. Smaller learning groups can work as a whole to encourage and foster learning. For example, group dyads can practice cognitive therapy skills in front of the group and receive feedback from colleagues on what they did well and what could be improved. A supportive atmosphere is necessary because therapists must feel safe and comfortable making mistakes in front of the group. If therapists feel group pressure to avoid mistakes, they will hesitate to try new approaches and new learning will be limited.

Guided Discovery/Empiricism

Cognitive therapy employs guided discovery and empirical investigative methods as the principal methods for client learning and change. Using these same principles to teach cognitive therapy to therapists reinforces the importance of data-based learning. Knowledge of previous empirical findings provides a foundation for cognitive therapy training programs. Students are encouraged and instructors are required to stay abreast of clinically relevant empirical research. The most successful clinical applications of cognitive therapy have been developed in parallel with empirical studies of the clinical phenomena treated. Cognitive therapy instructors learn about research by reading professional journals, attending research symposia at national and international cognitive therapy conferences, and often by conducting research themselves.

In addition to learning from empirical research, cognitive therapists add to their own personal competency by regularly investigating the benefits and shortcomings of clinical methods learned. Instructors encourage student use of empirical methods by setting up learning experiments for student therapists to complete. For example, students learning to use Automatic Thought Records can be assigned to first complete Thought Records for themselves. The instructor can guide discovery by questioning students about what they learned using Thought Records. These questions can include queries about a variety of factors such as what made it easy or difficult to notice automatic thoughts, what thoughts or emotions interfered with the task, what strategies helped the students, and how the experiences of these therapists might be similar or different from clients' experiences with this same assignment.

Following therapist practice of clinical methods and discussion of what was learned, therapists are asked to try the same methods with one or more clients to gather more information about the value and difficulties entailed in a specific clinical intervention. Practicing only a few new methods at a time facilitates student learning, especially if these methods are applied with several clients with the same diagnoses. Repeated practice with similar clients enhances therapist learning by allowing comparison of results from several closely spaced learning trials. Therapists with a full and diverse caseload can often create these learning circumstances by selecting two or three similar clients with which to practice particular cognitive therapy methods.

These experimental learning forays on the part of the student therapist will usually have a mixed clinical outcome; some clients will respond well to the interventions, others will not. The instructor or supervisor can encourage the learning therapist to use both positive and negative experiences to advance learning. A truly empirical stance on the part of the therapist consists of (1) formulating hypotheses (e.g., learning to use a Thought Record will help my depressed clients feel better), (2) conducting multiple experiments (e.g., teaching several depressed clients to use a Thought Record), (3) noting the outcome of these experiments (e.g., two clients benefited greatly from the Thought Record, one seemed to become more depressed in the process of learning the Thought Record), (4) analyzing these outcomes carefully (e.g., the client who did not find it helpful had a much more vegetative depression), (5) implementing further experiments (e.g., I could try more behavioral interventions with this client, or add medication), (6) reviewing the outcomes of these experiments (e.g., this third client is still quite depressed, but responding somewhat better to behavioral rather than cognitive interventions), and (7) drawing tentative conclusions (e.g., Thought Records seem helpful for most depressed clients; I will use behavioral and pharmacological approaches first with clients who have many vegetative symptoms) to be (8) further tested by additional clinical experiments.

Instructors foster therapist willingness to use this type of empirical approach if these methods are modeled in the teaching setting. Rather than didactically teaching "truths," instructors can summarize empirical findings and then devise learning experiments to see if and how these findings apply to the students' own experiences and clients. Students are encouraged to figure out why interventions are not always successful by examining the quality of the implementation of these interventions, characteristics of the client, and therapist beliefs and emotions that also influence treatment outcomes. Finally, students are taught that no clinical approach works perfectly with every client. The art and skill of therapy are best developed in a therapist who consistently analyzes and learns from both positive and negative client feedback and outcome.

Conceptualization

Another cornerstone of cognitive therapy instruction is teaching therapists to formulate a useful conceptualization of the client's problems. A cognitive therapy conceptualization will include beliefs (automatic thoughts, underlying assumptions, and schemas), emotional reactions, behavioral strengths and deficits, social factors that influence problems (both past and present), and consideration of biological factors. Persons (1989) recommends therapists look for the smallest number of explanatory elements that can account for all of the client's presenting problems. Thorough assessment of client beliefs is central to conceptualization in cognitive therapy, not because beliefs are considered the root cause of all problems, but because beliefs serve a powerful maintenance function for problematic behavioral and interpersonal difficulties (Padesky, 1994a).

A number of methods are used to teach case conceptualization to cognitive therapists. Often, beginning therapists are instructed to rely on empirically evaluated cognitive models to conceptualize client difficulties. For example, a client's panic disorder is conceptualized as the result of catastrophic misinterpretation of physical or mental sensations according to the model outlined by Clark (1986). Client depression is conceptualized as resulting from biopsychosocial stressors combined with negative cognitions about the self, world, and future (Beck et al., 1979). Therapists who adopt these template conceptualizations and follow the accompanying treatment protocols can be satisfied as long as these make sense to the client and treatment is successful.

Much of the time, however, clients present with more than one difficulty, requiring the therapist to combine or choose among generic conceptual models. Therefore, therapists must learn to develop individualized case conceptualizations. A number of training centers have developed case conceptualization forms to guide therapists in this process. These forms generally ask therapists to list a client's presenting problems, write a brief history of relevant events, describe the interpersonal process in therapy, and identify key underlying assumptions and schemas. This summary is used to write a brief treatment plan that is given to the supervisor for feedback. Written conceptualizations often are discussed with clients who may collaborate in their development.

Written conceptualization forms help the beginning cognitive therapist learn processes for constructing conceptualizations to guide treatment. More experienced cognitive therapists form written conceptualizations in collaboration with clients early in therapy, often as soon as the first or second session, with refinements added as therapy proceeds. Therapists are encouraged to discuss conceptualizations with clients as hypotheses to be evaluated through observation, data collection, and behavioral experiments. Cognitive therapy conceptualizations are descriptive and closely tied to understanding and explaining the client's day-to-day experiences.

Cognitive therapy instructors and supervisors are encouraged to model and illustrate a variety of case conceptualization methods for students. Students are encouraged to experiment with diagnostically based conceptualizations, written case conceptualization forms, and diagrams of client patterns to discover which approaches are most helpful.

Structure

Learning to do cognitive therapy in a structured fashion is often one of the most difficult tasks for therapists. Instructors model the use of structure in each teaching session by setting agendas, monitoring time usage, and seeking regular feedback from students on the learning pace followed. Students are encouraged to practice a more structured therapy approach within time-limited role-play assignments in which certain therapy tasks need to be accomplished. Role-play exercises are analyzed to find which strategies are effective for balancing structure, focus, and a positive therapy relationship.

Feedback from the "clients" in these role plays is usually very instructive. Therapists often believe that structure is disruptive to a good therapy relationship and client insight. As clients, therapists often discover that, compared with relatively unstructured interviewing methods, an empathic structured interview creates an atmosphere in which greater understanding from the therapist and more hope for improvement are experienced because a clearer treatment plan emerges.

Audio- and videotapes of therapists' sessions with actual clients are reviewed by the cognitive therapy instructor to assess whether the student therapist is adhering to a structured plan within the therapy hour. Therapists often need help learning to manage common impediments to structure such as agendas that are too complex for the time available, clients who have difficulty maintaining focus, and the demands of debriefing and developing homework assignments that can take more time than novice therapists allow. Discussion and role play of strategies for maintaining structure help develop a therapist's behavioral skills. In addition, therapist beliefs about the advantages and disadvantages of structure may need to be examined and tested using Thought Records and behavioral experiments.

Teaching Methods

While most cognitive therapy training programs strive to incorporate the principles outlined above, a variety of teaching methods are employed to accomplish these learning goals. Most programs use several of the teaching methods below. Ideally, therapists wishing to become competent cognitive therapists will sample all these learning methods en route.

Reading Materials

Cognitive therapists have written some of the most specific and wide-ranging topical descriptions of therapy in the history of psychotherapy. Therefore, students of cognitive therapy have no difficulty finding written references for almost any client population and set of problems. Cognitive therapy instructors facilitate student learning by selecting texts that combine the knowledge derived from empirical studies with clear and specific descriptions of their clinical applications.

Brief training programs sometimes use a single text that describes cognitive therapy applied to a variety of problems (cf. Freeman, Pretzer, Fleming, & Simon, 1990; Hawton, Salkovskis, Kirk, & Clark, 1989). Longer training programs usually ask students to study primary texts on cognitive therapy for specific problems such as depression (Beck et al., 1979), anxiety (Beck, Emery, & Greenberg, 1985), personality disorders (Beck et al., 1990), and other common clinical populations treated, such as couples (Baucom & Epstein, 1990; Dattilio & Padesky, 1990) or children (Kendall, 1991).

Cognitive therapy treatment manuals written for clients also facilitate therapist learning by providing a programmed text to use in therapy. A 12-chapter treatment manual written by Greenberger and Padesky (1995) teaches clients the basic cognitive therapy skills necessary for the treatment of many different client problems. Chapters teach how to identify emotions, identify automatic thoughts, use Thought Records to evaluate automatic thoughts, conduct behavioral experiments, and begin schema change methods. This client manual helps beginning cognitive therapists by providing written explanations for common cognitive therapy learning tasks.

Further, summaries, "hints," and troubleshooting guides in this client manual can be extremely helpful to a therapist learning to practice cognitive therapy. These written guidelines highlight key ideas and help solve common problems encountered in conducting cognitive therapy. A clinician's guide accompanies this client treatment manual and summarizes threatment protocols for a variety of cognitive therapy applications (Padesky with Greenberger, 1995). The clinician's guide also highlights common dilemmas faced by cognitive therapists, with recommendations about how collaboration and guided discovery can help resolve these difficulties.

Client treatment manuals also have been written for specific client problems such as depression (Burns, 1989; Eaves, Jarrett, & Basco, 1989), anxiety (Bourne, 1990), obsessive–compulsive disorder (Steketee & White, 1990), and relationship problems (Beck, 1988). Each of these client manuals provides a structured presentation of a cognitive therapy approach for treating these difficulties. Beginning cognitive therapists may find client workbooks a helpful addition to the therapy they conduct. Since workbooks provide explanations of cognitive therapy principles written in simple language, beginning therapists can model their own verbal explanations to clients on these written samples.

Clinical Demonstrations

Written texts and manuals describe treatment principles in detail. Clinical demonstrations illustrate therapeutic processes and, sometimes, artistry. For example, a cognitive therapy text will describe collaborative empiricism and perhaps even provide written therapist–client dialogues. Yet these illustrations leave much out. A clinical demonstration provides added information about pacing, vocal tone and inflection, nonverbal communication between therapist and client, and the development of interventions in "real therapy time."

Clinical demonstrations can be live, videotaped, or audiotaped and may involve clients or role plays. Each format has its advantages and disadvantages. Live demonstrations are useful when learning therapists want consultation with a particularly challenging client or diagnosis. A clinical instructor can meet with a selected client to illustrate interventions *in vivo*. Live demonstrations also can be done impromptu during classes or workshops to illustrate treatment principles or to respond to student questions. Students who are skeptical about the usefulness of cognitive therapy for particularly complex clients are often reassured by a live clinical demonstration that illustrates therapy principles applied under challenging circumstances.

Live clinical demonstrations can be provided by students as well as the instructor. It is helpful for therapists learning cognitive therapy to practice its tenets under the observation of other therapists who provide constructive feedback. Initially, students are most comfortable providing brief role-play demonstrations of particular therapeutic principles (e.g., 5 minutes of guided discovery). Eventually, it is helpful for students to provide and watch demonstrations of complete therapy sessions.

The "piggyback" supervision model (Padesky, 1993a) can be used to provide live clinical demonstrations when a group of therapists in a common clinical setting are learning cognitive therapy. This method involves therapy demonstrations conducted in rotation by each learning therapist. The most experienced therapist begins by conducting a cognitive therapy session observed live by the other therapists. After this session, the therapist group discusses the session, emphasizing learning for all group members. The first therapist continues his or her demonstration case with weekly discussions and critique of the sessions. After 2 or 3 weeks a second therapist begins treatment with a new client; sessions are similarly observed and critiqued by the learning group. Within a few months, each therapist provides clinical demonstrations for the group and each group member has the opportunity to observe several sessions per week accompanied by group discussion and analysis.

Clinical demonstrations also can be provided on videotape. Videotapes have the advantage of being shown either full-length to capture many of the advantages of live interviews or in an edited format to emphasize key learning points in a shorter period of time. In addition, videotaped interviews can be adapted flexibly to many teaching purposes. Therapists can watch videotaped segments and discuss them in relation to cognitive theory, case conceptualization, or interventions. An instructor can show a portion of a videotape and then ask students what choices they would make in the following minutes of the session. Videotaped role plays can illustrate several possible interventions and their outcomes with the same client in the same circumstances. Nonverbal aspects of cognitive therapy can be highlighted by watching a videotape of a session with the audio portion turned off.

Audiotaped demonstrations lack the visual portrayal of nonverbal therapy components, yet retain many of the other advantages of the videotape format. The main advantages of audiotaped demonstrations are increased portability and lower cost. Portability makes it easy for therapists to listen to audiotapes over and over again to enhance retention of therapy questioning patterns, pacing, methods for maintaining rapport, and other treatment principles that may be well-illustrated on a teaching audiotape. Audiotapes of student therapy sessions are used to analyze student strengths and weaknesses implementing particular cognitive therapy approaches with particular clients.

Classes and Workshops

Most therapists who practice cognitive therapy attend one or more cognitive therapy classes and workshops. Even advanced cognitive therapists attend workshops or listen to audiotapes of workshops to update skills and learn recent developments from clinician and researcher specialists. The structure and teaching methods used in these classes and workshops influence their learning value.

Classes may be as short as a few hours or meet regularly for 1 or more years. While most workshops are a few hours to 2 days in length, cognitive therapy is best learned in programs where learning occurs over a number of weeks, months, or years. Longer periods of instruction allow time to practice the therapy while still meeting with the instructor for questions and feedback. A number of established training programs exist in Australia, Canada, Europe, Great Britain, the United States, and South America where clinicians can participate in multiweek to yearlong training programs. Therapists who live great distances from such training centers often benefit from serial 1- and 2-day workshops or weeklong programs accompanied by ongoing supervision. A few extramural training programs exist in which therapists can receive training long-distance by attending weekend or weeklong training workshops periodically throughout a year and weekly telephone supervision.

Methods used to teach cognitive therapy in these programs are as varied as the topics taught. Cognitive therapy instructors usually prefer interactive teaching methods in classes and workshops, regardless of size. When teaching large groups of therapists, greater organization and creativity is necessary to engage the whole group in active learning processes. A few innovative teaching methods are highlighted here.

Imagery Exercises to Guide Discovery. Beck often uses imagery exercises to guide student discovery of key teaching points. For example, in an anxiety workshop (Beck & Padesky, 1984), Beck used guided imagery to help participants create vivid pictures of themselves as young children waiting at school for a ride home from parents who were quite late. Participants were instructed to note their thoughts and emotional reactions as time passed up to the time the parent eventually arrived, an hour late.

Following this imagination exercise, Beck questioned the audience about their emotional reactions while waiting for the parent (which varied from anger to happiness to terror) and the thoughts that accompanied these responses. He engaged the entire audience by asking individuals to describe their responses and other audience members to raise their hands if their experiences were similar. Using an overhead projector screen to write different moods next to a column of accompanying thoughts, Beck guided the audience to discover cognitive themes associated with particular emotions. Further questioning of the audience elicited information about the role of imagery in anxiety, the relevance of personal developmental history and schemas in relation to emotional vulnerability, and other theoretical points of interest.

Audience imagery exercises are a good way to generate the data necessary to construct learning points. Students are likely to recall these vivid learning experiences. Further, these exercises often parallel clinical methods used in therapy. After participation in imagery exercises, student therapists are asked to reflect on the power of creating vivid experiences in therapy, rather than simply intellectualizing about problems.

Using Socratic Questions with Groups. In therapy, Socratic questions are used to prompt active learning and to encourage a questioning, investigative attitude in the client. Socratic questions serve these same purposes with students. Beck's questions following the imagery exercise described above provide one example of Socratic questioning in a workshop. Instructors also intersperse questions into a lecture to encourage active learning. For example, an instructor might outline the cognitive theory for a particular problem and then ask workshop participants to identify treatment principles that follow from the theory.

As with all Socratic questioning, the level of questions asked should be appropriate to the knowledge base of those questioned (Padesky, 1993b). Beginning therapists can identify cognitive–affective connections but might have difficulty responding to questions that require independent formulation of a cognitive case conceptualization. Therapists with intermediate levels of cognitive therapy experience could respond to questions linking theory, case conceptualization, and applied treatment principles. Advanced therapists can be questioned about all levels of cognitive theory and therapy as applied to particularly challenging cases.

Group Demonstrations of Treatment Principles. The instructor can demonstrate treatment principles by applying them to an entire group. One useful group demonstration is to complete a Thought Record regarding a situation workshop participants have in common. For example, staff at a hospital were required to learn cognitive therapy and many were skeptical that this new approach would be helpful for severely depressed inpatients. As instructor, this author modeled group therapy by helping staff identify their feelings and negative automatic thoughts in the current situation, "learning to use cognitive therapy on the unit," recording and evaluating these reactions on a Thought Record.

Identification of negative automatic thoughts allowed staff members to express their skepticism and reluctance to learn cognitive therapy strategies. Through guided discovery, the instructor was able to help staff members begin to test out their negative beliefs. By the time the Thought Record was complete, the group had identified a number of alternative responses to their negative thoughts. More importantly, the group experienced *in vivo* the powerful effects cognitive therapy methods could have on emotional and cognitive responses to an event. By identifying their own negative, hopeless beliefs, staff experienced cognitive therapy from a perspective similar to that of the depressed inpatients they would help.

Experiential Exercises. To learn cognitive therapy, therapists must practice it. Therefore, most workshops and classes include experiential exercises in which participants apply the methods taught. For example, in a 2-day workshop on schema change interventions, the instructor demonstrated methods for schema identification by helping participant therapists identify their own schemas activated in target clinical situations (Padesky, 1994b). Once they identified schemas, individuals volunteered to participate in instructor-led demonstrations of schema change methods in front of the group. Workshop participants then practiced these same methods individually and in dyads with discussion of learning and stumbling points. Many therapists commented that intensive personal experience of the methods taught provided a much richer learning experience than provided by lecture and demonstration only.

Experiential workshop exercises often are conducted in dyads or small groups. In dyads, one therapist takes the client role and the other the therapist. If a small group is involved, some members are designated "therapist" and "client(s)," other members are consultants or observers. To enhance learning, instructors usually structure practice exercises for beginning to intermediate therapists. For example, therapists are assigned a therapy goal, a clinical method to practice, and a particular client situation for the role play. The client is instructed whether to enact a straightforward or more challenging clinical picture. The instructor(s) observes the small groups and provides consultation when requested. After a time-limited role play, the client gives the therapist feedback regarding what was or was not helpful. Then the larger group discusses what was learned in the role play and how to manage any obstacles encountered.

Beginning therapists often learn best from very structured, time-limited, and goal-oriented practice exercises. As cognitive therapists become more skilled, these role plays become more open ended, with greater therapist choice in goals, clinical methods, and level of client complexity. In this way, experiential exercises become more and more like actual therapy as therapist knowledge and experience increase. In advanced workshops, it is instructive to compare the results of different therapist choices with the same client situation.

COGNITIVE THERAPY SUPERVISION

Cognitive therapy supervision parallels the therapy itself. Supervisor and supervisee establish a supervision problem list, set goals, collaboratively conceptualize roadblocks to attaining these goals, and strategize to overcome these problems. Within each supervision session an agenda is set, new skills are taught, guided discovery is employed, and homework is assigned. The major teaching methods described above are often employed including clinical demonstrations, role plays, didactic instruction, Socratic questioning, behavioral experiments, and frequent use of case conceptualization.

Supervision Models

Supervision can include a variety of methods such as case discussion, video/audio/live observation, role-play demonstrations, and cotherapy. Supervision can emphasize a focus on mastery of cognitive therapy methods, case conceptualization, the client–therapist relationship, therapist reactions, and/or supervisory processes themselves (when the supervisor wishes supervision to improve supervisory skills and process). While most supervision includes a variety of methods and foci, the supervision grid in Table 13.1 provides a graphic outline of supervision options for purposes of discussion.

As Table 13.1 implies, within each supervision focus, learning can be achieved via any of the supervision modes. For example, a therapist attending supervision to learn cognitive therapy methods for treating panic disorder could learn these through discussion of a particular case, supervisor observation of treatment sessions, role plays in supervision, or enlistment of a cotherapist for the treatment itself, either the supervisor or a peer therapist. Similarly, any supervision method can advance learning about any super-

TABLE 13.1. Supervision Options Grid

		Mode				
		Case discussion	Video/audio/ live obser- vation	Role-play demon- stration	Supervisor– supervisee cotherapy	Peer cotherapy
Focus	Mastery of cognitive therapy methods					
	Case concept- ualization					
	Client–therapist relationship					
	Therapist reactions					
	Supervisory processes					

vision focus. For example, role-play demonstrations in supervision can emphasize learning cognitive therapy methods, case conceptualization, use of the client–therapist relationship, therapist reactions, or supervisory processes.

Supervision is conducted in both individual and group formats. The supervisee(s) sets an agenda to determine how time will be spent, including choice of supervision modes and foci. In group supervision, it is best if all group members participate each session, although one or two members may receive the majority of the supervision time in any given meeting. An advantage of group supervision is that group members help supervise each other. In this way, therapists learning cognitive therapy have an opportunity to reflect on the principles they are learning and discuss their application with colleagues.

Supervision Guidelines

While there are many supervisory options, a few principles can guide supervisory choices; (1) build on the supervisee's strengths; (2) choose modes and foci that help develop the next stage of competence; (3) build conceptualization skills so supervisees learn to help themselves, (4) when difficulties occur, use a supervisory road map to pinpoint the problem; and (5) pay attention to what is not discussed in supervision. These principles are illustrated with examples from the supervision models summarized in Table 13.1.

Build on the Supervisee's Strengths

Since guided discovery is central to cognitive therapy, supervision employs this same process. A supervisee's strengths provide a good starting point for guided discovery. For example, if a supervisee has good knowledge of cognitive therapy methods but poor conceptualization skills, the supervisor might ask the supervisee to role play a problem clinical situation (using a mode of supervision that is a strength). This role play could be followed by questions about how these interventions generally proceed (a focus on cognitive therapy method and process that is a strength) and how difficulties occur with this particular client. Then the supervisee could be asked to consider what client beliefs or interpersonal processes might be impeding progress (to begin to build case conceptualization skills).

In contrast, another supervisee might have good case conceptualization skills, yet poor knowledge of cognitive therapy methods. This supervisee might benefit from a initial focus on case conceptualization within a mode of case discussion. The supervisor could provide didactic instruction on therapy methods or elicit ideas from the supervisee by asking questions about how the case conceptualization might fit with cognitive theory and approaches. These discussions would be followed by role-play practice, perhaps with the supervisor initially modeling the methods that the supervisee needs to learn.

Choose Modes and Foci to Develop the Next Stage of Competence

As the preceding examples suggest, supervision begins within modes that emphasize a supervisee's strengths and then shifts to modes and foci that will develop new competencies. Any supervision mode can help develop new competencies. However, it is recommended that each supervision relationship include video, audio, or live observation of sessions because a supervisee's verbal summaries of sessions can describe, at best, only elements of the session within his or her current awareness and understanding. Observation of sessions alerts the supervisor to supervision needs the supervisee may not recognize.

The various foci in Table 13.1 also are used to enhance therapist competence. For beginning therapists, supervision time is usually spent mastering cognitive therapy methods, clinical processes, and case conceptualization skills. Intermediate therapists continue work in these areas with additional attention given to the client–therapist relationship. Advanced therapists ask advanced questions in these three areas and additionally benefit from therapist-focused supervision and even supervision-focused supervision.

Therapist-focused supervision involves identifying therapist emotions and beliefs activated during therapy. While this focus of supervision can be instructive to therapists of all skill levels, it is particularly useful for more advanced therapists learning about schema processes in cognitive therapy. The following vignette illustrates how this supervision focus might be explored with an advanced therapist:

THERAPIST: I'm really struggling in my work with Andy.

SUPERVISOR: What's a struggle for you?

THERAPIST: At the end of the session, he never wants to leave my office. And, unlike with other clients, I find myself letting him stay longer rather than setting a clear stopping time.

SUPERVISOR: What focus would you like to take in working on this: review of strategies for ending on time, case conceptualization, looking at your relationship with Andy, or focusing on your own reactions that might be playing a role?

THERAPIST: I know what to do and I think I have a pretty good case conceptualization. I'd like to understand my own reactions better because they surprise me; I'm not clear what's going on.

SUPERVISOR: Alright. Let's imagine it is the end of the hour and Andy is indicating he doesn't want to leave. Imagine it vividly and see if you can capture your thoughts and feelings.

THERAPIST: (*Imagines silently for a few minutes.*) I feel scared. I want to be helpful to him.

SUPERVISOR: Do any images or memories come to mind?

THERAPIST: How I feel is just like I felt when my mother was waiting for my dad to come home. He was a policeman and she always worried about him. She was anxious and wanted me there. I wanted to go play but felt like I should stay because she was scared. But being with her made me feel anxious.

SUPERVISOR: In this scene with your mother, what were your schemas about yourself?

THERAPIST: I'm responsible.

SUPERVISOR: About the world?

THERAPIST: I suppose, "Unpredictable things happen."

SUPERVISOR: About your mother?

THERAPIST: I'm not sure. I guess. . . . She needs me.

SUPERVISOR: And if you are not there?

THERAPIST: She'll fall apart.

SUPERVISOR: And if that happens?

THERAPIST: I'll be all alone.

SUPERVISOR: What feeling did you have when you said that?

THERAPIST: Scared.

SUPERVISOR: So, you see yourself as responsible and at risk of being alone if you are not supportive to your mother. Also, unpredictable things happen and others will fall apart if they do. Is that right?

THERAPIST: Pretty close. It's even a deeper belief that "if I stay close, I can prevent the bad thing from happening." I know that's illogical, but I think I believed that as a child.

SUPERVISOR: Do you see any way these reactions and beliefs might be related to this therapy dilemma with Andy?

THERAPIST: Yes. He has the same apprehensive silences my mother had. I also feel quite close to him and want him to feel more secure. He does have some rough things happening in his life right now and I think I'd like to protect him from those.

SUPERVISOR: And do you think Andy will fall apart in the face of these bad things?

THERAPIST: I'm not sure.

SUPERVISOR: Do you think spending extra time with him is protective in a good way?

THERAPIST: Hmm. I don't know. All I know is it feels risky at the time to end the session.

SUPERVISOR: Do you think there is a way to help Andy, without reflexively responding according to your childhood schemas?

THERAPIST: I know that's a straightforward question. But I really can't think of anything, so I agree my schemas must be interfering. What ideas do you have?

In this example, the therapist has enough knowledge of schemas that she can identify her own when asked to do so. Even with this knowledge, the supervisor needs to ask questions to help the supervisee identify key beliefs attached to emotional responses. Notice that there is a fine line between therapist-focused supervision and therapy. One way this supervisor maintains a supervision focus is to ask how these particular schemas and this particular developmental event relate to the therapy problem under discussion. In supervision, therapist emotional reactions, schemas, and developmental history are used to inform understanding of the dilemmas faced by a therapist conducting therapy; they are not explored for their own sake.

Build Conceptualization Skills

An ability to conceptualize client and therapy difficulties is critical to the development of therapist competency. Therefore, supervision aims to develop conceptualization ability rather than simply solving problems. Guided discovery can be used to foster analytical skills in supervisees following the stages outlined by Padesky (1993b):

1. *Begin with informational questions* such as, "How can I help you today?" "How would you prioritize your concerns?" "What mode or focus

of supervision do you think would be most helpful?" "What is happening or not happening in therapy that leads to your question?" "What are you doing that helps?" "At what point do your interventions break down?" "Do you have any idea what the problem is?" These questions require the supervisee to focus and define a problem area and encourage active participation in the supervision process. Further, they help educate the supervisee about areas of analysis that may be important to consider. In addition, they may elicit the information necessary to resolve the difficulty.

2. *Listen carefully to what the supervisee says or does not say.* Pay attention to how the supervisee describes the problem. What affect is present? Is the supervisee perplexed, ashamed, or anxious? Strong emotional responses may be clues that therapist beliefs are activated in the clinical situation or supervision and need to be addressed. Listen to assess the supervisee's level of understanding of the problem and the terms in which he or she is formulating it. For example, is he or she describing the problem as poor client motivation when the data suggests the client has skill deficits?

3. *Make frequent summaries and ask the supervisee to do the same.* Summaries provide an opportunity to mutually test your understanding of what has been discussed or role played. It is important to provide time in supervision to process feedback. Both supervisor and supervisee should write down helpful conclusions or hypotheses for future reference. Allow time for the supervisee to summarize what has been helpful or not. In turn, the supervisor can give feedback on what critical learning issues emerged from the supervisory session.

4. Finally, *ask analytical and synthesizing questions to foster the supervisee's conceptualization skills.* Basic synthesizing questions include, "How do you think this conceptualization might apply to the problem you had in the last session?" "So what might you do in the next session?" "If this doesn't have the desired result, what other options do you have? How do you predict this will affect the therapy relationship?" Therapists can be asked to draw their conceptual model on paper, linking beliefs, affect, behaviors, and situations.

Use a Supervisory Road Map for Locating Problems

Supervision is mostly filled with problems to be solved. The supervisor must assess what type of problem exists before choosing a strategy for addressing it. A five-stage decision tree can be helpful. A negative response to any of the first four questions indicates that supervision can begin at that level. The fifth question looks for more subtle sources of difficulty:

1. Is there a cognitive model for understanding and treating this client problem? If not, it is necessary to construct a cognitive model for conceptualization and treatment.

2. Is the cognitive model for conceptualization and treatment being

followed? If not, explore reasons for not doing so. Discuss advantages and disadvantages of cognitive or alternative conceptualizations and treatment plans.

3. Does the therapist have the knowledge and skill to properly implement the cognitive therapy treatment? If not, help the therapist learn these skills and knowledge.

4. Is the therapeutic response following expected patterns? If not, formulate hypotheses about why client response is different from expected. Consider client beliefs, skill deficits, emotional responses, interpersonal patterns, life circumstances, and developmental history. Also consider the factors in item 5 below.

5. What in the client conceptualization/therapy relationship/therapist response might be interfering with success? Include hypotheses about the therapist (beliefs, skill deficits, emotional responses, interpersonal patterns, life circumstances, developmental history), the therapy relationship (e.g., is it positive and collaborative?), the cognitive conceptualization (e.g., is something missing or inaccurate?), and the treatment plan (e.g., are there additional approaches that might help?).

Pay Attention to What Is Not Discussed

While important to address a supervisee's questions and concerns, it is also crucial to notice what is not discussed in supervision. Ongoing supervision should include a periodic review of a therapist's entire caseload. Otherwise, a few particularly troublesome cases may receive all supervisory help at the expense of other cases. Some supervisees will hesitate to discuss cases in which they feel particularly inept. Others may neglect to mention successful cases and thereby mislead the supervisor regarding areas of competency. Further, within case discussions it is important to note what information may be missing.

For example, one supervisee sought help for a client who was frequently noncompliant with homework tasks. The supervisee conceptualized the client as an extremely dependent woman who was unwilling to take on responsibilities. While the supervisee presented in great detail her hypotheses about why the client was not doing homework, the supervisor noted there was no mention of whether this client was responsible in any other areas of her life. When asked, the therapist noted that the client held two jobs. Further discussion revealed that the therapist felt critical of this client because she gave up a child for adoption 20 years earlier. The therapist concluded from this event that the client was "unwilling to bear her responsibilities."

Supervision helped this therapist see that her attitude toward the client was subtly judgmental and therefore harmful to the therapeutic relationship. The supervisor helped the therapist develop better understanding for her client's decision at age 17 to give her baby up for adoption. The therapist realized she was not considering her client's age and circumstances when the decision was made regarding her child. Once the therapist's reactions were examined, she was able to see her client as a responsible adult. This shift in perspective allowed the therapist to be open to other conceptualizations of the homework noncompliance. The therapist discussed the problem with the client with genuine curiosity rather than judgment and the therapy impasse was resolved.

If supervision seems constricted or overly narrow in focus, supervisor and supervisee can explore their emotional reactions and beliefs to discover what is impeding supervision. For example, although it is ideal to have collaboratory supervision relationships, some supervisors or supervisees adopt a more evaluative or judgmental tone that can negatively impact creative exploration and disclosure of cognitive therapy learning experiences by the supervisee.

COGNITIVE THERAPY FOR THERAPISTS

A final process that enhances the competency of cognitive therapists is participating in cognitive therapy as a client. To fully understand the process of the therapy, there is no substitute for using cognitive therapy methods on oneself. Most cognitive therapists use cognitive therapy in their own life at times. As described above, training programs and supervision often employ cognitive therapy methods to solve problems and enhance learning. It is also helpful for cognitive therapists to seek cognitive therapy when in need of psychotherapy.

Therapists, like most people, often enter therapy in a time of crisis. Cognitive therapy initiated during a crisis can be extended to include identification and exploration of schema issues that may maintain problem patterns. Others seek therapy for general self-improvement. Again, schema-focused therapy is immensely helpful for therapists wishing to understand patterns and make changes.

In regions or countries with only a few cognitive therapists, it can be difficult to identify a cognitive therapist who is not also a friend or colleague. Some therapists in these circumstances have chosen a therapist at some geographic distance and combined live sessions with telephone therapy. Other therapists form dyads or small groups for peer co-therapy. Therapists without access to another cognitive therapist could conduct structured manual-assisted self-therapy following procedures described in Greenberger and Padesky (1995) and Padesky with Greenberger (1995).

SUMMARY AND CONCLUSION

Athough cognitive therapy has well-defined conceptual models and treatment protocols, developing competent therapists is not a simple task. As cognitive therapy becomes more specified and sophisticated, therapists have more to learn in order to attain competency. Fortunately, the same processes and methods that characterize the therapy can be used to teach and supervise therapists.

Cognitive therapy instructors use the principles of collaboration, guided discovery, structure, and empirical investigation to ensure active student participation in learning programs. Supervisors build on therapists' strengths, choose supervisory methods that help develop therapist competency, and emphasize conceptualization skills to further promote therapist learning. Since the cognitive therapy field is dedicated to empirical research, cognitive therapists always need to improve competency based on new developments. Research on the relative merits of different teaching methods is in its infancy. The guidelines provided here are intended as a springboard for this research and further developments in the areas of training and supervision.

ACKNOWLEDGMENTS

I wish to thank participants of Camp Cognitive Therapy II, held in Dana Point, California, March 7–11, 1994, who helped devise the supervision grid in Table 13.1. Discussions during this weeklong workshop clarified many of the ideas in the supervision section of this chapter. As co-developer of every training program I've taught since 1983, Kathleen Mooney's creative insights are embedded throughout this chapter.

REFERENCES

American Psychiatric Association. (1994). *Diagnostic and statistical manual of mental disorders* (4th ed.). Washington, DC: Author.

Baucom, D., & Epstein, N. (1990). *Cognitive-behavioral marital therapy.* New York: Brunner/Mazel.

Beck, A. T. (1967). *Depression: Clinical, experimental, and theoretical aspects.* New York: Harper & Row. (Republished as *Depression: Causes and treatment.* Philadelphia: University of Pennsylvania Press, 1972.)

Beck, A. T. (1988). *Love is never enough.* New York: Harper & Row.

Beck, A. T. (1990, February). *Cognitive therapy of personality disorders.* Paper presented at the Cognitive Therapy of Personality Disorders, Inpatients, and Complex Marital Problems Conference, Newport Beach, CA.

Beck, A. T., Emery, G., & Greenberg, R. (1985). *Anxiety disorders and phobias: A cognitive perspective.* New York: Basic Books.

Beck, A. T., Freeman, A., Pretzer, J., Davis, D. D., Fleming, B., Ottavani, R., Beck, J., Simon, K. M., Padesky, C., Meyer, J., & Trexler, L. (1990). *Cognitive therapy of personality disorders.* New York: Guilford Press.

Beck, A. T., Hollon, S. D., Young, J. E., Bedrosian, R. C., & Budenz, D. (1985) Treatment of depression with cognitive therapy and amitriptyline. *Archives of General Psychiatry, 42,* 142–148.

Beck, A. T., & Padesky, C. A. (1984, November). *Cognitive therapy of anxiety and phobias.* Workshop presented at the meeting of the Association for the Advancement of Behavior Therapy, Philadelphia.

Beck, A. T., Rush, A. J., Shaw, B. F., & Emery, G. (1979). *Cognitive therapy of depression.* New York: Guilford Press.

Beck, A. T., Wright, F. D., Newman, C. F., & Liese, B. S. (1993). *Cognitive therapy of substance abuse.* New York: Guilford Press.

Beckham, E., & Watkins, J. (1989). Process and outcome in cognitive therapy. In A. Freeman, K. Simon, L. Beutler, & H. Arkowitz (Eds.), *Comprehensive handbook of cognitive therapy* (pp. 61–81). New York: Plenum Press.

Blackburn, I. M., Bishop, S., Glen, A. I. M., Whalley, J. J., & Christie, J. E. (1981). The efficacy of cognitive therapy in depression: A treatment trial using cognitive therapy and pharmacotherapy, each alone and in combination. *British Journal of Psychiatry, 139,* 181–189.

Bourne, E. J. (1990). *The anxiety and phobia workbook.* Oakland, CA: New Harbinger Press.

Burns, D. (1989). *The feeling good handbook: Using the new mood therapy in everyday life.* New York: William Morrow.

Butler, G., & Matthews, A. (1983). Cognitive processes in anxiety. *Advances in Behaviour Research and Therapy, 5,* 51–62.

Clark, D. M. (1986). A cognitive approach to panic. *Behaviour Research and Therapy, 24,* 461–470.

Dattilio, F. M., & Padesky, C. A. (1990). *Cognitive therapy with couples.* Sarasota, FL: Professional Resource Exchange.

Dobson, K., Shaw, B., & Vallis, T. (1985). Reliability of a measure of the quality of cognitive therapy. *British Journal of Clinical Psychology, 24,* 295–300.

Eaves, G. G., Jarrett, R. B., & Basco, M. R. (1989). *Cognitive treatment workbook.* Unpublished manuscript, Department of Psychiatry, University of Texas Southwestern Medical Center, Dallas.

Fairburn, C. G. (1985). Cognitive-behavioral treatment for bulimia. In D. M. Garner & P. E. Garfinkel (Eds.), *Handbook of psychotherapy for anorexia nervosa and bulimia* (pp. 160–192). New York: Guilford Press.

Freeman, A., Pretzer, J. L., Fleming, B., & Simon, K. M. (1990). *Clinical applications of cognitive therapy.* New York: Plenum Press.

Garner, D. M., & Bemis, K. M. (1982). A cognitive-behavioral approach to anorexia nervosa. *Cognitive Therapy and Research, 6,* 123–150.

Greenberger, D., & Padesky, C. A. (1995). *Mind over mood: A cognitive therapy treatment manual for clients.* New York: Guilford Press.

Hawton, K., Salkovskis, P. M., Kirk, J., & Clark, D. M. (1989). *Cognitive behavioural therapy for psychiatric problems: A practical guide.* New York: Oxford University Press.

Hollon, S., Mandell, M., Bemis, K., Derubeis, R., Emerson, M., Evans, M., & Kress, M. (1981). *Reliability and validity of the Young Cognitive Therapy Scale.* Unpublished manuscript, University of Minnesota, Minneapolis.

Kendall, P. C. (Ed.). (1991). *Child and adolescent therapy: Cognitive-behavioral procedures.* New York: Guilford Press.

Kingdon, D. G., & Turkington, D. (1994). *Cognitive-behavioral therapy of schizophrenia.* New York: Guilford Press.

Murphy, G. E., Simons, A. D., Wetzel, R. D., & Lustman, P. J. (1984). Cognitive therapy and pharmacotherapy singly and together in the treatment of depression. *Archives of General Psychiatry, 41,* 33–41.

Newman, C. F. (1994). Understanding client resistance: Methods for enhancing motivation to change. *Cognitive and Behavioral Practice, 1,* 47–69.

Padesky, C. A. (1988). Personality disorders: Cognitive therapy into the 90's. In C. Perris & M. Eisemann (Eds.), *Cognitive psychotherapy: An update. Proceedings of the Second International Conference on Cognitive Psychotherapy* (pp. 115–119). Umea, Sweden: DOPUU Press.

Padesky, C. A. (1993a). Staff and patient education. In J. H. Wright, M. E. Thase, A. T. Beck, & J. W. Ludgate (Eds.), *Cognitive therapy with inpatients: Developing a cognitive milieu* (pp. 393-413). New York: Guilford Press.

Padesky, C. A. (1993b, September). *Socratic questioning: Changing minds or guiding discovery?* Keynote address presented at the meeting of the European Congress of Behavioural and Cognitive Therapies, London.

Padesky, C. A. (1994a). Schema change processes in cognitive therapy. *Clinical Psychology and Psychotherapy, 1*(5), 267–278.

Padesky, C. A. (1994b, April). *Cognitive therapy for therapists: Gender-related beliefs and schema change processes.* Workshop presented at the meeting of the Association of Oregon Community Mental Health Programs, Gleneden Beach, OR.

Padesky, C. A., with Greenberger, D. (1995). *Clinician's guide to* Mind over Mood. New York. Guilford Press.

Perris, C. (1988). *Cognitive therapy with schizophrenic patients.* New York: Guilford Press.

Persons, J. (1989). *Cognitive therapy in practice: A case formulation approach.* New York: Norton.

Pretzer, J. L., & Fleming, B. (1989, December). Cognitive-behavioral treatment of personality disorders. *the Behavior Therapist, 12,* 105–109.

Raue, P. J., & Goldfried, M. R. (1994). The therapeutic alliance in cognitive-behavior therapy. In A. O. Horvath & L. S. Greenberg (Eds.), *The working alliance* (pp. 131–152). New York: Wiley.

Rush, A. J., Beck, A. T., Kovacs, M., & Hollon, S. D. (1977). Comparative efficacy of cognitive therapy and pharmacotherapy in the treatment of depressed outpatients. *Cognitive Therapy and Research, 1,* 17–37.

Safran, J. D., & Muran, J. C. (1995). Resolving therapeutic alliance ruptures: Diversity and integration. *In Session: Psychotherapy in Practice, 1,* 81–92.

Safran, J., & Segal, Z. (1990). *Interpersonal process in cognitive therapy.* New York: Basic Books.

Salkovskis, P. M. (1985). Obsessional–compulsive problems: A cognitive-behavioural analysis. *Behaviour Research and Therapy, 25,* 571–583.

Shaw, B. (1977). Comparison of cognitive therapy and behavior therapy in the treatment of depression. *Journal of Consulting and Clinical Psychology, 45,* 543–551.

Shaw, B. F. (1988, February). *Cognitive theory of depression: Where we are and where are we going?* Paper presented at the meeting of the Contemporary Psychological Approaches to Depression: Treatment, Research, and Theory, San Diego, CA.

Steketee, G. S., & White, K. (1990). *When once is not enough.* Oakland, CA: New Harbinger Press.

Thase, M. (1994, February). After the fall: Perspectives on cognitive-behavioral treatment of depression in the "post-Collaborative" era. *the Behavior Therapist, 2,* 48–51.

Vallis, T. M., Shaw, B. F., & Dobson, K. S. (1986). The Cognitive Therapy Scale: Psychometric properties. *Journal of Consulting and Clinical Psychology, 54,* 381–385.

Wright, J. H., & Davis, D. (1994). The therapeutic relationship in cognitive-behavioral therapy: Patient perceptions and therapist responses. *Cognitive and Behavioral Practice, 1,* 25–45.

Young, J., & Beck, A. T. (1980). *Cognitive therapy scale: Rating manual.* Unpublished manuscript, University of Pennsylvania, Philadelphia.

Young, J., Shaw, B. F., Beck, A.T., & Budenz, D. (1981). *Assessment of competence in cognitive therapy.* Unpublished manuscript, University of Pennsylvania, Philadelphia.

Chapter 14

Cognitive Therapy in the Treatment and Prevention of Depression

Steven D. Hollon
Robert J. DeRubeis
Mark D. Evans

In the several decades since it was first introduced, cognitive therapy for depression has won widespread acceptance in the clinical community. For the most part, this acceptance appears to be justified. Cognitive therapy has typically performed at least as well as alternative interventions, including pharmacotherapy, in terms of acute symptom reduction (Dobson, 1989), and there are indications that it may have an enduring effect not found with other approaches (Hollon, Shelton, & Loosen, 1991).

Nonetheless, not all studies have been supportive. In particular, cognitive therapy was no more effective than an inert pill placebo and somewhat less effective than pharmacotherapy alone among patients with more severe depressions in the National Institute of Mental Health Treatment of Depression Collaborative Research Program (NIMH TDCRP; Elkin et al., 1989). Moreover, there were only minimal indications of any preventive effect (Shea et al., 1992). Since this was a particularly visible trial, these findings have been widely interpreted as suggesting that cognitive therapy is not as effective as was first believed.

Despite its visibility, the NIMH study is not without flaws (Jacobson & Hollon, 1996a, 1996b). In this chapter, we argue that cognitive therapy is at least as effective as pharmacotherapy in the reduction of acute symptoms in outpatient samples and better able to reduce subsequent risk. We focus primarily on a controlled trial that we conducted with colleagues at the University of Minnesota and two participating clinical research sites to illustrate these points and draw contrasts between findings from this and other similar studies versus those from the NIMH TDCRP.

THE MINNESOTA
COGNITIVE–PHARMACOTHERAPY PROJECT

Overview and Introduction

In the late 1970s, Rush and colleagues published a study that suggested that cognitive therapy was superior to imipramine pharmacotherapy in the treatment of acute depression (Rush, Beck, Kovacs, & Hollon, 1977). In that study, depressed outpatients treated with up to 20 sessions of cognitive therapy over a 12-week period showed greater symptom reduction and were less likely to drop out of treatment than were comparable patients treated with imipramine pharmacotherapy. Moreover, there were indications (not all significant) of a preventive effect following treatment termination across a subsequent 1-year follow-up (Kovacs, Rush, Beck, & Hollon, 1981).

Although this study generated considerable enthusiasm for cognitive therapy, it was flawed in several respects. The fact that it was conducted at the site at which cognitive therapy was developed may have created a subtle form of bias favoring the psychosocial condition. Moreover, neither patients nor clinical evaluators were blind to treatment condition. Finally, and most critically, drug dosage levels were marginal by current standards and medication withdrawal was begun 2 weeks before the end of active treatment. Although this was done to ensure that patients treated pharmacologically were drug free at the time of the posttreatment assessment (patients assigned to cognitive therapy were to have terminated therapy at this point), this strategy probably led to a confounding of acute response with subsequent relapse. As shown in Figure 14.1, differences favoring cognitive therapy were more pronounced at week 10 (immediately prior to the beginning of medication withdrawal) than they were at posttreatment (week 12).

The Minnesota project was conceived as an effort to replicate and extend the findings from the study by Rush and colleagues (Rush et al., 1977), with a particular emphasis on correcting or modifying the problematic aspects of that earlier trial. First, the study was conducted at two sites (the St. Paul–Ramsey Medical Center and the Ramsey County Mental Health Clinic) that had no prior affiliation with cognitive therapy but that did have a history of participation in nationally funded pharmacological research (Prien et al., 1984). Second, all evaluations and reevaluations were conducted by independent clinicians not involved in the treatment of the patients they were interviewing. Moreover, all interviews were videotaped and any inadvertent breaks in the blind were edited out. These edited tapes were then rated by an additional set of evaluators and their judgments compared to those of the original interviewers to ensure that the occasional breaks in the blind did not bias the ratings of differential symptom change. Finally, pharmacotherapists were encouraged to be aggressive in their dosage strategies (some patients were taken as high as 450 mg/day of imipramine), plasma medication levels were monitored to ensure compliance and check absorp-

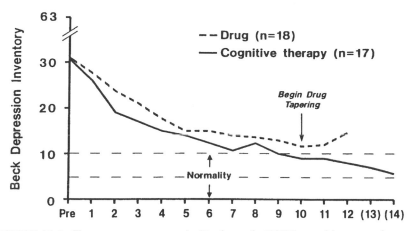

FIGURE 14.1. Treatment outcomes in Rush et al. (1977): weekly scores by group.

tion, and full dosage levels were continued through the end of the acute treatment period (12 weeks).

We were also interested in testing theories as to how therapy worked. Outcome research is particularly meaningful when approached in a manner that allows inferences to be tested with regard to which aspects of treatment are truly effective and what mechanisms are mobilized in the patient to produce that effect. As depicted in Figure 14.2, the respective treatment conditions (which together constitute the independent variable) typically consist of complex packages of components; with sufficient attention to measurement issues, these components can be described and differentiated from one another. Our group has long been involved in developing methods for assessing the components of therapy and has developed systems for differen-

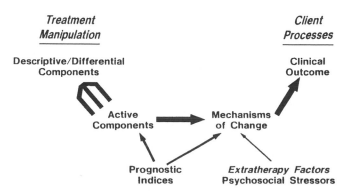

FIGURE 14.2. Model of the treatment outcome process. Adapted by Hollon et al. (1990, p. 118). Copyright 1990 by Plenum Publishing Corp. Adapted by permission.

tiating cognitive therapy from alternative interventions based on ratings of the actual treatment session (DeRubeis, Hollon, Evans, & Bemis, 1982; Hollon, Evans, Elkin, & Lowery, 1984). By applying these and other measures of treatment components to samples of therapy, we hoped to both describe and differentiate cognitive therapy from pharmacotherapy for depression.

If a treatment is effective, some of those components must be causally active in producing that result. These causally active components might be specific to the respective approaches (e.g., cognitive therapy could produce change by teaching patients how to recognize and test their maladaptive beliefs, whereas pharmacotherapy might produce change by producing changes at the synapse), or they might be nonspecific and shared by each approach (i.e., patients might get better because they confide in the therapist and acquire a renewed sense of optimism regarding change). We planned to assess both specific and nonspecific components of treatment and to relate each to ultimate outcome in an effort to determine whether cognitive therapy worked through the processes specified by theory (Beck, Rush, Shaw, & Emery, 1979).

Mechanisms represent those aspects of the patient that must be changed by the treatment to produce change in the outcomes of interest. Cognitive theory suggests that people become depressed, in part, because they possess negative cognitive schemas that become activated under conditions of stress (Beck, 1963, 1976). These schemas consist of both underlying assumptions (content) and maladaptive information-processing propensities (process). These proclivities serve as preexistent diatheses that lead to the production of specific negative automatic thoughts and negative expectations (e.g., "I'm a loser," "Nothing I do ever works out") that depress mood and undermine motivation for active coping under conditions of stress. As depicted in Figure 14.3, we reasoned that the disconfirmation of the more proximal negative expectations should play a central role in the amelioration of acute distress, whereas changes in more distal predispositions should be more important to the reduction of subsequent risk (Hollon & Garber, 1980). This model is consistent with and anticipated the more recent hopelessness theory of depression (Abramson, Metalsky, & Alloy, 1989).

Attention to the processes of therapy (both with respect to the components of treatment and the mechanisms of change within the patient) not only enriches what can be learned from the typical outcome trial, but also provides the most powerful context for testing theories of change. It is always difficult to test theories of mediation, but the inferential process can be made less ambiguous if change can be attributed to treatment. As we shall see, our design was not suited to test theories of mediation with respect to the reduction of acute distress (that is something we hope to address in a future study), but it did allow for tests of theories of the mediation of relapse prevention.

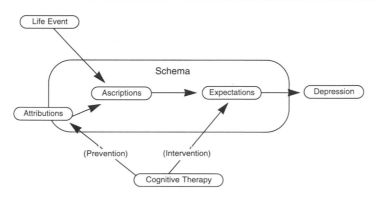

FIGURE 14.3. Cognition and change in cognitive therapy. Adapted from the Hollon et al. (1990, p. 123). Copyright 1990 by Plenum Publishing Corp. Adapted by permission.

Study Design

Our overall goal in the Minnesota project was to conduct a methodologically rigorous study in a clinically representative fashion. Patients were drawn from those people requesting treatment for depression from either of two outpatient treatment facilities in St. Paul, Minnesota. Prospective patients were referred to the project by referral coordinators in the respective agencies. All patients were screened by a clinical evaluator (typically a psychiatrist drawn from one of the participating facilities). Patients between the ages of 18 and 65 inclusive who met criteria for major depression and were free of schizophrenia, bipolar affective disorder, and current substance abuse were randomly assigned to one of four conditions: (1) cognitive therapy, (2) imipramine pharmacotherapy (without continuation), (3) imipramine pharmacotherapy with continuation, or (4) combined cognitive–pharmacotherapy. With the exceptions noted, the first two conditions essentially replicated the conditions in the study by Rush and colleagues (Rush et al., 1977). The medication continuation condition was included to provide a standard against which to compare prior cognitive therapy during the posttreatment follow-up. Treatment responders in that condition were continued on medication for the first year of the 2-year follow-up, since it had been shown that medication continuation is superior to medication withdrawal in the suppression of subsequent relapse (Prien & Kupfer, 1986). The combined treatment condition was included in order to determine whether combining two presumably active interventions improved on efficacy over either one alone; such a strategy was already beginning to gain widespread clinical acceptance despite the lack of supporting data.

At the time the project was designed, we did not think we needed to include an inert pill placebo. This is a decision we later came to regret. We reasoned that since cognitive therapy had proven superior to pharmacotherapy in the earlier trial by Rush and colleagues (Rush et al., 1977), we could anticipate differences between the two single modalities that would facilitate the interpretation of any findings with respect to combined treatment. We had not yet become aware that a major portion of the differences observed in Rush et al. (1977) favoring cognitive therapy was attributable to premature medication withdrawal in the pharmacotherapy condition. In all respects, including a pill placebo condition in our initial design would have strengthened the study and the inferences we could have drawn from it.

Patients who met all inclusion and exclusion criteria were randomly assigned to treatment. Patients assigned to cognitive therapy were seen for a maximum of twenty 50-minute sessions over a 12-week period; patients assigned to pharmacotherapy were seen weekly for about 30 minutes over that same 12-week interval. Patients assigned to combined treatment worked with a separate cognitive therapist and pharmacotherapist. This introduced a confound in terms of the amount of professional contact provided, but it was deemed representative of the way most people receive combined treatment in actual clinical settings.

Therapy was provided by professional staff at the two participating facilities. The cognitive therapists were four experienced psychotherapists (8–20 years experience); one was a male PhD psychologist, and two men and one woman were ACSW clinical social workers. None had extensive prior experience with cognitive therapy; training was provided by the authors over a 14-month period. Training included didactic presentations, role playing, and intensive supervision of practice cases. Ongoing 90-minute group supervision sessions were provided throughout the study, twice weekly during the initial two-thirds of the project and weekly thereafter. Our sense is that *ongoing* supervision is necessary in a project of this type; experienced therapists are particularly likely to revert to their previous approaches when dealing with difficult patients. In the NIMH study, minimal ongoing supervision was provided and differences in efficacy were evident across the sites (Elkin et al., 1989).

In the Minnesota study, selected therapy sessions were rated by training supervisors on both the Cognitive Therapy Scale (CTS; Young & Beck, 1980) and the Minnesota Therapy Rating Scale (MTRS; DeRubeis et al., 1982). These ratings were used to provide feedback to the therapists on an ongoing basis. Subsequent ratings were made by independent judges blind to treatment conditions and therapist using the Collaborative Study Psychotherapy Rating Scale (CSPRS; Hollon et al., 1984) and were used to provide ratings of treatment adherence. All sets of ratings showed that cognitive therapy could be clearly differentiated from pharmacotherapy and that there were no differences between cognitive therapy alone versus the cognitive component of combined treatment.

The pharmacotherapists were four male board-certified psychiatrists. Since all had previous experience in controlled drug trials, no formal training was provided before the project was begun. The pharmacotherapists met periodically under the supervision of the project medical director. The medication used was imipramine hydrochloride, provided in flexible daily dosages typically taken at bedtime. Protocol called for average daily dosages between 200 and 300 mg/day, with monitoring of plasma imipramine/desipramine levels. Dosage levels were raised for any patients with a plasma imipramine/desipramine level below 180 ng/ml; several patients had their dosages raised above 300 mg/day (to a high of 450 mg/day). Maximum daily dosages averaged 232 mg/day, with no differences between patients treated with medication alone versus those treated in the combined condition. Imipramine/desipramine levels averaged over 300 ng/ml at both weeks 6 and 12 for patients in the medication conditions; patients assigned to cognitive therapy alone had zero plasma levels. These values suggest that dosage levels were reasonable and appropriate and that pharmacotherapy was adequately conducted.

Three patients in combined treatment discontinued medications due to side effects; they were considered completers because they completed cognitive therapy. A fourth patient was largely noncompliant with cognitive therapy, but was considered a treatment completer because he completed pharmacotherapy. Although retaining such partial completers is somewhat controversial, our sense is that one of the advantages of combined treatment is that it increases the likelihood that each patient will receive a full course of at least one type of treatment.

The two medication-alone conditions were identical over the first 12 weeks of treatment. A 2-week medication withdrawal was begun immediately following the posttreatment reevaluation for all treatment responders in the medication–no continuation and combined conditions. Patients in the continuation medication condition stayed on study medications for the first year of the 2-year follow-up; dosage levels were not allowed to drop below half the maximum dosage during the acute treatment phase. Medications were withdrawn at the end of 1 year of continuation medication in accordance with the same schedule used for the other medication conditions. Patients receiving cognitive therapy (either alone or in combination) discontinued treatment prior to the 12-week posttreatment reevaluation.

Sample Characteristics and Response to Acute Treatment

A complete description of the sample and response to acute treatment is provided elsewhere (Hollon, DeRubeis, Evans, et al., 1992). In brief, the final sample consisted of 107 patients and was predominantly female (80%), white (91%), and middle-aged. Twenty-six percent were single, 32% were married or cohabitating, and 42% were separated, divorced, or widowed. Sixty-two percent of the sample was employed outside of the home. The sample as a whole was characterized by a moderate level of education and was drawn predominantly from middle- and lower-middle-class socioeconomic strata. Sixty-four percent of the sample met criteria for recurrent depression and 24% for "double depression." Sixty-four percent met research diagnostic criteria (RDC) for endogenicity; 33% had a history of previous hospitalization and 39% had made at least one suicide attempt. On the whole, the sample could be characterized as moderately to severely depressed, and representative of the kinds of depressed patients found in clinical outpatient settings.

Of the 107 patients initially assigned to treatment, 43 (40%) failed to complete 12 weeks of active treatment. Although there were no differences in the overall rates of attrition, patients were more likely to refuse cognitive therapy alone (because they wanted medications) and they were more likely to drop out of pharmacotherapy (because of problems with side effects). Nine patients were withdrawn from treatment by the project medical director because of complications, all but one from the medication conditions. Included among the patients "withdrawn" were two who died as a consequence of suicide attempts involving study medication. On the whole, these patterns suggest that there was no particular bias in favor of cognitive therapy on the part of the patients and that medications were more likely to elicit problematic reactions that precluded continuation or that threatened patients' safety.

Figure 14.4 depicts change over time in levels depression among treatment completers on the clinician-rated Hamilton Rating Scale for Depression (HRSD; Hamilton, 1960). All treatment conditions showed massive and clinically meaningful reductions in acute symptoms across treatment, with the bulk of the change occurring during the first 6 weeks (scores for the two drug-only groups are combined, since they were treated identically during the acute treatment phase). There was some indication of superior response among patients assigned to combined treatment, but those differences were not significant and were at least partially attributable to a tendency for nonresponders to be more likely to drop out of that condition (Hollon, DeRubeis, Evans, et al., 1992). Patterns of response on the HRSD were essentially replicated on several other self-report and clinician-rated measures of depression. As shown, the sample as a whole was at least moderately depressed at intake, with the typical patient moving into the high end of the normal range by the end of treatment. About half of the patients who completed treatment in either single modality evidenced a full response, versus about three-quarters of the completers in the combined condition.

On the whole, these findings suggest that the two single modalities were comparably effective for the typical depressed outpatient. But one might ask whether pharmacotherapy was superior to cognitive therapy among more severely depressed patients, as was suggested by the NIMH study (Elkin et al., 1989). Figure 14.5 shows this was not the case. Patients were defined as being high severity if they scored 20 or above at intake on the HRSD, the same criterion applied in the NIMH study. As can be seen, there was no evidence that high-severity patients did any better in pharmacotherapy than they did in cognitive therapy. We also conducted additional analyses based on even more restrictive definitions of severity (our sample was some-

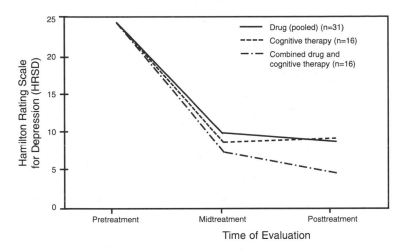

FIGURE 14.4. Change in depression by condition among treatment completers (HRSD). From Hollon, DeRubeis, Evans, et al. (1992, p. 778). Copyright by the American Medical Association. Reprinted by permission.

what more severely depressed than that studied in the NIMH trial) and other measures of depression and general adjustment; none provided any indication of superior response to pharmacotherapy among high-severity patients (see Hollon, DeRubeis, Evans, et al., 1992, for an extended report). Thus, there was no indication from our Minnesota study that cognitive therapy is in any way less effective than pharmacotherapy among more severely depressed outpatients.

On the whole, we suspect that cognitive therapy's poor showing among more severely depressed patients in the NIMH study was an anomaly that will not replicate (Jacobson & Hollon, 1996a). None of the other studies comparing cognitive therapy to pharmacotherapy in clinical samples have ever reported differential response as a function of severity (Blackburn, Bishop, Glen, Whalley, & Christie, 1981; Murphy, Simons, Wetzel, & Lustman, 1984; Rush et al., 1977). Moreover, findings in the NIMH study were not even robust across sites. In the NIMH study, differences favoring pharmacotherapy over cognitive therapy among more severely depressed patients were evident at only one of the three sites; at a second site, cognitive therapy did at least as well as pharmacotherapy with such patients and there were too few severely depressed patients at the third site to support separate analyses (Elkin et al., 1989). A similar pattern of site differences was evident for interpersonal psychotherapy.

As previously described, only minimal supervision was provided on an ongoing basis during the study proper in the NIMH trial. Given the nature of the respective sites (Oklahoma had an extensive history with cognitive therapy prior to participation in the NIMH study, whereas the other two

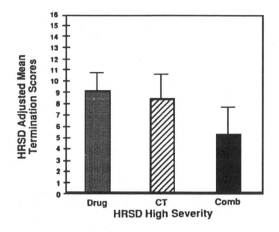

FIGURE 14.5. Posttreatment depression by condition among high-severity treatment completers (Hamilton Rating Scale for Depression [HRSD]). From Hollon, DeRubeis, Evans, et al. (1992, p. 779). Copyright 1992 by the American Medical Association. Reprinted by permission.

sites did not), we are concerned that cognitive therapy was not adequately operationalized at all three sites and that this was most detrimental with more severely depressed patients (Jacobson & Hollon, 1996b). The fact that drug–placebo differences were robust across the two sites with sufficient numbers of severely depressed patients makes it unlikely that there were important differences in the nature of the patient populations. Although the NIMH study is the largest and, in many respects, the best controlled of the existing comparative trials, it is important to recognize that the relatively poorer performance of cognitive therapy among more severely depressed patients was restricted to a single site and may have reflected inadequate operationalization of the approach (Jacobson & Hollon, 1996b). We eagerly await the publication of the full findings from the NIMH study, particularly with respect to linking site to outcome and presenting scores on the competency measures by site and therapist for both the training phase and the study proper.

Prevention of Relapse

All patients in the Minnesota project were followed across a subsequent 2-year posttreatment follow-up. With the exception of patients assigned to the medication continuation condition, patients in all other conditions who showed at least a partial response were withdrawn from treatment at the start of that period (after 12 weeks of active treatment). Patients in the continuation medication condition were kept on study medications for the first year of the 2-year follow-up, then withdrawn from medications. Patients who failed to respond to initial treatment were provided with whatever treatment was clinically indicated; typically, cognitive therapy was added for nonresponders to pharmacotherapy alone, and drugs were added for nonresponders to cognitive therapy alone. Medications were changed for patients in combined treatment.

All treatment responders were asked to refrain from seeking additional treatment during the follow-up in the absence of a clinical relapse. Patients were asked to return to the clinic every 6 months during the follow-up for a clinical interview. In addition, all patients were contacted monthly by phone and asked to complete a self-report measure of depression; any patient who showed an increment in symptoms of depression or who reported considering a return to treatment was brought back into the clinic within 7 days for an additional interview. Patients were judged to have relapsed who evidenced scores of 16 or above for 2 consecutive weeks on the Beck Depression Inventory (BDI; Beck, Ward, Mendelson, Mock, & Erbaugh, 1961); all who could be reinterviewed also showed elevations of 12 or above on the HRSD (Evans et al., 1992).

As shown in Figure 14.6, patients treated to remission with cognitive therapy (either alone or in combination) were less likely to relapse following treatment termination than were patients withdrawn from medications. Patients continued on study medications also were protected against relapse. Prior cognitive therapy was at least as effective as continuation medication at preventing subsequent relapse; differences between continuation medication versus medication withdrawal closely paralleled those reported in the continuation literature (Prien & Kupfer, 1986). It is unlikely that the high rate of relapse shown by the medication–no continuation patients was simply an artifact of medication withdrawal, since patients in combined treatment were withdrawn at exactly the same time in accordance with exactly the same schedule, as were medication continuation patients at the end of the first year of follow-up. In neither of these circumstances did patients who were withdrawn from medications evidence a "rebound." Because premature return to treatment can confound the results of naturalistic follow-ups, we also considered the effect of incorporating additional treatment into the definition of relapse; doing so only enhanced the differences favoring prior cognitive therapy over medication withdrawal (see Evans et al., 1992, for a more complete report). These findings strongly suggest that cognitive therapy reduces risk for relapse following treatment termination and that it is at least as effective in that regard as continuing the patient on medications.

Moreover, these findings are consistent with those of other naturalistic studies of subsequent course following treatment termination in similar comparisons between cognitive therapy and pharmacotherapy (Blackburn, Eunson, & Bishop, 1986; Kovacs et al., 1981; Simons, Murphy, Levine, & Wetzel, 1986). Despite differences in definitions of response and relapse, patients treated to remission with cognitive therapy have typically been about half as likely to relapse following treatment termination as patients treated to remission pharmacologically. The lone exception was again the NIMH

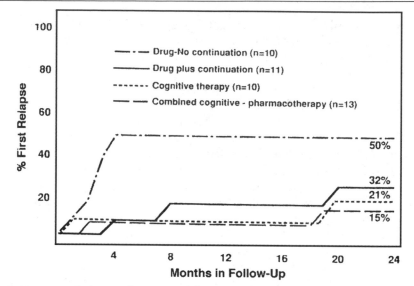

FIGURE 14.6. Relapse after successful treatment. From Evans et al. (1992, p. 805). Copyright 1992 by the American Medical Association. Reprinted by permission.

study; although patients treated to remission with cognitive therapy were less likely to relapse than patients treated to remission pharmacologically, the magnitudes of the difference were not as great as in the other trials, and the differences were not significant (Shea et al., 1992). As with regard to acute response, it would be of interest to examine rates of relapse as a function of treatment site; if cognitive therapy was less than adequately implemented at the Pittsburgh site (and possibly Washington), then an advantage for cognitive therapy approaching that found in other studies would be expected at the Oklahoma site.

On the whole, findings from the naturalistic follow-up studies suggest that cognitive therapy has an enduring effect that survives the end of treatment. Although no competent pharmacotherapist nowadays would withdraw medications so soon following initial response, comparisons of cognitive therapy with medication–no continuation conditions have demonstrated that prior cognitive therapy has the capacity to reduce subsequent risk. Moreover, this preventive capacity appears to be at least as effective as continuation medications, the current standard of treatment. Since not all patients can or should stay on medications indefinitely, finding a prophylactic effect for cognitive therapy is potentially quite exciting. Although these findings are not conclusive, they do suggest a potential advantage for cognitive therapy that deserves exploration in subsequent studies.

Active Ingredients of Cognitive Therapy

Cognitive theory suggests that cognitive therapy works by virtue of helping patients learn to test systematically their beliefs and to modify maladaptive information-processing proclivities (Beck, 1964, 1970; Beck et al., 1979). If that is the case, then theoretically specified therapist behaviors should both be elevated in cognitive therapy over other approaches and more highly correlated with subsequent change than more general and nonspecific aspects of the therapy process. As previously noted, random subsets of therapy sessions from both cognitive therapy and pharmacotherapy were rated by independent judges on several measures of treatment process.

Figure 14.7 depicts scores for both cognitive therapy and pharmacotherapy sessions on the MTRS (DeRubeis et al., 1982) and the CTS (Young & Beck, 1980). The MTRS consists of four factors, including dimensions representing therapist behaviors specific to cognitive therapy, nonspecific interpersonal aspects of the therapeutic relationship, therapist directiveness, and therapist behaviors specific to interpersonal psychotherapy. As can be seen, cognitive-therapists engaged in more specific cognitive-behavioral strategies and provided more supportive nonspecific interpersonal relationships than did the pharmacotherapists. Both types of therapists were directive and neither engaged in strategies specific to interpersonal psychotherapy. Scores on the CTS, which can also be factored into theoretically specific and general nonspecific factors, paralleled those on the MTRS and further indicated that

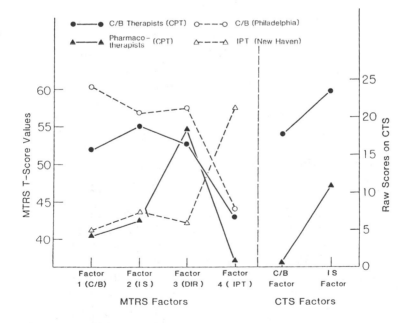

FIGURE 14.7. Components of change in cognitive therapy and pharmacotherapy. C/B, cognitive-behavioral; CPT, Cognitive–Pharmacotherapy Project; CTS, Cognitive Therapy Scale; DIR, therapist directiveness; IPT, therapist behaviors specific to interpersonal psychotherapy; IS, nonspecific interpersonal aspects of the therapeutic relationship; MTRS; Minnesota Therapy Rating Scale. Adapted from Hollon et al. (1990, p. 119). Copyright 1990 by Plenum Publishing Corp. Adapted by permission.

the overall level of cognitive therapy delivered was adequate. Thus, ratings of therapy sessions indicated that cognitive therapy could be differentiated from pharmacotherapy on the basis of actual therapist behaviors and that those behaviors were largely consistent with what would have been expected in each modality.

In a separate sample, DeRubeis and Feeley (1990) have shown that levels of theoretically specified behaviors early in therapy predicted subsequent change in depression; the quality of the interpersonal relationship was more a consequence than a cause of change in depression. In an as-yet-unpublished study, they have essentially replicated this pattern of findings on tapes from the Minnesota project using a second set of raters not involved in the training of the study therapists and a more advanced tape-rating system developed for the NIMH study (CSPRS; Hollon et al., 1984). These findings suggest that it is the theoretically specific aspects of cognitive therapy that carry the weight of change in that approach.

Mediation of Response and the Prevention of Relapse

Cognitive theory further predicts that cognitive therapy produces change in depression by changing cognition (Beck, 1963, 1976; Beck et al., 1979). However, as previously discussed, different aspects of cognition are likely to play different roles in the causal chain leading to depression, with more distal and stable cognitive predispositions (also known as "depth" cognitions) interacting with negative life events to produce more proximal and transient changes in expectations and self-perceptions (also known as "surface" cognitions) that lead to the onset of depression (Abramson et al., 1989; Hollon & Garber, 1980). We further hypothesized that once a person was depressed, it was the process of disconfirmation of those negative expectations and automatic self-referential thoughts that was critical to the alleviation of distress (treatment), whereas the modification of more distal underlying dysfunctional attitudes and information-processing propensities should be more central to the reduction of subsequent risk (prevention) (Hollon & Garber, 1980).

We therefore included two measures of "surface" cognitions, the Hopelessness Scale (HS; Beck, Weissman, Lester, & Trexler, 1974), a measure of general expectations, and the Automatic Thoughts Questionnaire (ATQ; Hollon & Kendall, 1980), a measure of specific negative ruminations. We also included two measures of "depth" cognitions, the Dysfunctional Attitude Scale (DAS; Weissman & Beck, 1978), a measure of underlying attitudes believed to sit close to the core of depressotypic schema, and the Attributional Styles Questionnaire (ASQ; Seligman, Abramson, Semmel, & von Baeyer, 1979), a measure of the propensity to make internal, global, and stable attributions (e.g., blame the self) for negative life events.

All patients completed both sets of measures at intake, midtreatment (6 weeks), and posttreatment (12 weeks). We predicted that changes in expectations and automatic thoughts would be more highly correlated with subsequent change in depression in cognitive therapy than in pharmacotherapy, whereas changes in dysfunctional attitudes and attributional style would mediate cognitive therapy's relapse prevention effect. As shown in Figure 14.8, these predictions were at least partially confirmed with respect to acute response; change in expectations (as measured by the HS) was more highly correlated with subsequent change in depression in cognitive therapy than in pharmacotherapy. This finding is consistent with that observed by Rush and colleagues in their earlier trial (Rush, Kovacs, Beck, Weissenburger, & Hollon, 1981). The same pattern also held for the two measures of "depth" cognitions (the DAS and ASQ), but not for the measure of automatic thoughts (ATQ), which behaved more like a state-dependent consequence of change in depression than a mechanism.

As shown in Figure 14.9, pharmacotherapy produced as much change in expectations as did cognitive therapy; it was only in the temporal pattern of change in which differences between cognitive therapy and pharmacotherapy were evident. As we have noted elsewhere, nonspecificity (with respect to the construct of interest) does not rule out mediation (Hollon, DeRubeis, & Evans, 1987). It is quite possible for cognitive therapy to work through cognitive change to produce changes in depression and yet produce no greater change in thinking than pharmacotherapy, so long as changes in depression, however produced, also have an influence on cognition. Since pharmacotherapy was as effective as cognitive therapy at producing changes

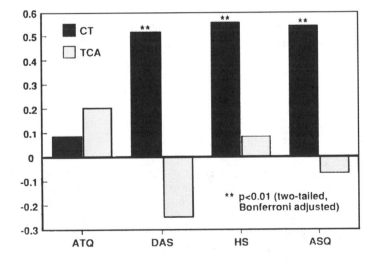

FIGURE 14.8. Prediction of late change in depression from early cognitive change for each treatment group. ASQ, Attributional Styles Questionnaire; ATQ, Automatic Thoughts Questionnaire; CT, cognitive therapy; DAS, Dysfunctional Attitude Scale; HS, Hopelessness Scale; TCA, tricyclic antidepressants.

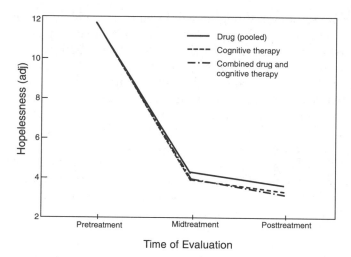

FIGURE 14.9. Changes in hopelessness as a function of differential treatment.

in depression, and since levels of hopelessness are known to rise and fall with levels of depression, it is quite possible that changes in expectations led to changes in cognitive therapy, whereas changes in depression led to changes in expectations in pharmacotherapy.

What is needed is a study that measures both expectations and depression on a repeated basis over time and that includes a minimal treatment control in addition to separate cognitive and pharmacotherapy conditions. Such a design would permit the application of sophisticated causal modeling strategies sensitive to the temporal order of effects (Baron & Kenny, 1986). Our decision not to include a minimal treatment control in the Minnesota study was as much a problem for the ascertainment of mediation as it was for the interpretation of treatment effects; because both treatment conditions were comparably effective, there was relatively little variance in outcome to predict (and such variance as was available was probably more closely related to preexistent differences in capacity to respond than to factors related to treatment).

Nonetheless, our findings were consistent with the notion that change in cognition (especially expectations) mediates change in depression in cognitive therapy, but not in pharmacotherapy. However, they also suggest that change in expectations is not a sufficient mediator of change; rather, since treatment type moderated the relation between change in expectations and subsequent change in depression, there must be some other process (or processes) that interacts with change in cognition to produce change in depression in cognitive therapy. Elsewhere, we have speculated that this "missing" process may be exposure to corrective learning experiences provided by cognitive therapy (DeRubeis et al., 1990).

If our design was less than wholly adequate for testing theories of mediation with respect to the reduction of acute distress (treatment), it was closer to the ideal with respect to the identification of the mechanisms behind cognitive therapy's preventive effect. Whereas the two single modalities produced comparable reductions in symptoms during active treatment, cognitive therapy was associated with a far greater reduction in subsequent risk following treatment termination than was pharmacotherapy. This meant that the medication–no continuation condition could be used as a control for prior cognitive therapy for the purposes of modeling mediation. It also meant that any purported mediator would have to show specificity of change, since there was now a treatment "effect" to explain. Neither of the two measures of "surface" cognitions (the HS or the ATQ) met this requirement. As shown in Figure 14.10, the ASQ did (as did the DAS, to a lesser extent), at least when analyses were restricted to patients who responded to the respective interventions. It is also of interest that the bulk of the change in attributional styles occurred during the latter portion of therapy, well after the bulk of the change in depression. This is not at all the pattern observed for changes in hopelessness (or automatic thoughts) depicted in Figure 14.9, which showed a pattern similar to that depicted for syndrome depression (see Figure 14.3), but exactly what would be expected if therapists dealt first with the disconfirmation of specific automatic thoughts and expectations in the early stages of therapy and addressed more generic beliefs and information-processing propensities only as treatment progressed.

According to Baron and Kenny (1986), the following conditions must be met if change in cognition can be said to mediate cognitive therapy's relapse prevention effect. First, cognitive therapy must produce a greater reduction in risk than pharmacotherapy. As previously described, this condition was

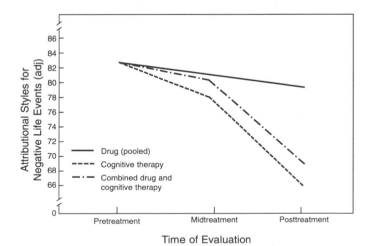

FIGURE 14.10. Changes in attributional style as a function of differential treatment.

met (see Evans et al., 1992). Second, cognitive therapy must produce greater change in cognition than does the alternative treatment; as just noted, this was the case for the measures of "depth" cognitions (the ASQ and, to a lesser extent, the DAS), but not the measures of "surface" cognition (DeRubeis et al., 1990). Third, changes in the cognitive variable must covary with the reduction in risk, even when "treatment" is held constant (in essence, relapse must be regressed simultaneously on the purported cognitive mediator and treatment type). As reported elsewhere, this condition was also met, but only with respect to the ASQ and only when the quality of execution of cognitive therapy was substituted for treatment condition (Hollon, Evans, & DeRubeis, 1990). This latter finding is consistent with the notion that cognitive therapy works by virtue of focusing on changing cognitions, since measures of specific therapist behaviors proved more "powerful" than simple categorization with regard to type of treatment. Changes on the DAS were consistent with the notion of mediation, but not significant.

Thus, despite small sample sizes, there were indications that changes in attributional styles (and to a lesser extent, dysfunctional attitudes) mediated cognitive therapy's relapse preventive effect. These findings are suggestive only and clearly require replication, but they were predicted a priori (Hollon & Garber, 1980) and they are consistent with a growing body of evidence that different aspects of cognition play differing roles in the onset and remediation of depression (see Hollon, 1992). For example, unpublished data suggest that depression secondary to Cushing's syndrome is associated with clinical elevations in "surface" cognitions such as negative expectations and automatic thoughts, but relatively normal levels of "depth" cognitions, particularly attributional styles. Similarly, work in progress by Alloy and Abramson suggests that attributional styles and dysfunctional attitudes play a predispositional role in the onset of depression, interacting with negative life events to produce increments in hopelessness that then lead to subsequent depression. Although the case is far from proven, the existing data are consistent with the notion that cognitive therapy works by virtue of producing change in cognitions. Moreover, it appears that the reduction of acute distress is more closely linked with the disconfirmation of negative expectations that stand "downstream" in the causal chain, while the reduction of subsequent risk is more closely associated with the modification of stable underlying predispositions.

DIRECTIONS FOR FUTURE RESEARCH

Although these findings are intriguing, they clearly stand in need of replication and extension. For example, although we think the existing data are most consistent with the notion that cognitive therapy is at least as effective as pharmacotherapy in the reduction of acute distress, we are troubled by the fact that cognitive therapy yielded unimpressive results in the NIMH study, the most ambitious and best controlled study in the literature. Although we think that cognitive therapy was less than adequately implemented at some sites in that study, leading us to discount the suggestion that it might be less effective than pharmacotherapy for more severely depressed patients, the question should ultimately be resolved on empirical grounds. What is needed is a study that compares adequately executed cognitive therapy to clinically representative pharmacotherapy in the context of a pill placebo control; demonstration of a "true" drug effect would make more interpretable any lack of differences between cognitive therapy and pharmacotherapy.

This is exactly the design that we hope to execute in a collaborative project between our two sites. In that study, cognitive therapists at the University of Pennsylvania would be drawn from the Center for Cognitive Therapy, ensuring real expertise with that approach, whereas cognitive therapists at Vanderbilt University would be trained *de novo* at that site, allowing us to assess the generalizability of training. Pharmacotherapists would be drawn from the pharmacology clinics operated by the Departments of Psychiatry at each site, ensuring that they are experienced with and invested in that modality. Patients would be drawn from persons seeking treatment from the pharmacology clinics (or the larger Departments of Psychiatry), increasing the likelihood that the sample selected will be representative of patients seeking treatment for depression. We plan to pay careful attention to initial level of severity. Although we do not expect to see differential response to cognitive therapy versus pharmacotherapy as a function of severity, we do expect differences between drug versus placebo to be limited to the more severely depressed patients, as was found in the NIMH study (Elkin et al., 1989).

This same study would also attempt to replicate and extend the finding that cognitive therapy prevents relapse following treatment termination. Half of the responders to pharmacotherapy alone would be withdrawn onto a pill placebo at the end of active treatment, whereas the other half would be continued on study medication. Previous studies of this kind, including our own Minnesota trial, have typically not withdrawn patients from active medication in a double-blind fashion; although we think it is unlikely, it is possible that cognitive therapy's apparent prophylactic effect is an artifact of patient expectations. If prior cognitive therapy can reduce the rate of relapse relative to that shown by patients withdrawn onto a pill placebo in a double-blind fashion, it will be difficult to dismiss its prophylactic effect.

Finally, in this same study, we hope to replicate and extend earlier findings that cognitive therapy works through theoretically specified components to produce changes in cognitive mechanisms that mediate its effects on depression, both with respect to the reduction of acute distress and the prevention of subsequent relapse. Measures of both "surface" and "depth" cognitions shall again be included and related to both measures of specific and nonspecific treatment components and subsequent symptom change.

The inclusion of minimal treatment pill placebo controls in both the active treatment and continuation phases will allow the application of sophisticated causal modeling strategies to test for mediation with respect to both response and the prevention of relapse. Moreover, we plan to assess not only changes in existing cognitive proclivities, but also the acquisition of coping skills (Barber & DeRubeis, 1992) in order to determine whether cognitive therapy works via reversing existing defects (accommodation) or enhancing coping skills (compensation) (see Barber & DeRubeis, 1989).

As excited as we are by the possibility that cognitive therapy may have an enduring effect, we recognize that the naturalistic follow-ups on which this claim is based are particularly susceptible to the confounding effects of differential retention. In the typical controlled outcome trial, only about 70% of all patients initially assigned actually complete treatment, and only about 70% of those who complete show a sufficient response to justify treatment termination. This means that only about half of the patients initially randomized to treatment can actually provide data relevant to the question of whether successful treatment reduces subsequent risk. With such massive "attrition," it is possible that preexistent differences in risk could be misinterpreted as a prevention effect; that is, if high-risk patients are more likely to drop out of (or fail to respond to) cognitive therapy than pharmacotherapy, then the pool of responding completers entering the follow-up from cognitive therapy could be at considerably lower risk for relapse than the pool of responding completers entering the follow-up from pharmacotherapy.

The possibility that acute treatment could operate as a "differential sieve" to systematically undermine initial randomization does not require poor research design on the part of the investigators; it is simply a fact of life that is the inevitable consequence of the nature of the question asked (we found no evidence of differential retention in our Minnesota study, but cannot be sure that we did not overlook some important confound). Moreover, not a lot can be done about it, other than to minimize attrition and to maximize response. Lavori (1992) has recommended including all patients initially assigned to treatment in the subsequent analyses, but that simply begs the question, since it is not clear how such patients are to be coded for purposes of analysis (it hardly seems appropriate to assume that a patient who fails to complete or respond to treatment should be counted as having relapsed).

One possible strategy is to turn conventional outcome logic on its head and provide all dropouts and nonresponders to the respective single modalities with a common second treatment. The typical treatment outcome study uses randomization to maximize the likelihood that potential confounds are comparably distributed across the groups. Since differential retention, if it occurs, should differentially segregate high- versus low-risk patients into dropout/nonresponder versus completing responder pools, providing a common second treatment for all patients who fail to complete or respond to their first treatment should maximize the chance of unmasking the generation of systematic bias. This is exactly the strategy that we plan to follow in the study already described.

Second, because the risk of differential retention is greatest when treatment conditions are maximally dissimilar, anything that can be done to minimize irrelevant differences between the treatments should minimize the risk of systematically unmatching the treatment conditions. This means that it is preferable to operationalize cognitive therapy in the form of combined treatment whenever the question of interest involves the reduction of subsequent risk, since patients treated with combined treatment differ from patients treated with pharmacotherapy alone only with respect to the presence of cognitive therapy, not the absence of pharmacotherapy. This is the strategy we plan to pursue in a second study designed to determine whether cognitive therapy's preventive effect extends to the prevention of recurrence following recovery from the index episode. Although we are quite excited by the indications that cognitive therapy may reduce risk for relapse, we recognize that there is a growing consensus that relapse, the return of symptoms associated with the treated episode, needs to be distinguished from recurrence, the onset of a wholly new episode (Frank et al., 1991). The majority of the instances of differential symptom return evident in the naturalistic follow-up studies suggesting a prophylactic effect for cognitive therapy have occurred in the first 6 months following initial remission, well within the period of risk for relapse rather than recurrence. If cognitive therapy were only to prevent relapse and not recurrence, it would be of little importance clinically, since current pharmacological practice has moved toward medicating patients for up to a year beyond initial remission. In order to determine whether cognitive therapy's prophylactic effect extends to the prevention of recurrence, it will be necessary to protect patients brought to remission pharmacologically with an extended period of continuation medication, at least until they are past the period of risk for relapse.

That is exactly the study that we hope to do as the second of two sequential collaborative projects. We plan to assign patients randomly to either pharmacotherapy or combined treatment and treat them to the point of full recovery (i.e., until they have been symptom free for at least 6 consecutive months). At that point, all recovered patients will be withdrawn from treatment and followed across a subsequent 3-year follow-up period. If cognitive therapy is truly prophylactic (as we expect it to be), it should be associated with a lower rate of recurrence than that observed for patients previously treated with pharmacotherapy alone. As in our other studies, we plan to carefully monitor the quality of treatment execution and change in cognition and relate each to initial response and subsequent recurrence.

Finally, we are currently involved in a test of primary prevention involving cognitive therapy under the direction of Martin Seligman at the University of Pennsylvania. This project involves identifying euthymic college students at risk for depression due to elevated attributional styles, providing half with a brief workshop in which they are taught the basic skills of cognitive therapy, and then following the full sample across a subsequent 3-year interval (see Hollon, DeRubeis, & Seligman, 1992, for an expanded discussion). As in the other studies, we plan to assess purported cognitive mechanisms across treatment and test them for status with respect to mediation. We predict that cognitive therapy will prevent the onset of depression in this at-risk sample and that it will do so by virtue of producing change in attributional style. Although it is still too early to tell whether cognitive therapy is having the predicted effect with respect to subsequent onset, findings to date suggest that it can reduce cognitive propensities presumed to contribute to risk.

SUMMARY AND CONCLUSIONS

Although far from conclusive, the existing findings suggest that cognitive therapy is as effective as pharmacotherapy in the reduction of acute distress, and that it is better able to reduce subsequent risk, at least when it is done in an adequate fashion. The majority of the studies in the literature are consistent with these interpretations. Only the NIMH study stands as an outlier, and questions can be raised about the adequacy with which cognitive therapy was implemented in that trial. These very questions underscore the importance of maintaining quality control over the implementation of treatment; when cognitive therapy is adequately implemented, it appears to perform quite well. Moreover, there are indications that cognitive therapy works by virtue of changing beliefs and information-processing proclivities and that different aspects of cognition play different roles in the process of change. This is as predicted by theory, thus increasing our confidence in our understanding of the approach.

It is clear that cognitive therapy has emerged as a major approach to the treatment of depression. Moreover, evidence for its efficacy has evolved in the context of a body of research that supports the validity of the larger cognitive theory of depression. The success of the therapy and the insights into the nature and causes of depression it has provided stand as a testament to Aaron T. Beck, its founder and primary theoretician.

REFERENCES

Abramson, L. Y., Metalsky, G. I., & Alloy, L. B. (1989). Hopelessness depression: A theory-based subtype of depression. *Psychological Review, 96,* 358–372.

Barber, J. P., & DeRubeis, R. J. (1989). On second thought: Where the action is in cognitive therapy for depression. *Cognitive Therapy and Research, 13,* 441–457.

Barber, J. P., & DeRubeis, R. J. (1992). The Ways of Responding: A scale to assess compensatory skills taught in cognitive therapy. *Behavioral Assessment, 14,* 93–115.

Baron, R. M., & Kenny, D. A. (1986). The moderator–mediator variable distinction in social psychological research: Conceptual, strategic, and statistical considerations. *Journal of Personality and Social Psychology, 51,* 1173–1182.

Beck, A. T. (1963). Thinking and depression: I. Idiosyncratic content and cognitive distortions. *Archives of General Psychiatry, 9,* 324–333.

Beck, A. T. (1964). Thinking and depression: 2. Theory and therapy. *Archives of General Psychiatry, 10,* 561–571.

Beck, A. T. (1970). Cognitive therapy: Nature and relation to behavior therapy. *Behavior Therapy, 1,* 184–200.

Beck, A. T. (1976). *Cognitive therapy and the emotional disorders.* Madison, CT: International Universities Press.

Beck, A. T., Rush, A. J., Shaw, B. F., & Emery, G. (1979). *Cognitive therapy of depression.* New York: Guilford Press.

Beck, A. T., Ward, C. H., Mendelson, M., Mock, J., & Erbaugh, J. (1961). An inventory for measuring depression. *Archives of General Psychiatry, 4,* 561–571.

Beck, A. T., Weissman, A., Lester, D., & Trexler, L. (1974). The measurement of pessimism: The Hopelessness Scale. *Journal of Consulting and Clinical Psychology, 42,* 861–865.

Blackburn, I. M., Bishop, S., Glen, A. I. M., Whalley, L. J., & Christie, J. E. (1981). The efficacy of cognitive therapy in depression: A treatment trial using cognitive therapy and pharmacotherapy, each alone and in combination. *British Journal of Psychiatry, 139,* 181–189.

Blackburn, I. M., Eunson, K. M., & Bishop, S. (1986). A two-year naturalistic follow-up of depressed patients treated with cognitive therapy, pharmacotherapy and a combination of both. *Journal of Affective Disorders, 10,* 67–75.

DeRubeis, R. J., Evans, M. D., Hollon, S. D., Garvey, M. J., Grove, W. M., & Tuason, V. B. (1990). How does cognitive therapy work: Cognitive change and symptom change in cognitive therapy and pharmacotherapy for depression. *Journal of Consulting and Clinical Psychology, 58,* 862–869.

DeRubeis, R. J., & Feeley, M. (1990). Determinants of change in cognitive therapy for depression. *Cognitive Therapy and Research, 14,* 469–482.

DeRubeis, R. J., Hollon, S. D., Evans, M. D., & Bemis, K. M. (1982). Can psychotherapies for depression be discriminated? A systematic investigation of cognitive therapy and interpersonal therapy. *Journal of Consulting and Clinical Psychology, 50,* 744–756.

Dobson, K. S. (1989). A meta-analysis of the efficacy of cognitive therapy for depression. *Journal of Consulting and Clinical Psychology, 57,* 414–419.

Elkin, I., Shea, M. T., Watkins, J. T., Imber, S. D., Sotsky, S. M., Collins, J. F., Glass, D. R., Pilkonis, P. A., Leber, W. R., Docherty, J. P., Fiester, S. J., & Parloff, M. B. (1989). NIMH Treatment of Depression Collaborative Research Program: I. General effectiveness of treatments. *Archives of General Psychiatry, 46,* 971–982.

Evans, M. D., Hollon, S. D., DeRubeis, R. J., Piasecki, J. M., Grove, W. M., Garvey, M. J., & Tuason, V. B. (1992). Differential relapse following cognitive therapy and pharmacotherapy for depression. *Archives of General Psychiatry, 49,* 802–808.

Frank, E., Prien, R. F., Jarrett, R. B., Keller, M. B., Kupfer, D. J., Lavori, P. W., Rush, A. J., & Weissman, M. M. (1991). Conceptualization and rationale for consensus definitions of terms in major depressive disorders: Remission, recovery, relapse, and recurrence. *Archives of General Psychiatry, 48,* 851–855.

Hamilton, M. (1960). A rating scale for depression. *Journal of Neurological and Neurosurgical Psychiatry, 23,* 56–61.

Hollon, S. D. (1992). Cognitive models of depression from a psychobiological perspective. *Psychological Inquiry, 3,* 250–253.

Hollon, S. D., DeRubeis, R. J., & Evans, M. D. (1987). Causal mediation of change in treatment for depression: Discriminating between nonspecificity and noncausality. *Psychological Bulletin, 102,* 139–149.

Hollon, S. D., DeRubeis, R. J., Evans, M. D., Wiemer, M. J., Garvey, M. J., Grove, W. M., & Tuason, V. B. (1992). Cognitive therapy and pharmacotherapy for depression: Singly and in combination. *Archives of General Psychiatry, 49,* 774–781.

Hollon, S. D., DeRubeis, R. J., & Seligman, M. E. P. (1992). Cognitive therapy and the prevention of depression. *Applied and Preventive Psychology, 1,* 89–95.

Hollon, S. D., Evans, M. D., & DeRubeis, R. J. (1990). Cognitive mediation of relapse prevention following treatment for depression: Implications of differential risk. In R. E. Ingram (Ed.), *Contemporary psychological approaches to depression* (pp. 117–136). New York: Plenum Press.

Hollon, S. D., Evans, M. D., Elkin, I., & Lowery, A. (1984, May). *System for rating therapies for depression.* Paper presented at the Annual Meeting of the American Psychiatric Association, Los Angeles.

Hollon, S. D., & Garber, J. A. (1980). A cognitive–expectancy theory of therapy for helplessness and depression. In J. Garber & M. E. P. Seligman (Eds.), *Human helplessness: Theory and applications* (pp. 173–195). New York: Academic Press.

Hollon, S. D., & Kendall, P. C. (1980). Cognitive self-statements in depression: Development of an automatic thoughts questionnaire. *Cognitive Therapy and Research, 4,* 383–396.

Hollon, S. D., Shelton, R. C., & Loosen, P. T. (1991). Cognitive therapy and pharmacotherapy for depression. *Journal of Consulting and Clinical Psychology, 59,* 88–99.

Jacobson, N. S., & Hollon, S. D. (1996a). Cognition behahvior therapy vs. pharmacotherapy: Now that the jury's returned its verdict, it's time to present the rest of the evidence. *Journal of Consulting and Clinical Psychology, 64,* 74–80.

Jacobson, N.S., & Hollon, S. P. (1996b). Prospects for future comparisons between drugs and psychotherapy: Lessons from the CBT vs. pharmacotherapy exchange. *Journal of Consulting and Clinical Psychology, 24,* 104–108.

Kovacs, M., Rush, A. J., Beck, A. T., & Hollon, S. D. (1981). Depressed outpatients treated with cognitive therapy or pharmacotherapy. *Archives of General Psychiatry, 38,* 33–39.

Lavori, P. W. (1992). Clinical trials in psychiatry: Should protocol deviation censor patient data? *Neuropsychopharmacology, 6,* 39–48.

Murphy, G. E., Simons, A. D., Wetzel, R. D., & Lustman, P. J. (1984). Cognitive therapy and pharmacotherapy, singly and together in the treatment of depression. *Archives of General Psychiatry, 41,* 33–41.

Prien, R. F., & Kupfer, D. J. (1986). Continuation drug therapy for major depressive episodes: How long should it be maintained? *American Journal of Psychiatry, 143,* 18–23.

Prien, R. F., Kupfer, D. J., Mansky, P. A., Small, J. G., Tuason, V. B., Voss, C. B., & Johnson, W. E. (1984). Drug therapy in the prevention of recurrences in unipolar and bipolar affective disorders. *Archives of General Psychiatry, 41,* 1096–1104.

Rush, A. J., Beck, A. T., Kovacs, M., & Hollon, S. D. (1977). Comparative efficacy of cognitive therapy and pharmacotherapy in the treatment of depressed outpatients. *Cognitive Therapy and Research, 1,* 17–37.

Rush, A. J., Kovacs, M., Beck, A. T., Weissenburger, J., & Hollon, S. D. (1981). Differential effects of cognitive therapy and pharmacotherapy in the treatment of depressed outpatients. *Journal of Affective Disorders, 3,* 221–229.

Seligman, M. E. P., Abramson, L. Y., Semmel, A., & von Baeyer, C. (1979). Depressive attributional style. *Journal of Abnormal Psychology, 88,* 242–247.

Shea, M. T., Elkin, I., Imber, S. D., Sotsky, S. M., Watkins, J. T., Collins, J. F., Pilkonis, P. A., Beckham, E., Glass, D. R., Dolan, R., & Parloff, M. B. (1992). Course of depressive symptoms over follow-up: Findings from the National Institute of Mental Health Treatment of Depression Collaborative Research Program. *Archives of General Psychiatry, 49,* 782–787.

Simons, A. D., Murphy, G. E., Levine, J. L., & Wetzel, R. D. (1986). Cognitive therapy and pharmacotherapy for depression: Sustained improvement over one year. *Archives of General Psychiatry, 43,* 43–48.

Weissman, A., & Beck, A. T. (1978, November). *Development and validation of the Dysfunctional Attitude Scale: A preliminary investigation.* Presented at the annual meeting of the American Educational Research Association, Toronto, Ontario.

Young, J. E., & Beck, A. T. (1980). *Development of an instrument for rating cognitive therapy: The Cognitive Therapy Scale.* Philadelphia: University of Pennsylvania.

Chapter 15

Panic Disorder:
From Theory to Therapy

David M. Clark

In the 1960s and early 1970s substantial improvements in the effectiveness of psychological treatments for a variety of emotional disorders were achieved by behavior therapists who focused on the systematic application of conditioning principles. However, by the mid-1970s the limitations of an exclusively behavioral approach to therapy were becoming increasingly evident. Clinicians and researchers interested in further enhancing the effectiveness of short-term treatments started to explore the value of incorporating cognitive models and procedures into behavior therapy. Many writers, including Albert Bandura, Albert Ellis, Richard Lazarus, Michael Mahoney, and Donald Meichenbaum, made major contributions to the ensuing "cognitive revolution," but the writer who has probably had the greatest impact on clinical theorizing and treatment is Aaron T. Beck. Why is this? Such a question rarely has a simple answer. Many factors are likely to have been involved. His charm, his endless enthusiasm, his ability to identify and encourage promising young researchers, his initial focus on depression rather than anxiety, and his tendency to ignore rather than fight his critics are all likely to have contributed. In addition, one suspects that part of his influence also results from the fact that he has not only generated original ideas about the role of cognition in emotional disorders, but in his work on depression he also outlined an overall approach to psychotherapy research that seems particularly well-suited to identifying effective treatment procedures and persuading the clinical and academic community to use them. This chapter briefly summarizes the approach and then outlines the way it has been used to understand and treat another condition: panic disorder.

THE BECKIAN APPROACH TO PSYCHOTHERAPY RESEARCH

The approach Beck and colleagues (Beck, Rush, Shaw, & Emery, 1979) adopted in depression has five main elements.

1. *Specification of a simple clinical model that places cognition at the center of the disorder.* The term "clinical model" is here used to denote a model in which the main processes are expressed in everyday language rather than in the more precise, technical terms that characterize many models in cognitive psychology (see Teasdale, 1988). The advantage of such a model is the ease with which it suggests specific clinical procedures. The disadvantage is that it can be more difficult to test because it is not always clear how to operationalize key terms in a way that allows them to be precisely measured and manipulated.

2. *Experimental investigations of the model.* Beck's first book on depression (Beck, 1967) contained an impressive set of correlational and experimental findings supporting his model. His lead in subjecting the theory to empirical investigation encouraged others (e.g., Hammen, 1988; Teasdale, 1983) to do the same, producing a substantial body of experimental investigations.

3. *A detailed account of the factors that prevent cognitive change in the absence of treatment.* In depression the main factors highlighted by Beck et al. (1979) were withdrawal from everyday activities, logical errors, and dysfunctional assumptions that biased information processing.

4. *Carefully chosen treatment procedures that specifically targeted the factors preventing cognitive change.* These included scheduling activities that would give patients a sense of mastery or pleasure, and training in identifying and testing negative automatic thoughts, logical errors, and dysfunctional assumptions.

5. *Controlled trials evaluating the effectiveness of the therapy.* These are of course crucial for the general acceptance and application of a new treatment. Beck and colleagues wisely delayed publication of their cognitive therapy for depression treatment manual until a major outcome trial (Rush, Beck, Kovacs, & Hollon, 1977) establishing the effectiveness of the approach had been published. Numerous additional trials have since been published (see Hollon & Beck, 1994, for a recent review).

PANIC ATTACKS AND PANIC DISORDER

The essential feature of panic disorder is the occurrence of panic attacks. DSM-IV (American Psychiatric Association, 1994) defines a panic attack as a sudden onset period of intense fear or discomfort associated with at least four symptoms, which include breathlessness, palpitations, dizziness, trembling, a feeling of choking, nausea, derealization, chest pain, and paresthesias. Defined this way, occasional panic attacks are common in all anxiety disorders (Barlow et al., 1985). The diagnosis of panic disorder, however, is reserved for a subset of individuals who experience *recurrent* panic attacks, at least some of which come on unexpectedly. That is to say, the attacks are not always triggered by entering phobic situations or by anticipating doing so. Individuals diagnosed as panic disorder with agoraphobia can identify certain situations in which they think attacks are particularly likely to occur, or would be especially catastrophic, and tend to avoid these situations. Individuals diagnosed as panic disorder without agoraphobia tend not to be able to identify such situations and show no gross situational avoidance.

The apparently "out-of-the-blue" nature of some panic attacks lead many biologically oriented researchers to suggest that panic disorder might best be understood as a neurochemical disorder. However, several investigators (Beck, Emery, & Greenberg, 1985; Clark, 1986, 1988; Ehlers & Margraf, 1989; Margraf, Ehlers, & Roth, 1986; Salkovskis, 1988) have argued that panic disorder is best understood in cognitive terms.

THE COGNITIVE THEORY OF PANIC DISORDER

The cognitive theory of panic states that

> individuals who experience recurrent panic attacks do so because they have a relatively enduring tendency to interpret certain bodily sensations in a catastrophic fashion. The sensations that are misinterpreted are mainly those involved in normal anxiety responses (e.g., palpitations, breathlessness, dizziness, paresthesias) but also include some other sensations. The catastrophic misinterpretation involves perceiving these sensations as much more dangerous than they really are and, in particular, interpreting the sensations as indicative of an *immediately* impending physical or mental disaster — for example, perceiving a slight feeling of breathlessness as evidence of impending cessation of breathing and consequent death, perceiving palpitations as evidence of an impending heart attack, perceiving a pulsing sensation in the forehead as evidence of a brain haemorrhage, or perceiving a shaky feeling as evidence of impending loss of control and insanity. (Clark, 1988, p. 149)

The suggested sequence of events that occurs in panic attacks is shown in Figure 15.1. External stimuli (such as a department store for an agoraphobic) and internal stimuli (bodily sensations, thoughts, images) can both provoke panic attacks. The sequence that culminates in an attack starts with the stimuli being interpreted as a sign of impending danger. This interpretation produces a state of apprehension, which is associated with a wide range of bodily sensations. If these anxiety-produced sensations are interpreted in a catastrophic fashion (impending insanity, death, loss of control, etc.) a further increase in apprehension occurs, producing more bodily sensations, leading to a vicious circle that culminates in a panic attack. The cognitive theory accounts both for panic attacks that are preceded by elevated anxiety and for panic attacks that are not and instead appear out of the blue. For both types of attack it is argued that the critical event is the misinterpretation of certain bodily sensations. In attacks preceded by height-

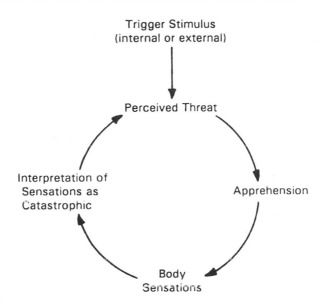

Trigger Stimulus
(internal or external)

Perceived Threat

Interpretation of
Sensations as
Catastrophic

Apprehension

Body
Sensations

FIGURE 15.1. The suggested sequence of events in a panic attack. From Clark (1986, p. 463). Copyright 1986 by Pergamon Press. Reprinted by permission.

ened anxiety, the sensations are often a consequence of the preceding anxiety, which in turn is due to anticipating an attack *or* some other anxiety-evoking event unrelated to panic. In attacks that are not preceded by heightened anxiety, the misinterpreted sensations are initially caused by a different emotional state (anger, excitement, disgust) or by innocuous events such as exercising (breathlessness, palpitations), drinking too much coffee (palpitations), or standing up quickly after sitting (dizziness). In such attacks patients frequently fail to distinguish between the triggering bodily sensations and the subsequent panic and so perceive the attack as having no cause and coming out of the blue.

When applying the cognitive theory to individual patients, it is often useful to distinguish between the first panic attack and the subsequent development of repeated attacks and panic disorder. Community surveys (Brown & Cash, 1990; Margraf & Ehlers, 1988; Norton, Dorward, & Cox, 1986; Wilson et al., 1991) indicate about 7–28% of the normal population will experience an occasional unexpected panic attack. It is unlikely that there is a single explanation for these relatively common, but occasional, autonomic events. Stressful life events, hormonal changes, illness, caffeine, drugs, and a variety of transient medical conditions could all produce occasional perceived autonomic changes. However, the cognitive theory assumes that individuals only go on to develop the rarer condition of repeated panic attacks and panic disorder (approximately 3–5% of the general population; Wittchen & Essau, 1991) if they develop a tendency to interpret these perceived autonomic events in a catastrophic fashion. Such a tendency could either be a consequence of learning experiences that predate the first attack (e.g., observing one's parents panicking or modeling illness-related behavior; Ehlers, 1993) or could arise as a consequence of the way the patient, physicians, and significant others respond to the first attack.

EXPERIMENTAL INVESTIGATIONS OF THE COGNITIVE MODEL

The cognitive theory of panic can in principle account for the main clinical features of panic disorder (Clark, 1986). However, this does not necessarily mean the theory is correct. In order to evaluate the theory, it is necessary to subject its predictions to appropriate investigation. Clark (1986, 1988) outlined four central predictions that can be derived from the theory.

1. Panic patients will be more likely to interpret bodily sensations in a catastrophic fashion than individuals who do not experience panic attacks.
2. Procedures that activate catastrophic misinterpretations of bodily sensations will produce an increase in anxiety and panic in panic disorder patients.
3. Panic attacks can be prevented by reducing patients' tendency to interpret bodily sensations in a catastrophic fashion.
4. Sustained improvement after the end of any treatment (whether psychological or pharmacological) will depend on cognitive change having occurred during the course of therapy.

The first prediction is concerned with establishing that panic disorder patients think in the way required by the theory. However, demonstrating that patients think as required by the theory does not in itself establish that the thinking plays a causal role in the production of attacks. Logically, the negative thinking could be just an epiphenomenon. To illustrate this point, consider epilepsy. Epileptic attacks are an alarming experience. After having suffered an attack many epileptics develop a characteristic set of fearful thoughts about the attacks. However, no one would argue that these thoughts have a primary causal role in epilepsy. Instead, the epileptic attacks are the result of spontaneously occurring neural activity. Some biological theorists would make similar statements about the cognitions that accompany panic attacks. To discount the epiphenomena argument one must go beyond correlational observations and manipulate the putative cause. The second and third predictions are concerned with establishing causation by manipulating misinterpretations of bodily sensations and seeing whether these manipulations have the predicted effects on the occurrence of panic. The fourth prediction concerns the clinically important topic of relapse following treatment.

Prediction 1

The first direct test of prediction 1 was reported by McNally and Foa (1987). A modified version of a questionnaire originally developed by Butler and Mathews (1983) was used to compare DSM-III agoraphobia with panic patients and nonpatient controls in terms of the extent to which they interpreted ambiguous events in a negative way. Two classes of ambiguous events were included. "Internal stimuli" consisted of descriptions of bodily sensations that the cognitive theory predicts will be more likely to be misinterpreted by panic patients (e.g., "You notice your heart beating quickly and pounding. Why?"). "External stimuli" consisted of potentially threatening external events (e.g., "You wake with a start in the middle of the night, thinking you heard a noise, but all is quiet. What do you think woke you up?"). Subjects were asked to write down the first explanation that came to mind for each event. After writing their response to the open-ended question, subjects turned the page and rank ordered three explanations with respect to the likelihood of their coming to mind in a similar situation. One explanation was negative and the remaining two were neutral or positive. Analysis of both open-ended responses and rank-order data indicated that agoraphobia with panic patients were more likely than controls to interpret both internal and external stimuli in a negative fashion.

In a subsequent study, Harvey, Richards, Dziadosz, and Swindell (1993) administered McNally and Foa's (1987) questionnaire to DSM-III-R (American Psychiatric Association, 1987) panic disorder patients, social phobics, and nonpatient controls. The comparison between panic disorder patients and nonpatient controls replicated McNally and Foa's finding of a significant difference for both internal and external events. The comparison between panic disorder patients and social phobics revealed evidence for a more specific cognitive abnormality. In particular, panic patients were significantly more likely to choose negative interpretations of internal events than social phobics but the two patient groups did not differ in the likelihood of choosing a negative interpretation for external events. This pattern of results suggests anxiety disorders may have a general effect on threat interpretation and, in addition, panic disorder is associated with a specifically enhanced tendency to interpret internal events in a negative fashion.

Clark, Salkovskis, Öst, et al. (1996) replicated and extended Harvey et al.'s findings. The Interpretations Questionnaire was modified to exclude anxiety responses (e.g., "I am having a panic attack") from the experimenter-provided interpretations and belief ratings were included. Consistent with prediction 1, patients with panic disorder were more likely to interpret ambiguous autonomic sensations as signs of immediately impending physical or mental disaster, and were more likely to believe these interpretations, than other anxiety disorder patients (social phobics and generalized anxiety disorder) and nonpatients. In addition, the likelihood of interpreting ambiguous autonomic sensations as signs of immediately impending disaster reduced with successful treatment and the degree of change in interpretations discriminated between treatments which varied in their impact on panic.[1]

Prediction 2

Ehlers, Margraf, Roth, Taylor, and Birbaumer (1988) used a false heart rate feedback task to test the prediction that conditions likely to activate patients' catastrophic interpretations of bodily sensations will lead to increased anxiety in panic patients. During the course of a laboratory experiment, panic disorder patients and normal controls were given false auditory feedback indicating a sudden increase in heart rate. Because patients are prone to misinterpret cardiac changes, it was predicted that panic patients would show a greater increase in anxiety during the false feedback, and this is what happened. Compared to normal controls, panic disorder patients showed significantly greater increases in self-reported anxiety, heart rate, skin conductance, and blood pressure.

Clark et al. (1988) used another cognitive manipulation to activate catastrophic misinterpretations and obtained essentially similar results to those reported by Ehlers et al. (1988). Panic patients and normal controls were asked to read out loud a series of pairs of words. In the crucial conditions, the pairs of words consisted of various combinations of bodily sensations and catastrophes (e.g., palpitations–dying, breathless–suffocate, numbness–stroke, dizziness–fainting, chest tight–heart attack, unreality–insane). As these combinations represent the sort of thoughts that panic patients are prone to have and believe during attacks, it was predicted that panic patients would show greater increases in anxiety and panic while reading the pairs of words. This is indeed what happened. Panic disorder patients, recovered panic disorder patients (treated with cognitive therapy), and normal controls were asked to rate their anxiety before and after reading the cards and also to rate whether they experienced an increase in any of the 12 DSM-III (American Psychiatric Association, 1980) panic symptoms. On the basis of this information, it was determined that 10 out of 12 (83%) panic patients, but no recovered patients or normal controls, had a panic attack while reading the cards.

Prediction 3

Several studies have tested the prediction that reducing patients' tendency to misinterpret bodily sensations will prevent panic attacks. Early research in panic established that a range of pharmacological agents (sodium lactate, yohimbine, carbon dioxide, isoproterenol, caffeine) can reliably induce a state that is perceived as similar to natural panic attacks in panic disorder patients but rarely does so in nonpanic patients or normal controls. Biological theorists interpreted these findings as evidence that panic can be directly induced by biochemical changes and that panic disorder is due to a neurochemical disturbance. In contrast, cognitive theorists have argued that these pharmacological agents do not have a direct panic-inducing effect but, instead, induce panic because patients misinterpret the pharmacologically induced bodily sensations. To test prediction 3, and to distinguish between the cognitive and biological accounts of pharmacological panic inductions, Rapee, Mattick, and Murrell (1986); Sanderson, Rapee, and Barlow (1989); Clark (1993); and Clark, Salkovskis, Anastasiades, et al. (1996) investigated whether or not purely cognitive manipulations could block pharmacologically induced panic.

Rapee et al. (1986) used a preinhalation instructional manipulation to influence patients' interpretation of the sensations induced by a single inhalation of 50% carbon dioxide/50% oxygen. One-half of the panic disorder patients were allocated to a no-explanation condition in which minimal information about the procedure was provided. The other half were given a more detailed explanation in which all possible sensations were described and attributed to the effects of the gas. A manipulation check confirmed that the detailed explanation group had less catastrophic cognitions during the inhalation than the no-explanation group. As predicted by cognitive theory, the detailed explanation group also reported significantly less panic than the no-explanation group.

Sanderson et al. (1989) studied carbon dioxide inhalation. Prior to receiving a 20-minute inhalation of 5% carbon dioxide in air, panic disorder patients were shown a dial and told that turning this dial would reduce carbon dioxide flow if a nearby light was illuminated but not otherwise. In fact, the dial had no effect on carbon dioxide flow. During the infusion, the light came on for half the patients (illusion-of-control group) but was not illuminated for the remaining subjects (no-illusion-of-control group). As predicted, patients in the illusion-of-control group were significantly less likely to panic, even though they did not use the dial and received as much carbon dioxide as the no-illusion group.

Clark, Salkovskis, Anastasiades, Middleton, and Gelder (1996) studied sodium lactate infusions. Panic disorder patients were randomly allocated to one of two preinfusion instruction sets (experimental or control). The experimental instructions were designed to prevent patients from misinterpreting lactate-induced sensations. Consistent with cognitive theory, patients' self-reports, physiological monitoring, and judgments by a blind assessor indicated that patients given the experimental instructions were significantly less likely to panic than patients given the control instructions, even though the amount of lactate infused was the same in both groups.

Prediction 4

Clark et al. (1994) tested prediction 4 by examining end-of-treatment and follow-up data in their trial of psychological (cognitive therapy or applied relaxation) and pharmacological (imipramine) treatments for panic disorder. Two analyses provided support for prediction 4. First, when the data from all patients were examined, misinterpretation of bodily sensations at the end of treatment was a significant predictor of panic/anxiety at follow-up, and this relationship remained significant when panic/anxiety at the end of treatment was partialed out. Second, within patients who were panic free at the end of treatment, there was a significant correlation between misinterpretation of bodily sensations at the end of treatment and subsequent relapse.

FACTORS THAT PREVENT COGNITIVE CHANGE IN THE ABSENCE OF TREATMENT

If panic attacks occur because patients have distorted beliefs about certain bodily sensations, we must ask, what maintains this negative thinking style? As Seligman (1988) pointed out, in the absence of treatment many panic patients persist in maintaining distorted beliefs about bodily sensations despite numerous apparent disconfirmations of those beliefs. For example, a patient who is concerned that he might be having a heart attack during a panic may persist in this belief despite having had hundreds of attacks in which he did not die and numerous visits to emergency rooms during which he was reassured that his heart was normal.

Cognitive theorists (Clark, 1988; Ehlers & Margraf, 1989; Salkovskis, 1988) have suggested that at least two processes are involved in maintaining such patients' distorted beliefs. First, because the patients are frightened of certain sensations, they may become hypervigilant and repeatedly scan their body for signs of danger. This internal focus of attention would allow them to notice sensations that many other people would not be aware of. Once noticed, these sensations could be taken as further evidence of the presence of some serious physical or mental disorder. Second, various types of avoidance behavior are likely to prevent patients from disconfirming their negative beliefs. This could be true not only for patients with marked phobic avoidance (panic disorder with agoraphobia) but also for those without such gross situational avoidance (panic disorder without agoraphobia). As Salkovskis (1988, 1991) pointed out, such patients often engage in subtle forms of avoidance (safety behaviors) that could maintain their negative beliefs. For example, a patient preoccupied with the idea she is suffering from cardiac disease might avoid exercise and rest whenever she notices a palpitation. She may then believe this avoidance has prevented her from experiencing a fatal heart attack. However, because she has no cardiac disease, the avoidance is more likely to have simply maintained her somatic preoccupation.

Ehlers and colleagues have reported a series of studies that provide support for the role of interoception in the maintenance of panic disorder. In one study (Ehlers & Breuer, 1992, Experiment 2) subjects were given a heartbeat perception task in which they had to silently count their heartbeats without taking their pulse. Consistent with the hypothesis that panic disorder is characterized by enhanced awareness of bodily sensations, panic disorder patients were more accurate in their heartbeat perception than infrequent panickers, simple phobics, or normal controls. In a subsequent study (Ehlers, 1995), a longitudinal design was used to determine whether or not enhanced cardiac awareness contributes to the persistence of panic disorder. Patients who had a history of panic disorder but were in remission when tested in the laboratory were followed up 1 year later and asked whether or not they had experienced any further panic attacks during the follow-up period. As predicted, patients who reported a reoccurrence of their panic attacks had demonstrated significantly better heart rate perception during the initial laboratory test than patients who did not experience a reoccurrence.

Salkovskis, Clark, and Gelder (1996) provided evidence that panic patients engage in safety behaviors of the sort which *could* maintain their negative beliefs. Panic disorder patients completed the Agoraphobic Cognitions Questionnaire (Chambless, Caputo, Bright, & Gallagher, 1984), which assesses thoughts experienced during a panic attack, and a Behaviors Questionnaire, which assesses their behavior during a panic. Correlational analyses revealed a series of meaningful links between cognitions and behavior. For example, patients who reported thinking that they might be having a heart attack rested and slowed down their breathing during a panic; patients who thought they might be about to faint leaned against solid objects; and patients who thought they might be going insane made strenuous efforts to control their thinking.

To determine whether these safety behaviors prevent disconfirmation of panic patients' negative beliefs about bodily sensations, it is necessary to experimentally manipulate the safety behaviors. Salkovskis (1995) has recently reported preliminary results from a study in which patients with panic disorder and agoraphobia had equivalent periods of exposure to a feared situation while either maintaining their usual safety behaviors or dropping them. As predicted, the drop-safety-behaviors condition led to a significantly larger decrease in negative beliefs and produced a significantly greater improvement in anxiety in a subsequent behavior test.

SPECIALIZED TREATMENT PROCEDURES

Cognitive theory suggests that it should be possible to treat naturally occurring panic attacks by helping patients to identify and change their misinterpretations of bodily sensations. Several cognitive-behavioral treatment packages that attempt to achieve these goals have been devised, the most prominent of which are the Oxford-based Cognitive Therapy Package, developed by Clark, Salkovskis, Beck, and colleagues (Clark, 1989: Salkovskis & Clark, 1991), and the closely related, but independently derived,

Albany-based Panic Control Treatment (PCT), devised by Barlow and colleagues (Barlow & Cerny, 1988; Barlow & Craske, 1989).

The Cognitive Therapy Package uses a wide range of cognitive and behavioral procedures to help patients change their misinterpretations of bodily sensations and to modify the processes that tend to maintain the misinterpretations. The cognitive techniques include using review of a recent panic attack to derive the vicious circle model, identifying and challenging patients' evidence for their misinterpretations, substituting more realistic interpretations, and restructuring images. The behavioral procedures include inducing feared sensations (by hyperventilation, by reading pairs of words representing feared sensations and catastrophes, or by focusing attention on the body) in order to demonstrate the true cause of the panic symptoms, and dropping safety behaviors (such as holding onto solid objects when feeling dizzy) and entering feared situations in order to allow patients to disconfirm their negative predictions about the consequences of their symptoms.

The way in which these various procedures are interwoven in therapy is illustrated by the following case example. The patient was a 40-year-old man who had been suffering from panic disorder for one and a half years and was currently experiencing approximately three panic attacks per week. His main thoughts in the attacks (with belief ratings) were: "I'll have a heart attack (100%)," "I'll have a stroke (100%)," "I'm about to die (100%)," "I'll faint (50%)," and "I'll go crazy (40%)." The main feared sensations were palpitations, a tight and heavy feeling in the chest, blurred vision, dry throat, dizziness, tingling in the fingers, breathlessness, and feelings of unreality. Safety behaviors used during panic attacks included monitoring his heart (to see whether it was going too fast *or* too slow), trying to distract himself, taking paracetamol, taking deep breaths, and leaving the situation. The main activities avoided through fear of having a panic attack were sex and exercise.

Treatment was given in two sessions as part of an experimental series investigating ways of delivering brief treatment. Session 1 lasted 4 hours (with a coffee break) and session 2 lasted 1 hour. Session 1 started with patient and therapist reviewing a recent panic attack and deriving the vicious circle model (see Figure 15.2). The most prominent thought in the panic attack was "My heart will stop and I will die." The notion of two alternative possibilities was then introduced. The first possibility, which the patient favored, was that there was something seriously wrong with his heart and that he is genuinely in danger of dying during a panic attack. The alternative was that the problem was his *belief* that he was having a heart attack. In order to start the process of determining which of these ideas was correct, the therapist focused on the patient's safety behaviors and inquired how distraction and taking paracetamol might stop a heart attack. On reflection, the patient agreed that neither procedure was likely to stop an actual heart attack but both would be good ways of distracting him from his negative thoughts and that this might be the reason they seem to help during an at-

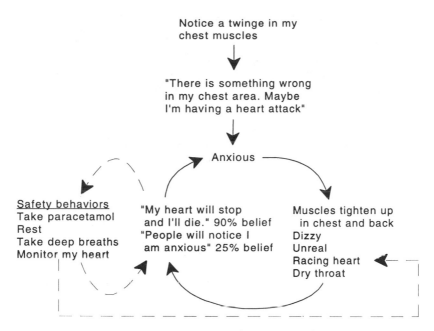

FIGURE 15.2. A specific panic attack.

tack. The patient was then encouraged to breathe the way he normally breathes during a panic attack. To his surprise, he found that the deep breathing he did to control his symptoms actually produced dizziness and a racing heart. A graph of Ehlers and Breuer's (1992) demonstration of enhanced cardiac awareness in panic disorder patients was then used to show that another of his safety behaviors (monitoring his heart) was probably causing some of the symptoms that he took as evidence for cardiac disease. By this stage the patient's belief that during a panic he might be having a heart attack had declined from 100% to 60%. It was agreed that one of the main things maintaining the belief was the patient's marked avoidance of exercise and the safety behaviors he engaged in during an attack. Both prevented him from discovering whether a feeling of breathlessness and chest pain would actually lead to a heart attack.

In view of this point, it was decided that the most helpful thing to do next would be to use exercise to produce marked cardiac sensations and then to not engage in any safety behaviors. The therapist and patient therefore alternated sprinting and jogging around a local football field. At the start of the exercise the patient had a 50% belief that he would have a heart attack. Midway through, when he was very out of breath, the belief had dropped to 35%; toward the end after he had managed to abandon all his safety behaviors the belief dropped to 5%.

Next the therapist and patient returned to the office and summarized the evidence for and against the alternative beliefs (see Table 15.1) and con-

TABLE 15.1. Evidence for the Two Alternative Explanations

"There is something seriously wrong with my heart"	"My problem is my belief that there is something wrong with my heart."
1. "I hear my heart thumping sometimes, even in my ear, *but* because of my fears I focus on my body and that makes me notice it. When I notice it I get anxious and that makes it louder because my heart beats are bigger."	1. "I think I am dying in a panic attack and that thought makes me anxious, producing many more sensations and setting up a vicious circle."
2. "I have chest and rib tightness throughout the day, *but* cardiac patients don't. They get chest pain (often crushing and more localized) during heart attacks. It is muscle tension due to work stress. It is mild after a good night's sleep and easier on weekends. It is worst after a stressful day at work."	2. "Distraction sometimes helps. That makes sense if the problem is my thoughts. It does not make sense if the problem is a heart attack. The same argument applies to leaving the situation. That would not stop a heart attack but it makes me feel more comfortable and undermines the negative thoughts."
3. "I occasionally get tingling in my fingertips, *but* this is a common symptom of anxiety. Also deep breathing—which I do when I *think* there is something wrong—causes tingling."	3. "I get symptoms most often at the end of the day, when I have come to expect them and have time to dwell on them."
	4. "I have proved to myself that there is nothing wrong with my heart with vigorous exercise. All that happens is that my heart beats faster and pumps harder, as it should do in order to supply my muscles with the energy they need."

solidated the cognitive model by reviewing a series of "out-of-the-blue" panic attacks, identifying the trigger for the mild sensation that invariably started these attacks, and then deriving a generic vicious circle that encompassed all of the patient's attacks (see Figure 15.3). Finally, the remaining evidence for the thought "I'll faint in a panic attack" was reviewed. The patient had never fainted during an attack and his main evidence that he might was the dizziness he experiences in attacks. The earlier exercise involving reproducing the way he breathes in an attack had demonstrated that his breathing pattern was partly responsible for the dizziness. The physiology of fainting was then discussed with the therapist explaining a blood pressure drop is necessary and that blood pressure increases in a panic attack. This final piece of information reduced the belief he might faint in a panic to 0%.

Homework involved listening to the audiotape of the therapy session and making notes, a daily exercise program, and instruction about how to change his behavior if he experienced another episode of chest pain, dizziness, and feelings of unreality. In order to demonstrate that this was not dangerous, he should avoid controlling his breathing, not distract himself, and stay in the situation. He mentioned that he often heard his heart beat-

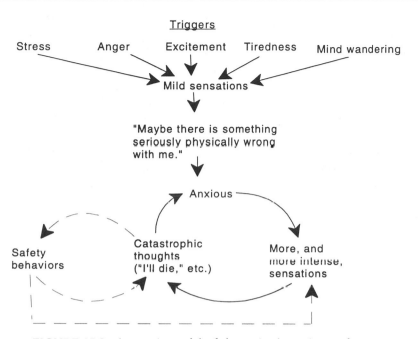

FIGURE 15.3. A generic model of the patient's panic attack.

ing in his ear while lying in bed. As he took this as evidence for cardiac abnormality, he was instructed to ask his wife whether she ever heard her heart when in a similar situation.

The second treatment session took place 3 weeks later. During the intervening period the patient had not had a full-blown attack but had had a small number of limited symptom attacks which he had used as an opportunity to drop safety behaviors and test out the consequences of the sensations. His belief that he might have a heart attack during a panic had dropped to 10% and his total belief score on a modified version of the Agoraphobic Cognitions Questionnaire was also 10%. The assignment to ask his wife about her sensations had helped as she reported often noticing her heart when lying quietly in bed. The main part of the session was devoted to identifying the patient's remaining evidence for his cardiac concern. He pointed out that he tends to notice chest tightness when he is ready to go to bed or during a quiet moment after a lot of stress at work (phones ringing, appointments, etc.). He had tended to see this as evidence that there might be something wrong with his heart because even activities involving reduced cardiac effort were associated with chest pain. However, questioning from the therapist helped him to see that the fact that his pain rarely occurred during exercise or stressful events, but instead occurred at quiet moments when he could focus on his body, was inconsistent with a cardiac abnormality but fitted the idea that stress at work made much of his upper body tense, but he only noticed this when able to rest and focus on his body. Following this discussion, his belief that he might have a heart attack during a panic declined to 0% and he experienced no further attacks.

CONTROLLED TRIALS EVALUATING THE EFFECTIVENESS OF COGNITIVE THERAPY

Five trials have investigated full cognitive therapy for panic disorder. Beck et al. (1992) allocated panic patients to 12 weeks of cognitive therapy or 8 weeks of supportive therapy. When assessed at comparable time points (4 and 8 weeks), patients given cognitive therapy had improved significantly more than those given supportive therapy, indicating that the effectiveness of cognitive therapy is not entirely attributable to nonspecific therapy factors. In addition, the gains achieved in treatment were maintained at the 1-year follow-up.

Clark et al. (1994) compared cognitive therapy with an alternative active psychological treatment and with a pharmacological intervention. Panic disorder patients were randomly allocated to cognitive therapy, applied relaxation, imipramine (mean 233 mg/day), or a 3-month wait followed by allocation to treatment. During treatment patients had up to 12 sessions in the first 3 months and up to three booster sessions in the next 3 months. Imipramine was gradually withdrawn after 6 months. All treatments included homework assignments involving self-exposure to feared situations. Comparisons with waiting list showed all three treatments were effective. Comparisons between treatments showed that at 3 months cognitive therapy was superior to both applied relaxation and imipramine. Between 3 and 6 months imipramine treated patients continued to improve while those who had received cognitive therapy or applied relaxation showed little change. As a consequence, at 6 months cognitive therapy did not differ from imipramine and both were superior to applied relaxation. Imipramine was gradually withdrawn after the 6-month assessment. Between 6 and 15 months, 40% of imipramine patients relapsed compared with only 5% of cognitive therapy patients. At 15 months cognitive therapy was again superior to both applied relaxation and imipramine.

Öst, the originator of applied relaxation, has also compared cognitive therapy and applied relaxation (Öst & Westling, 1995). Assessments were at pretreatment, posttreatment, and 1-year follow-up. Pretreatment to posttreatment comparisons indicated that cognitive therapy and applied relaxation were both associated with substantial improvements in panic frequency, panic-related distress/disability, and generalized anxiety. In the initial report (Öst & Westling, 1995) there were no significant differences between the treatments. However, L. G. Öst (personal communication, September 1995) has pointed out that each of the four therapist's initial training case in cognitive therapy had been included. Only 1 of 4 (25%) of the training cases became panic free but 13 of 15 (87%) of subsequent cognitive therapy cases became panic free and achieved high end-state function at the end of treatment. When the data were reanalyzed excluding the four cognitive therapy training cases, there is a significant difference between cognitive therapy and applied relaxation in terms of the percentage of patients achieving high end-state function at posttreatment: 13 of 15 (87%) for cognitive therapy versus 8 of 17 (47%) for applied relaxation. For both treatments the gains made during therapy were maintained at the 1-year follow-up.

Arntz and van den Hout (1996) have recently reported an independent evaluation of cognitive therapy and applied relaxation. Their group was not involved in the development of either treatment. Therapists were given specialist training in cognitive therapy from Clark and Salkovskis and specialist training in applied relaxation from Öst. Assessments were at pretreatment, posttreatment, and 1-month and 6-month follow-ups. A significantly greater proportion of cognitive therapy patients achieved panic-free status at the end of treatment and this difference was maintained at both follow-ups.

Finally, Margraf and Schneider (1991) conducted a component analysis of cognitive therapy. The full cognitive treatment (which combines cognitive and behavioral procedures) was compared with an intervention involving cognitive procedures alone and an intervention involving situational and interoceptive exposure without explicit cognitive restructuring. Comparison with a waiting-list control group indicated that all three treatments were highly effective. Most measures showed no significant differences, although combined treatment was superior to exposure on an intention-to-treat analysis of the percentage of patients who became panic free. In all three groups treatment gains were fully maintained at the 1-year follow-up. Change in panic-related cognitions was a significant predictor of immediate improvement in all three treatments, suggesting that the cognitive and behavioral procedures both have their effects through the common mechanism of cognitive change.

Table 15.2 summarizes the five trials reviewed above. In each trial the therapists were provided with some training from the Oxford group. Taken together, the five trials indicate that properly conducted cognitive therapy is a highly effective treatment for panic disorder, with intention-to-treat analyses indicating 74% to 94% of patients becoming panic free and these gains being maintained at follow-up. It is also clear that the effects of the treatment are not entirely due to nonspecific therapy factors, as three studies (Beck et al., 1992; Clark et al., 1994; Arntz & van den Hout, 1996) have found cognitive therapy to be superior to an equally credible alternative psychological treatment, and reanalysis of a fourth (Öst & Westling, 1995) suggests the same pattern of results. One study (Clark et al., 1994) compared cognitive therapy with imipramine in adequate dose. Cognitive therapy was superior to imipramine early in treatment and again at 1-year follow-up. Finally, the treatment seems to travel well as the results obtained with cog-

TABLE 15.2. Controlled Trials of (Full) Cognitive Therapy for Panic Disorder

Study	Treatments	Percentage (number) of panic-free patients	
		Posttreatment	Follow-up
Beck et al. (1992)	1. CT	94 (16/17)	77 (13/17)[b]
	2. ST	25 (4/16)[a]	—
Clark et al. (1994)	1. CT	86 (18/21)	76 (16/21)[c]
	2. AR	48 (10/21)	43 (9/21)[c]
	3. IMP	52 (11/21)	48 (10/21)[c]
	4. WL	7 (1/16)	—
Öst and	1. CT	74 (14/19)	89 (17/19)[c]
Westling (1995)[d]	2. AR	58 (11/19)	74 (14/19)[c]
Arntz and	1. CT	78 (14/18)	78 (14/18)
van den Hout	2. AR	47 (9/19)	47 (9/19)
(1996)	3. WL	28 (5/18)	—
Margraf and	1. Combined (CT)	91 (20/22)[e]	—
Schneider (1991)	2. Pure CT	73 (16/22)[e]	—
	3. Pure Exp	52 (11/21)[e]	—
	4. WL	5 (1/20)	—
Total across all studies for CT		85 (82/97)	80 (60/75)

Note. Intention-to-treat analysis includes dropouts as well as completers. Dropouts are coded as still panicking. CT, cognitive therapy; ST, supportive therapy; AR, applied relaxation; IMIP, imipramine; Exp, interoceptive and situational exposure; WL, waiting list.
[a]At 8 weeks, which is the end of supportive therapy. At this time 71% of CT patients were panic free.
[b]One-year follow-up.
[c]Percentage of patients panic free at follow-up and who received no additional treatment during the follow-up period.
[d]The figures for CT are conservative as they *include* the therapists' four training cases.
[e]Four-week follow-up.

nitive therapy are remarkably consistent across five countries (England, Germany, Netherlands, Sweden, and the United States).

The excellent results obtained with the full cognitive therapy package have encouraged researchers to investigate whether it might be possible to obtain similar results with a briefer form of the treatment. If so, more patients could potentially benefit from it. The studies of full treatment described above had a total of 12–16 sessions. The first group to report an evaluation of a briefer version was Black, Wesner, Bowers, and Gabel (1993). These investigators devised their own brief (eight-session) version of cognitive therapy which included additional psychological procedures specifically devised by the investigators (W. Bowers, personal communication, July 13, 1993). The Oxford group had no involvement in therapist training or in the modification of treatment content. Panic disorder patients were randomly allocated to brief cognitive therapy, fluvoxamine, or placebo medication. Main assessments were at pretreatment and 8 weeks later. No follow-up was reported. Response to fluvoxamine was superior to brief cognitive therapy on a number of measures in a completers analysis. However, the unusually high dropout rate (40%[2] for brief cognitive therapy compared to between 0% and 5% in the studies of full cognitive therapy reviewed above) suggests that the investigators' modifications severely interfered with treatment acceptability.

Clark, Salkovskis, Hackmann, Wells, and Gelder (1995) have recently reported a more successful attempt to produce a brief version of cognitive therapy. The total number of sessions was reduced to seven by devising a series of self-study modules covering the main stages in therapy. Patients read the self-study modules and completed the homework outlined in the modules before discussing an area with their therapist. In this way, the therapist was able to devote more attention to misunderstandings and problems. Panic disorder patients were randomly allocated to brief cognitive therapy, full cognitive therapy, or waiting list. Brief and full cognitive therapy were both superior to no treatment and did not differ from each other. In addition, the substantial improvement observed with both treatments was as large as that obtained in the Oxford group's previous trial (Clark et al., 1994), which used the same selection criteria.

Five studies have investigated the effectiveness of Barlow and colleagues' PCT and have established that it is also a highly effective treatment for panic disorder. Barlow, Craske, Cerny, and Klosko (1989) compared PCT with another cognitive treatment, with progressive muscle relaxation, and with a waiting-list control. Both cognitive treatments were consistently superior to waiting list and were more effective than relaxation at reducing panic frequency. Klosko, Barlow, Tassinari, and Cerny (1990) compared PCT with alprazolam, placebo, and a waiting-list control. PCT was superior to alprazolam,[3] placebo, and waiting list. The percentages of patients who became panic free on alprazolam and placebo were similar to the Cross-National Collaborative Panic Study (1992), but alprazolam was not significantly different from placebo, perhaps because of the very small sample size in the latter condition.

Shear, Pilkonis, Cloitre, and Leon (1994) compared PCT with a specially devised nonprescriptive treatment. PCT appeared to be slightly less successful than in the preceding two studies and did not differ significantly from nonprescriptive treatment. In discussing the study, Shear et al. (1994) point out that PCT may not have been delivered optimally as therapist adherence ratings were lower than expected. An additional possible explanation for a lack of difference between treatment is a design confound. The first three sessions in the nonprescriptive treatment were identical to those in PCT and may have accounted for much of the common outcome variance. Unfortunately, it is not possible to assess this suggestion as the investigators did not conduct an assessment after the third session.

Finally, Craske , Maidenberg, and Brystritsky (1995) investigated a brief (four-session) version of PCT. Panic disorder patients were randomly allocated to four sessions of PCT or four sessions of nondirective supportive therapy. Brief PCT was more effective than nondirective supportive therapy in reducing panic and phobic fear, suggesting that it has a specific effect. However, the overall panic-free rate at the end of treatment (53%) was relatively low, suggesting that a number of patients would have benefited from more treatment sessions.

CRITICISMS OF THE COGNITIVE THEORY

The 1986 exposition of the cognitive theory of panic (Clark, 1986) has attracted considerable attention, being listed by the Institute for Scientific Information as the world's second most highly cited psychology article for the period 1986 to 1990 (Garfield, 1992). It would be strange if a theory that has attracted so much attention had not also attracted some criticism. In this section I list, and hopefully rebut, the most cogent of the criticisms.

The Sequence of Events in a Panic Attack

Wolpe and Rowan (1988) reported the results of an interview covering the perceived sequence of events in a panic attack. We are not told the questions the 10 panic disorder patients were asked, but they generally reported that the first thing they noticed was a bodily sensation, next an increase in anxiety, and then a catastrophic thought about impending physical or mental harm to themselves. Wolpe and Rowan appear to believe this sequence of events is inconsistent with the cognitive theory, perhaps because they think the key cognition should come first. On the contrary, the 1986 paper made it clear that a bodily sensation can only be misinterpreted if it has been experienced. For this reason, the theory *predicts* that a bodily sensation would be one of the first things noticed in an attack. The observation that anxiety starts to increase before the key catastrophic thought occurs is also consistent with the model. Indeed the vicious circle in the original paper (Clark, 1986, Fig. 1, p. 463) shows this exact sequence. The specific examples of the vicious circle given above (Figures 15.2 and 15.3) make it clear why this happens.

A Conditioning Theory of Panic Disorder

Wolpe and Rowan (1988) point out that many individuals experience an occasional panic attack but do not develop full-blown panic disorder. They argue that the occasional attacks have a multitude of both physical and psychological causes, but that an individual only develops recurrent attacks (and hence panic disorder) if he or she conditions to the first attack. In particular, they propose that for these individuals the initial mild physical stimuli that precede the attack become conditioned stimuli with the attack itself being the unconditioned stimulus. For example, a patient who subsequently develops panic and agoraphobia might go into a store and feel very hot and dizzy, so much so that she thinks she might be fainting and sits down to prevent collapse. Prior to this peak of symptoms she is likely to have noticed milder symptoms, say, slight dizziness and speeding of the heart. In Wolpe and Rowan's account these initial symptoms become the conditioned stimulus (CS) with the final symptoms, which are construed by the patient as a collapse or near miss, being the unconditioned stimulus (US). McNally (1994) has pointed out that this account is problematic as conditioning refers to relationships between distinct stimuli, but in this account the bodily sensations linked to a panic episode appear to be CS, conditioned response (CR), US, and unconditioned response (UR), and it is not clear how you decide which is which. This is a serious problem. However, it may not matter because I wish to suggest that even if Wolpe and Rowan's account could be considered valid in conditioning terms, it is not an alternative to the cognitive account. Wolpe and Rowan argue their account is different because what is learned is different and that the learning, because it is based on conditioning, is impervious to pure cognitive interventions.

I would suggest they are mistaken on both counts. First, although traditional accounts of classical conditioning emphasized the importance of temporal contiguity between the CS and US, modern accounts (Davey, 1987; Rescorla, 1988) indicate that conditioning mainly only occurs if the CS tells the subject something new about the occurrence of the US. This leads to the view that what is learned during conditioning is a contingency of the form, if the CS occurs then the US will occur (with a given probability). If we apply this to the patient example above, we deduce that what the patient would have learned if she had conditioned à la Wolpe and Rowan is "a slight feeling of dizziness and speeded heart means I am in danger of collapsing." This is, of course, an example of a catastrophic misinterpretation of bodily sensations. Second, if we view this interpretation as the result of conditioning, there is no reason to suppose that it would be impervious to cognitive intervention. There are now numerous examples of the modification of CR strength by the provision of information or other "nonassociative" maneuvers (see Davey, 1987). Third, the experiments by Rapee et al. (1986), Sanderson et al. (1989), and Clark, Salkovskis, Anastasiades, et al. (1996) discussed above clearly demonstrate that panic can be reduced by information alone.

Noncognitive Panics?

Rachman, Levitt, and Lopatka (1987) asked a group of 20 panic disorder patients to complete three to five behavior tests. At the completion of each test they completed the DSM-III-R checklist of panic symptoms and a panic cognition checklist. Fourteen patients reported at least one "panic or near miss" and two of these failed to endorse any of the thoughts on the cognition checklist when thinking about the panic afterwards. It has been suggested that these failures of report indicate that the cognitive theory may not apply to all panic disorder patients, or at least not to all of their attacks. While this is a possible interpretation of the data, I do not think it is a compelling argument. First, the checklist omitted two key catastrophic thoughts: "I'm dying" and "I'm going mad." Second, other analyses indicated that the noncognitive panics were milder than the cognitive panics in the sense that they were accompanied by less physical symptoms. Indeed, as "near misses" also appear to have been included as panics, it is not clear that any of the noncognitive panics were full-blown attacks. Third, the checklist was filled in after the event and it is possible patients simply forgot some of their thoughts. This would not be surprising, especially as the relevant episodes were relatively mild and hence the cognitive theory would suppose the thoughts were transient and not strongly believed.

Although the Rachman et al. (1987) data are not compelling evidence for the existence of panic patients whose attacks are not based on misinterpretation of bodily sensations, one should specify how one would recognize such individuals if they do exist. It would be necessary to give any candidates the well-established measures of panic cognition and show that they are negative on all of them. This would help get around the problem of measurement error associated with individual indices. Well-validated self-report measures include the Agoraphobic Cognitions Questionnaire (Chambless et al., 1984) and the Body Sensations Interpretation Questionnaire (Clark, Salkovskis, Öst, et al., 1996). Clark (1988, p.76) pointed out that in some patients who have experienced repeated attacks the "catastrophic misinterpretations may be so fast and automatic that patients may not always be aware of them." Given this possibility, one might recommend that the researcher consider also using some of the priming tasks (Clark et al., 1988; Cloitre, Shear, Cancienne, & Zeitlin, 1994) that have been shown to distinguish panic patients from controls.

Nocturnal Panic

Some patients who experience frequent daytime panic attacks also report being woken from sleep, apparently in the midst of a panic attack. Klein and Klein (1989, p. 186) argue that the existence of nocturnal panic is inconsistent with the cognitive theory. However, a year earlier Clark (1988, p. 75) explicitly addressed this issue and explained how the cognitive theory deals with such attacks. To quote:

> Sleep studies (Oswald, 1966) have shown that we monitor the external world for personally significant sounds while asleep and tend to have our sleep disturbed or woken by such sounds. It seems reasonable to suppose that we also monitor our *internal* environment for significant events. If this is the case, then an individual who is concerned about his or her heart might have a panic at

tack triggered by a palpitation which is detected and misinterpreted during sleep. He or she would then wake up in a state of panic.

Mellman and Uhde (1989) and Hauri, Friedman, and Ravaris (1989) recorded a total of 14 nocturnal panics in the sleep laboratory. None were associated with rapid-eye-movement (REM) sleep, indicating that patients were not dreaming. This point has also been viewed by Klein and Klein (1989) as contrary to the cognitive account. However, it is in fact the pattern of results that one would expect on the basis of cognitive theory. This is because patients will only misinterpret bodily sensations if they don't have available at that moment a compelling alternative explanation for the sensations. A dream would often provide such an explanation. For example, "My heart is racing because I am being chased through Trafalgar Square by a tiger." The point that patients only misinterpret bodily sensations if they do not have available an alternative explanation which *they can believe* also explains the common clinical observation that panic patients often do not panic in genuinely stressful situations such as a job interview (see Clark, 1988, p. 78).[4]

Limited Symptom Attacks

Klein and Klein[5] (1989, pp. 185–186) erroneously infer that cognitive theory implies that all attacks should be full blown. Their argument seems to be based on the assumption that negative thoughts will always be held with complete conviction. However, negative thoughts are no different from other thoughts; at different times and in different contexts they are believed with widely different degrees of conviction and can be easy or remarkably difficult to dismiss. Limited symptom attacks occur in contexts where any misinterpretations of bodily sensations that are triggered are only modestly believed and easy to dismiss. A large number of variables, some of which are biological (see Clark, 1988, p. 85), influence believability and ease of dismissal.[6]

SUMMARY AND CONCLUSIONS

Over the last 15 years the Beckian approach to psychopathology has been applied to the understanding and treatment of panic disorder. A cognitive model of panic disorder consistent with the main clinical features of the condition has been developed. Experimental investigations have supported the proposed role of misinterpretations of bodily sensations in the production of panic attacks and have provided support for the two main processes which are said to maintain misinterpretations in the absence of treatment. A specialized form of cognitive therapy has been developed to modify patients' misinterpretations of bodily sensations. Controlled trials indicate that this specialized form of cognitive therapy is a specific, and highly effective, treatment for panic disorder.

ACKNOWLEDGMENTS

David M. Clark is a Wellcome Trust Principal Research Fellow. The research described in this chapter was supported by grants from the Medical Research Council of the United Kingdom, The Wellcome Trust, and the North Atlantic Treaty Organization.

NOTES

1. In contrast to the positive findings obtained by McNally and Foa (1987), Harvey et al. (1993), and Clark et al. (1996), Ahmad, Wardle, and Hayward (1992) failed to find evidence for an enhanced tendency to misinterpret bodily sensations in patients with panic and agoraphobia. Ahmad et al. (1992) used their own Health Knowledge Questionnaire to assess individuals' predictions of illness in relation to symptoms that could be experienced during anxiety episodes. Agoraphobic patients' responses did not differ from those of nonpatient controls. Inspection of Ahmad et al.'s items reveals an obvious explanation for this negative finding. The cognitive theory specifies that panic attacks result from patients' tendency to interpret their *own* symptoms as signs that they are about to die, go mad, lose control, and so forth. However, none of Ahmad et al.'s items were self-referent. Unlike the Interpretations Questionnaire, the Health Knowledge Questionnaire did not ask patients about their interpretations of their own symptoms. Instead, it asked them about their interpretations of *someone else's* symptoms, an issue not relevant to the cognitive theory of panic disorder.

2. The dropout rate reported here is slightly higher (40% vs. 36%) than that given in the original paper, which contains a typographic error (D. W. Black, personal communication, October 5, 1994).

3. In the original paper, the authors did not report that PCT was superior to alprazolam, however in a subsequent correction (Barlow & Brown, 1995) they point out that significantly more patients achieved panic-free status with PCT than with alprazolam.

4. Craske and Freed (1995) have recently reported a study that appears to provide experimental support for a cognitive account of nocturnal panic.

5. Klein and Klein (1989) outline several other criticisms not reproduced here as they have already been rebutted by McNally (1994).

6. Although an obvious point to most cognitive theorists, it is perhaps worth mentioning that the cognitive theory of panic, like almost all cognitive theories of emotional disorders, is concerned with idiosyncratic meaning. That is to say, a catastrophic interpretation of a bodily sensation will only produce a panic attack if that individual views the predicted outcome as personally catastrophic. For example, an elderly person who is severely handicapped after suffering many strokes and who welcomes the prospect of death is unlikely to panic in response chest pain, breathlessness, and the thought "I'm having a heart attack."

REFERENCES

Ahmad, T., Wardle, J., & Hayward, P. (1992). Physical symptoms and illness attributions in agoraphobia and panic. *Behaviour Research and Therapy, 30,* 493–500.

American Psychiatric Association. (1980). *Diagnostic and statistical manual of mental disorders* (3rd ed.). Washington, DC: Author.

American Psychiatric Association. (1987). *Diagnostic and statistical manual of mental disorders* (3rd ed., rev.). Washington, DC: Author.

American Psychiatric Association. (1994). *Diagnostic and statistical manual of mental disorders* (4th ed.). Washington, DC: Author.

Arntz, A., & van den Hout, M. (1996). Psychological treatments of panic disorder without agoraphobia: Cognitive therapy versus applied relaxation. *Behaviour Research and Therapy, 34,* 113–121.

Barlow, D. H., & Brown, T. A. (1995). Correction to Klosko et al. (1990). *Journal of Consulting and Clinical Psychology, 63,* 830.

Barlow, D. H., & Cerny, J. A. (1988). *Psychological treatment of panic.* New York: Guilford Press.

Barlow, D. H., & Craske, M. G. (1989). *Mastery of your anxiety and panic.* Albany, NY: Graywind.

Barlow, D. H., Craske, M. G., Cerny, J. A., & Klosko, J. S. (1989). Behavioral treatment of panic disorder. *Behavior Therapy, 20,* 261–282.

Barlow, D. H., Vermilyea, J., Blanchard, E. B., Vermilyea, B. B., Di Nardo, P. A., & Cerny, J. A. (1985). The phenomenon of panic. *Journal of Abnormal Psychology, 94,* 320–328.

Beck, A. T. (1967). *Depression: Clinical, experimental and theoretical aspects.* New York: Hoeber.

Beck, A. T., Emery, G., & Greenberg, R. L. (1985). *Anxiety disorders and phobias.* New York: Basic Books.

Beck, A. T., Rush, A. J., Shaw, B. F., & Emery, G. (1979). *Cognitive therapy of depression.* New York: Guilford Press.

Beck, A. T., Sokol, L., Clark, D. A., Berchick, B., & Wright, F. (1992). Focused cognitive therapy of panic disorder: A crossover design and one year follow-up. *American Journal of Psychiatry, 147,* 778–783.

Black, D. W., Wesner, R., Bowers, W., & Gabel, J. (1993). A comparison of fluvoxamine, cognitive therapy, and placebo in the treatment of panic disorder. *Archives of General Psychiatry, 50,* 44–50.

Brown, T. A., & Cash, T. F. (1990). The phenomenon of non-clinical panic: Parameters of panic, fear, and avoidance. *Journal of Anxiety Disorders, 4,* 15–29.

Butler, G., & Mathews, A. (1983). Cognitive processes in anxiety. *Advances in Behaviour Research and Therapy, 5,* 51–62.

Chambless, D. L., Caputo, G. C., Bright, P., & Gallagher, R. (1984). Assessment of fear of fear in agoraphobics: The Body Sensations Questionnaire and the Agoraphobic Cognitions Questionnaire. *Journal of Consulting and Clinical Psychology, 52,* 1090–1097.

Clark, D. M. (1986). A cognitive approach to panic. *Behaviour Research and Therapy, 24,* 461–470.

Clark, D. M. (1988). A cognitive model of panic. In S. Rachman & J. Maser (Eds.), *Panic: Psychological perspectives.* Hillsdale: Erlbaum.

Clark, D. M. (1989). Anxiety states: Panic and generalized anxiety. In K. Hawton, P. Salkovskis, J. Kirk, & D. M. Clark (Eds.), *Cognitive behaviour therapy for psychiatric problems: A practical guide.* Oxford, UK: Oxford University Press.

Clark, D. M. (1993). Cognitive mediation of panic attacks induced by biological challenge tests. *Advances in Behaviour Research and Therapy, 15,* 75–84.

Clark, D. M., Salkovskis, P. M., Anastasiades, P., Middleton, H., & Gelder, M. G. (1996). *Cognitive mediation of sodium lactate induced panic attacks.* Manuscript in preparation.

Clark, D. M., Salkovskis, P. M., Gelder, M., Koehler, C., Martin, M., Anastasiades, P., Hachmann, A., Middleton, H., & Jeavons, A. (1988). Tests of a cognitive theory of panic. In I. Hand & H. U. Wittchen (Eds.), *Panic and phobias 2*. Berlin: Springer-Verlag.

Clark, D. M., Salkovskis, P. M., Hackmann, A., Middleton, H., Anastasiades, P., & Gelder, M. (1994). A comparison of cognitive therapy, applied relaxation and imipramine in the treatment of panic disorder. *British Journal of Psychiatry, 164,* 759–769.

Clark, D. M., Salkovskis, P. M., Hackmann, A., Wells, A., & Gelder, M. G. (1995, July 10–15). *A comparison of standard and brief cognitive therapy for panic disorder*. Paper presented at the World Congress of Behavioural and Cognitive Therapies. Copenhagen, Denmark.

Clark, D. M., Salkovskis, P. M., Öst, L. G., Breitholz, E., Koehler, K. A., Westling, B., Jeavons, A., & Gelder, M. G. (1996). *Misinterpretation of body sensations in panic disorder*. Manuscript submitted for publication.

Cloitre, M., Shear, M. K., Cancienne, J., & Zeitlin, S. B. (1994). Implicit and explicit memory for catastrophic associations to bodily sensation words in panic disorder. *Cognitive Therapy and Research, 18,* 225–240.

Craske, M. G., & Freed, S. (1995). Expectations about arousal and nocturnal panic. *Journal of Abnormal Psychology, 104,* 567–575.

Craske, M. G., Maidenberg, E., & Brystritsky, A. (1995). Brief cognitive-behavioral versus nondirective therapy for panic disorder. *Journal of Behavior Therapy and Experimental Psychiatry, 26,* 113–120.

Cross-National Collaborative Panic Study, Second Phase Investigators. (1992). Drug treatment of panic disorder: Comparative efficacy of alprazolam, imipramine and placebo. *British Journal of Psychiatry, 160,* 191–202.

Davey, G. C. L. (1987). An integration of human and animal models of Pavlovian conditioning: associations, cognitions and attributions. In G. Davey (Ed.), *Cognitive processes and Pavlovian conditioning in humans*. Chichester, UK: Wiley.

Ehlers, A. (1993). Somatic symptoms and panic attacks: A retrospective study of learning experiences. *Behaviour Research and Therapy, 31,* 269–278.

Ehlers, A. (1995). A one-year prospective study of panic attacks: Clinical course and factors associated with maintenance. *Journal of Abnormal Psychology, 104,* 164–172.

Ehlers, A., & Brever, P. (1992). Increased cardiac awareness in panic disorder. *Journal of Abnormal Psychology, 101,* 371–382.

Ehlers, A., & Margraf, J. (1989). The psychophysiological model of panic attacks. In P. M. G. Emmelkamp, W. T. A. M. Everaerd, F. Kraaimaat, & M. J. M. van Son (Eds.), *Fresh perspectives on anxiety disorders*. Amsterdam: Swets & Zeitlinger.

Ehlers, A., Margraf, J., Roth, W. T., Taylor, C. B., & Birbaumer, N. (1988). Anxiety produced by false heart rate feedback in patients with panic disorder. *Behaviour Research and Therapy, 26,* 1–11.

Garfield, E. (1992). A citationist perspective on psychology. Part 1: Most-cited papers, 1986–1990. *APS Observer, 5*(6), 8–9.

Hammen, C. (1988). Depression and cognitions about personal stressful life events. In L. B. Alloy (Ed.), *Cognitive processes in depression*. New York: Guilford Press.

Harvey, J. M., Richards, J. C., Dziadosz, T., & Swindell, A. (1993). Misinterpretation of ambiguous stimuli in panic disorder. *Cognitive Therapy and Research, 17,* 235–248.

Hauri, P. J., Friedman, M., & Ravaris, C. L. (1989). Sleep in patients with spontaneous panic attacks. *Sleep, 12,* 323–337.

Hollon, S. D., & Beck, A. T. (1994). Cognitive and behavior therapies. In A. E. Bergin & S. L. Garfield (Eds.), *Handbook of psychotherapy and behavior change.* New York: Wiley.

Klein, D. F., & Klein, H. M. (1989). The nosology, genetics, and theory of spontaneous panic and phobia. In P. Tyrer (Ed.), *Psychopharmacology of anxiety.* New York: Oxford University Press.

Klosko, J. S., Barlow, D. H., Tassinari, R., & Cerny, J. A. (1990). A comparison of alprazolam and behavior therapy in the treatment of panic disorder. *Journal of Consulting and Clinical Psychology, 58,* 77–84.

Margraf, J., & Ehlers, A. (1988). Panic attacks in non-clinical subjects. In I. Hand & H. U. Wittchen (Eds.), *Panic and phobias 2.* Berlin: Springer-Verlag.

Margraf, J., Ehlers, A., & Roth, W. T. (1986). Biological models of panic disorder and agoraphobia: A review. *Behaviour Research and Therapy, 24,* 553–567.

Margraf, J., & Schneider, S. (1991, November 26). *Outcome and active ingredients of cognitive-behavioral treatments for panic disorder.* Paper presented at the Annual Conference of the Association for Advancement of Behavior Therapy, New York.

McNally, R. J., & Foa, E. B. (1987). Cognition and agoraphobia: Bias in the interpretation of threat. *Cognitive Therapy and Research, 11,* 567–581.

McNally. R. J. (1994). *Panic disorder: A critical analysis.* New York: Guilford Press.

Mellman, T. A., & Uhde, T. W. (1989). Electroencephalographic sleep in panic disorder: A focus on sleep-related panic attacks. *Archives of General Psychiatry, 46,* 178–184.

Norton, G. R., Dorward, J., & Cox, B. J. (1986). Factors associated with panic attacks in nonclinical subjects. *Behavior Therapy, 17,* 239–252.

Öst, L. G., & Westling, B. (1995). Applied relaxation vs. cognitive therapy in the treatment of panic disorder. *Behaviour Research and Therapy, 33,* 145–158.

Oswald, I. (1966). *Sleep.* Harmondsworth, UK: Penguin.

Rachman, S., Levitt, K., & Lopatka, C. (1987). Panic: The links between cognitions and bodily sensations—I. *Behaviour Research and Therapy, 25,* 411–424.

Rapee, R., Mattick, R., & Murrell, E. (1986). Cognitive mediation in the affective component of spontaneous panic attacks. *Journal of Behavior Therapy and Experimental Psychiatry, 17,* 245–253.

Rescorla, R. A. (1988). Pavlovian conditioning: It's not what you think it is. *American Psychologist, 43,* 151–160.

Rush, A. J., Beck, A. T., Kovacs, M., & Hollon, S. D. (1977). Comparative efficacy of cognitive therapy and pharmacotherpy in the treatment of depressed outpatients. *Cognitive Therapy and Research, 1,* 17–37.

Salkovskis, P. M. (1988). Phenomenology, assessment and the cognitive model of panic. In S. Rachman & J. Mascr (Eds.), *Panic: Psychological perspectives.* Hillsdale, NJ: Erlbaum.

Salkovskis, P. M. (1991). The importance of behaviour in the maintenance of anxiety and panic: A cognitive account. *Behavioural Psychotherapy, 19,* 6–19.

Salkovskis, P. M. (1995, July 10–15). *Cognitive approaches to health anxiety and obsessional problems: Some unique features and how this affects treatment.* Paper presented at the World Congress of Behavioural and Cognitive Therapies, Copenhagen, Denmark.

Salkovskis, P. M., & Clark, D. M. (1991). Cognitive therapy for panic disorder. *Journal of Cognitive Psychotherapy, 5,* 215–226.

Salkovskis, P. M., Clark, D. M., & Gelder, M. G. (1996). Cognition–behaviour links in the persistence of panic. *Behaviour Research and Therapy, 34,* 453–458.

Sanderson, W. C., Rapee, R. M., & Barlow, D. H. (1989). The influence of an illusion of control on panic attacks induced via inhalation of 5.5% carbon dioxide enriched air. *Archives of General Psychiatry, 46,* 157–162.

Seligman, M. E. P. (1988). Competing theories of panic. In S. Rachman & J. D. Maser (Eds.), *Panic: Psychological perspectives.* Hillsdale, NJ: Erlbaum.

Shear, M. K., Pilkonis, P. A., Cloitre, M., & Leon, A. C. (1994). Cognitive behavioural treatment compared with non-prescriptive treatment of panic disorder. *Archives of General Psychiatry, 51,* 395–401.

Teasdale, J. D. (1983). Negative thinking in depression: Cause, effect, or reciprocal relationship? *Advances in Behaviour Research and Therapy, 5,* 3–26.

Teasdale, J. D. (1988). Cognitive models and treatments for panic: A critical evaluation. In S. Rachman & J. D. Maser (Eds.), *Panic: Psychological perspectives.* Hillsdale, NJ: Erlbaum.

Wilson, K. G., Sandler, L. S., Asmundson, G. H. G., Derrick, K., Larsen, B. A., & Ediger, J. M. (1991). Effects of instructional sets on self-reports of panic attacks. *Journal of Anxiety Disorders, 5,* 43–63.

Wittchen, H. U., & Essau, C. A. (1991). The epidemiology of panic attacks, panic disorder and agoraphobia. In J. R. Walker, G. R. Norton, & C. A. Ross (Eds.), *Panic disorder and agoraphobia.* Monterey, CA: Brooks/Cole.

Wolpe, J., & Rowan, V. C. (1988). Panic disorder: A product of classical conditioning. *Behaviour Research and Therapy, 26,* 441–450.

Chapter 16

Cognitive Approaches to the Psychopathology and Treatment of Social Phobia

Dianne L. Chambless
Debra A. Hope

Social phobia is characterized by the desire to perform well in situations involving interaction with or observation by others, coupled with the fear that one will fail and, as a result, will meet with embarrassment, rejection, or negative evaluation. Under this general label, there are meaningful subtypes. The *Diagnostic and Statistical Manual of Mental Disorders,* third edition, revised (DSM-III-R; American Psychiatric Association, 1987) recognizes two: specific social phobia which concerns fear of a discrete phobic situation such as public speaking or eating in public, and generalized social phobia, the fear of most social interactions. These subtypes are not arcane distinctions. A growing body of research (e.g., Heimberg, Hope, Dodge, & Becker, 1990) indicates that people with generalized social phobia are more disabled by their disorder, more likely to be depressed, and have a poorer treatment outcome (e.g., Brown, Heimberg, & Juster, 1995; Chambless, Glass, & Tran, 1993).

Social phobia, especially the generalized type, is often complicated by comorbid Axis I disorders, most frequently other anxiety disorders and dysthymia, but also alcoholism (Feske, Perry, Chambless, Renneberg, & Goldstein, in press; Schneier, Johnson, Hornig, Liebowitz, & Weissman, 1992). The most common comorbid disorder is avoidant personality disorder (e.g., Feske et al., in press). Indeed, the overlap between generalized social phobia and avoidant personality is so great that a number of authors have questioned whether they can be meaningfully distinguished and have suggested that avoidant personality is but the extreme end of generalized social phobia (e.g., Herbert, Hope, & Bellack, 1992). Overall this research indicates that social phobics with avoidant personality have the most severe social anxiety and are also most likely to be depressed (e.g., Tran & Chambless, 1995);

345

there is also some evidence that their treatment outcome is less favorable (e.g., Feske et al., in press; but see Brown et al., 1995; Hope, Herbert, & White, 1995).

Social phobia is a prevalent disorder. Estimates from the Epidemiologic Catchment Area Study (a randomized sample of four U.S. cities) are that 2.4% of the U.S. population meet diagnostic criteria at some point in their lives, although few get treatment (Schneier et al., 1992). Social phobia develops early on. Many report lifelong problems, whereas for others the onset is in adolescence (Schneier et al., 1992). Given the marked distress and disability associated with social phobia (see Turner & Beidel, 1989), especially the generalized form, it is surprising that research in this anxiety disorder has only burgeoned of late.

In the remainder of this chapter we will review the literature on the cognitive psychopathology of social phobia and its treatment by cognitive-behavioral therapy. Social anxiety is prevalent among patients with a variety of psychiatric disorders other than social phobia (e.g., schizophrenia). To ensure that studies included in our review concerned social phobia itself, we limited our scope to those investigations using DSM-III or DSM-III-R criteria for a diagnosis of social phobia and those in which, by the description of the sample, it seemed clear that DSM criteria would have been met had they been in use.

COGNITIVE THEORY OF SOCIAL PHOBIA

Beck and Emery (1985) propose that the core of social phobia is the fear of having one's inadequacies exposed in front of others, of being shamed. Alert for danger, socially phobic people are hypersensitive to the possibility of evaluation and thus form a vigilant cognitive set for rejection. Their sense of vulnerability is further increased by doubts that they have sufficient skills to win the approval of others, rigid rules they construct about social behavior, and exaggerations about the consequences of failure. Beck and Emery suggest that, feeling vulnerable to the threat of failure in front of evaluators, socially phobic people may freeze or go blank (a reflex inhibitory action) or experience high autonomic arousal. Paradoxically, these responses increase the likelihood that one's performance will actually be inadequate and create a vicious circle. Finally, they may avoid social situations to minimize the likelihood of evaluation and rejection, thus depriving themselves of the opportunity to test the validity of their beliefs. How well does this model fit with current research on the psychopathology of social phobia? The remainder of this section will be devoted to research addressing this question.

Tests of the cognitive theory of social phobia have been conducted following a number of methodological approaches. Researchers have examined the *content* of social phobics' thoughts as well as their *cognitive processes*.

Findings from research on processes (e.g., attention, memory) are presumed to reflect the operation of schemas, cognitive structures that are hypothesized to direct and organize these processes.

Thought Content

Self-Statements and Probability Estimates

Studies on the content of social phobics' cognitions consistently show the negative orientation of their thinking and their distorted self-perceptions. For example, using a modified version of the Social Interaction Self-Statement Test (SISST; Glass, Merluzzi, Biever, & Larsen, 1982), Dodge, Hope, Heimberg, and Becker (1988) asked 28 social phobics to rate the frequency with which they had positive and negative thoughts about social interactions with the opposite sex. Subjects who reported a higher rate of negative thoughts were more severely phobic on self-report and clinicians' ratings of severity. Using the SISST administered after role plays and collecting thoughts specific to those interactions (the standard method for this scale), Turner, Beidel, and Larkin (1986) found social phobics and nonclinical socially anxious subjects both reported a higher rate of negative thinking and a lower rate of positive thinking after social interactions and a speech than did subjects without social anxiety.

Stopa and Clark (1993) asked 12 social phobics to engage in a conversation with a confederate and later to imagine several interactions. After each real or imagined interaction, they were asked to report the thoughts they had during the interactions, to "think aloud." These thoughts were later categorized by judges. In addition, subjects completed a thought questionnaire about social situations and endorsed thoughts that were common for them as well as the degree to which they believed these thoughts. Responses of social phobics were compared to those of 12 clients with other anxiety disorders, and 12 nonclinical subjects. Social phobics reported more negative thoughts during think aloud periods and on the questionnaire than did the control subjects. Moreover, they indicated they believed these thoughts more than nonclinical subjects. Somewhat surprisingly, social phobics' thoughts after the conversation with the confederate were distinguished by their focus on negative *self*-evaluation, whereas one might have expected their thoughts to center more on negative evaluation from the confederate. This finding is consistent with research by Strauman (1989) who determined that social phobics, compared to those with major depressive disorder, were particularly characterized by a discrepancy between the way they perceived themselves to be and the way they thought they ought to be, which Strauman terms the actual/ought discrepancy. Thus, in social interaction, social phobics' thoughts may be dominated by their perceived failure to achieve what they themselves believe to be acceptable standards of behavior.

Heimberg, Bruch, Hope, and Dombeck (1990) studied 49 social phobics' thoughts in the context of Schwartz and Garamoni's (1989) States of Mind (SOM) theory. According to SOM theory, healthy thinking is demonstrated by a proportion of Positive:Positive + Negative thoughts equaling .618 (range of .56–.68). Schwartz and Garamoni suggest that exclusively positive thinking is not realistic and that preponderantly negative thinking is dysfunctional. Categorizing social phobics' written thoughts after an individualized behavioral challenge test (e.g., a conversation with a confederate or a brief speech), Heimberg, Bruch, et al. (1990) found an average SOM ratio of .28, which Schwartz and Garamoni consider extremely negative. Chambless et al. (1993) reported a less negative average ratio of .50 derived from the SISST, a self-report questionnaire of thoughts completed by 53 social phobics after each of three standardized behavioral challenges. According to Schwartz and Garamoni, this score represents an internal dialogue of conflict characterized by indecision and doubt and typical of mildly anxious people. This categorization conflicts with the clinical nature of the sample but may result from averaging SOMs across several situations, not all of which may have been particularly pertinent to a given client. In contrast, Heimberg et al. collected their data after an individually designed challenge.

Finally, Lucock and Salkovskis (1988) have shown that social phobics not only have negative thoughts about interactions that have just taken place, but they also hold negative expectations for the future. Compared to nonclinical controls, 12 social phobics given a questionnaire about the subjective probability of positive and negative events rated negative social events, but not other negative events, as being more probable and positive events of all types as being less probable.

Self-Perceptions

The research reviewed so far indicates that social phobics' thinking is highly negative, which is consistent with cognitive theory. It does not, however, show that their thinking is distorted, which would require that it be not only negative but also erroneous. If social phobics are as inept as they think, then their perceptions might be distressing, but accurate. The results of several studies bear on this question; the findings are mixed. Tran and Chambless (1995) had 44 social phobics (27 with generalized social phobia) participate in social interaction role plays with a confederate and deliver a brief speech. Both clients and observers rated clients' skill after each role play. Following the conversations clients were significantly more critical about their performances than were the observers, regardless of subtype. No differences were observed on the speech ratings. These data provide some support for the notion that social phobics are needlessly hard on themselves, but it is possible that people in general are more critical of their own performance than observers are. The remaining two studies to be reviewed address this question.

Stopa and Clark (1993) had both subjects and observers rate subjects' performance during a conversation with a confederate. Observers did rate social phobics more negatively than anxious and nonclinical controls, but the social phobics rated themselves even more negatively than observers did. This discrepancy was significantly larger than that for the controls. Rapee and Lim (1992) asked social phobics and nonclinical controls to give a brief public speech. They rated themselves after their own speeches and also rated other subjects after those persons spoke. Both social phobics and observers rated the phobics more negatively than nonclinical subjects on specific speech behaviors (e.g., clear voice). Global ratings (e.g., generally spoke well) revealed a different pattern. Here observers gave the two groups equivalent ratings, but social phobics rated themselves more harshly than did nonclinical subjects.

Overall these data suggest that social phobics are partly right. In a highly anxiety-provoking situation, their performance suffers in comparison to people without social anxiety. Whether this is actually a skill deficit or reflects disruption from anxiety cannot be determined by these data. On the other hand, these findings also indicate that social phobics are unduly pessimistic where their own performance is concerned, in that they rate themselves even more negatively than others do. Interestingly, Rapee and Lim (1992) found social phobics were not pancritical; their overly harsh criticism was reserved for themselves and did not extend to their ratings of the performance of others.

Cognitive Processes

Data based on self-report questionnaires are open to the criticism that clients' responses may be biased. For example, clients' reports of high levels of negative thoughts in social situations might reflect nothing more than their attempt to explain to the experimenters, clinicians, or themselves why they are anxious. Moreover, important aspects of schema operations are not accessible to introspection or self-report. Accordingly, it is important to add to the wealth of self-report data with information collected via other paradigms. Research on cognitive processes provides this additional perspective.

Being hypothetical constructs, schemas are not observable. Researchers who examine cognitive operations attempt to indirectly establish that social phobics have a schema for social threat by borrowing the laboratory methodology of experimental cognitive psychologists. They examine processes such as attention and memory that are hypothesized to be affected by schema operations.

Reaction Time

One of the most common paradigms in current use for research on anxiety disorders is a modification of the Stroop color-naming task. The original

Stroop task requires subjects to label aloud the ink colors of words presented to them while ignoring the words themselves. This is somewhat tricky because the words are the names of colors other than the ink used for that particular word. Thus, for example, the subject is charged with saying "red" when presented with the word *blue,* written in red ink. This task reliably proves to be more difficult than color-naming a string of XXXs of the same size in that subjects' reaction time in providing the correct response is slower. Modified for research on anxiety, the task involves color-naming words thought to represent the clinical subjects' anxiety schema (e.g., *humiliation* for a social phobic). Subjects' response time to schema-relevant words is then compared to response time to a set of neutral words matched for length and frequency of use in the language or to a set of schema-irrelevant threat words (e.g., those drawn from the concerns of another anxious group). Slowed reaction time has been interpreted as evidence of schema-driven effects on perception, as researchers reason that attentional resources are attracted by the schema-congruent words, thereby distracting the subject from the color-naming task. Thus, this task may be construed as a laboratory analogue of the vigilance for social threat which, according to Beck and Emery (1985), is characteristic of social phobics.

Stroop responses have been examined in three samples of socially phobic clients. Hope, Rapee, Heimberg, and Dombeck (1990) compared responses of 16 people with social phobia and 15 with panic disorder. As hypothesized, people with social phobia took longer to color-name words associated with social failure (e.g., *stupid, failure*) than neutral words. The panic control group did not (although they did respond more slowly to panic-related threat words). Socially phobic clients did not respond more slowly to words related to panic schemas (e.g., *insane, deadly*). These data suggest that, for people with social phobia, attentional deployment is driven by very specific concerns having to do with negative evaluation and inadequacy and not by anxious concerns in general. Moreover, they support Beck and Emery's (1985) general thesis that anxiety patients with different disorders are guided by different and predictable schemas. These basic findings were replicated in the same laboratory by Mattia, Heimberg, and Hope (1993) who compared 28 social phobics' responses to social threat, panic threat, and neutral control words with responses of 47 nonclinical volunteers. Once again social phobics were distinguished by their especially slow reaction time to social threat words. Finally, McNeil et al. (1995) demonstrated that clients with different subtypes of social phobia can be distinguished by their response to Stroop threat words. Those with generalized social phobia responded more to general social phobia threat words than clients with public speaking phobia alone. The subtype groups were equivalent in their response to threat words concerning public speaking and concerning negative social evaluation, highlighting the importance of anticipated negative evaluation in the psychopathology of social phobia.

Based on data derived from a different reaction time paradigm, Cloitre,

Heimberg, Holt, and Liebowitz (1992) proffered another explanation for reaction time data that may also be extended to Stroop research findings. These authors presented social phobics with two tasks requiring responses to lists of words—social threat, positive (e.g., *delighted*), and neutral. In the first task, clients made lexical decisions in response to each word (i.e., Is this a word?) In the second task, they made semantic decisions (Is this a feeling word?). The latter task is believed to require deeper cognitive processing. In both cases the dependent variable was reaction time, and in both cases social phobics, but not normal control subjects, responded more slowly to social threat words than to positive or neutral words. Cloitre et al. (1992) suggest that these data may reflect the phobic subjects' freezing in response to threatening stimuli, resulting in performance decrements on tasks where speed is the criterion. This interpretation might also be extended to Stroop data. Social phobics' slower response in color-naming social threat words might not reflect greater attention to those words but freezing in response to threatening cues. Such a response is made more likely by the approach to the Stroop test used in this research to date. Both Mattia et al. (1993) and Hope et al. (1990) presented social threat words in blocks of similar words rather than showing them individually, interspersed with neutral words.[1] Reading one threat word after another might build an anxious, inhibitory response in phobic clients. Recall that Beck and Emery (1985) propose that freezing in response to social cues, especially those hinting of negative evaluation or shame, is characteristic of social phobics.

Asmundson and Stein (1994) pointed out that the difficulty with interpreting Stroop data arises from the paradigm's confounding measurement of attention and reaction time. Do social phobics respond more slowly to social threat cues because their attention is drawn to or held by threat, or because their ability to respond is disrupted by their reaction to the threat? A laboratory paradigm devised by MacLeod, Mathews, and Tata (1986) for research on generalized anxiety disorder, and applied by Asmundson and Stein to social phobia, permits these two processes to be teased apart. In this procedure clients watch for a dot on a computer screen and respond by pressing a button when they see it. The dot follows the presentation of various words, some of which are threat words. Thus, the cue to which the clients respond is neutral. Asmundson and Stein demonstrated that when the dot appeared in a location that had been occupied by a social threat word immediately before, the socially phobic clients responded to the dot more quickly than if a neutral word or panic threat word had been in the same area of the computer screen. Normal control subjects showed no such bias. In this case the social phobics' reaction time was facilitated by social threat cues. Accordingly, one can rule out the possibility that freezing in response to threat accounts for the differential response, making it highly likely that greater attention to the threat cue explains social phobics' enhanced response. As with the Stroop research, the attention effect was only observed for social threat words and not for panic (physical) threat words, indicating specificity of response.

Memory

Research on patients with depression has consistently shown that depressed persons have an enhanced memory for negative events (Dalgleish & Watts, 1990). Studies on memory are now being conducted with anxious patients as well, and initial findings indicate that panic patients have enhanced memory for panic threat words (e.g., Becker, Rinck, & Margraf, 1994). The data on memory effects for social phobia are only beginning to emerge.

In two studies comparing responses of 33 social phobics to 21 non-clinical subjects, Rapee, McCallum, Melville, Ravenscroft, and Rodney (1994) tested whether social phobics show enhanced memory for negative events. In one study subjects were asked to relate memories triggered by social versus neutral cues. Social phobics recalled no more negative memories than nonclinical subjects. In the second study, social phobics failed to show enhanced memory for negative pseudofeedback after an imagined speech. The results of the second study might be challenged on the grounds of external validity (is feedback about an imagined speech a potent enough stimulus to evoke a differential response?). However, the findings of the autobiographical memory study challenge a common notion in cognitive therapy with social phobics, to wit that they have a mental filter through which they strain out positive experiences and retain negative ones in their memories. In two additional studies with separate samples of social phobics versus nonclinical controls, Rapee et al. (1994) examined whether social phobics would show enhanced memory for the kind of social threat words used in the reaction time experiments compared to panic threat words, neutral words, and positive words. In neither study did social phobics show a greater implicit or explicit memory bias for social threat words than nonclinical controls.

Stopa and Clark (1993) conducted a final memory study with the sample already described above. They hypothesized that social phobics would be distracted by their negative internal dialogue during the conversation with the confederate and would therefore have more difficulty remembering the conversation itself, as well as objects worn by the confederate, and objects and sounds in the room where the conversation took place. Although social phobics certainly reported having more negative thoughts during the conversation, there was no evidence that these thoughts interfered with their memory for events.

Treatment Implications

The available self-report and laboratory data support the hypothesis that social phobics think negatively about themselves in social situations. They anticipate social failure, perceive their social performance negatively, and may be preoccupied with self-evaluation in social situations. They are hyper-alert to cues concerning social failure and rejection and are unusually likely to freeze in response to such cues. However, no evidence to date indicates that they are more likely to remember threatening cues or experiences than the average person once these have passed.

Extensions to clinical work from these data must be very tentative, but these findings may indicate that cognitive therapy would most usefully focus on social phobics' initial perceptions and evaluations of themselves in social situations and the likelihood that they will focus on the most threatening cues in a social situation. The data also suggest that clinicians need to be aware that social phobics are somewhat accurate when they believe that they have not performed well in front of others, perhaps in part because they freeze in response to the social threats that they are particularly likely to notice. This makes social phobia rather different from, for example, panic disorder. It is clear after a panic attack that a client's prediction that she would die was incorrect. The socially phobic man who thinks his date found him anxious and fumbling for words may well be right, even if he exaggerates the extent of his problem and of her negative evaluation.

COGNITIVE-BEHAVIORAL TREATMENT

Research on cognitive-behavioral treatment (CBT) of social phobia is burgeoning. We use the term CBT rather than cognitive therapy because, with rare exception, the cognitive treatments tested for social phobia have included systematic behavioral components such as social skills training or exposure. Under the general CBT rubric, several varieties have been tested, most notably Self-Instructional Training (SIT; Meichenbaum, 1975), Rational Emotive Therapy (RET; Ellis, 1962), Anxiety Management Training (AMT; Suinn & Richardson, 1971), and Beck and Emery's cognitive therapy (1985), as developed specifically for social phobia by Heimberg and colleagues (Heimberg, 1991; Heimberg & Becker, 1984). In this section we will examine the efficacy data for CBT as well as those findings that point to possible mechanisms of change.

Effectiveness of CBT

At the most basic level, we need to know whether CBT works better than no treatment at all or, even better from a methodological perspective, whether it is more effective than a credible placebo. To address this question, we will review a number of individual studies and also present in Table 16.1 the results of a descriptive meta-analytic summary of 12 published and 2 unpublished investigations of CBT. As the effect size, we calculated Smith and Glass's delta (1977). To include the broadest number of studies possible, we used crude pretest–posttest effect size according to the following formula: $(M_{pretest} - M_{posttest}) / SD_{pretest}$. This summary includes of necessity only those studies for which authors provided means and standard deviations

TABLE 16.1. Cognitive-Behavioral Treatment for Social Phobia:
Pre–Post Treatment Effect Sizes

Study	Group	Social phobia	FNE	Cog.
Butler et al. (1984)	EXP/GAMT	0.62	0.56	—
Chambless et al. (1993)	CBGT	0.62	0.64	1.32
Clark & Agras (1991)	CBGT	0.50	—	1.67
Gelernter et al. (1991)	CBGT	1.15	—	—
Heimberg et al. (1985)	CBGT	1.21	0.78	0.69
Heimberg, Dodge, et al. (1990)	CBGT	0.73	0.76	—
Hope (1989)	CBGT	0.57	0.41	1.20
Hope et al. (1995)	CBGT	0.97	0.84	—
Jerremalm et al. (1986)	SIT	0.94	—	—
Mattick & Peters (1988)	CBGT + EXP	0.71	0.74	0.47
Mattick et al. (1989)	CBGT + EXP	1.79	1.59	1.21
Scholing & Emmelkamp (1993a)	CBT	.96	—	.84
Scholing & Emmelkamp (1993b)	CBT	1.81	—	1.01
Stravynski et al. (1982)	SST + RET	1.53	1.00	0.55
Weighted average		.94	.70	1.03

Note. Cog., cognitive measure; CBGT, cognitive-behavioral group treatment; EXP, exposure; FNE, fear of negative evaluation scale; GAMT, group anxiety management training; RET, rational emotive therapy; SIT, self-instructional training; SST, social skills training.

in their reports. The variables for the analysis were the major questionnaire or evaluator rating measures of social phobia for a given study; if there was more than one, these were composited to yield one effect size for each study. The summary effect size is weighted by sample size. In the case of the follow-up data (Table 16.2), two effect sizes were discrepant from the remainder and were not included in the weighted average of the effect sizes. In Figure 16.1, we present the weighted average effect size for the subset of 8 studies in which a control group (waiting list, pill placebo, or supportive psychotherapy) was included along with the contrasting weighted average effect size

TABLE 16.2. Cognitive-Behavioral Treatment for Social Phobia: Pretreatment–Follow-Up Treatment Effect Sizes

Study	FU	Group	Social phobia	FNE	Cog.
Butler et al. (1984)	6 mo.	EXP/GAMT	0.91	0.92	—
Chambless et al. (1993)	6 mo.	CBGT	0.71	0.95	1.20
Clark & Agras (1991)	1 mo.	CBGT	3.09[a]	—	—
Gelernter et al. (1991)	2 mo.	CBGT	1.08	—	—
Heimberg et al. (1985)	6 mo.	CBGT	1.41	1.10	—
Heimberg, Dodge, et al. (1990)	6 mo.	CBGT	1.15	1.07	—
Hope et al. (1995)	12 mo.	CBGT	0.86	1.03	—
Mattick & Peters (1988)	3 mo.	CBGT + EXP	0.95	0.95	0.68
Mattick et al. (1989)	3 mo.	CBGT + EXP	1.22	1.41	1.11
Scholing & Emmelkamp (1993a)	3 mo.	CBT	1.01	—	0.85
Scholing & Emmelkamp (1993b)	3 mo.	CBT	1.73	—	0.47
Stravynski et al. (1982)	6 mo.	SST + RET	4.80[a]	1.23	1.49
Weighted average			1.05	1.03	0.95

Note. FU, length of follow-up. Other abbreviations as in Table 16.1.
[a]Outlier, not included in the weighted average.

for the control groups (Butler, Cullington, Munby, Amies, & Gelder, 1984; Clark & Agras, 1991; Heimberg, Dodge, et al., 1990; Hope, 1989; Jerremalm, Jansson, & Öst, 1986; Mattick, Peters, & Clarke, 1989; Scholing & Emmelkamp, 1993a, 1993b).

Treatments included in Table 16.1 were from 5 to 16 sessions in duration. In most studies treatment was provided in groups. In three studies the investigators used individual sessions (Butler et al., 1984; Jerremalm et al., 1986; Scholing & Emmelkamp, 1993a), whereas in two clients were treated in either an individual or a group format (Scholing & Emmelkamp, 1993b; Stravynski, Marks, & Yule, 1982). It is often assumed that group treatment is more effective for social phobia because of the ease of conducting exposure and social skills training in that format. Only Scholing and Emmelkamp (1993b) and Lucas and Telch (1993) have reported randomized

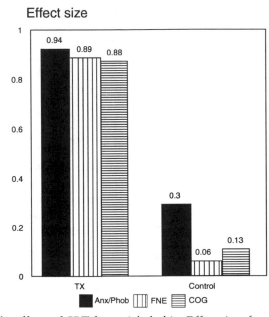

FIGURE 16.1. The effects of CBT for social phobia: Effect sizes for eight studies comparing CBT to a control group on measures of social phobia and anxiety, fear of negative evaluation, and negative thinking.

comparison trials of individual versus group CBT. In these studies the treatments were equally effective. Clearly this is a question of considerable practical significance, and more data addressing this point would be very helpful.

Attesting to the efficacy of CBT for social phobia, the effect sizes for change on measures of social phobia, fear of negative evaluation, and maladaptive cognitions are all large at posttest and are even larger at follow-up. The effect sizes in Figure 16.1, showing the average difference in effects for CBT versus control conditions (pill placebo, education and support, and waiting list), clearly demonstrate the superiority of CBT to control conditions.

Comparisons with No Treatment

Four controlled studies speak to the efficacy of CBT versus baseline or a no-treatment control group.[2] Stravynski (1983) conducted a multiple baseline across-settings design investigation of the benefits of exposure, social skills training, and cognitive modification for a socially phobic man who vomited in anxiety-provoking situations. In general the patient's anxiety in a given phobic situation declined when and only when that particular situation was targeted for treatment, meaning that the treatment rather than passage of time was responsible for the change. The patient's anxiety and vomiting were relieved by treatment, and he had maintained his improvement at the 2-year follow-up. Jerremalm et al. (1986) compared 10–12 sessions of SIT plus exposure homework to a waiting-list control. Subjects were divided into physiological and cognitive reactors.[3] Regardless of classification, clients who received SIT improved more than waiting-list clients on questionnaire and behavioral ratings of social phobia. Among cognitive reactors, those in the SIT group also reported more change on behavior test anxiety. Butler et al. (1984) contrasted the effects of seven sessions of exposure plus AMT to waiting list. The 15 treated clients were clearly more improved than waiting-list clients on measures of social phobia, satisfaction with the number of social contacts in their lives, and behavior test anxiety. Finally, Hope (1989) compared the effects of 12 weeks on a waiting list to Heimberg's (1991) group CBT. Clients who received CBT improved more on most measures of social phobia than waiting-list subjects who demonstrated minimal change between assessment points.

In three studies CBT has been compared to a psychological or pill placebo condition. Heimberg, Dodge, et al. (1990) examined the effects of 12 sessions of group CBT versus an equal amount of group educational-supportive therapy. The educational-supportive group provided controls for attention, group contact, education about social phobia, and expectancy effects and thus constituted a rigorous basis for comparison. Subjects rated the control treatment equal to CBT in credibility and were as likely to finish the educational-supportive group as were CBT subjects. At both posttest and 6-month follow-up, independent evaluators rated CBT clients as more improved than the control group clients. At posttest evaluators rated 75% of the former versus 40% of the latter as clinically significantly improved. At follow-up CBT clients also reported less anxiety on the behavioral test. There were no differences on observer ratings of behavior test anxiety at either time point, nor were there differences observed on analyses of the self-report questionnaires. The latter finding is hard to interpret in that the authors followed a data analytic strategy that was probably unfortunate. They combined all questionnaire data, regardless of the construct measured, in one multivariate analysis of variance. Actual differences may be obscured by such an approach, for example, if one treatment was better on measures of social phobia, but not on other measures such as depression.

In a recent brief report, Lucas and Telch (1993) have provided a replication of the Heimberg et al. (1990) study in which they used the same treatment manuals. Clients who received group CBT were significantly more likely to meet criteria for reliable change (see Jacobson & Truax, 1991) on the Social Phobia and Anxiety Inventory than were clients in the educational-supportive control group. Tests of continuous outcome measures are obscured by a similar multivariate strategy to that used by Heimberg et al. (1990). The CBT group tended to show more change on the behavioral test measures, but not on the heterogeneous group of self-report measures.

In 1993 Heimberg, Salzman, Holt, and Blendall published 5-year follow-up data for a subset of 19 of the original group of clients who could be located and agreed to participate. For both treatment groups, clients willing to participate were more likely to have been treatment responders at posttest, thereby probably inflating improvement rates at follow-up. Again independent evaluators rated CBT clients as less socially phobic as well as less impaired by their phobias than were control group clients. Of the CBT clients 89% were clinically significantly improved versus 44% of the control group. Additionally the CBT group had lower scores on two of four self-report measures of social phobia and were rated as less anxious and more skilled on the behavior test by judges, although not by themselves. Overall the set of studies based on Heimberg's approach (1991) indicates that CBT is more effective than a stringent control condition on critical measures of social phobia, and that the results may be well-maintained out to 5-year follow-up.

Clark and Agras (1991) reported treatment outcome for an unusual sample in this literature: All patients were musicians with performance anxiety who underwent very brief treatment. Patients were randomly assigned to five sessions of group CBT + placebo, the tranquilizer buspirone, CBT + buspirone, or placebo alone. At posttest, CBT + placebo[4] subjects were better than placebo alone on judges' ratings of the quality of a behavior test musical performance but not on questionnaire or self-report behavior test data. At 1-month follow-up, one measure was collected, the Personal Report of Confidence as a Performer (PRCP). The CBT + placebo group was superior to placebo alone at this time point. The authors speculate that, given their very brief treatment program, subjects needed time to incorporate what they had learned and the changes they had made before these were reflected in a self-report measure such as the PRCP. This explanation fits with the pattern of the PRCP data, but examination of the means for other measures suggests that the low power the authors had for comparisons (seven subjects per cell) played a role in the lack of differences between groups, for the CBT + placebo group consistently fared better than placebo alone.

In summary, the substantial effect sizes in Tables 16.1 and 16.2, and the results of controlled investigations (see Figure 16.1) indicate that CBT is an effective treatment for social phobia and that its impact is more significant than that of credible placebo or supportive therapies. While important, these findings do not tell us whether CBT is as effective or is more effective than other active treatments. We turn to this issue next.

Comparisons with Other Treatments

In this section we examine the 12 controlled studies in which CBT was contrasted to another active treatment. Given the dearth of data on nonbehavioral psychosocial treatments of social phobia, this review will be limited to pharmacological interventions and to several behavioral interventions.

Pharmacotherapy

The design of the study by Clark and Agras (1991) on musical performance anxiety has been described above and the problems with low power noted. There were no significant differences between CBT + placebo and buspirone-treated subjects at posttest, and buspirone did not add to the effectiveness of CBT. By follow-up the CBT + placebo group was superior to all other groups, including the buspirone alone and buspirone + CBT groups, on outcome. However, drug group clients had been withdrawn from medication by this time. These data indicate that brief CBT + placebo has more lasting effects than brief pharmacotherapy.

A more extensive study contrasting pharmacological treatment to CBT was conducted by Gelernter et al. (1991). These authors provided 12 sessions of group CBT following the Heimberg and Becker manual (1984). Drug group subjects received either the monoamine oxidase inhibitor (MAOI) phenelzine or the high-potency benzodiazepine alprazolam. All groups received weekly homework assignments for exposure to phobic situations. Power was improved over the Clark and Agras study (1991), although it was still low for comparisons among active treatments (14–17 per cell). After 12 weeks patients received a posttest, were withdrawn from any medication, and were seen again at 2-month follow-up. There were no significant between-group effects at posttest or follow-up on measures of social phobia.

As this review shows, comparisons of CBT with pharmacotherapy are very limited. We conclude that CBT appears to be as effective as pharmacological interventions but that more research is necessary for a more definitive answer.

Exposure

CBT has most extensively been compared to exposure without cognitive modification with mixed results. In one of the earliest studies, Biran, Augusto, and Wilson (1981) examined the results of three single cases, two of which were treated with cognitive restructuring (five sessions) followed by exposure (five sessions), whereas the third control subject got exposure alone. All had severe fear of writing in front of others. Change on behavioral test avoidance occurred when and only when the clients received exposure. Cognitive restructuring without exposure during or between sessions led to no change. Change on fear was inconsistent and therefore difficult to interpret.

Gelernter et al. (1991) included a fourth group beyond the three described in the pharmacotherapy section. This group received pill placebo but, like the other conditions in that study, were also asked to complete weekly exposure homework assignments. Placebo plus exposure homework was as effective as CBT and as pharmacotherapy. These findings may speak to the power of exposure homework (perhaps combined with expectations of better performance and lower anxiety due to the placebo), but an alternative explanation must be ruled out first. Gelernter et al. conducted standard 2-hour CBT sessions but included 10 patients per group. In our experience with the same treatment manual, this is almost twice the number of patients who can be adequately treated in a 2-hour session.

Several other groups of investigators have obtained results consistent with Gelernter et al. (1991) despite having conducted more adequate trials of CBT. Hope (1989) also followed the Heimberg (1991) 12-session treatment manual. Exposure-only subjects (n = 11) role-played in group and also discussed material from the educational-supportive condition of the Heimberg, Dodge, et al. (1990) study to fill time CBT subjects (n = 18) spent in cognitive restructuring. Although the results varied according to measure, on the whole the exposure-only group improved more than the CBT group on important measures of social phobia. Although the treatment was supervised by Heimberg, Hope noted that the CBT outcome was inferior in this study to that typical of other subjects at Heimberg's center. Hope suggested that the group process may have been disrupted in the CBT groups. These groups had a higher dropout rate (28%) than usual. This rate was higher, although not to a statistically significant degree, than the 9% in the exposure-alone group. One CBT group in particular was disrupted by an unusually hostile member who eventually was removed from the group, a rare occurrence in our experience.

Mattick et al. (1989) compared brief group CBT (six sessions) to group exposure. Posttest was followed by another assessment 3 months later. The authors contrasted the average of posttest and follow-up data for the two groups. There was little evidence of statistically significant differential change. However, note that the power was too low to detect any but large effects (n = 10 or 11 per group), and that the CBT group consistently changed more, if not significantly more, than the exposure-alone group.

Scholing and Emmelkamp (1993a, 1993b) reported the results of two trials in which they compared RET plus exposure homework instructions (they label this "integrated treatment") to exposure alone. In the first study (1993a) subjects had specific fears of trembling, blushing, or sweating in front of others. Exposure and CBT were compared after 8 sessions. (CBT clients ultimately received a total of 16 sessions of treatment. The data in the tables reflect change over all 16 sessions.) Clients in the second study (1993b) had generalized social phobia. Contrasts in this study were made after 16 sessions of treatment. In neither study was there any trend to suggest that CBT was more effective than exposure alone despite, in the case of the study on generalized social phobia, a reasonable sample size and provision of more sessions of CBT than was typical of earlier trials.

In contrast to the studies described in the previous paragraph, in two investigations CBT proved more effective than exposure alone. In a second study Mattick and colleagues (Mattick & Peters, 1988) once again compared six sessions of CBT to six sessions of exposure alone, but with a more generous sample size (total n = 51). CBT clients improved more on self-report and behavioral measures of phobia. Differences were especially apparent at 3-month follow-up due to continued improvement in the CBT group and slight losses in the exposure group. Exposure-alone clients (47%) were twice as likely to request additional treatment at follow-up as were CBT clients (24%). Butler et al. (1984) examined the effects of AMT (distraction, relaxation, and rational self-talk) plus exposure homework to exposure homework plus a credible psychological placebo for 30 clients. After seven sessions, the AMT group was superior to the exposure-alone group on some, but not most, measures of social phobia. However, by 6-month follow-up the AMT group was more improved than the exposure-alone group on four of six major outcome measures. Moreover, in the year after treatment, 40% of the exposure-alone group requested additional treatment versus none of the AMT group. Interpretation of the Butler et al. data for our present purposes is somewhat unclear. Although the AMT package definitively boosted treatment efficacy, it is a heterogeneous set of procedures, and we cannot know whether the rational self-talk or some other procedure (e.g., relaxation) was responsible for the enhanced power of treatment.

Other Behavior Therapy

Stravynski et al. (1982) contrasted the effects of individual or group social skills training (SST) to those of SST plus cognitive modification procedures similar to RET. Subjects were 22 generalized social phobics with avoidant personality disorder who received twelve 90-minute sessions of treatment. Results from self-report and assessor-rated measures were comparable; in no case was SST plus cognitive modification more effective than SST alone. Although the power for this experiment was low, the pattern of the results does not suggest that the augmented treatment would have proved more successful with a larger sample. However, examination of the means for the standardized questionnaires indicates that this sample of patients may have been unusual for social phobics. Patients started treatment below the normal sample mean (15.47, Watson & Friend, 1969) on the Fear of Negative Evaluation (FNE) Scale and relatively close to the normal sample mean (9.11, Watson & Friend, 1969) on the Social Avoidance and Distress (SAD) Scale. Both their mean FNE scores and their SAD scores were substantially lower than in other studies of generalized social phobia. (For example, M for the 0–28 SAD scale was 10.3–11.1 in Stravynski et al.'s [1982] study vs. 21.5 in Chambless et al.'s [1993] sample; M for the 0–30 FNE scale was 12.6–13.3 vs. 25.1.) Given the absence of structured diagnostic interviewing with clearly established criteria and of evidence of reliability of diagnostic assessment in this study, these data raise some question about the possibly unusual nature of this sample.

In the final study to be discussed, Jerremalm et al. (1986) compared the effects of SIT to applied relaxation for 20 socially phobic clients classified as cognitive or physiological reactors. Clients received 10–12 sessions of treatment. SIT clients were instructed to carry out exposure homework; applied relaxation clients participated in role plays during several sessions but apparently were not assigned exposure homework. For both cognitive and physiological reactors SIT proved more effective than applied relaxation on the major questionnaire measure of social phobia, although not on the behavioral test. These data may suggest that CBT is more effective than a less explicitly cognitive approach. However, this conclusion cannot be clearly drawn because amount of exposure was confounded with treatment. Because exposure is itself an effective treatment, and the SIT group got homework exposure instructions when the applied relaxation group apparently did not, we cannot rule out the competing hypothesis that SIT was superior because of the exposure instructions.

Cognitive Therapy without Exposure

We noted previously that most investigators have tested the effects of cognitive-behavioral therapy for social phobia. In this section, we review the handful of studies in which cognitive therapy without behavioral elements (e.g., exposure) was examined.

Employing brief group treatment (six sessions), Emmelkamp, Mersch, Vissia, and van der Helm (1985) contrasted the effects of RET, SIT, and *in vivo* exposure. The two cognitive therapy conditions received neither therapist-assisted exposure nor instructions for *in vivo* exposure homework. On the whole, the cognitive treatments were as effective as exposure at posttest or 1-month follow-up. These results are echoed in several other studies by Emmelkamp's research group.

Mersch, Emmelkamp, Bogels, and van der Sleen (1989) contrasted RET to SST. In this study 37 clients received SST or RET. In neither group were clients instructed to carry out exposure homework. Unlike the Stravynski et al. (1982) study, in this case clients in the cognitive therapy condition did not participate in role plays during sessions or receive any other SST. Naturally SST clients role-played extensively during treatment sessions. Behavioral as well as self-report assessment data were collected. Treatment benefits were comparable in the two conditions at posttest and at follow-up. Further subgroup analyses were conducted to determine whether cognitive reactors would respond better to RET and behavioral reactors to SST. This proved not to be the case.

The pair of studies by Scholing and Emmelkamp (1993a, 1993b) have been introduced in the previous section. The design of these studies allows the comparison of RET without exposure homework or within-session role plays to the combination of RET and exposure homework and to exposure homework alone after 8 sessions, although not after the full 16 sessions clients ultimately received. (Clients in the RET-alone condition received exposure after 8 sessions.) RET alone proved as effective as the other two conditions.

The study by Mattick et al. (1989) has also been introduced in the previous section. Of interest here is a third group included in that research: six sessions of group cognitive restructuring with antiexposure instructions. This condition was included for theoretical reasons; obviously cognitive-behavioral therapists rarely caution their clients against entering phobic situations. Clients were told to put off deliberate exposure until they had changed their negative thoughts. Not surprisingly, when faced with a behavioral avoidance test at posttest and follow-up (data from these two points were combined for analysis), clients in the cognitive therapy–antiexposure group behaved more fearfully than those in the CBT group. However, on the whole this group fared as well as the exposure-only and CBT clients.

Summary

Overall the studies reviewed clearly indicate that CBT is an effective treatment for social phobia but not that it is more beneficial than other behavioral treatments. Although occasionally investigators do find CBT to be superior to other treatments, most do not. No obvious factors account for the variable results across investigations. Often investigations can be faulted for insufficient power for comparisons between active treatments or for treatment that may have been too brief to be adequate for the delivery of CBT. Nonetheless, investigation of the patterns of the data does not suggest that low power or insufficient treatment length was consistently responsible for the null statistical findings.

Although it seems that cognitive therapy does not add to the effectiveness of behavior therapy, neither does behavior therapy in the form of exposure add to the benefits of cognitive therapt. According to the results of four investigations of this question, at least in brief treatment (six to eight sessions), cognitive restructuring without explicit exposure instructions is as effective as cognitive therapy + exposure and as exposure alone. Given the difficulties in conducting *in vivo* exposure treatment of social phobia (see Butler, 1985), these data are of practical significance, particularly if they are replicated in a longer trial in which treatment is extended until a more clinically satisfactory response is obtained. Until that time, we would encourage clinicians at least to include explicit exposure homework instructions in their treatment plans.

Effects of CBT on Cognitive Variables

In the review above we have focused on the effects of CBT on measures of social phobia. Given its explicit focus on changing cognitions, one might expect that CBT should differentially affect measures of socially phobic thinking. Is this the case? The answer to this question is made difficult by the scant attention paid to cognitive assessment of social phobia outcome in many studies. However, some general conclusions may be drawn. Examination of the uncontrolled effect sizes in Tables 16.1 and 16.2 indicates that CBT has a very substantial impact on measures of cognition, and the data for the controlled studies represented in Figure 16.1 demonstrate this result is greater than for control conditions.

Studies Using Measures of Rational Thinking

In the earlier studies of social phobia outcome, investigators often used the Irrational Beliefs Test (IBT; Jones, 1969) or the FNE (Watson & Friend, 1969) as measures of cognition. However, the FNE is best thought of as a measure of a specific component of social anxiety and not a measure of cognition per se. Characterization of the IBT as a measure of cognition has also been criticized on the grounds that it poorly discriminates between anxiety and cognitions (e.g., Smith & Zurawski, 1983). At any rate, it was certainly not constructed to measure cognitions of social phobics in any specific sense. With these caveats in mind, we review the studies in which the IBT or the kindred Rational Behavior Inventory (Shorkey & Whiteman, 1977) were used in this section. Data on the FNE were considered under social phobia outcome.

In the earliest study to use the IBT, Heimberg, Becker, Goldfinger, and Vermilyea (1985) reported no significant change with treatment for clients in their study; however, the sample size ($n = 7$) was very small. Mattick and colleagues (Mattick & Peters, 1988; Mattick et al., 1989) contrasted the effects of exposure alone versus exposure plus cognitive restructuring on this measure. Neither study reported superior results for the combined condition. Mattick et al. (1989) also included a pure cognitive restructuring group that received neither within- nor between-session exposure instructions. This group improved more during the 3-month follow-up interval than exposure-treated clients on the IBT. These findings may suggest that a group of clients receiving more thorough cognitive therapy were more able to continue to challenge their irrational beliefs during the follow-up period. However, because Mattick et al. (1989) do not present data to show whether the treatment groups were equivalent at posttest on this or other variables (data analyzed were averages of post- and follow-up assessments), it is equally possible that the cognitive therapy alone group lagged behind the others at posttest and merely caught up during the follow-up period.

Results comparable to those of the Mattick and Peters study (1988) were reported in two additional investigations. Stravynski et al. (1982) found cognitive modification added nothing to the effects of SST on the IBT, and Mersch et al. (1989) found RET to be no more beneficial in effecting change on the Rational Behavior Inventory than was SST without cognitive modification. However, between posttest and 6-week follow-up, clients classified by Mersch et al. as cognitive reactors improved more on this inventory if they had received RET, again suggesting that CBT may show its greatest effects on cognition after formal treatment has ended. This interpretation is buttressed by the findings reported by Emmelkamp, Mersch, Vissia, and van der Helm (1985) on the IBT. When these authors contrasted the effects of SIT and RET considered together versus exposure *in vivo,* they found no superiority for CBT at posttest. Yet after 1 month with no additional treatment, CBT-treated clients were superior to exposure-treated clients on this variable.

Social Anxiety Self-Statement Questionnaires

Jerremalm et al. (1986) developed a Thought Index of positive and negative thoughts to be used after a behavioral interaction task. This was employed in their own study as well as in that of Mersch et al. (1989). Jerremalm et al. (1986) reported that clients treated with SIT improved significantly more than those on a waiting list. Among clients classified as cognitive reactors, SIT clients also improved more than those who received applied relaxation training. In contrast Mersch et al. (1989) noted no greater change with RET than with SST at posttest or follow-up for cognitive or physiological reactors. Unfortunately, results from these studies are quite tenuous because the thought index proved to have poor test–retest reliability. Psychometric data are lacking for the Self-Statement Questionnaire, a measure used by Clark and Agras (1991) to assess music performance–related positive and negative thoughts. Minimally described, this questionnaire appears to have been developed specifically for this investigation and to be a general report of thinking patterns rather than one tied specifically to the behavioral assessment occasions. Change at posttest on this measure was not superior in the groups that received brief CBT + placebo versus a tranquilizer alone. Follow-up data were not collected.

In four studies investigators have used reliable and validated measures of socially anxious cognitions. These include the SISST and a Dutch measure, the Social Cognition Inventory (van Kamp & Klip, 1981, as cited by Scholing & Emmelkamp, 1993a, 1993b). The former is intended to be completed on the basis of a specific preceding interaction but in the case of the Heimberg, Dodge, et al. (1990) investigation, was altered to be a general measure of socially anxious thinking, more like the Social Cognition Inventory. In an uncontrolled treatment study, Chambless et al. (1993) reported results for 50 social phobics who received 10–11 sessions of Heimberg's group CBT (Heimberg, 1991). Cognitions were measured with the SISST after each of three behavioral tests and analyzed according to the States of Mind (SOM) ratio. As a whole, clients changed from an internal dialogue of conflict (.50) to a positive dialogue (.60), hypothesized by Schwartz and Garamoni (1989) to be the healthiest thinking pattern. At 6-month follow-up the SOM (.56) remained in the positive dialogue range. Although these results support the hypothesis that CBT leads to change on the SISST, this change may not be unique to CBT. Heimberg, Dodge, et al. (1990) found equivalent change on their altered version of the SISST with the educational-supportive group control condition as with CBT. Similarly, Gelernter et al.

(1991) found exposure, whether combined with placebo or active medication, was as effective as Heimberg's group CBT in altering SISST-reported cognitions after a behavior test. Comparable results were obtained with tests using the more general Social Cognition Inventory. In two studies Scholing and Emmelkamp (1993a, 1993b) found no superiority for RET over exposure alone after 8 or 16 sessions of treatment or at 3-month follow-up.

Thought Listing

In two samples the investigators have used thought listing as their cognitive outcome measure. Subsequent to a behavioral interaction task or speech, clients are asked to list the thoughts they had during the behavioral test, and these are later categorized by judges. This procedure, which has considerable face validity, allows for a less constrained as well as less prompted measure of cognition than the questionnaire formats. Data obtained via the two different methods may yield different patterns of results (Glass & Arnkoff, 1993).

Comparing the effects of Heimberg's group CBT to waiting-list and to exposure alone, Hope (1989) reported that, at posttest, CBT subjects had changed more on cognitions than waiting-list subjects and exposure-only clients, but the differences were not statistically significant. In their comparison of group CBT to educational-supportive therapy, Heimberg, Dodge, et al. (1990) also found no differences at posttest on amount of change on the thought-listing measure. However, by 6-month follow-up the CBT clients reported less negative and more positive thoughts than the control group clients. Again, differences in favor of CBT were more apparent at follow-up than immediately after treatment. In a reanalysis of these data according to the SOM model, Bruch, Heimberg, and Hope (1991) reported that CBT-treated clients had moved from the internal dialogue of conflict range at posttest to the positive dialogue range at follow-up. By contrast, educational-supportive condition clients were similarly characterized at posttest, but by follow-up had worsened and reported a mean SOM in the negative monologue range. Regardless of treatment group assignment, clients who were rated as improved at follow-up by an independent assessor had a more positive SOM than unimproved clients. As would be predicted, the average SOM for improved clients was in the positive dialogue range, reflecting a healthy thinking pattern according to Schwartz and Garamoni's (1989) model.

Other Measures

Only two studies provide data other than self-reports of thoughts. In an uncontrolled investigation of a small sample, Lucock and Salkovskis (1988) found that social phobics who had undergone eight sessions of group CBT demonstrated reductions in their inflated estimates of the likelihood of negative social events. Mattia et al. (1993) have reported the only analysis of change with treatment on a laboratory-based measure of social phobia schema activity. These authors assessed change on the Stroop test of response to social threat words for 29 social phobics treated either with the MAOI phenelzine, pill placebo, or Heimberg's (1991) group CBT. Clients were classified as responders or nonresponders at posttest by independent evaluators. Relative to nonresponders, treatment responders showed a decreased Stroop interference response at posttest. Results were not broken out separately for the CBT group alone. Like the results reported by Bruch et al. (1991), these data indicate that cognitive change is associated with treatment improvement.

Summary

Overall, the pattern of the results described above indicates that improvement on cognitive aspects of social phobia is to be expected with CBT and that clients who show greater cognitive change will be more improved on social phobia symptoms as well. Whether the relationship of cognitive change to treatment outcome is causal, as cognitive theory proposes, or correlational cannot be determined from the findings to date. Unfortunately, social phobia researchers have yet to apply data analytic models that allow approximations to tests of causality (see Baron & Kenny, 1986).

Although it seems plausible that CBT would lead to greater cognitive change than other treatments, in general this does not seem to be the case.[5] When CBT did prove superior in effecting cognitive change, this typically occurred in studies where CBT was the more effective treatment for social phobia symptoms in general. Accordingly, we cannot rule out the possibility that the greater cognitive change in these studies followed symptom improvement rather than led to it. (For a further discussion of these issues, see Chambless & Gillis, 1993.) Differences in favor of CBT, when found, were more likely to occur at follow-up than immediately after treatment, emphasizing the importance of collecting follow-up data, which not all investigators have done. Reasons why CBT is superior in an occasional study but not others are not readily apparent.

CLINICAL APPLICATION: A CASE STUDY

Sherri was a 37-year-old single woman who had worked in a skilled office position for the same employer since graduating from college 15 years prior to seeking treatment. Sherri sought treatment because of the anxiety she experienced in social situations, especially in situations involving unfamiliar people or potential dating partners. Although she remembered being somewhat shy her entire life, Sherri dated the onset of her anxiety to age 9 or 10 when she believed it became significantly worse.

Her anxiety was characterized by sweating, nausea, mild depersonalization, and mild trembling. She worried that she did not know how to act appropriately in social situations and that others would think poorly of her if she said the wrong thing or failed to appear "correct" in some way. She reported feeling very self-conscious because she believed she was overweight despite the fact her weight appeared to be within the normal range. She also worried that her clothing was outmoded and that she did not know how to pick out stylish clothing. Sherri's social life was limited to occasional social activities with a few coworkers with whom she was particularly comfortable, nearly always at their initiation. In addition to the social anxiety, Sherri reported a history of mild, recurrent depressive episodes secondary to the social isolation caused by the anxiety. Sherri was interviewed using the Anxiety Disorders Interview Schedule–Revised (ADIS-R; DiNardo & Barlow, 1988) and received a primary diagnosis of social phobia, generalized type. She did not meet criteria for any other Axis I or II disorders. On the self-rated 0–4 interference in functioning rating included in the ADIS-R Sherri rated herself a 4, indicating that she believed the social phobia was "disabling." The ADIS-R interviewer rated the severity of the social phobia as "markedly disturbing/disabling" but not severe or incapacitating.

Cognitive-Behavioral Group Therapy

Sherri was treated according to the procedures outlined in Heimberg's (1991) treatment manual for cognitive-behavioral group therapy (CBGT) for social phobia. CBGT consists of three primary components—cognitive restructuring, simulated exposures to feared situations in the context of the therapy group, and homework assignments for *in vivo* exposure. Groups consist of five to seven clients and two therapists. CBGT groups meet for 2–2.5 hours weekly for 12 weeks. Detailed explanations of CBGT procedures are available from Heimberg (1991) and Hope and Heimberg (1993) but will be reviewed briefly below.

Prior to starting treatment, group members meet individually with one of the therapists to construct a fear and avoidance hierarchy and to become familiar with basic CBGT procedures. Once the group convenes, the first two sessions are largely didactic. After a discussion of ground rules and detailed presentation of the CBT model, the remainder of session 1 and all of session 2 are devoted to a series of exercises to teach basic cognitive restructuring skills. By the end of the second session, clients should have developed basic skills to perceive and report their automatic thoughts, identify cognitive distortions in their automatic thoughts, use a questioning approach to challenge the automatic thoughts, and develop a rational response that summarizes these challenges to combat that automatic thought when it occurs. Sessions 3–11 of CBGT are devoted to graduated role-played exposures to feared situations with the cognitive procedures fully integrated into the exposure as will be seen below. Session 12 consists of final exercises to consolidate gains as formal treatment ends and a social hour.

Sherri's Initial Sessions of CBGT

Sherri received treatment in exchange for her participation in an ongoing psychopathology study. Sherri was one of a group of seven social phobics with a male–female therapist team. During the initial two didactic sessions of CBGT, Sherri appeared to accept the cognitive model readily and to understand the basic cognitive restructuring skills. However, she made only modest attempts to self-monitor her automatic thoughts between sessions, despite the therapists' encouragement to do so. In the third session, two other group members completed their first in-session therapeutic exposures. Sherri spoke up frequently in assisting other group members' cognitive restructuring and gave helpful, supportive feedback after the exposures. Sherri was scheduled for her first exposure during session 4 but was absent due to illness.

Session 5

Sherri's first therapeutic exposure occurred in the fifth session and revolved around a part-time job she had recently taken to deliver coupon books door-to-door. She took the job for two primary reasons: She needed the extra money, and she thought it would provide an opportunity to exercise regularly as the job required extensive walking. She was scheduled to make her first deliveries in the upcoming week but was very anxious that she would be seen by and possibly have to talk with people out working in their yards.

As the diagnostic interview and earlier group sessions had shown, Sherri was extremely self-conscious about her appearance and constantly monitored how she thought she appeared to others. Thus, in this situation, Sherri's primary automatic thought was "They'll think I look 'dorky' [awkward and unsophisticated]." The group helped her identify the cognitive distortion in this automatic thought as mind reading (believing others have formed a negative opinion despite little or no evidence that they have) (Burns, 1980; Persons, 1989). Through Socratic questioning and the group's assistance, Sherri was able to see that she had no idea what the people she might meet would think of her and, because she was unlikely to see them again, their opinions of her were relatively unimportant. She developed the following rational response to use during the exposure: "This isn't a beauty contest, and I am primarily doing this to get physically fit." This rational response encouraged Sherri to focus her attention on the personal benefits of the job instead of her self-conscious thoughts about her current appearance. The rational response was written on an easel to cue Sherri to use it to help control her anxiety during the exposure.

Because any one encounter with someone while Sherri delivered coupon books would be very brief, the therapists used the procedures outlined by Hope (1993) and Hope and Heimberg (1993) for staging exposures to brief situations. This technique involves repeated occurrences of the brief situation. In Sherri's case, each group member and one of the therapists stood around the perimeter of the group room as if they were a series of people out working in their yards. Sherri's exposure consisted of approaching each person and handing him or her a coupon book with a short explanation of what it was. Sometimes the person engaged her in a brief conversation. Other times the person simply thanked her and turned away. As she finished with each person, she simply moved on to the next individual as if she had walked to the next house. The therapists assisted Sherri in setting a behavioral goal for the exposure of saying hello to each person at the minimum.

As is customary in CBGT, Sherri was prompted approximately once per minute throughout the exposure for anxiety ratings on the 0–100 Subjective Units of Discomfort Scale (SUDS), higher numbers indicating greater anxiety. At each SUDS prompt, she also repeated her rational response aloud. Over the course of the 5-minute role play, Sherri approached nine people with the following SUDS ratings: 20, 35, 40, 30, 30, 25.

In the debriefing that followed the exposure, two major points became clear. First, Sherri had been worried about starting the deliveries for several days, but the situation was much less anxiety-provoking than anticipated once she began the role-played exposure. Although Sherri had been unable to report it when the therapists elicited automatic thoughts prior to the exposure, Sherri had been thinking that the encounters with people in their yards would require extended conversations. It quickly became apparent during the role play that the weather and the coupon books were two obvious conversation topics, and that few people would be interested in continuing to talk beyond that. Second, Sherri learned from the exposure that the encounters were relatively anonymous, not unlike dozens of other brief interactions people have every week with delivery persons and salesclerks. Not only do people rarely think about the person to whom they are talking, but also they are unlikely to even remember the conversation a few hours later. Sherri concluded by stating that the exposure had been helpful, and that she was much less concerned about starting the deliveries in the upcoming week.

Sherri's homework assignment for session 5 involved completing the cognitive restructuring exercises on her own before beginning the deliveries and saying hello to at least two people while making the deliveries. She successfully completed this assignment with only mild levels of anxiety.

Session 6

Sherri did not participate in an exposure in session 6, but she assisted in other group members' cognitive restructuring. Her new behavioral homework assignments addressed the problem of her limited social network and the fact that it did not include anyone from outside of work. The therapists discussed with her the importance of expanding her social network. Sherri believed this would be difficult, however, given her limited financial resources. This resulted in a homework assignment to explore low-cost options to meet new people. The group started her on the assignment by brain-storming the first two items on her list—(1) checking the newspaper for free cultural events in which she might be interested and (2) calling the volunteer bureau about opportunities to volunteer a few hours a month. Sherri was to find four more strategies or places to meet people.

Sherri worked diligently on her homework for session 6 and brought in a longer list of possible ways to meet new people than had been assigned. She was surprised that her limited financial circumstances were less problematic than she had believed. Her list included attending the adult singles group at a local church she had visited several years earlier, taking an inexpensive arts and crafts class at the local community college, and taking a different part-time job that would allow her to meet people instead of her current delivery job which involved working alone. Sherri decided to explore the adult singles group first.

Session 7

Sherri completed her second exposure in session 7. She reported to the group that she had been invited to a coworker's housewarming party the next weekend. Although she sometimes accepted this type of invitation, she usually spent the entire evening with a small group of people she knew well from work. Because her primary treatment goal involved reducing her fears in dating situations, Sherri agreed to do an exposure around having a conversation with an unfamiliar man at the housewarming party. Prior to the exposure, Sherri reported the following automatic thoughts: "We won't have much to talk about," "He'll think I'm not attractive," "He might be a jerk," and "He'll think my clothes are weird."

Because self-consciousness about her appearance was a recurrent theme for Sherri and represented one of the primary reasons she avoided social situations, the therapists focused the cognitive restructuring on the automatic thought "He'll think I'm not attractive." With the group's help, mind reading and all-or-nothing thinking (Sherri felt she had to be gorgeous to be considered attractive) (Burns, 1980; Persons, 1989) were identified as the cognitive distortions in the automatic thought. The therapists and other group members helped Sherri see that she would probably not know whether he found her attractive. Furthermore, she did not yet know whether she would be interested in him either. Thus the best strategy was to have a conversation in order to get acquainted because, until then, there was no way to know whether either of them would be interested in having any further contact. Sherri developed the rational response of "I'm here to have fun and meet people, not to impress him" to counter her primary automatic thought.

The male cotherapist served as the role player for the exposure because the other male members of the group had severe dating fears themselves or were too young for Sherri to see them as potential dating partners. Sherri's behavioral goal for the exposure was to get to know two things about her conversation partner. The role play was staged so that the therapist was standing on one side of the room as if he were milling around at a party. Sherri approached him and started the 6-minute conversation. Sherri reported very little anxiety during the exposure (SUDS = 10, 20, 20, 15, 15, 10, 10) and displayed excellent social skills.

In the debriefing after the exposure, Sherri once again stated that the anticipation of the conversation was worse than the conversation itself, as had occurred in the previous exposure in session 5. However, she also attempted to discount the experience by stating that the cotherapist was easy to talk to, especially because she felt she already knew him. The therapists redirected her to focus on her behavioral goal of learning two things about him and the fact that she was able to list eight things she had learned. Group members praised her excellent conversation skills and pointed out that her sense of humor and pleasant interpersonal style would likely make a positive impression on most people. For homework, Sherri agreed to attend the housewarming and start a conversation with at least one man with whom she was unacquainted. A greeting and one further comment would be minimally sufficient. The next week she reported that she had successfully completed the assignment with a moderate amount of anxiety, and that the conversation had lasted 2–3 minutes.

Starting in midtreatment, CBGT clients receive a second, ongoing homework assignment to complete a small *in vivo* exposure every day as a way to make facing their fears more routine. For Sherri this assignment involved greeting someone everyday to whom she would not normally speak. On work days, this was defined as someone who worked outside of her department. During the first week, she spoke with someone on 3 days. Therapists' exploration with Sherri of the poor compliance with the daily assignment is described below.

Session 8

Sherri was not scheduled for an in-session exposure for session 8. She served as a role player for another group member's exposure. While negotiating a homework assignment for the upcoming week, Sherri reported that she had been invited to join several female coworkers who were planning to go dancing. Sherri had sometimes joined them on previous occasions but always refused any invitations to dance because of her self-consciousness about her appearance. She agreed to join her coworkers and dance at least once if asked. The therapists reminded her of the importance of completing the cognitive restructuring exercises on her own before the event. The next week, Sherri reported that she had completed the assignment despite high anxiety. She had used a modified version of the rational response from session 7 ("I'm here to have fun, not to impress anyone") to help control her anxiety. However, she reported that she continued to think about people looking at her and making negative judgments about her appearance.

Before reassigning the daily homework to greet people with whom she did not normally speak, the therapists attempted to determine why she had done so only 3 of 7 days the previous week. The therapists were unable to discover any obstacles to completion of the assignment every day so they simply reemphasized the importance of daily attempts, and Sherri agreed to try again. The next session Sherri reported speaking to someone on 6 days and that she had not found an opportunity to do so on one of the weekend days. As is often reported by group members completing similar assignments, Sherri expressed surprise at how responsive people were to her greetings and that, on occasion, a brief conversation developed.

Session 9

For her third in-session exposure, the therapists decided to enact a similar situation to the session 7 exposure but to utilize a new role player with whom Sherri was unacquainted in order to make the situation more realistic. A research assistant who was approximately Sherri's age was recruited to role-play a man in a nightclub who starts a conversation with Sherri before asking her to dance. Sherri's primary automatic thought was "I'll be so self-conscious I won't be able to talk to him." This was identified as fortune telling (treating a future possibility as if it were already an established fact) and disqualifying the positive (discounting previous successes such as the numerous times she had demonstrated excellent conversation skills, even when experiencing significant anxiety) (Burns, 1980; Persons, 1989). With the group's help, Sherri was able to recognize that it was unlikely she would be unable to talk at all. Furthermore, the group pointed out that she had consistently experienced less anxiety in the actual situation than she anticipated beforehand.

Sherri's subjective anxiety was moderately high at the beginning of the conversation (SUDS = 65) but decreased somewhat over the next 5 minutes (50, 45, 40, 40, 40). She exceeded her behavioral goal of asking two questions by asking four questions of her conversation partner. Once again the group gave extensive positive feedback on her excellent conversation skills. The group concurred with the role player that the conversation had seemed realistic and typical of what would happen in such a setting. During the debriefing, Sherri asked the role player if she "looked okay." Since the role player was unaware of her concerns about her appearance, his genuine surprise that she would feel the need to ask such a question provided convincing evidence that she was overly concerned about her appearance.

For homework, the therapists sought an assignment that would allow Sherri to continue to receive evidence that her poor image of her physical appearance was unwarranted. Sherri did not have any social events in the next week, and she was not sure any of her coworkers would be available to go some place where there would be dancing. Consequently, the therapists explored other possible situations that would evoke Sherri's thoughts about her appearance. Sherri indicated that she ran for exercise several times a week, and that she usually did so after dark or some place with few people because she was anxious about being seen by others. Sherri agreed to run in her neighborhood during daylight hours. Once again the therapists emphasized the importance of challenging her automatic thoughts before going out to run using the procedures learned in group. The subsequent week Sherri reported that she was less anxious each time she went out and that she was beginning to believe that she must not look "too fat or stupid" because people who saw her seemed to pay only passing attention. Sherri also reported continued success that week with the daily assignment to greet people.

Session 10

Sherri was not scheduled for an in-session exposure in the 10th session. For homework, she agreed to continue running in daylight hours and to continue the daily greetings. She had attended the adult singles group at the church a couple of times and was thinking about attending an upcoming social outing with that group. She agreed to make the appropriate calls to get the details on the outing so she could attend later in the month. She successfully completed all three assignments.

Sessions 11 and 12

Sherri was unexpectedly out of town and missed session 11. Although she had participated in only three in-session exposures, she had made substantial progress toward her treatment goals. Therefore, the therapists decided to have Sherri participate in a group exercise that was relevant to all of the members rather than complete another individual exposure in the final session of group. The exercise involved having group members take turns complimenting each other while the person receiving the compliment writes it on the easel using the first person. The person receiving the compliment must thank the speaker without disqualifying the compliment. For example, one group member said that she thought Sherri genuinely cared about other people. Sherri wrote "I genuinely care about others" on the easel. This exercise served three purposes. First, as part of disengaging from the group process, it gave group members an opportunity to express appreciation for help they had received from other members. Second, writing the compliments in the first person forced the group members to cognitively process positive information about themselves that was likely to be inconsistent with the negative self-schema with which they started the group. Third, since group members took the sheets of paper home with them, they had powerful evidence to challenge negative self-appraisals that may have arisen in future cognitive restructuring that they continued on their own.

    Sherri received numerous compliments about her interpersonal style and courage in facing her fears as well as appreciation for things she had said that had been helpful to another group member. As is often the case for this exercise, two group members took the opportunity to compliment an aspect of her physical appearance, knowing that such statements would be particularly important to Sherri.

The remainder of session 12 was devoted to discussing how to consolidate and further treatment gains, followed by a social time with cake and soft drinks to allow group members to say good-byes.

Evaluation of Treatment Efficacy

Following the final session of CBGT, group members usually meet individually with one of the cotherapists for a final discussion of progress in group and consideration of the need for further treatment. Sherri readily agreed with the therapists that further treatment was not warranted, although she would need to continue to work on her own. When asked to rate on a 0–4 scale how much the social phobia interfered with her functioning, Sherri rated herself a 1, indicating mildly distressed but not at all disabled. Note that prior to treatment, Sherri rated herself a 4 on this scale. Sherri reported to the therapists that she believed her social fears had reduced considerably over the course of therapy. She spoke at length about how the reduction in self-consciousness about her appearance had improved her day-to-day life. For example, she enjoyed being able to leave her house for activities such as grocery shopping without excessive concern over her hair, clothing, and makeup. Her increased comfort in daily interactions with coworkers made work less stressful, allowed her to get involved in a wider variety of duties, and caused other staff to see her as friendlier and more open. In fact, several people who did not know she had been in treatment commented to Sherri that she seemed "different." As will be seen below, this subjective self-report is supported by improvement on more objective measures, although improvement on the latter is surprisingly less dramatic.

An abbreviated version of Sherri's fear and avoidance hierarchy appears in Table 16.3. Each hierarchy item was rated on three 0–100 scales—fear, behavioral avoidance, and fear of negative evaluation by others. The hierarchy was completed and initial ratings made prior to the first session. Posttreatment ratings were obtained in the individual follow-up appointment with one of the therapists after session 12. The pretreatment ratings were not available to Sherri or the therapist when the posttreatment ratings were completed. Examination of the ratings revealed meaningful reductions on all three scales across the six items. However, some particularly difficult situations such as a first date and attending a large party with unfamiliar people continued to generate significant fear. Two of the three situations demonstrating the most dramatic change were ones addressed directly with role-played and *in vivo* exposures—conversations with potential dating partners and with other strangers. It is notable that the third situation in which

TABLE 16.3. Selected Items from Sherri's Fear and Avoidance Hierarchy:
Pretreatment and Posttreatment Ratings

Situation	Assessment point	Fear	Avoidance	Evaluation
Conversation with an unfamiliar	Pretreatment	95	100	100
attractive man	Posttreatment	40	50	60
First date with someone	Pretreatment	90	50	98
	Posttreatment	80	55	80
Having a new hair stylist at	Pretreatment	70	90	92
the beauty shop	Posttreatment	30	50	75
Attending a large party with	Pretreatment	85	75	75
mostly unfamiliar people	Posttreatment	70	50	50
Talking with a stranger — not	Pretreatment	50	55	55
potential dating partner	Posttreatment	5	30	20
Being on a date other than	Pretreatment	50	50	40
the first one	Posttreatment	25	10	20

Note. Ratings are of fear, avoidance, and fear of negative evaluation by others. All ratings are
on 0–100 scales with higher numbers signifying greater fear or more extensive avoidance.

fear and avoidance decreased substantially, going to a new hair stylist, was
never discussed in group. This situation is often particularly difficult for
social phobics such as Sherri who are excessively self-conscious about their
physical appearance. Improvement in this situation demonstrates generalization to nontarget situations as well as probable change in her core irrational belief about the unacceptability of her physical appearance.

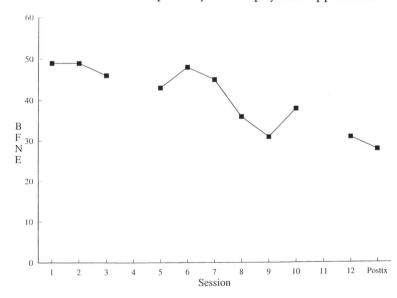

FIGURE 16.2. Session-by-session Brief Fear of Negative Evaluation Scale scores for Sherri.

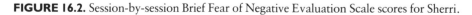

The second objective measure available to evaluate the success of Sherri's treatment is session-by-session Brief Fear of Negative Evaluation Scale (BFNE; Leary, 1983) scores. The BFNE is a 12-item version of the Watson and Friend (1969) FNE scale discussed earlier in the chapter. The BFNE uses a 5-point response format with possible scores ranging from 12 to 60. For the purposes of ongoing assessment in CBGT, the instructions were modified to ask clients to make ratings based on the previous week rather than how they generally feel. As shown in Figure 16.2, Sherri's BFNE score was 49 at the beginning of treatment and remained fairly stable until session 8 when it decreased significantly. Sherri's final BFNE score, 1 week after treatment during the posttreatment clinical interview, was 28. Change on the BFNE is particularly encouraging because previous research has suggested that improvement on the original FNE is associated with positive long-term treatment outcome for social phobics (Mattick & Peters, 1988; Mattick et al., 1989).

CONCLUSION

Our understanding of social phobia has grown considerably since it was first recognized officially in 1980 (DSM-III, American Psychiatric Association, 1980). The negative self-statements and biased attentional processes predicted by Beck and Emery's (1985) cognitive model of social phobia have been substantiated by research. A growing literature clearly demonstrates that CBT is an effective treatment for social phobia leading to decreases in social anxiety and avoidance, in fear of negative evaluation, and in laboratory and self-report cognitive measures. Despite arguments that the strong cognitive features of social phobia make it especially well suited to CBT (Butler, 1985), CBT has rarely been found to be more effective than other active treatments. Such differences as exist are more likely to surface at follow-up. On the other hand, CBT was clearly not less effective than other beneficial therapies and may be more readily applied to social phobia than exposure (see Butler, 1985).

Relatively few investigators have employed reliable and valid measures for cognitive assessment. However, the data extant indicate that change on cognitive measures is related to improvement with treatment. We encourage researchers in this area to pay closer attention to cognitive assessment and particularly to include laboratory-based measures of cognition in addition to self-report. Laboratory measures are less likely to be biased by a possible perceived demand to report rational thinking after treatment. Such experimental demand might be especially influential for CBT clients because of the particular emphasis placed on reducing negative thinking throughout treatment with this approach.

Continuing research on cognitive change in social phobia is important given the ample evidence for the importance of cognitive factors in the psychopathology of this disorder. It may well be that change in cognition is critical to treatment improvement, although CBT as currently practiced might not be the only way, or even a superior way, to effect that change (see Bandura, Adams, & Beyer, 1977). In addition, more attention needs to be paid to increasing the benefit clients receive from CBT. Although CBT is effective, a substantial number of clients fail to achieve normal levels of functioning after treatment (see Chambless et al., 1993; Lucas & Telch, 1993).

ACKNOWLEDGMENTS

We wish to thank Marty Gillis for her assistance with the meta-analytic summary, Gillian Butler and James Herbert for providing data for the meta-analysis, and Aaron T. Beck for his valuable comments. This chapter was prepared while Dr. Chambless was a visiting professor at the Center for Psychotherapy Research at the University of Pennsylvania. She acknowledges the Center's support with gratitude.

NOTES

1. Whether McNeil et al. (1995) followed this same procedure is difficult to discern from their report, although it is clear that they used lists of words, rather than individual words, on the computer screen.

2. Heimberg, Becker, Goldfinger, and Vermilyea (1985) conducted their study according to a multiple baseline across subjects design. Unfortunately, because their subjects' baselines were often descending or unstable before the clients started treatment, it is difficult to ascribe improvements clearly to treatment as opposed to the effects of repeated measurement. Accordingly, we have included their pretest–posttest data in the meta-analysis as an uncontrolled study but do not consider their work in this section. Further, we have not discussed waiting-list comparisons reported by Mattick et al. (1989) and by Scholing and Emmelkamp (1993a, 1993b), although their data are included in Figure 16.1. In their statistical analysis, these authors combined several treatment groups, only one of which was CBT, for comparison with the waiting-list group.

3. In this study, as in some others, clients were categorized according to their type of fear reaction, typically in response to an exposure to the feared stimulus, for example, a staged social interaction. Subjects who showed a marked heart rate response but little evidence of negative thinking were labeled physiological reactors, whereas those with little heart rate increase but a high rate of negative thinking were labeled cognitive reactors. Other categorizations are possible. For example, in a study to be described later, Mersch, Emmelkamp, Bogels, and van der Sleen (1989) compared cognitive reactors to behavioral reactors, with the latter defined as demonstrating relatively poor social skills on eight brief staged social interactions.

4. Strictly speaking, CBT + placebo is not the same as CBT. As has been cogently discussed by Hollon and DeRubeis (1981), for various reasons CBT + placebo may well be less effective than CBT alone.

5. Note that such a hypothesis does not necessarily follow from cognitive theory. Rather, cognitive theory would predict that it is crucial to change maladaptive cognitions, but that various interventions (even pharmacotherapy) might be used to achieve this goal (Beck, personal communication, October 5, 1994).

REFERENCES

American Psychiatric Association. (1980). *Diagnostic and statistical manual of mental disorders* (3rd ed.). Washington, DC: Author.

American Psychiatric Association. (1987). *Diagnostic and statistical manual of mental disorders* (3rd ed., rev.). Washington, DC: Author.

Asmundson, G. J. G., & Stein, M. B. (1994). Selective processing of social threat in patients with generalized social phobia: Evaluation using a dot-probe paradigm. *Journal of Anxiety Disorders, 8,* 107–117.

Bandura, A., Adams, N. E., & Beyer, J. (1977). Cognitive processes mediating behavioral change. *Journal of Personality and Social Psychology, 35,* 125–139.

Baron, R. M., & Kenny, D. A. (1986). The moderator–mediator variable distinction in social psychological research: Conceptual, strategic, and statistical considerations. *Journal of Personality and Social Psychology, 51,* 1173–1182.

Beck, A. T., & Emery, G. (1985). *Anxiety disorders and phobias: A cognitive perspective.* New York: Basic Books.

Becker, E., Rinck, M., & Margraf, J. (1994). Memory bias in panic disorder. *Journal of Abnormal Psychology, 103,* 396–399.

Biran, M., Augusto, F., & Wilson, G. T. (1981). In vivo exposure vs. cognitive restructuring in the treatment of scriptophobia. *Behaviour Research and Therapy, 19,* 525–532.

Brown, E. J., Heimberg, R. G., & Juster, H. R. (1995). Social phobia subtype and avoidant personality disorder: Effect on severity of social phobia, impairment, and outcome of cognitive-behavioral treatment. *Behavior Therapy, 26,* 467–486.

Bruch, M. A., Heimberg, R. G., & Hope, D. A. (1991). States of Mind Model and cognitive change in treated social phobics. *Cognitive Therapy and Research, 15,* 429–441.

Burns, D. D. (1980). *Feeling good: The new mood therapy.* New York: Morrow.

Butler, G. (1985). Exposure as a treatment for social phobia: Some instructive difficulties. *Behaviour Research and Therapy, 23,* 651–657.

Butler, G., Cullington, A., Munby, M., Amies, P., & Gelder, M. (1984). Exposure and anxiety management in the treatment of social phobia. *Journal of Consulting and Clinical Psychology, 52,* 642–650.

Chambless, D. L., & Gillis, M. M. (1993). Cognitive therapy of anxiety disorders. *Journal of Consulting and Clinical Psychology, 61,* 248–260.

Chambless, D. L., Glass, C. R., & Tran, G. Q. (1993, November). Effects of avoidant personality and subtype on outcome of cognitive-behavioral treatment of social phobia. In D. Chambless (Chair), *Social phobia and avoidant personality disorder.* Symposium presented at the annual meeting of the Association for Advancement of Behavior Therapy, Atlanta.

Clark, D. B., & Agras, W. S. (1991). The assessment and treatment of performance anxiety in musicians. *American Journal of Psychiatry, 148,* 598–605.

Cloitre, M., Heimberg, R. G., Holt, C. S., & Liebowitz, M. R. (1992). Reaction time to threat stimuli in panic disorder and social phobia. *Behaviour Research and Therapy, 30,* 609–617.

Dalgleish, T., & Watts, F. N. (1990). Biases of attention and memory in disorders of anxiety and depression. *Clinical Psychology Review, 10,* 589–604.

DiNardo, P. A., & Barlow, D. H. (1988). *The Anxiety Disorders Interview Schedule–Revised.* Albany, NY: Graywind Publications.

Dodge, C. S., Hope, D. A., Heimberg, R. G., & Becker, R. E. (1988). Evaluation of the Social Interaction Self-Statement Test with a social phobic population. *Cognitive Therapy and Research, 12,* 211–222.

Ellis, A. (1962). *Reason and emotion in psychotherapy.* New York: Lyle Stuart.

Emmelkamp, P. M. G., Mersch, P.-P., Vissia, E., & van der Helm, M. (1985). Social phobia: A comparative evaluation of cognitive and behavioural interventions. *Behaviour Research and Therapy, 23,* 365–369.

Feske, U., Perry, K. J., Chambless, D. L., Renneberg, B., & Goldstein, A. J. (in press). Avoidant personality disorder as a predictor of treatment outcome among generalized social phobics. *Journal of Personality Disorders.*

Gelernter, C. S., Uhde, T. W., Cimbolic, P., Arnkoff, D. B., Vittone, B. J., Tancer, M. E., & Bartko, J. J. (1991). Cognitive-behavioral and pharmacological treatments for social phobia: A controlled study. *Archives of General Psychiatry, 48,* 938–945.

Glass, C. R., & Arnkoff, D. B. (1993). Validity issues in self-statement measures of social phobia and social anxiety. *Behaviour Research and Therapy, 32,* 255–267.

Glass, C. R., Merluzzi, T. V., Biever, J. L., & Larsen, K. H. (1982). Cognitive assessment of social anxiety: Development and validation of a self-statement questionnaire. *Cognitive Therapy and Research, 6,* 37–55.

Heimberg, R. G. (1991). *Cognitive-behavioral treatment of social phobia in a group setting: A treatment manual.* Unpublished manuscript, Department of Psychology, State University of New York at Albany.

Heimberg, R. G., & Becker, R. E. (1984). *Cognitive-behavioral treatment of social phobia in a group setting: A treatment manual.* Unpublished manuscript, Department of Psychology, State University of New York at Albany.

Heimberg, R. G., Becker, R. E., Goldfinger, K., & Vermilyea, J. A. (1985). Treatment of social phobia by exposure, cognitive restructuring, and homework assignments. *Journal of Nervous and Mental Disease, 173,* 236–245.

Heimberg, R. G., Bruch, M. A., Hope, D. A., & Dombeck, M. (1990). Evaluating the States of Mind Model: Comparison to an alternative model and effects of method of cognitive assessment. *Cognitive Therapy and Research, 14,* 543–557.

Heimberg, R. G., Dodge, C. S., Hope, D. A., Kennedy, C. R., Zollo, L. J., & Becker, R. E. (1990). Cognitive behavioral group treatment for social phobia: Comparison with a credible placebo control. *Cognitive Therapy and Research, 14,* 1–23.

Heimberg, R. S., Hope, D. A., Dodge, C. S., & Becker, R. E. (1990). DSM-III-R subtypes of social phobia: Comparison of generalized and public speaking phobics. *Journal of Nervous and Mental Disease, 178,* 172–179.

Heimberg, R. G., Salzman, D. G., Holt, C. S., & Blendall, K. (1993). Cognitive behavioral group treatment for social phobia: Effectiveness at five-year follow-up. *Cognitive Therapy and Research, 17,* 325–339.

Herbert, J. D., Hope, D. A., & Bellack, A. S. (1992). Validity of the distinction between generalized social phobia and avoidant personality disorder. *Journal of Abnormal Psychology, 101,* 332–339.

Hollon, S. D., & DeRubeis, R. J. (1981). Placebo–psychotherapy combinations: Inappropriate representations of psychotherapy in drug–psychotherapy comparative trials. *Psychological Bulletin, 90,* 467–477.

Hope, D. A. (1989). *Cognitive-behavioral group treatment for social phobia: How important is the cognitive component?* Unpublished doctoral dissertation, Department of Psychology, State University of New York at Albany.

Hope, D. A. (1993). Conducting exposure-based treatments with social phobics. *the Behavior Therapist, 16,* 7–12.

Hope, D. A., & Heimberg, R. G. (1993). Social phobia and social anxiety. In D. H. Barlow (Ed.), *Clinical handbook of psychological disorders: A step-by-step treatment manual* (2nd ed., pp. 99–136). New York: Guilford Press.

Hope, D. A., Herbert, J. D., & White, C. (1995). Diagnostic subtype, avoidant personality disorder, and efficacy of cognitive behavioral group therapy for social phobia. *Cognitive Therapy and Research, 9,* 399–419.

Hope, D. A., Rapee, R. M., Heimberg, R. G., & Dombeck, M. J. (1990). Representations of the self in social phobia: Vulnerability to social threat. *Cognitive Therapy and Research, 14,* 177–189.

Jacobson, N. S., & Truax, P. (1991). Clinical significance: A statistical approach to defining meaningful change in psychotherapy research. *Journal of Consulting and Clinical Psychology, 59,* 12–19.

Jerremalm, A., Jansson, L., & Öst, L.-G. (1986). Cognitive and physiological reactivity and the effects of different behavioral methods in the treatment of social phobia. *Behaviour Research and Therapy, 24,* 171–180.

Jones, R. G. (1969). A factored measure of Ellis' irrational belief system, with personality and adjustment correlates *Dissertation Abstracts International, 29,* 4379B–4380B.

Leary, M. R. (1988). A brief version of the Fear of Negative Evaluation Scale. *Personality and Social Psychology Bulletin, 9,* 371–375.

Lucas, R. A., & Telch, M. J. (1993, November). *Group versus individual treatment of social phobia.* Paper presented at the meeting of the Association for Advancement of Behavior Therapy, Atlanta.

Lucock, M. P., & Salkovskis, P. M. (1988). Cognitive factors in social anxiety and its treatment. *Behaviour Research and Therapy, 26,* 297–302.

MacLeod, C., Mathews, A. M., & Tata, P. (1986). Attentional bias in emotional disorders. *Journal of Abnormal Psychology, 95,* 15–20.

Mattia, J. L., Heimberg, R. G., & Hope, D. A. (1993). The revised Stroop colournaming task in social phobics. *Behaviour Research and Therapy, 31,* 305–313.

Mattick, R. P., & Peters, L. (1988). Treatment of severe social phobia: Effects of guided exposure with and without cognitive restructuring. *Journal of Consulting and Clinical Psychology, 56,* 251–260.

Mattick, R. P., Peters, L., & Clarke, J. C. (1989). Exposure and cognitive restructuring for social phobia: A controlled study. *Behavior Therapy, 20,* 3–23.

McNeil, D. W., Ries, B. J., Taylor, L. J., Boone, M. L., Carter, L. E., Turk, C. L., & Lewin, M. R. (1995). Comparison of social phobia subtypes using Stroop tests. *Journal of Anxiety Disorders, 9,* 47–57.

Meichenbaum, D. (1975). Self-instructional methods. In F. H. Kanfer & A. P. Goldstein (Eds.), *Helping people change* (pp. 357–391). Elmsford, NY: Pergamon Press.

Mersh, P. P. A., Emmelkamp, P. M. G., Bogels, S. M., & van der Sleen, J. (1989). Social phobia: Individual response patterns and the effects of behavioural and cognitive interventions. *Behaviour Research and Therapy, 27,* 421–434.

Persons, J. B. (1989). *Cognitive therapy in practice: A case formulation approach.* New York: W. W. Norton.

Rapee, R. M., & Lim, L. (1992). Discrepancy between self- and observer ratings of performance in social phobics. *Journal of Abnormal Psychology, 101,* 728–731.

Rapee, R. M., McCallum, S. L., Melville, L. F., Ravenscroft, H., & Rodney, J. M. (1994). Memory bias in social phobia. *Behaviour Research and Therapy, 32,* 89–99.

Schneier, F. R., Johnson, J., Hornig, C. D., Liebowitz, M. R., & Weissman, M. M. (1992). Social phobia: Comorbidity and morbidity in an epidemiologic sample. *Archives of General Psychiatry, 49,* 282–288.

Scholing, A., & Emmelkamp, P. M. G. (1993a). Cognitive and behavioural treatments of fear of blushing, sweating or trembling. *Behaviour Research and Therapy, 31,* 155–170.

Scholing, A., & Emmelkamp, P. M. G. (1993b). Exposure with and without cognitive therapy for generalized social phobia: Effects of individual and group treatment. *Behaviour Research and Therapy, 31,* 667–681.

Schwartz, R. M., & Garamoni, G. L. (1989). Cognitive balance and psychopathology: Evaluation of an information processing model of positive and negative states of mind. *Clinical Psychology Review, 9,* 271–294.

Shorkey, C. T., & Whiteman, V. L. (1977). Development of the Rational Behavior Inventory: Initial validity and reliability. *Educational and Psychological Measurement, 37,* 527–534.

Smith, M. L., & Glass, G. V. (1977). Meta-analysis of psychotherapy outcome studies. *American Psychologist, 32,* 752–760.

Smith, T. W., & Zurawski, R. M. (1983). Assessment of irrational beliefs: The question of discriminant validity. *Journal of Clinical Psychology, 39,* 976–979.

Stopa, L., & Clark, D. M. (1993). Cognitive processes in social phobia. *Behaviour Research and Therapy, 31,* 255–267.

Strauman, T. J. (1989). Self-discrepancies in clinical depression and social phobia: Cognitive structures that underlie emotional disorders? *Journal of Abnormal Psychology, 98,* 14–22.

Stravynski, A. (1983). Behavioral treatment of psychogenic vomiting in the context of social phobia. *Journal of Nervous and Mental Disease, 171,* 448–451.

Stravynski, A., Marks, I., & Yule, W. (1982). Social skills problems in neurotic outpatients. *Archives of General Psychiatry, 39,* 1378–1385.

Suinn, R. M., & Richardson, F. (1971). Anxiety management training: A nonspecific behavior therapy program for anxiety control. *Behavior Therapy, 2,* 498–510.

Tran, G .Q., & Chambless, D. L. (1995). Psychopathology of social phobia: Effects of subtype and of avoidant personality disorder. *Journal of Anxiety Disorders, 6,* 489–501.

Turner, S. M., & Beidel, D. C. (1989). Social phobia: Clinical syndrome, diagnosis, and comorbidity. *Clinical Psychology Review, 9,* 3–18.

Turner, S. M., Beidel, D. C., & Larkin, K. T. (1986). Situational determinants of social anxiety in clinic and nonclinic samples: Physiological and cognitive correlates. *Journal of Consulting and Clinical Psychology, 54,* 523–527.

Watson, D., & Friend, R. (1969). Measurement of social–evaluative anxiety. *Journal of Consulting and Clinical Psychology, 33,* 448–456.

Chapter 17

The Current Status
of Cognitive-Behavioral Models
# of Anorexia Nervosa
and Bulimia Nervosa

Kelly M. Vitousek

Models based on Beck's insights about psychopathology and therapy were proposed independently and almost simultaneously for bulimia nervosa (Fairburn, 1981) and anorexia nervosa (Garner & Bemis, 1982). These observers were certainly not the first to comment on the prominence of distorted beliefs in the eating disorders (e.g., Bruch, 1973, 1978; Crisp & Fransella, 1972; Russell, 1979; Selvini-Palazzoli, 1971; Ushakov, 1971), but they presented the first systematic cognitive-behavioral analyses of anorexic and bulimic psychopathology and described comprehensive treatment programs derived from these accounts.

In the 15 years that have elapsed since the models were detailed, both have had a pervasive influence on clinical practice in the eating disorder field. Surveys of psychologists and physicians attending international eating disorder conferences in 1988 and 1990 indicated that between 88% and 92% of respondents considered cognitive-behavioral treatment, either alone or in combination with psychodynamic treatment, to be indicated for anorexic patients, while 85% to 94% concurred with reference to bulimics (Herzog, Keller, Strober, Yeh, & Pai, 1992). These apparently equivalent levels of acceptance do not reflect the empirical status of the two applications: Cognitive-behavioral therapy for bulimia nervosa has garnered extensive support through controlled treatment trials, while the efficacy of the corresponding approach to anorexia nervosa has yet to be established.

Both approaches have also exerted major effects on the direction of research on the psychopathology of the eating disorders. The dominant cognitive-behavioral emphasis has influenced successive revisions of diagnostic criteria for bulimia nervosa (American Psychiatric Association, 1987) and anorexia nervosa (American Psychiatric Association, 1994), and is strongly represented in the most widely used assessment devices (Z. Cooper & Fairburn, 1987; Garner, Olmsted, & Polivy, 1983). Most recently, the models have generated a series of basic research studies on information processing in the eating disorders (Vitousek & Hollon, 1990).

STATUS OF THE THEORETICAL MODELS

Reduced to its essence, the cognitive-behavioral model holds that anorexic and bulimic symptoms are maintained by a characteristic set of overvalued ideas about the personal implications of body shape and weight. These attitudes have their origins in the interaction of stable individual characteristics (such as perfectionism, asceticism, and difficulties in affect regulation) with sociocultural ideals for female appearance. Once formed, the beliefs influence the individuals who hold them to engage in stereotypic eating and elimination behaviors, to be responsive to eccentric reinforcement contingencies, to process information in accordance with predictable cognitive biases, and, eventually, to be affected by physiological sequelae that also serve to sustain disordered beliefs and behaviors.

A detailed explication of the hypothesized elements and their interactions is far beyond the scope of this chapter. The comprehensive cognitive model of anorexia nervosa is outlined in Garner and Bemis (1982, 1985) and Garner (1986a); cognitive-behavioral theories of bulimia nervosa are discussed in Fairburn, Cooper, and Cooper (1986), Garner (1986b), and Wilson (1989). For extended considerations of specific components, the reader is referred to Vitousek and Ewald (1993) on individual variables; to Garner, Garfinkel, and Olmsted (1983) and Stice (1994) on sociocultural influences; to Casper and Davis (1977) on precipitating stressors; to Slade (1982) and Bemis (1983) on positive and negative reinforcement; to Vitousek and Ewald (1993) and Vitousek and Orimoto (1993) on the functional bases for eating disordered behavior; to Vitousek and Hollon (1990) on schematic processing; and to Garner, Rockert, Olmsted, Johnson, and Coscina (1985), Kaplan and Garfinkel (1993), Laessle, Schweiger, and Pirke (1988), and Wilson (1991) on the physical and psychological effects of dieting, purging, and semistarvation.

Many of the initiating and maintaining variables identified in these multidimensional causal models are in no sense distinctively "cognitive-behavioral" in that they would be endorsed by virtually all contemporary accounts of the etiology of these conditions. The most distinctive features of cognitive-behavioral theories are their emphases on the status of beliefs and values about weight as the central and primary psychopathological elements, and on the automatic (and functional) influence of biased information processing on the perceptions, thoughts, affect, and behavior of affected individuals. Cognitive theorists must assume the responsibility of examining whether these specific postulates make an incremental contribution to the understanding, prediction, and resolution of eating disorder phenomena.

Cognitive-behavioral models have tended to stress the close correspondence between the belief systems of anorexics and bulimics (Fairburn & Garner, 1988), suggesting that the superficially dissimilar symptom patterns these patients manifest are all traceable to an excessive reliance on weight and shape as bases for self-evaluation. The assumption of uniformity in core psychopathology is supported by the strong resemblance between these groups on attitudinal inventories, and is consistent with the observation that individual subjects frequently qualify for both diagnoses, either simultaneously or successively (Vandereycken & Pierloot, 1983). It is possible that the symptoms demarcating the boundaries between these groups, including the attainment of subnormal weight status and the presence or absence of binge eating episodes, result from independent variables that are unrelated to the common cluster of weight-related beliefs, such as biological intolerance for hunger or displacement below setpoint weight.

Alternatively, it may be that differences between eating disorder subtypes are also represented on the level of cognitive schemas about weight. For example, Vitousek and Hollon (1990) speculate that anorexics may be distinguished by a preference for simplicity, certainty, and a "New Year's resolution" cognitive style. Individuals with these characteristics may be particularly likely to welcome the emergence and eventual dominance of monolithic cognitive structures about weight precisely *because* of their potent schematic properties—their power to reduce ambiguity, facilitate judgments and predictions, and provide an inclusive set of premises from which specific rules can be deduced. Bulimics may be primarily responsive to the perceived social contingencies for thinness and fatness, while anorexics construct more complex associative networks linking weight status to a wider range of intrinsically reinforcing states (Vitousek, Orimoto, & Ewald, 1995). The greater heterogeneity in background variables, personality features, and general adjustment associated with bulimia nervosa may also correspond to a greater diversity in the motives for and functions of eating disordered behavior within this subgroup (Vitousek & Manke, 1994).

Assessment of Self-Statements and Beliefs

Abundant evidence indicates that subjects with concerns about eating and weight differ from others in the tendency to endorse items on measures of irrational beliefs, depressogenic attributional styles, and processing errors (e.g., Fremouw & Heyneman, 1983; Goebel, Spalthoff, Schulze, & Florin, 1989; Poulakis & Wertheim, 1993; Ruderman, 1986; Schlesier-Carter, Hamilton, O'Neil, Lydiard, & Malcolm, 1989; Steiger, Fraenkel, & Leichner, 1989; Steiger, Goldstein, Mongrain, & Van der Feen, 1990; Strauss & Ryan, 1988). Because of the extremely high rates of comorbidity between the eating disorders and the depressive and anxiety disorders, however, these data do little more than reconfirm Beck's most basic observations about the relationship between psychopathology and distorted thinking styles (Beck, 1976). Cognitive models of anorexia nervosa and bulimia nervosa must be supported by evidence that individuals with these disorders hold distinctive beliefs in the domains of weight, shape, and food, and are particularly prone to reasoning errors in these content domains.

Both attitudinal inventories and interview schedules confirm that clinical subjects differ from normal controls (and, typically, from obese, restrained, and dieting controls) in the stated drive for thinness and concern for body shape and weight (e.g., Z. Cooper & Fairburn, 1987; Garner, Olmsted, & Polivy, 1983). The most sensitive instrument for assessing the complex specific psychopathology of anorexia and bulimia nervosa is a semistructured interview schedule, the Eating Disorder Examination, which yields individual profiles on five key elements: Bulimia, Restraint, Eating Concern, Shape Concern, and Weight Concern (Z. Cooper, Cooper, & Fairburn, 1989; Z. Cooper & Fairburn, 1987; Fairburn & Cooper, 1993; Rosen, Vara, Wendt, & Leitenberg, 1990; Wilson & Smith, 1989).

Self-statement inventories have also verified that anorexics and bulimics espouse characteristic irrational ideas about the magical properties of food and the implications of body weight. In the initial cognitive model of anorexia nervosa, Garner and Bemis (1982) speculated that after symptom onset a host of derivative beliefs emerge from the central anorexic premise about the importance of thinness: for example, that self-control in diverse areas is predicated on the control of eating and weight; that small increments in weight will progress inexorably to obesity; that ingested sugar will be converted instantly into stored fat; that vomiting and laxative-induced diarrhea purify the body. Self-statement inventories composed of similar items have been found to differentiate bulimics and/or anorexics from normal controls (e.g., Clark, Feldman, & Channon, 1989; Dritschel, Williams, & Cooper, 1991; Franko & Zuroff, 1992; Goldberg et al., 1980; Mizes, 1990; Mizes & Klesges, 1989; Phelan, 1987; Scanlon, Ollendick, & Bayer, 1986; Schulman, Kinder, Gleghorn, Powers, & Prange, 1986; Thompson, Berg, & Shatford, 1987). Some have additionally been demonstrated to decrease over the course of treatment, predict response to treatment, and correlate with other indices of eating disorder symptomatology (for a review, see Mizes & Christiano, 1995).

Numerous investigations have been conducted to examine relationships between daily events, hunger, affect, and cognition across the binge–purge cycle in bulimia nervosa. In most of these studies, subjects have been instructed to self-monitor the targeted variables in naturalistic settings, either upon occurrence, at fixed time intervals, or in response to signals from a paging device (P. Cooper & Bowskill, 1986; Davis, Freeman, & Solyom, 1985; Davis, Freeman, & Garner, 1988; Elmore & de Castro, 1990; Johnson & Larson, 1982; Lingswiler, Crowther, & Stevens, 1987, 1989; Rebert, Stanton, & Schwarz, 1991; Schlundt, Johnson, & Jarrell, 1985; Zotter

& Crowther, 1991). A few have collected responses during laboratory eating sessions (Chiodo & Latimer, 1986; Kaye, Gwirtsman, George, Weiss, & Jimerson, 1986; Williamson, Kelley, Davis, Ruggiero, & Veitia, 1985). Other studies have asked subjects to characterize their bulimic episodes retrospectively (J. Cooper et al., 1988; Hsu, 1990; Steinberg, Tobin, & Johnson, 1990).

Such investigations have confirmed that negative mood states tend to precede the binge–purge cycle; some report a decrease in anxiety and/or anger but typically not in depression following completion of the episode. Regrettably, most of these studies have emphasized affective ratings; few have collected or analyzed this potentially rich source of self-statement data in informative ways. In Hsu's (1990) questionnaire study, bulimics indicated that dichotomous self-statements such as "Now that I've done it, I might as well go all the way" frequently preceded binge episodes. Other common themes included self-condemnation, bewilderment at loss of control, and resolutions to "be good" tomorrow. The self-monitoring study conducted by Lingswiler et al. (1989) also found that dichotomous cognitions were reported prior to eating episodes by both bulimic and binge-eating subjects. Using a different methodology, Zotter and Crowther (1991) obtained few instances of dichotomous thinking, but found that bulimics were more likely than normal or dieting controls to record negatively toned and distorted cognitions about food and weight.

Although recent attempts to assess cognitive content in anorexia and bulimia nervosa are encouraging, progress has been hampered by the failure to address a number of critical methodological and conceptual issues. Self-report may be particularly vulnerable to bias and distortion with this population for a number of reasons (Vitousek, Daly, & Heiser, 1991). Because anorexics are typically invested in preserving their egosyntonic symptomatology, they may deliberately falsify information as part of a defensive stance; paradoxically, a tendency to overcompliance may also influence anorexics to conform to the subtly communicated biases of therapists or researchers. Finally, the capacity to give an accurate account of private experience may be further restricted by the effects of starvation, which can contribute to a diminished capacity for abstraction and general impoverishment of thought content.

Another problem concerns the inadequate conceptualization of theoretical issues in most cognitive assessment research within this domain. Self-statement measures are typically heterogeneous compilations of the kinds of peculiar ideas anorexic and bulimic clients verbalize in psychotherapy; rarely are inventories designed to test hypotheses about specific aspects of the cognitive model. Rather than using this scattershot approach to scale development, it might prove more informative to derive items from an organized model that specifies the perceptions, evaluations, attributions, and expectations theoretically crucial to the maintenance of these syndromes (Vitousek & Orimoto, 1993).

Finally, it should be noted that the assessment of self-statements about eating and weight has marked limitations as a means of testing the comprehensive cognitive model. No controversy surrounds the proposition that the thought *content* of subjects who worry about eating and weight is distinguishable from the thought content of subjects who are indifferent to such matters (Vitousek & Hollon, 1990). Ultimately, however, we need to learn not simply what our clients think *about*, but what causes them to formulate their erroneous ideas, how such beliefs affect their experience of the world, and why they become extraordinarily resistant to efforts to persuade them to think anything else.

Assessment of Schematic Processing

Cognitive processing paradigms offer distinct advantages in the study of the eating disorders. Because they often employ test strategies that subjects are unable to decode and use dependent variables that are difficult to falsify, they can minimize or eliminate the dependency on self-report. They can also help investigators move beyond cognitive content to explore the processes through which beliefs develop, proliferate, and become autonomous.

Vitousek and Hollon (1990) outlined 10 general strategies for the investigation of information processing in the eating disorders. They suggested that individuals with these conditions may differ from others in the following ways: (1) the ease and speed with which food- and weight-related stimuli are processed; (2) the elaboration of meaning around the construct of weight; (3) the intrusion of weight-related content into unrelated or ambiguous situations; (4) the possession of differentiated knowledge structures in connected domains; (5) an enhanced memory for schema-consistent information; (6) the ability to retrieve schema-relevant behavioral evidence; (7) the degree of confidence in judgments and predictions about food and weight; (8) the specific relevance of weight concerns for the self; (9) the level of cognitive and affective involvement in weight-related events; and (10) the resistance to counterschematic information.

In view of the prominence of cognitive constructs in dominant theories of anorexia and bulimia nervosa, surprisingly little research has been done on the nature and operation of domain-specific schemas (M. Cooper & Fairburn, 1992a; Mahamedi & Heatherton, 1993; Mizes & Christiano, 1995; Vitousek & Hollon, 1990). A sharp increase in activity over the past few years has yielded some data bearing on 5 of the 10 hypotheses outlined above, and many other information-processing studies are currently in progress or under review.

The most extensively researched parameter is the *speed of processing* of disorder-relevant content, studied almost exclusively through adaptations of the Stroop paradigm (Stroop, 1935). Presumably because of its considerable popularity in the general cognitive psychopathology field, the Stroop technique has been widely disseminated—and perhaps prematurely accepted—as a measure of the interference in information processing caused by schema-based conflict or anxiety.

The disorder-relevant stimuli used in these investigations have varied; most employ lists of both food- and weight- or shape-related words, sometimes segregated on separate cards and sometimes mixed together to form a single array. The conflict cards concerning food have included items such as "chocolate" and "cake"; typically, stimuli are matched for graphomorphemic features and frequency of word use to neutral words ("catalogue," "chat") that appear on a corresponding control card. Target cards concerning weight and shape include items such as "flabby" and "fat," which are paired with neutral words listed on a separate control card.

Almost all published studies have reported that anorexic and/or bulimic subjects (and sometimes restrained or dieting subjects) do manifest delayed response times when asked to name the ink colors of food- and/or weight-related word sets relative to normal subjects and relative to their own responses when neutral stimuli are presented (Ben-Tovim, Walker, Fok, & Yap, 1989; Ben-Tovim & Walker, 1991; Channon, Hemsley, & de Silva, 1988; M. Cooper, Anastasiades, & Fairburn, 1992; M. Cooper & Fairburn, 1992b; M. Cooper & Fairburn, 1993; Fairburn, Cooper, Cooper, McKenna, & Anastasiades, 1991; Green, McKenna, & de Silva, 1994; Long, Hinton, & Gillespie, 1994; Mahamedi & Heatherton, 1993; Perpina, Hemsley, Treasure, & de Silva, 1993; Wilson, 1989). The results appear to be strongest for food-related stimuli when these can be examined separately, with more equivocal results obtained for anorexics when weight-related words are presented (Ben-Tovim et al., 1989; Channon et al., 1988; Green et al., 1994; Perpina et al., 1993). Neither familiarity with the procedure (Walker, Ben-Tovim, Jones, & Bachok, 1992) nor variations in the order of card presentation (M. Cooper et al., 1992) appear to affect the magnitude of interference; however, habituation may occur to some target stimuli within the course of an assessment session (Green et al., 1994; Green & Rogers, 1993).

The theoretically preferred explanation of this effect would be that eating disordered subjects are manifesting an attentional bias toward threatening stimuli—perhaps, that the more elaborated fear structures associated with focal concerns require more cognitive processing capacity, and thus compete with the cognitive resources available for color naming (Foa, Feske, Murdock, Kozak, & McCarthy, 1991). It has been hoped that this effect might also prove useful for several clinical and research purposes. Since the absolute differences between pathological and control groups appear to be fairly modest and the overlap in distributions considerable, the test is unlikely to have diagnostic utility (Ben-Tovim et al., 1989); however, it might be valuable as an index of the degree of food/weight preoccupation that is not dependent on self-report. Some evidence indicates that disruptions in processing disappear with clinical recovery (Ben-Tovim et al., 1989; M. Cooper & Fairburn, 1994), although the technique does not appear to provide a means of examining the mechanisms of treatment, since alternative modalities do not produce differential effects on Stroop times at posttest (M. Cooper & Fairburn, 1994).

Unfortunately, it is not clear that this application of the Stroop task can yield the theoretical or clinical answers that investigators anticipated it could provide (Huon, 1995; Mizes & Christiano, 1995; Vitousek & Ewald, 1993; Vitousek & Orimoto, 1993). None of the studies with clinical samples reported to date has ruled out the possibility that hunger or chronic deprivation is the most parsimonious explanation for observed disruptions in processing, which, as noted above, are most marked for food-related stimuli. Channon and Hayward (1990) confirmed that normal subjects also show delayed processing times when the food Stroop is administered after a 24-hour period of fasting. Lavy and van den Hout (1993) also reported an attentional bias for food stimuli in fasting normal subjects relative to some but not all control stimulus sets. The investigators hypothesized that the computerized presentation of single items in their research minimized the effects of food-related rumination, which could have accounted for the stronger disruption effect in the card format used by Channon and Hayward (1990) and most other researchers in this area.

Green and Rogers (1993) found interference effects on both food and shape stimulus sets for restrained eaters and dieters. (Restrained eaters are identified within normal samples on the basis of cutoff scores or a median split on measures of dietary restraint, developed by Herman and Mack, 1975; Stunkard and Messick, 1985; and Van Strien, Frijters, Bergers, & Defares, 1986.) Overduin, Jansen, and Louwerse (1995) reported that restrained subjects recorded longer latencies to food but not shape stimuli relative to control words. M. Cooper and Fairburn (1992b) detected interference on a mixed array for dieters with a history of eating disorder symptoms but not for normal dieters.

Another relevant investigation has been described by Schmidt and Telch (1991) using a sample of restrained eaters. These subjects produced slower response times to food and body shape stimuli compared to unrestrained eaters; however, the use of a dietary preload yielded effects opposite to those hypothesized. It had been anticipated that the consumption of a milk shake by restrained subjects would result in an even greater delay in processing because of the increased salience of food and weight concerns. In fact, there was a trend toward *reduced* interference for both restrained and unrestrained subjects who received a preload. The investigators concluded that food consumption may have decreased response times to food words by alleviating hunger, noting that "from an evolutionary perspective, it makes sense for sated individuals to spend less of their attentional time on dietary stimuli."

Contradictory data on interference with and without dietary preloading of restrained subjects has been reported in other investigations. Several studies failed to find interference effects for food stimuli (Long et al., 1994; Mahamedi & Heatherton, 1993; Ogden & Greville, 1993) or shape stimuli

(Long et al., 1994; Mahamedi & Heatherton, 1993; Ogden & Greville, 1993; Overduin et al., 1995) for high-restraint subjects in the absence of a dietary preload. In fact, in two of these investigations, restrained subjects showed *decreased* latencies to food and/or shape stimuli relative to control stimuli (Long et al., 1994; Mahamedi & Heatherton, 1993). In one pair of studies, both unrestrained and restrained subjects who had consumed a milk shake showed more interference for shape words, with the effect especially pronounced for the restrained sample; neither showed interference for food stimuli (Mahamedi & Heatherton, 1993). Using a different Stroop procedure with similar stimuli, Ogden and Greville (1993) found interference to both food and shape words for restrained subjects given a high calorie preload. Overduin et al. (1995) found food interference but not shape interference for restrained subjects whether or not they received a small "appetizer" preload; unrestrained subjects showed interference for food stimuli only after receiving the preload.

The results of some of these studies suggest that, in the eating disorders, the Stroop task may indeed be assessing state-like salient concerns instead of or in addition to more stable attentional biases, just as temporary concerns about health evoked by the imminent prospect of surgery can produce Stroop response patterns similar to those obtained with anxiety disorder samples (Cook, Jones, & Johnston, 1989).

As the Stroop research on restrained eaters suggests, it is also unclear whether either food or weight interference effects measure any sort of core psychopathology specific to the clinical eating disorders. As noted above, food and/or shape interference is found in some investigations using subclinically symptomatic subjects or nonpreloaded restrained eaters (Green & Rogers, 1993; Overduin et al., 1995; Perpina et al., 1993; Schmidt & Telch, 1991; Wilson, 1989). Unselected normal control subjects display longer latencies to target words than to control words in some studies, even when the discrepancy is significantly less than that recorded for clinical subjects. In view of the prevalence of weight concern in contemporary society, Green and Rogers (1993) caution that there may be "an attentional bias toward eating and body shape-related matters among probably a substantial proportion of the non-eating-disordered female population" (p. 517). One study that assessed cross-sectional samples of 9- to 14-year-olds suggested that for girls interference to food stimuli begins at age 11 and to body stimuli at age 14, while remaining absent for boys throughout these developmental periods (Green & McKenna, 1993).

Some of the inconsistencies in the eating disorder Stroop data may be attributable to technical variations in materials, procedures, and analyses Huon, 1995). Many studies have presented cards in a fixed order, allowing for the possibility of practice or fatigue effects. Only a few research groups have assembled control stimuli from a common semantic category to parallel the single content areas from which target stimuli are selected (Green & McKenna, 1993; Green et al., 1994; Green & Rogers, 1993; Lavy & van den Hout, 1993; Overduin et al, 1995). Several have used computer technology that can permit the presentation of single stimuli to separate automatic attentional biases from postattentional ruminations and to allow the detection of fine-grained habituation effects (Green et al., 1994; Green & Rogers, 1993; Lavy & van den Hout, 1993; Overduin et al., 1995). The capacity to present stimuli individually also makes it possible to use priming strategies to assess whether constructs such as achievement and virtue are linked within organized cognitive structures to weight and shape concerns, as cognitive-behavioral models hypothesize (Orimoto, 1996). Unless future investigations are thoughtfully designed to examine specific hypotheses about the mechanisms underlying the disruption effect, it is questionable whether the Stroop paradigm will contribute substantially to the understanding of eating disorder psychopathology (Huon, 1995; Vitousek & Hollon, 1990).

Another processing paradigm has been used to examine whether domain-relevant stimuli interfere with the ease and speed with which subjects reallocate attention to nondominant response sets during the course of simple tasks (Newman et al., 1993). Compared to normal subjects, bulimics responded more slowly to peripherally presented task-relevant stimuli when these followed body-related words such as "scale" or "figure" (or affective words such as "sad" or "anxious") than when they appeared after neutral words; intermediate effects were obtained for symptomatic normal controls. The authors suggested that the motivationally significant stimuli disrupted subjects' capacity for control processing, extending the latency of shifts out of a dominant response set for centrally located material.

The second parameter listed by Vitousek and Hollon (1990) for examining weight-related self-schemas, the *elaboration of meaning,* is particularly crucial for cognitive models of the eating disorders. The theories of Garner and Bemis for anorexia nervosa and Fairburn for bulimia nervosa contend that eating disordered individuals attach rich and extreme connotations to the events of weight gain and weight loss and to the states of fatness and thinness. Although no published research has described the use of the multidimensional scaling technique recommended by Vitousek and Hollon (1990) for this population, a number of studies have employed a related psychometric technique, the repertory grid test, to examine the personal constructs of anorexic patients (Button, 1983; Crisp & Fransella, 1972; Fransella & Button, 1983; Fransella & Crisp, 1979; Mottram, 1985). The collective findings of these investigations suggest that anorexics are disposed to organize their perceptions around a monolithic system related to weight, to attach a broad range of meaning to weight, and to construe themselves and others in extreme terms.

A recent study confirmed these conclusions with large samples of anorexic, bulimic, restrained, and unrestrained subjects (Butow, Beumont, & Touyz, 1993). Subjects provided constructs concerning eating situations and self-and-other elements, which were then used to form two standardized repertory grids completed by separate samples. Individuals with eating disorders employed extreme, rule-bound concepts of weight to describe eating situations, and extended these constructs broadly to situations for which most control subjects thought them inapplicable. Both patient groups characterized themselves in overwhelmingly negative terms. Anorexics, who had already attained a low weight status, expressed ambivalence about the relationship between weight and self-esteem, while bulimics associated thinness with a host of positive self-attributes. Butow et al. (1993) concluded that "these findings support the contention of Garner and Bemis (1982) that constricted, black and white thinking is a fundamental problem in dieting disorders" (p. 326), noting that patients exhibited both the assumptions that cognitive models identify as causally related to anorexia and bulimia and the thinking errors hypothesized to keep these assumptions in place.

The parameter of *intrusiveness of eating and weight content into unrelated or ambiguous situations* has been examined through self-report questionnaires and experimental paradigms. The Body Shape Questionnaire (P. Cooper, Taylor, Cooper, & Fairburn, 1987), the Feelings of Fatness Questionnaire (Roth & Armstrong, 1993), and subscales of the Eating Disorder Examination (Z. Cooper & Fairburn, 1987) all include items that measure the projection of concerns about eating and weight into a wide range of situations, and have been found to differentiate anorexics, bulimics, and/or weight-preoccupied subjects from normal control subjects.

Schotte, McNally, and Turner (1990) used a dichotic listening paradigm to examine biased attention to weight cues. Bulimic subjects detected the target word "fat" more often than neutral material when these were presented on the unattended channel. In addition, there was a tendency for bulimics to exhibit greater physiological reactivity to the weight-related cue.

Jackman, Williamson, Netemeyer, and Anderson (1995) compared the interpretation of ambiguous body-related sentences by female athletes high and low in weight preoccupation. For example, one sentence read: "After exercising for two hours at a health club, you catch a glimpse of the shape of your hips as you pass by a mirror." All subjects were instructed to interpret the sentences as referring to themselves. In a recognition memory task, weight-preoccupied subjects recalled the sentences as having contained connotations of fatness (e.g., "you get a glimpse of your large hips"), while the comparison group remembered them as thinness-related (e.g., "you get a glimpse of your toned hips"). No group differences were found in the interpretation of ambiguous sentences that referred to health or athletic performance.

Jackman et al. (1995) concluded that weight-preoccupied individuals manifest an interpretive bias that is specific to weight-related stimuli. It should be noted, however, that although the groups did not differ significantly in body mass index (BMI), the weight-preoccupied sample was slightly heavier (BMI = 23.21) than the unconcerned group (BMI = 21.86). This discrepancy would correspond to a difference of approximately 10 lbs. at a height of 5′4″. Because subjects were told to imagine *themselves* in each situation, it is possible that those in the weight-preoccupied group were expressing their own likely reaction (and perhaps that of others, in a society that sets stringent weight standards for women) to the objectively somewhat larger proportions of the bodies they would be viewing in a mirror, rather than displaying a bias in processing.

Vitousek, Ewald, Yim, and Manke (1995) adapted an ambiguous stimuli paradigm from research with clinically anxious subjects (Mathews, Richards, & Eysenck, 1989) to examine the hypothesis that eating disordered individuals would manifest differential attentiveness toward those meanings of homophones and homographs that were related to their specific psychopathology. As predicted, anorexics and bulimics were more likely than normal or subclinical control subjects to attend to the food and weight meanings of homophones (words that are pronounced the same, but have multiple meanings and spellings, such as "weight/wait") and homographs (words that have a single spelling but multiple meanings, such as "pound" or "light"). On posttest questionnaires, however, clinical subjects reported more awareness of the study's concealed purpose than did controls, and some acknowledged intentional avoidance of eating or weight responses. The nature of the experiment had been disguised from all subjects with a false rationale and some distractor tasks, but it appeared possible that anorexics and bulimics were "tipped off" by the logical assumption that they had been included in the study because of their symptomatic status. To examine this possibility, an additional control group was primed before the experimental session with the knowledge that the study concerned the eating disorders. These normal subjects produced responses similar to those of clinical subjects and, like clinical subjects, more often discerned the purpose of the investigation. It appears that this paradigm measures the influence of contextual cues instead of (or in addition to) more stable and meaningful differences in information processing—and provides a cautionary tale about the delicacy of theoretically nontransparent cognitive assessment tasks.

The parameter of *memory for schema-consistent information* was assessed in an investigation using obese, restrained, and unrestrained subjects along with a small sample ($N = 6$) of anorexic patients (King, Polivy, & Herman, 1991). Subjects were given a description of a fictitious female in an essay containing descriptive statements about her behavior or characteristics in each of four categories: weight, eating/food, age, and sewing/fashion. After a filler task, subjects were asked to reproduce the essay as completely as possible. Restrained subjects recalled more items from the combined weight-and-food categories than unrestrained subjects. A separate comparison of obese and anorexic subjects revealed that both groups recalled significantly more weight-and-food items than items from other categories, but did not differ from one another. While contextual priming does not appear to have been a factor influencing the obtained differences between restrained and unrestrained eaters, it is unclear whether it contributed to the effect for obese and anorexic subjects, and the small and unequal sample sizes precluded more informative comparative analyses. It does appear that selective memory for schema-consistent information as measured by this experimental paradigm was not a distinctive feature of the psychopathology of clinical eating disorder subjects.

Cognitive and affective involvement in eating- and weight-related domains has been examined through a variety of techniques. Hypothesized bidirectional relationships between affective states and weight perception or eating behavior (Streigel-Moore, McAvay, & Rodin, 1986; Vitousek & Hollon, 1990) have been assessed in a number of mood induction studies, principally using restrained rather than clinically disordered subjects. One study failed to detect increased body concern in restrained subjects following exposure to a failure experience (Eldredge, Wilson, & Whaley, 1990); however, in another investigation using a normal sample, negative mood induction led to greater overestimation of body size and greater body dissatisfaction, with the effect most pronounced for subjects with higher initial levels of shape concern (Taylor & Cooper, 1992). Two studies determined that restrained but not unrestrained subjects consumed more food while watching a horror film or, to a lesser extent, a comedy film than while viewing a travelogue (Cools, Schotte, & McNally, 1992; Schotte, Cools, & McNally, 1990). The sole induction study that included clinical subjects reported that bulimics in whom negative mood had been induced showed more heart rate deceleration when viewing slides of forbidden foods, an effect that was not obtained with restrained controls (Laberg, Wilson, Eldredge, & Nordby, 1991). No published studies have as yet attempted the clinically more perilous procedure of providing false feedback about weight changes to measure effects on such variables as mood shifts and susceptibility to the induction of negative affect.

One study that could be subsumed under the heading of self-statement research or the investigation of cognitive processing involved collecting the thoughts of anorexics, bulimics, normal dieters, symptomatic dieters, and nondieters during and after brief exposure to three behavioral situations (M. Cooper & Fairburn, 1992a). Subjects were instructed to "think aloud" during self-weighing, while standing in front of a full-length mirror, and while consuming a chocolate candy. After each of these procedures, they also completed a thoughts checklist. Groups did not differ on the total number of thoughts expressed concerning themes of food, weight, and shape (an unsurprising result in view of the focus implicit in each test situation), but were clearly discriminable in the emotional valence of reported cognitions. The eating-, weight-, and shape-related thoughts of anorexics and bulimics were significantly more negative than those of normal controls, with the two dieting groups intermediate. Anorexics also differed significantly from dieters in the frequency of negative thoughts about eating, while bulimics were more likely than dieters to report negative thoughts about weight and appearance. The observation that the thoughts checklist yielded similar findings but did not significantly differentiate between clinical and symptomatic dieters suggested that the think-aloud procedure was more sensitive to core psychopathology, perhaps because of its temporal concurrence with the focal situations and perhaps because it required production rather than endorsement of self-statements.

M. Cooper and Fairburn (1992a) concluded from their findings that cognitive theorists may have been incorrect in the assumption that weight concerns are equally prominent and similarly represented in anorexic and bulimic populations. They speculated that the apparently appropriate emphasis on weight and shape concerns in cognitive-behavioral therapy for bulimia nervosa might explain the demonstrated efficacy of this approach, while a redirection of focus toward eating concerns might be necessary for the attainment of equivalent success in the treatment of anorexia nervosa.

As will be discussed in a subsequent section, however, it is more accurate to describe cognitive therapy for anorexia nervosa as unexamined rather than unsuccessful; moreover, it is not clear that a reformulation of cognitive theory or therapy for the condition is warranted on the basis of Cooper and Fairburn's results. It seems probable that differences in the relative satisfaction of anorexics and bulimics with their current body weight (which is, by definition, subnormal in anorexia and typically average or slightly above average in bulimia) account for the relative negativity of their reactions to viewing their mirror images and measuring their weights. Differences in the tendency to shun "forbidden foods" altogether (in the case of restricting anorexia nervosa) or consume them frequently if erratically (in the case of bulimia) can explain the intensity of subjects' reactions to the experimental eating situation. Just as the stronger effects for food stimuli in Stroop research with anorexics may reflect the influence of hunger rather than more specific and essential features of the disorder, these think-aloud data may be revealing some of the secondary *consequences* of anorexic and bulimic patterns rather than illuminating the primary cognitive elements that underlie them. Distorted beliefs about food are certainly conspicuous among the concerns that cognitive therapists must (and do) address in treating anorexic clients, but they are not equated with core psychopathology — which, in the case of both anorexia and bulimia, is postulated to be founded on overvalued ideas about weight and its implications for the self. As noted earlier, weight-related self-schemas may not be identical in these complexly related disorders; however, discrepancies in the salience of food cues or levels of satisfaction with current weight status are probably not the best markers of any fundamental differences that do exist.

STATUS OF THE TREATMENT MODELS

The principles of cognitive-behavioral therapy for anorexia nervosa and bulimia nervosa are derived from the approach delineated by Beck and his coworkers (Beck, Rush, Shaw, & Emery, 1979); however, conventional cognitive strategies have been adapted to address the specific features of these disorders. For anorexia nervosa, these features include the egosyntonic nature of symptoms and the prominence of deficits in self-concept; for both disorders, they include idiosyncratic beliefs related to weight and food, and the interaction between physical and psychological factors. Some of these distinctive features are briefly reviewed below; for more extended descriptions of cognitive therapy for anorexia nervosa, the interested reader is referred to Garner (1986a); Garner and Bemis (1982, 1985); Pike, Loeb, and Vitousek (1996); and Vitousek and Ewald (1993), while applications for bulimia nervosa are detailed in Fairburn (1985); Fairburn and Cooper (1989); Fairburn, Marcus, and Wilson (1993); Garner (1986b); Hsu, Santhouse, and Chesler (1991); and Pike et al. (1996).

Because anorexics are typically unwilling clients, resistant to treatment in the fundamental sense that they would prefer not to participate in it at all, considerable attention must be focused on engaging them as active participants during the crucial initial phase of treatment. Garner and Bemis (1982, 1985) suggest that the guiding principle of collaborative empiricism makes the cognitive-behavioral approach particularly suitable for this wary and resistant population. Clients are not impelled to concede the irrationality of cherished values, but are asked to join the therapist in taking a closer look at the *means* they have chosen to secure them and the full range of *consequences* that result. The establishment of a sound, supportive therapeutic relationship is viewed as essential for success in this endeavor, since its quality profoundly influences clients' willingness to confront the terrifying prospect of weight gain.

Garner and Bemis (1982, 1985; Bemis, 1988) note that the suitability of this therapeutic style for anorexia nervosa was recognized long before their own endorsement of Beck's principles—by a clinician who espoused a very different etiological model. The influential psychodynamic writer Hilde Bruch (1973, 1978) maintained that traditional forms of therapy were "singularly ineffective," "useless even when correct," and perhaps "harmful, even fatal" when applied to anorexia nervosa. She indicated that she had found herself devising a new approach to treatment out of clinical necessity, which she described in the following terms: "[With anorexic patients] psychotherapy is a process during which erroneous assumptions and attitudes are recognized, defined, and challenged so that they can be abandoned" (Bruch, 1978, p. 143). She contended that "it is important to proceed slowly and to use concrete small events or episodes for illustrating certain false assumptions or illogical deductions . . . using relatively small events as they come up" (p. 144). She described this "fact-finding treatment" as "the constructive use of ignorance, using the word ignorance in the way a scientist might use it. . . . [Patient and therapist] should be true collaborators in the search for unknown factors" (Bruch, 1973, p. 338).

Such a description is recognizable as a remarkably apt characterization of Beck's cognitive therapy—a correspondence that is particularly striking in view of the pronounced differences in theoretical orientation. Unfortunately, Bruch did not elaborate further on how therapists might actually implement the general strategy she proposed. Beck, however, had detailed a rich variety of specific techniques derived from the same guiding principle of collaborative empiricism. Garner and Bemis (1982, 1985) maintain that many of these are readily translatable to the eating disordered population, with some improvisations for the unique problems these patients present.

A substantial portion of the first few sessions of cognitive therapy may be devoted to helping the anorexic client develop an exhaustive list of both the "pros" and the "cons" of her eating disorder, phrased in her own terms (Vitousek & Orimoto, 1993).[1] The therapist explicitly acknowledges that weight loss confers some significant perceived benefits (often including a sense of self-control, purity, and accomplishment) that will be missed, and emphasizes that therapy will be unsuccessful if the client is not ultimately compensated for these losses. At the same time, the therapist begins to articulate a theme that will recur throughout treatment: that many of the confessed disadvantages of the disorder (such as depression, irritability, and food preoccupation) are inextricably connected to restrictive dieting and suboptimal weight, and it is not within the client's power to eliminate them selectively while retaining the benefits she associates with the attainment of her thin ideal. The *functional* emphasis inherent in this exercise reflects one of the most distinctive features of cognitive therapy for anorexia nervosa.

For both anorexia nervosa and bulimia nervosa, the normalization of eating and weight is viewed as a prerequisite to the conduct of effective psychotherapy, as well as to eventual successful outcome. Clients who are starving or engaging in chaotic eating behavior are unable to participate fully in the therapeutic process; therefore, efforts to improve nutritional and weight status are an integral part of the clinical agenda from the inception of treatment.

Extensive self-monitoring of food intake and associated affect and cognition is used to identify binge precipitants and idiosyncratic dietary rules, and, in the later stages of therapy, serves as the basis for more elaborate analyses of dysfunctional beliefs. Initially, clients are encouraged to eat in a "mechanical" fashion according to prescribed guidelines for the composition, quantity, and spacing of meals, rather than to attempt to interpret the signals of hunger and satiety that have become confused by their belief systems and disorganized or restrictive patterns of intake. "Forbidden foods" that have been avoided because of fears that they will cause weight gain or precipitate binge-eating episodes are reintroduced into the daily diet. Much as the elicitation of physical sensations cuing panic serves as the basis for restructuring catastrophic misinterpretations in the cognitive treatment of panic disorder (Clark, 1986), exposure to the experiences of eating differently and weighing more provides a wealth of material for cognitive-behavioral interventions in the eating disorders.

The treatment manuals referenced above describe a wide range of cognitive and behavioral techniques that can be used toward the modification of distorted beliefs about food, weight, and shape. These include the provision of psychoeducational material about the effects of dieting, starvation, and purgative tactics; the evaluation of automatic thoughts and information-processing errors on dysfunctional thought records; the analysis of cues and chains supporting the binge–purge cycle; coping and self-control strategies for high-risk situations; *in vivo* exercises; prospective hypothesis testing; challenging the bases for sociocultural pressures about weight and shape; and development of alternative standards for self-evaluation and self-reinforcement. Relapse prevention techniques tailored to the vulnerabilities of these clients are practiced prior to treatment termination (Fairburn, Marcus, & Wilson, 1993; Orimoto & Vitousek, 1992).

The usual course of cognitive-behavioral therapy for bulimia nervosa is 10–20 sessions over a 3- to 6-month period. The recommended duration of therapy for anorexia nervosa is considerably longer—often 1–2 years of weekly sessions, with more intensive treatment in the first several months. This extended course is necessary in part to accommodate the greater resistance of anorexic clients to the change process, as well as to accomplish weight restoration in the early phase of intervention. In addition, cognitive-behavioral therapy for bulimia nervosa is typically restricted to the focal symptomatology of eating and weight concerns; the later stages of treatment in anorexia nervosa shift the emphasis to general problems such as perfectionism and interpersonal concerns, making more extensive use of cognitive restructuring techniques for the modification of higher-order beliefs. It is not clear whether these disparities in the recommended depth and breadth of cognitive-behavioral therapy address fundamental distinctions between the two disorders or simply reflect the slightly different theoretical orientations of the specialists who developed the respective approaches.

Empirical Findings for Anorexia Nervosa

Although the cognitive-behavioral method appears to be fairly widely used in the treatment of anorexia nervosa, there is no compelling evidence for its efficacy. Since the approach was described in detail more than a dozen years ago (Garner & Bemis, 1982), the persistent lack of data is increasingly embarrassing for a modality with a stated commitment to empiricism—but it is, at least, nothing singular for the field. Astonishingly, only five controlled studies of psychotherapy of any kind have been reported for anorexia nervosa, with generally unimpressive results. Drug trials have also been rare, and for the most part disappointing (Walsh, 1991). All commentators agree that the early weight-restoration phase of treatment, which usually occurs in the hospital, is vital but in some senses trivial; all concur that the real therapeutic challenge comes during the prolonged second phase, typically individual and/or family therapy on an outpatient basis. Yet, while the former has been extensively studied (Bemis, 1987), the latter remains almost un-examined.

Several reasons can be advanced to explain this curious gap in the literature, which contrasts sharply with the state of research on bulimia nervosa. Anorexia nervosa is a rarer condition, and the common expedient of assembling bulimic samples through solicitation is not available to the anorexia specialist, since most anorexics shun treatment. The longer recommended course of therapy both increases the likelihood of subject attrition (which will further reduce sample size and undo randomization) and places investigators reinforced for publication frequency on a schedule of dysfunctionally deferred gratification. The "crisis" phase of short-term weight restoration also seems to distract research attention from the extended course of therapy that must follow. Moreover, the first stage is appealingly direct and specific; the issues that must be addressed subsequently are heterogeneous, and clinician–researchers seem to have more difficulty formulating the therapeutic task for the middle and late phases of intervention.

Perhaps one more reason should be added from the perspective of a recovered anorexic who was apparently well versed in the state of research concerning her disorder: "It is difficult not to gain the impression from the literature on anorexia nervosa that individual therapy has been devalued because (among other reasons) psychotherapists do not like anorexics and anorexics do not like psychotherapists" (MacLeod, 1982, p. 122).

A few systematic case studies of cognitive-behavioral therapy for anorexia nervosa have been reported (P. Cooper & Fairburn, 1984; Garner, 1988; Peveler & Fairburn, 1989). The only controlled trial published to date yielded equivocal evidence for the relative efficacy of the approach (Channon, de Silva, Hemsley, & Perkins, 1989). In this investigation, behavioral and cognitive-behavioral therapy conditions were compared with an unspecified treatment-as-usual cell. After 6 months of active treatment and at 6- and 12-month follow-up, all groups were significantly improved; few differences were obtained between conditions. No group could be considered clinically recovered by the end of the study period. The cognitive modality appeared more acceptable to clients and was associated with higher rates of compliance, a finding that the authors noted was of some interest because of the notorious difficulty of engaging anorexics in treatment.

Unfortunately, a number of methodological problems make it difficult to draw clear conclusions from the Channon et al. (1989) trial. Sample size was small (eight per cell); as subject availability is a predictable problem with this population, it would have been preferable to increase power by reducing the comparison to two rather than three alternative modalities. The restricted number of subjects also led to some apparent inequalities in cell composition, although significant pretreatment differences could not be detected with this sample size; for example, 12% of the behaviorally treated versus 50% of the cognitively treated subjects had been hospitalized previously, and the mean age of onset was 21 and 16 years, respectively. The duration of treatment was limited (18 sessions followed by 6 booster sessions) and was markedly discrepant from that recommended by Garner and Bemis (1982, 1985). Means on dependent measures were provided only for the pretest assessment point; at posttest and follow-up, significant differences alone were reported, of which there were, unsurprisingly, very few due to the low power of analyses. The first author served as the sole therapist for both behavioral and cognitive conditions, and the sole evaluator of clinical status.

Finally, while the investigators stated that the cognitive condition was patterned after the recommendations of Garner and Bemis, it is not clear how closely it conformed to specified procedures. It appears that the primary focus of the cognitive-behavioral treatment was the identification and challenge of specific irrational beliefs about food and weight. In discussing the failure of this condition to demonstrate incremental benefit over the behavioral treatment, Channon et al. (1989) suggested that in the future it might be "more appropriate to focus on the relative importance of thinness as a life goal relative to other goals . . . rather than attempting to modify individual cognitions" (p. 534). Since the former is precisely what Garner and Bemis advocate on both practical and theoretical grounds, it is surprising that this crucial component of cognitive therapy for anorexia nervosa was apparently omitted from a test of the method's utility.

Empirical Findings for Bulimia Nervosa

The state of knowledge concerning the efficacy of cognitive-behavioral therapy for bulimia nervosa is dramatically more advanced, and the evidence favoring the approach increasingly compelling. More than 15 comparative trials have been reported; in each instance, the cognitive-behavioral condition has proven equal or superior to every modality with which it has been compared (for reviews, see Abbott & Mitchell, 1993; Agras, 1993; Cox & Merkel, 1989; Craighead & Agras, 1991; Fairburn, 1988a; Fairburn, Agras, & Wilson, 1992; Fairburn & Hay, 1992; Freeman & Munro, 1988; Garner, 1987; Garner, Fairburn, & Davis, 1987; Hollon & Beck, 1994; Laessle, Zoettl, & Pirke, 1987; Mitchell, Raymond, & Specker, 1993; Rosen, 1987; Wilson, 1993; Wilson & Fairburn, 1993).

Despite considerable variability across studies, the method typically yields an 80% reduction in the frequency of bingeing and purging, with approximately half of treated clients reporting the elimination of bulimic episodes. The most recent and carefully designed studies have obtained decreases in binge frequency of from 73% to 93%, with vomiting frequency reduced from 77% to 94%; between 51% and 71% of subjects are free of binge episodes at the end of treatment, and 36–56% no longer induce vomiting (Wilson & Fairburn, 1993). Although many published trials include limited follow-up data, those that have examined subjects 1–6 years after intervention generally find excellent maintenance of treatment gains. In view of these impressive findings, several reviewers have concluded that cognitive-behavioral therapy must be regarded as the current treatment of choice for bulimia nervosa (Craighead & Agras, 1991; Fairburn, 1988a; Wilson & Fairburn, 1993).

The most sophisticated treatment trial in the literature was described in a series of reports by Fairburn and his colleagues (Fairburn, Jones, et al., 1991; Fairburn, Jones, Peveler, Hope, & O'Connor, 1993; Fairburn, Peveler, Jones, Hope, & Doll, 1993). A total pool of 75 subjects was randomly assigned to receive 19 sessions of behavioral therapy, cognitive-behavioral therapy, or interpersonal psychotherapy. The comparison between behavioral and cognitive-behavioral therapies represented a dismantling study intended to examine the effectiveness of techniques such as self-monitoring, stimulus control, and dietary planning in isolation from attention to attitudes about food, weight, and shape. The interpersonal therapy condition was included to compare the influence of a nonspecific treatment whose efficacy has been documented with a different psychiatric population (unipolar depression) to an established modality specifically tailored to the symptoms of bulimia nervosa. As implemented in the Fairburn, Jones, et al. study, interpersonal therapy did not include any direct focus on attitudes about weight and shape and did not attempt to change eating behavior.

All three treatments were equally effective in reducing binge episodes and alleviating symptoms of general psychiatric distress; however, cognitive-behavioral therapy appeared superior on some indices. The full treatment package had significantly greater effects on concerns about weight and shape than the simplified behavioral intervention. Compared to interpersonal therapy, it again proved more effective in modifying weight concerns and produced greater reductions in the frequency of vomiting.

Data collected after a 1-year closed follow-up period revealed some surprising trends (Fairburn, Jones, et al., 1993). Subjects in the behavioral condition were doing so poorly that nearly half had dropped out or had been withdrawn from the study. The high attrition rate precluded a formal analysis of the relative efficacy of this modality, but contributes to the impression that this dismantled subset of techniques is markedly less effective than standard cognitive-behavioral treatment. In contrast, subjects treated with interpersonal therapy continued to improve after termination, and by 12 months had caught up to the cognitive-behavioral condition on every index of outcome.

The finding that cognitive-behavioral treatment outperformed the behavioral intervention is consistent with the postulated mechanisms of change in the dominant cognitive-behavioral model; however, the unanticipated efficacy of interpersonal therapy at follow-up raises important questions for theoretical accounts of bulimia nervosa. Since interpersonal therapy did not address food or weight issues directly, through what mechanisms did it exert its beneficial effects on the focal symptoms of this disorder? In addition, how did a modality lacking any emphasis on relapse prevention prove so successful in maintaining—indeed, enhancing—treatment gains?

Fairburn and colleagues speculated that the decrease in bulimic behavior achieved through interpersonal therapy may have been mediated through effects on negative self-evaluation. They noted that "the patients who respond seem to develop an increased sense of self-worth and competence and, as a result, their tendency to evaluate themselves largely in terms of their weight lessens in intensity" (Fairburn, 1988a, p. 641). Improvements in eating behavior were hypothesized to follow from these basic changes in self-concept. The temporal patterns of improvement in various domains of functioning across the cognitive-behavioral and interpersonal cells supported the assumption that these treatments operated through different mediating mechanisms, and was inconsistent with the alternative hypothesis that bulimia nervosa responds to any credible psychological intervention (Fairburn, Jones, et al., 1993).

The most extended outcome evaluation of cognitive-behavioral therapy for bulimia nervosa was recently reported by Fairburn et al. (1995). This 3- to 11-year follow-up combined subjects participating in the study described above with subjects who had been randomly assigned in an earlier trial to cognitive-behavioral therapy or a focal psychotherapy (Fairburn, Kirk, O'Connor, & Cooper, 1986). The investigators interviewed 89 of the 99 subjects entered into the two trials, after an average period of nearly 6 years. Those who had received focal therapy during the first study were grouped with those given interpersonal therapy during the second because of the similarity between the approaches and the lack of discernible differences in outcome.

In general, the findings of this long-term follow-up assessment continued the pattern evident at 1-year posttreatment. The gains made by former patients who had participated in cognitive-behavioral or interpersonal therapy were largely maintained and were substantially equivalent, while those who had received behavioral therapy had deteriorated further. Significantly more of those in the behavioral condition (86%) met criteria for some form of eating disorder (typically Eating Disorder Not Otherwise Specified), compared to those in the cognitive-behavioral (37%) or interpersonal (28%) conditions, and fewer were free of bulimic episodes. Only a few indices differentiated subjects in the other two conditions from each other. A significantly larger percentage (74%) of those who had participated in cognitive-behavioral therapy obtained global Eating Disorder Examination scores within one standard deviation of the mean for young women, compared to 55% of those in the interpersonal cell and 33% of those in the behavioral cell. There were no differences in the proportion of subjects who had sought additional psychological treatment after termination.

If the results of comparative psychotherapy trials suggest that the cognitive-behavioral approach may be equivalent or slightly superior to other short-term psychotherapies, it appears consistently more effective than current pharmacological regimens for bulimia nervosa. Most reviewers would endorse the conclusion of Mitchell, Raymond, and Specker (1993) that "the results of drug trials are at the same time encouraging and somewhat disheartening" (p. 236), in that antidepressants reliably produce more improvement than placebo but are associated with high rates of attrition, residual symptomatology, and relapse (Fairburn & Hay, 1992; Mitchell & de Zwaan, 1993; Walsh, 1991). Cognitive-behavioral therapy has proven superior to medication conditions in two comparative treatment studies, with the combination of both modalities producing only modest incremental benefits on some outcome indices (Agras et al., 1992; Mitchell et al., 1990).

Several reviewers have suggested that antidepressant drugs and cognitive-behavioral therapy may exert their effects on bulimic behavior through directly opposite mechanisms (Craighead & Agras, 1991; Fairburn et al., 1992; Wilson, 1993). Medication may facilitate dietary restraint by suppressing appetite, while cognitive techniques seek to decrease restraint by encouraging subjects to consume regular, ample meals and reintroduce avoided foods into their diets. Studies have confirmed that imipramine-treated subjects continue to restrict their caloric intake after intervention, while those participating in cognitive-behavioral therapy increase the consumption of nonpurged calories significantly more (Rossiter, Agras, & Losch, 1988; Rossiter, Agras, Losch, & Telch, 1988). This difference may explain the better maintenance of treatment gains following cognitive-behavioral therapy, since restrained eating is often cited as an important causal variable in the development and maintenance of bulimic symptoms.

Recent applications of cognitive-behavioral treatment to subjects qualifying for the provisional DSM-IV diagnosis of binge eating disorder (American Psychiatric Association, 1994) suggest that it yields lower rates of improvement and higher rates of relapse in this population, while comparing favorably with waiting-list conditions and similarly to interpersonal therapy (Telch, Agras, Rossiter, Wilfley, & Kenardy, 1990; Wilfley et al., 1993). One study found cognitive-behavioral treatment superior to a weight loss program in reducing binge frequency over a 3-month period; however, after the weight loss program was continued for *all* subjects for an additional 6 months (supplemented by desipramine for some), there was only a nonsignificant trend for a higher percentage of subjects formerly treated with cognitive-behavioral therapy to have eliminated binge episodes (Agras et al., 1994). Across all groups, abstinence rates were low and weight losses modest. The apparently refractory nature of binge eating behavior in overweight individuals is consistent with the finding that indices of vulnerability to obesity (including weight variability, body mass index, premorbid obesity, and paternal obesity) sometimes predict poor outcome in bulimia nervosa (Fairburn et al., 1995; Garner, 1987).

With the efficacy of cognitive-behavioral therapy for bulimia nervosa established as at least comparable to the best available alternatives, researchers are beginning to investigate more narrowly focused questions about its optimal form and duration, suitability for different patient subgroups, and mechanisms of action. Fairburn (1988b) has cautioned against a premature crystallization of the treatment program he originated. He notes that the standard cognitive-behavioral course is neither necessary for all patients—some of whom respond to briefer and more cost-effective interventions—nor sufficient for the substantial minority who experience unresolved bulimic symptomatology (Fairburn & Hay, 1992; Wilson & Fairburn, 1993).

Different groups of investigators have experimented with abbreviated versions of Fairburn's standard treatment package, with mixed and inconclusive results. Two uncontrolled series obtained remission rates substantially below those reported for the full regimen with 8–10 sessions of individual (Fahy & Russell, 1993) or group therapy (Blouin et al., 1994). In one comparative trial, a shortened version administered in a group format fared poorly compared to typical results (and comparably to a behavior therapy condition) (Wolf & Crowther, 1992); in another, eight individual sessions yielded more characteristic rates of symptom remission (and outperformed behavior therapy and attention-placebo conditions) (Thackwray, Smith, Bodfish, & Meyers, 1993). Self-help manuals outlining the cognitive-behavioral approach produced symptom reduction and remission rates that approximated those of clinician-administered programs in one uncontrolled series (P. Cooper, Coker, & Fleming, 1994), but were associated with less impressive results in a second (Schmidt, Tiller, & Treasure, 1993).

Since none of these studies randomly assigned clients drawn from the same subject pool to complete or condensed versions of cognitive-behavioral treatment, it is impossible to interpret the conflicting findings evident across them. The sole systematic comparison of different treatment intensities examined a somewhat idiosyncratic variant of cognitive therapy (Mitchell, Pyle, et al., 1993). It concluded that once-a-week group cognitive-behavioral therapy was less effective than a more intensive group cognitive-behavioral format (or either of two abstinence-oriented interventions); however, the generalizability of this finding is questionable in view of the poor response of subjects to what should represent the "typical case" of session scheduling for cognitive-behavioral treatment.

Investigators have not yet isolated mode-specific predictors of outcome that could allow therapists to match clients to the programs from which they would be most likely to benefit. The different temporal courses of response to cognitive-behavioral and interpersonal therapy in the Fairburn, Jones, et al. (1993) trial certainly suggest that these treatments work through separate mechanisms; however, it is not clear whether they are selectively effective with different subgroups of patients or facilitate improvement through alternative means in the same set of treatment responders. In the former case, a greater proportion of subjects might be expected to profit if these two effective strategies were combined. Even if the latter were correct, it is possible that a blend of the "direct" and "indirect" tactics they employ might support more complete or durable symptom remission in clients who obtain some improvement from either.

Fairburn (1994) contends that the modalities are incompatible; rather than attempting to conjoin them in therapy sessions, he is examining the effects of interpersonal therapy supplemented with a self-help manual that outlines cognitive-behavioral strategies. This variant may be advantageous for a number of technical reasons, but the premise on which it is based appears neither clinically nor theoretically clear. If clients are able to reconcile conflicting approaches on their own when these are delivered in separate formats, it is not apparent why it should be more difficult for them to so with therapeutic guidance.

Alternative ways of incorporating the presumed active components of both interpersonal and cognitive-behavioral therapy into a single program can be conceptualized. If the rationale or strategies of interpersonal therapy are deemed inconsistent with an emphasis on the modification of specific beliefs and behaviors, a cognitive-behavioral approach can be fully consonant with the exploration of relationship patterns and the facilitation of basic changes in self-concept. Although Fairburn's own effective adaptation of cognitive-behavioral principles for bulimia nervosa is restricted to focal symptomatology, specifications of cognitive therapy for other disorders—including depression and anorexia nervosa—characteristically extend to a broader range of content, particularly in the later phases of treatment. Since the distinctive style and emphases of the cognitive approach are continued throughout the treatment course, it cannot be assumed to work through the same mechanisms as interpersonal therapy, even when addressing similar problems—or to be more, less, or equally powerful in resolving them. Nonetheless, there is no clear reason to avoid trying a broader spectrum variant of cognitive-behavioral therapy that sequentially focuses on disorder-specific and more generalized self and interpersonal issues, given the evidence that modalities separately targeting each of these are effective in the treatment of bulimia nervosa.

CONCLUSION

Substantial progress has been made over the past 15 years in examining the validity and utility of cognitive-behavioral models of the eating disorders. In spite of the prevalence of weight concern and dieting in the general female population, numerous investigations confirm that anorexics and bulimics are distinguishable from the "dissatisfied well" by the content, intensity, and valence of their beliefs about weight, shape, and food. Techniques for gathering self-report data are gradually becoming more sophisticated, making use of semistructured interviews and creative assessment strategies to gain better access to the subtleties of distorted cognition in these subjects.

Data on information processing in the eating disorders have accumulated at an accelerating rate over the past 5 years. Although the shift in emphasis from descriptive to experimental psychopathology is welcome, it is not clear that such research has as yet contributed significantly to our understanding of core issues in anorexia and bulimia. Early results generally support the hypotheses outlined by Vitousek and Hollon (1990); however, investigations have been limited in scope and are sometimes technically and theoretically unsophisticated. A majority of studies rely on a single technique to examine one parameter of information processing, the speed of response in tasks involving domain-relevant stimuli. Investigators' affinity for the Stroop paradigm may have more to do with its familiarity and ease of administration than with any assumptions about its relevance as a measure of key constructs of the cognitive model. Results have been inconsistent, particularly with reference to the essential comparison groups of restrained, dieting, or temporarily food-deprived subjects. Moreover, it is not apparent that the strategies applied to date can deliver on their promise to bypass distortion in self-report by presenting nontransparent tasks that are invulnerable to censorship or manipulation by subjects.

The field must also be wary of an inclination to misinterpret data collected at this level (Vitousek & Hollon, 1990). To clinical researchers frustrated by the fallibility of the self-reported evidence on which they must ordinarily rely, the prospect of collecting data through more respectably "scientific" techniques is beguiling. The results of cognitive processing research are sometimes accepted as uncontaminated indices of fundamental psychopathology inaccessible through more prosaic means. Alternative explanations that attribute the same findings to secondary or superficial aspects of symptomatology are not consistently entertained.

The data obtained to date do suggest that more refined experimental strategies may eventually clarify the role of biased attention and memory in the maintenance of anorexia nervosa and bulimia nervosa. Perhaps the most distinctive hypothesis of cognitive theory for the eating disorders is likely to prove the most difficult to operationalize: that dominant schemas about weight not only exert automatic effects on information processing, but also serve a valued *function* for individuals who have an urgent need for their simplifying and organizing properties.

Cognitive-behavioral therapy is solidly established as the current treatment of choice for bulimia nervosa. The most interesting question for the next generation of research concerns the identification of the therapeutic mechanisms through which this modality and other effective forms of therapy operate (Wilson & Fairburn, 1993). Eventually, such knowledge may allow clinicians to match clients to the treatments from which they are most likely to benefit, and enable researchers to develop even more succesful intervention programs combining the active components of different modalities.

At present, cognitive-behavioral treatment for anorexia nervosa can be advocated only with reference to the appeal of its comprehensive theoretical and therapeutic model; to clinical impressions of its applicability; or, by extrapolation, to data on the effectiveness of a related approach with a kindred disorder. None of these grounds is compelling; however, in the absence of strong empirical support for any alternative psychological or pharmacological approach, they are sufficient to justify the inclusion of this modality in the three comparative trials presently in progress.

ACKNOWLEDGMENTS

Portions of this chapter appeared previously in Vitousek and Orimoto (1993). Copyright 1993 by Academic Press, Inc. Adapted by permission. The former name of the author is Kelly M. Bemis.

NOTE

1. Because the great majority of anorexics and bulimics are female, female pronouns are used throughout the chapter to refer to individuals with these disorders.

REFERENCES

Abbott, D. W., & Mitchell, J. E. (1993). Antidepressants versus psychotherapy in the treatment of bulimia nervosa. *Psychopharmacology Bulletin, 29,* 115–119.

Agras, W. S. (1993). Short-term psychological treatments for binge eating. In C. G. Fairburn & G. T. Wilson (Eds.), *Binge eating: Nature, assessment, and treatment* (pp. 270–286). New York: Guilford Press.

Agras, W. S., Rossiter, E. M., Arnow, B., Schneider, J. A., Telch, C. F., Raeburn, S. D., Bruce, B., Perl, M., & Koran, L. M. (1992). Pharmacologic and cognitive-behavioral treatment for bulimia. *American Journal of Psychiatry, 149,* 82–87.

Agras, W. S., Telch, C. F., Arnow, B., Eldredge, K., Wilfley, D. E., Raeburn, S. D., Henderson, J., & Marnell, M. (1994). Weight loss, cognitive-behavioral, and desipramine treatments in binge eating disorder: An additive design. *Behavior Therapy, 25,* 225–238.

American Psychiatric Association. (1987). *Diagnostic and statistical manual of mental disorders* (3rd ed., rev.). Washington, DC: Author.

American Psychiatric Association. (1994). *Diagnostic and statistical manual of mental disorders* (4th ed.). Washington, DC: Author.

Beck, A. T. (1976). *Cognitive therapy and the emotional disorders.* New York: International Universities Press.

Beck, A. T., Rush, A. J., Shaw, B. F., & Emery, G. (1979). *Cognitive therapy of depression.* New York: Guilford Press.

Bemis, K. M. (1983). A comparison of functional relationships in anorexia nervosa and phobia. In P. L. Darby, P. E. Garfinkel, D. M. Garner, & D. V. Coscina (Eds.), *Anorexia nervosa: Recent developments in research* (pp. 403–415). New York: Alan R. Liss.

Bemis, K. M. (1987). The present status of operant conditioning for the treatment of anorexia nervosa. *Behavior Modification, 11,* 432–463.

Bemis, K. M. (1988). The evolution of cognitive-behavioral therapy for anorexia nervosa and bulimia nervosa. *International Cognitive Therapy Newsletter, 4*(3), 11–14.

Ben-Tovim, D. I., & Walker, M. K. (1991). Further evidence for the Stroop Test as a quantitative measure of psychopathology in eating disorders. *International Journal of Eating Disorders, 10,* 609–613.

Ben-Tovim, D. I., Walker, M. K., Fok, D., & Yap, E. (1989). An adaptation of the Stroop test for measuring shape and food concerns in eating disorders: A quantitative measure of psychopathology? *International Journal of Eating Disorders, 6,* 681–687.

Blouin, J. H., Carter, J., Blouin, A. G., Tener, L., Schnare-Hayes, K., Zuro, C., Barlow, J., & Perez, E. (1994). Prognostic indicators in bulimia nervosa treated with cognitive-behavioral group therapy. *International Journal of Eating Disorders, 15,* 113–123.

Bruch, H. (1973). *Eating disorders: Obesity, anorexia nervosa, and the person within.* New York: Basic Books.

Bruch, H. (1978). *The golden cage: The enigma of anorexia nervosa.* Cambridge, MA: Harvard University Press.

Butow, P., Beumont, P., & Touyz, S. (1993). Cognitive processes in dieting disorders. *International Journal of Eating Disorders, 14,* 319–329.

Button, E. (1983). Personal construct theory and psychological well-being. *British Journal of Medical Psychology, 56,* 313–321.

Casper, R. C., & Davis, J. M. (1977). On the course of anorexia nervosa. *American Journal of Psychiatry, 134,* 974–977.

Channon, S., de Silva, P., Hemsley, D., & Perkins, R. (1989). A controlled trial of cognitive-behavioural and behavioural treatment of anorexia nervosa. *Behaviour Research and Therapy, 27,* 529–535.

Channon, S., & Hayward, A. (1990). The effect of short-term fasting on processing of food cues in normal subjects. *International Journal of Eating Disorders, 9,* 447–452.

Channon, S., Hemsley, D., & de Silva, P. (1988). Selective processing of food words in anorexia nervosa. *British Journal of Clinical Psychology, 22,* 137–138.

Chiodo, J., & Latimer, P. R. (1986). Hunger perceptions and satiety responses among normal-weight bulimics and normals to a high-calorie, carbohydrate-rich food. *Psychological Medicine, 16,* 343–349.

Clark, D. A., Feldman, J., & Channon, S. (1989). Dysfunctional thinking in anorexia and bulimia nervosa. *Cognitive Therapy and Research, 13,* 377–387.

Clark, D. M. (1986). A cognitive approach to panic. *Behaviour Research and Therapy, 24,* 461–470.

Cook, J. A. M., Jones, N., & Johnston, D. W. (1989). The effects of imminent minor surgery on the cognitive processing of health and interpersonal threat words. *British Journal of Clinical Psychology, 28,* 281–282.

Cools, J., Schotte, D. E., & McNally, R. J. (1992). Emotional arousal and overeating in restrained eaters. *Journal of Abnormal Psychology, 101,* 348–351.

Cooper, J. P., Morrison, T. L., Bigman, O. L., Abramowitz, S. I., Levin, S., & Krener, P. (1988). Mood changes and affective disorder in the bulimic binge–purge cycle. *International Journal of Eating Disorders, 7,* 469–474.

Cooper, M. J., Anastasiades, P., & Fairburn, C. G. (1992). Selective processing of eating-, shape-, and weight-related words in persons with bulimia nervosa. *Journal of Abnormal Psychology, 101,* 352–355.

Cooper, M. J., & Fairburn, C. G. (1992a). Thoughts about eating, weight and shape in anorexia nervosa and bulimia nervosa. *Behaviour Research and Therapy, 30,* 501–511.

Cooper, M. J., & Fairburn, C. G. (1992b). Selective processing of eating, weight, and shape related words in patients with eating disorders and dieters. *British Journal of Clinical Psychology, 31,* 363–365.

Cooper, M. J., & Fairburn, C. G. (1993). Demographic and clinical correlates of selective information processing in patients with bulimia nervosa. *International Journal of Eating Disorders, 13,* 109–116.

Cooper, M. J., & Fairburn, C. G. (1994). Changes in selective information processing with three psychological treatments for bulimia nervosa. *British Journal of Clinical Psychology, 33,* 353–356.

Cooper, P. J., & Bowskill, R. (1986). Dysphoric mood and overeating. *British Journal of Clinical Psychology, 25,* 155–156.

Cooper, P. J., Coker, S., & Fleming, C. (1994). Self-help for bulimia nervosa: A preliminary report. *International Journal of Eating Disorders, 16,* 401–404.

Cooper, P. J., & Fairburn, C. G. (1984). Cognitive behaviour therapy for anorexia nervosa: Some preliminary findings. *Journal of Psychosomatic Research, 28,* 493–499.

Cooper, P. J., Taylor, M. J., Cooper, Z., & Fairburn, C. G. (1987). The development and validation of the Body Shape Questionnaire. *International Journal of Eating Disorders, 6,* 485–494.

Cooper, Z., Cooper, P. J., & Fairburn, C. G. (1989). The validity of the Eating Disorder Examination and its subscales. *British Journal of Psychiatry, 154,* 807–812.

Cooper, Z., & Fairburn, C. G. (1987). The Eating Disorder Examination: A semistructured interview for the assessment of the specific psychopathology of eating disorders. *International Journal of Eating Disorders, 6,* 1–8.

Cox, G. L., & Merkel, W. T. (1989). A qualitative review of psychosocial treatments for bulimia. *Journal of Nervous and Mental Disease, 177,* 77–84.

Craighead, L. W., & Agras, W. S. (1991). Mechanisms of action in cognitive-behavioral and pharmacological interventions for obesity and bulimia nervosa. *Journal of Consulting and Clinical Psychology, 59,* 115–125.

Crisp, A. H., & Fransella, F. (1972). Conceptual changes during recovery from anorexia nervosa. *British Journal of Medical Psychology, 45,* 395–405.

Davis, R., Freeman, R. J., & Garner, D. M. (1988). A naturalistic investigation of eating behavior in bulimia nervosa. *Journal of Consulting and Clinical Psychology, 56,* 273–279.

Davis, R., Freeman, R., & Solyom, L. (1985). Mood and food: An analysis of bulimic episodes. *Journal of Psychiatric Research, 19,* 331–335.

Dritschel, B., Williams, K., & Cooper, P. F. (1991). Cognitive distortions amongst women experiencing bulimic episodes. *International Journal of Eating Disorders, 10,* 547–555.

Eldredge, K., Wilson, G. T., & Whaley, A. (1990). Failure, self-evaluation, and feeling fat in women. *International Journal of Eating Disorders, 9,* 37–50.

Elmore, D. K., & de Castro, J. M. (1990). Self-rated moods and hunger in relation to spontaneous eating behavior in bulimics, recovered bulimics, and normals. *International Journal of Eating Disorders, 9,* 179–190.

Fahy, T. A., & Russell, G. F. M. (1993). Outcome and prognostic variables in bulimia nervosa. *International Journal of Eating Disorders, 14,* 135–145.

Fairburn, C. G. (1981). A cognitive behavioural approach to the management of bulimia. *Psychological Medicine, 11,* 707–711.

Fairburn, C. G. (1985). Cognitive-behavioral treatment for bulimia. In D. M. Garner & P. E. Garfinkel (Eds.), *Handbook of psychotherapy for anorexia nervosa and bulimia* (pp. 160–192). New York: Guilford Press.

Fairburn, C. G. (1988a). The current status of psychological treatments for bulimia nervosa. *Journal of Psychosomatic Research, 32,* 635–645.

Fairburn, C. G. (1988b). The uncertain status of the cognitive approach to bulimia nervosa. In K. M. Pirke, & W. Vandereycken, & D. Ploog (Eds.), *The psychobiology of bulimia nervosa* (pp. 129–136). Berlin: Springer-Verlag.

Fairburn, C. G. (1994). Interpersonal psychotherapy for bulimia nervosa. *The Clinical Psychologist, 47,* 21–22.

Fairburn, C. G., Agras, W. S., & Wilson, G. T. (1992). The research on the treatment of bulimia nervosa: Practical and theoretical implications. In G. H. Anderson & S. H. Kennedy (Eds.), *The biology of feast and famine: Relevance to eating disorders* (pp. 318–340). New York: Academic Press.

Fairburn, C. G., & Cooper, P. J. (1989). Eating disorders. In K. Hawton, P. Salkovskis, J. Kirk, & D. M. Clark (Eds.), *Cognitive behaviour therapy for psychiatric problems: A practical guide* (pp. 277–314). Oxford, UK: Oxford University Press.

Fairburn, C. G., Cooper, P. J., Cooper, M. J., McKenna, F. P., & Anastasiades, P. (1991). Selective information processing in bulimia nervosa. *International Journal of Eating Disorders, 10,* 415–422.

Fairburn, C. G., & Cooper, Z. (1993). The Eating Disorder Examination (12th ed.). In C. G. Fairburn & G. T. Wilson (Eds.), *Binge eating: Nature, assessment, and treatment* (pp. 317–360). New York: Guilford Press.

Fairburn, C. G., Cooper, Z., & Cooper, P. J. (1986). In K. D. Brownell & J. P. Foreyt (Eds.), *Handbook of eating disorders: Physiology, psychology, and treatment of obesity, anorexia, and bulimia* (pp. 389–404). New York: Basic Books.

Fairburn, C. G., & Garner, D. M. (1988). Diagnostic criteria for anorexia nervosa and bulimia nervosa: The importance of attitudes to shape and weight. In D. M. Garner & P. E. Garfinkel (Eds.), *Diagnostic issues in anorexia nervosa and bulimia nervosa* (pp. 36–55). New York: Brunner/Mazel.

Fairburn, C. G., & Hay, P. J. (1992). The treatment of bulimia nervosa. *Annals of Medicine, 24,* 297–302.

Fairburn, C. G., Jones, R., Peveler, R. C., Carr, S. J., Solomon, R. A., O'Connor, M. E., Burton, J., & Hope, R. A. (1991). Three psychological treatments for bulimia nervosa. *Archives of General Psychiatry, 48,* 463–469.

Fairburn, C. G., Jones, R., Peveler, R. C., Hope, R. A., & O' Connor, M. (1993). Psychotherapy and bulimia nervosa: Longer-term effects of interpersonal psychotherapy, behavior therapy, and cognitive behavior therapy. *Archives of General Psychiatry, 50,* 419–428.

Fairburn, C. G., Kirk, J., O'Connor, M., & Cooper, P. J. (1986). A comparison of two psychological treatments for bulimia nervosa. *Behaviour Research and Therapy, 24,* 629–643.

Fairburn, C. G., Marcus, M. D., & Wilson, G. T. (1993). Cognitive-behavioral therapy for binge eating and bulimia nervosa: A comprehensive treatment manual. In C. G. Fairburn & G. T. Wilson (Eds.), *Binge eating: Nature, assessment, and treatment* (pp. 361–404). New York: Guilford Press.

Fairburn, C. G., Norman, P. A., Welch, S. L., O'Connor, M. E., Doll, H. A., &

Peveler, R. C. (1995). A prospective study of outcome in bulimia nervosa and the long-term effects of three psychological treatments. *Archives of General Psychiatry, 52,* 304–312.

Fairburn, C. G., Peveler, R. C., Jones, R., Hope, R. A., & Doll, H. A. (1993). Predictors of 12-month outcome in bulimia nervosa and the influence of attitudes to shape and weight. *Journal of Consulting and Clinical Psychology, 61,* 696–698.

Foa, E. B., Feske, U., Murdock, T. B., Kozak, M. J., & McCarthy, P. R. (1991). Processing of threat-related information in rape victims. *Journal of Abnormal Psychology, 100,* 156–162.

Franko, D. L., & Zuroff, D. C. (1992). The Bulimic Automatic Thoughts Questionnaire: Initial reliability and validity data. *Journal of Clinical Psychology, 48,* 505–509.

Fransella, F., & Button, E. (1983). The "construing" of self and body size in relation to maintenance of weight in anorexia nervosa. In P. L. Darby, P. E. Garfinkel, D. M. Garner, & D. V. Coscina (Eds.), *Anorexia nervosa: Recent developments in research* (pp. 107–116). New York: Alan R. Liss.

Fransella, F., & Crisp, A. H. (1979). Comparisons of weight concepts in groups of neurotic, normal, and anorexic females. *British Journal of Psychiatry, 134,* 79–86.

Freeman, C. P. L., & Munro, J. K. M. (1988). Drug and group treatments for bulimia/bulimia nervosa. *Journal of Psychosomatic Research, 32,* 647–660.

Fremouw, W. J., & Heyneman, N. E. (1983). Cognitive styles and bulimia. *the Behavior Therapist, 6,* 143–144.

Garner, D. M. (1986a). Cognitive therapy for anorexia nervosa. In K. D. Brownell & J. P. Foreyt (Eds.), *Handbook of eating disorders: Physiology, psychology, and treatment of obesity, anorexia, and bulimia* (pp. 301–327). New York: Basic Books.

Garner, D. M. (1986b). Cognitive therapy for bulimia nervosa. *Adolescent Psychiatry, 13,* 358–390.

Garner, D. M. (1987). Psychotherapy outcome research with bulimia nervosa. *Psychotherapy and Psychosomatics, 48,* 129–140.

Garner, D. M. (1988). Anorexia nervosa. In M. Hersen & C. G. Last (Eds.), *Child behavior therapy casebook* (pp. 263–276). New York: Plenum Press.

Garner, D. M., & Bemis, K. M. (1982). A cognitive-behavioral approach to anorexia nervosa. *Cognitive Therapy and Research, 6,* 123–150.

Garner, D. M., & Bemis, K. M. (1985). Cognitive therapy for anorexia nervosa. In D. M. Garner & P. E. Garfinkel (Eds.), *Handbook of psychotherapy for anorexia nervosa and bulimia* (pp. 107–146). New York: Guilford Press.

Garner, D. M., Fairburn, C. G., & Davis, R. (1987). Cognitive-behavioral treatment of bulimia nervosa. *Behavior Modification, 11,* 398–431.

Garner, D. M., Garfinkel, P. E., & Olmsted, M. P. (1983). An overview of the sociocultural factors in the development of anorexia nervosa. In P. L. Darby, P. E. Garfinkel, D. M. Garner, & D. V. Coscina (Eds.), *Anorexia nervosa: Recent developments in research* (pp. 65–82). New York: Alan R. Liss.

Garner, D. M., Olmsted, M. P., & Polivy, J. (1983). Development and validation of a multidimensional eating disorder inventory for anorexia nervosa and bulimia. *International Journal of Eating Disorders, 2,* 15–34.

Garner, D. M., Rockert, W., Olmsted, M. P., Johnson, C., & Coscina, D. V. (1985). Psychoeducational principles in the treatment of bulimia and anorexia nervosa. In D. M. Garner & P. E. Garfinkel (Eds.), *Handbook of psychotherapy for anorexia nervosa and bulimia* (pp. 513–572). New York: Guilford Press.

Goebel, M., Spalthoff, G., Schulze, C., & Florin, I. (1989). Dysfunctional cognitions, attributional style, and depression in bulimia. *Journal of Psychosomatic Research, 33,* 747–752.

Goldberg, S. C., Halmi, K. A., Eckert, E. D., Casper, R. C., Davis, D. M., & Roper, M. (1980). Attitudinal dimensions in anorexia nervosa. *Journal of Psychiatric Research, 15,* 239–251.

Green, M. W., & McKenna, F. P. (1993). Developmental onset of eating related color-naming interference. *International Journal of Eating Disorders, 13,* 391–397.

Green, M. W., McKenna, F. P., & De Silva, M. S. L. (1994). Habituation patterns to colour-naming of eating-related stimuli in anorexics and non-clinical controls. *British Journal of Clinical Psychology, 33,* 499–508.

Green, M. W., & Rogers, P. J. (1993). Selective attention to food and body shape words in dieters and restrained nondieters. *International Journal of Eating Disorders, 14,* 515–517.

Herman, C. P., & Mack, D. (1975). Restrained and unrestrained eating. *Journal of Personality, 43,* 647–660.

Herzog, D. B., Keller, M. B., Strober, M., Yeh, C., & Pai, S.-Y. (1992). The current status of treatment for anorexia nervosa and bulimia nervosa. *International Journal of Eating Disorders, 12,* 215 220.

Hollon, S. D., & Beck, A. T. (1994). Cognitive and cognitive-behavioral therapies. In S. L. Garfield & A. E. Bergin (Eds.), *Handbook of psychotherapy and behavior change: An empirical analysis* (4th ed., pp. 428–466). New York: Wiley.

Hsu, L. K. G. (1990). Experiential aspects of bulimia nervosa: Implications for cognitive behavioral therapy. *Behavior Modification, 14,* 50–65.

Hsu, L. K. G., Santhouse, R., & Chesler, B. E. (1991). Individual cognitive behavioral therapy for bulimia nervosa: The description of a program. *International Journal of Eating Disorders, 10,* 273–283.

Huon, G. F. (1995). The Stroop color-naming task in eating disorders: A review of the research. *Eating Disorders: The Journal of Treatment and Prevention, 3,* 124–132.

Jackman. L. P., Williamson, D. A., Netemeyer, R. G., & Anderson, D. A. (1995). Do weight-preoccupied women misinterpret ambiguous stimuli related to body size? *Cognitive Therapy and Research, 19,* 341–355.

Johnson, C., & Larson, R. (1982). Bulimia: An analysis of moods and behavior. *Psychosomatic Medicine, 44,* 341–351.

Kaplan, A. S., & Garfinkel, P. E. (1993). *Medical issues and the eating disorders: The interface.* New York: Brunner/Mazel.

Kaye, W. H., Gwirtsman, H. E., George, D. T., Weiss, S. R., & Jimerson, D. C. (1986). Relationship of mood alterations to bingeing behavior in bulimia. *British Journal of Psychiatry, 149,* 479–485.

King, G. A., Polivy, J., & Herman, C. P. (1991). Cognitive aspects of dietary restraint: Effects on person memory. *International Journal of Eating Disorders, 12,* 221–228.

Laberg, J. C., Wilson, G. T., Eldredge, K., & Nordby, H. (1991). Effects of mood on heart rate reactivity in bulimia nervosa. *International Journal of Eating Disorders, 10,* 169–178.

Laessle, R. G., Schweiger, U., & Pirke, K. M. (1988). Depression as a correlate of starvation in patients with eating disorders. *Biological Psychiatry, 23,* 719–725.

Laessle, R. G., Zoettl, C., & Pirke, K. M. (1987). Metaanalysis of treatment studies for bulimia. *International Journal of Eating Disorders, 6,* 647–653.

Lavy, E. H., & van den Hout, M. A. (1993). Attentional biases for appetitive cues:

Effects of fasting in normal subjects. *Behavioural and Cognitive Psychotherapy, 21,* 297–310.

Lingswiler, V. M., Crowther, J. H., & Stevens, M. A. P. (1987). Emotional reactivity and eating in binge eating and obesity. *Journal of Behavioral Medicine, 10,* 287–299.

Lingswiler, V. M., Crowther, J. H., & Stevens, M. A. P. (1989). Affective and cognitive antecedents to eating episodes in bulimia and binge eating. *International Journal of Eating Disorders, 8,* 533–539.

Long, C. G., Hinton, C., & Gillespie, N. K. (1994). Selective processing of food and body size words: Application of the Stroop test with obese restrained eaters, anorexics, and normals. *International Journal of Eating Disorders, 15,* 279–283.

MacLeod, S. (1982). *The art of starvation: A story of anorexia and survival.* New York: Schocken.

Mahamedi, F., & Heatherton, T. F. (1993). Effects of high calorie preloads on selective processing of food and body shape stimuli among dieters and nondieters. *International Journal of Eating Disorders, 13,* 305–314.

Mathews, A., Richards, A., & Eysenck, M. (1989). Interpretation of homophones related to threat in anxiety states. *Journal of Abnormal Psychology, 98,* 31–34.

Mitchell, J. E., & de Zwaan, M. (1993). Pharmacological treatments of binge eating. In C. G. Fairburn & G. T. Wilson (Eds.), *Binge eating: Nature, assessment, and treatment* (pp. 250–269). New York: Guilford Press.

Mitchell, J. E., Pyle, R. L., Eckert, E. D., Hatsukami, D., Pomeroy, C., & Zimmerman, R. (1990). A comparison study of antidepressants and structured intensive group psychotherapy in the treatment of bulimia nervosa. *Archives of General Psychiatry, 47,* 149–157.

Mitchell, J. E., Pyle, R. L., Pomeroy, C., Zollman, M., Crosby, R., Seim, H., Eckert, E. D., & Zimmerman, R. (1993). Cognitive-behavioral group psychotherapy of bulimia nervosa: Importance of logistical variables. *International Journal of Eating Disorders, 14,* 277–287.

Mitchell, J. E., Raymond, N., & Specker, S. (1993). A review of the controlled trials of pharmacotherapy and psychotherapy in the treatment of bulimia nervosa. *International Journal of Eating Disorders, 14,* 229–247.

Mizes, J. S. (1990). Criterion-related validity of the Anorectic Cognitions Questionnaire. *Addictive Behaviors, 15,* 153–163.

Mizes, J. S., & Christiano, B. A. (1995). Assessment of cognitive variables relevant to cognitive behavioral perspectives in anorexia nervosa and bulimia nervosa. *Behaviour Research and Therapy, 33,* 95–105.

Mizes, J. S., & Klesges, R. C. (1989). Validity, reliability, and factor structure of the Anorectic Cognitions Questionnaire. *Addictive Behaviors, 14,* 589–594.

Mottram, M. A. (1985). Personal constructs in anorexia. *Journal of Psychiatric Research, 19,* 291–295.

Newman, J. P., Wallace, J. F., Strauman, T. J., Skolaski, R. L., Oreland, K. M., Mattek, P. W., Elder, K. A., & McNeely, J. (1993). Effects of motivationally significant stimuli on the regulation of dominant responses. *Journal of Personality and Social Psychology, 65,* 165–175.

Ogden, J., & Greville, L. (1993). Cognitive changes to preloading in restrained and unrestrained eaters as measured by the Stroop task. *International Journal of Eating Disorders, 14,* 185–195.

Orimoto, L. (1996). *Schematic processing of body weight, shape, and self-referent attributes in the eating disorders: A comparison of anorexic, bulimic, depressed, dieting, and nondieting women.* Unpublished doctoral dissertation, University of Hawaii, Honolulu.

Orimoto, L., & Vitousek, K. B. (1992). Anorexia nervosa and bulimia nervosa. In P. H. Wilson (Ed.), *Principles and practice of relapse prevention* (pp. 85–127). New York: Guilford Press.

Overduin, J., Jansen, A., & Louwerse, E. (1995). Stroop interference and food intake. *International Journal of Eating Disorders, 18,* 227–285.

Perpina, C., Hemsley, D., Treasure, J., & de Silva, P. (1993). Is the selective information processing of food and body words specific to patients with eating disorders? *International Journal of Eating Disorders, 14,* 359–366.

Peveler, R. C., & Fairburn, C. G. (1989). Anorexia nervosa in association with diabetes mellitus: A cognitive-behavioural approach to treatment. *Behaviour Research and Therapy, 27,* 95–99.

Phelan, P. W. (1987). Cognitive correlates of bulimia: The Bulimic Thoughts Questionnaire. *International Journal of Eating Disorders, 6,* 593–607.

Pike, K. M., Loeb, K., & Vitousek, K. (1996). Cognitive behavioral therapy for anorexia nervosa and bulimia nervosa. In J. K. Thompson (Ed.), *Body image, eating disorders, and obesity: An integrative guide for assessment and treatment* (pp. 253–302). Washington, DC: American Psychological Association.

Poulakis, Z., & Wertheim, E. H. (1993). Relationships among dysfunctional cognitions, depressive symptoms, and bulimic tendencies. *Cognitive Therapy and Research, 17,* 549–559.

Rebert, W. M., Stanton, A. L., & Schwarz, R. M. (1991). Influence of personality attributes and daily moods on bulimic eating patterns. *Addictive Behaviors, 16,* 497–505.

Rosen, J. C. (1987). A review of behavioral treatments for bulimia nervosa. *Behavior Modification, 11,* 464–486.

Rosen, J. C., Vara, L., Wendt, S., & Leitenberg, H. (1990). Validity studies of the Eating Disorder Examination. *International Journal of Eating Disorders, 9,* 519–528.

Rossiter, E. M., Agras, W. S., & Losch, M. (1988). Changes in self-reported food intake in bulimics as a consequence of antidepressant treatment. *International Journal of Eating Disorders, 7,* 779–783.

Rossiter, E. M., Agras, W. S., Losch, M., & Telch, C. F. (1988). Dietary restraint of bulimic subjects following cognitive-behavioural or pharmacological treatment. *Behaviour Research and Therapy, 26,* 495–498.

Roth, D., & Armstrong, J. (1993). Feelings of Fatness Questionnaire: A measure of the cross-situational variability of body experience. *International Journal of Eating Disorders, 14,* 349–358.

Ruderman, S. (1986). Bulimia and irrational beliefs. *Behaviour Research and Therapy, 24,* 193–197.

Russell, G. F. M. (1979). Bulimia nervosa: An ominous variant of anorexia nervosa. *Psychological Medicine, 9,* 429–448.

Scanlon, E., Ollendick, T. H., & Bayer, K. (1986). *The role of cognitions in bulimia: An empirical test of basic assumptions.* Paper presented at the annual meeting of the Association for the Advancement of Behavior Therapy, Chicago.

Schlesier-Carter, B., Hamilton, S. A., O'Neil, P. M., Lydiard, B., & Malcolm, R. (1989). Depression and bulimia: The link between depression and bulimic cognitions. *Journal of Abnormal Psychology, 98,* 322–325.

Schlundt, D. G., Johnson, W. G., & Jarrell, M. P. (1985). A naturalistic functional analysis of eating behaviour in bulimia and obesity. *Advances in Behaviour Research and Therapy, 7,* 149–162.

Schmidt, N. B., & Telch, M. J. (1991). *Selective processing of body shape and food cues in high and low restraint subjects.* Poster presented at the annual meeting of the Association for the Advancement of Behavior Therapy, New York.

Schmidt, U., Tiller, J., & Treasure, J. (1993). Self-treatment of bulimia nervosa: A pilot study. *International Journal of Eating Disorders, 13,* 273–277.

Schotte, D. E., Cools, J., & McNally, R. J. (1990). Film-induced negative affect triggers overeating in restrained eaters. *Journal of Abnormal Psychology, 99,* 317–320.

Schotte, D. E., McNally, R. J., & Turner, M. L. (1990). A dichotic listening analysis of body weight concern in bulimia nervosa. *International Journal of Eating Disorders, 9,* 109–113.

Schulman, R. G., Kinder, B. N., Gleghorn, A., Powers, P. S., & Prange, M. (1986). The development of a scale to measure cognitive distortions in bulimia. *Journal of Personality Assessment, 50,* 630–639.

Selvini-Palazzoli, M. (1971). Anorexia nervosa. In S. Arieti (Ed.), *World biennial of psychiatry and psychotherapy* (Vol. 1, pp. 197–218). New York: Basic Books.

Slade, P. (1982). Towards a functional analysis of anorexia nervosa and bulimia nervosa. *British Journal of Clinical Psychology, 21,* 167–179.

Steiger, H., Fraenkel, L., & Leichner, P. P. (1989). Relationship of body image distortion to sex-role identification, irrational cognitions, and body weight in eating-disordered females. *Journal of Clinical Psychology, 45,* 61–65.

Steiger, H., Goldstein, C., Mongrain, M., & Van der Feen, J. (1990). Description of eating-disordered, psychiatric, and normal women along cognitive and psychodynamic dimensions. *International Journal of Eating Disorders, 9,* 129–140.

Steinberg, S., Tobin, D., & Johnson, C. (1990). The role of bulimic behaviors in affect regulation: Different functions for different patient subgroups? *International Journal of Eating Disorders, 9,* 51–55.

Stice, E. (1994). Review of the evidence for a sociocultural model of bulimia nervosa and an exploration of the mechanisms of action. *Clinical Psychology Review, 14,* 633–661.

Strauss, J., & Ryan, R. M. (1988). Cognitive dysfunction in eating disorders. *International Journal of Eating Disorders, 7,* 19–27.

Striegel-Moore, R., McAvay, G., & Rodin, J. (1986). Psychological and behavioral correlates of feeling fat in women. *International Journal of Eating Disorders, 5,* 935–947.

Stroop, J. R. (1935). Studies of interference in serial verbal reactions. *Journal of Experimental Psychology, 18,* 643–662.

Stunkard, A. J., & Messick, S. (1985). The three-factor eating questionnaire to measure dietary restraint, disinhibition, and hunger. *Journal of Psychosomatic Research, 29,* 71–83.

Taylor, M. J., & Cooper, P. J. (1992). An experimental study of the effect of mood on body size perception. *Behaviour Research and Therapy, 30,* 53–58.

Telch, C. F., Agras, W. S., Rossiter, E. M., Wilfley, D., & Kenardy, J. (1990). Group cognitive-behavioral treatment for the nonpurging bulimic: An initial evaluation. *Journal of Consulting and Clinical Psychology, 58,* 629–635.

Thackwray, D. E., Smith, M. C., Bodfish, J. W., & Meyers, A. W. (1993). A comparison of behavioral and cognitive-behavioral interventions for bulimia nervosa. *Journal of Consulting and Clinical Psychology, 61,* 639–645.

Thompson, D. A., Berg, K. M., & Shatford, L. A. (1987). The heterogeneity of bulimic symptomatology: Cognitive and behavioral dimensions. *International Journal of Eating Disorders, 6,* 215–234.

Ushakov, G. K. (1971). Anorexia nervosa. In J. G. Howells (Ed.), *Modern perspectives in adolescent psychiatry* (pp. 274–289). Edinburgh: Oliver & Boyd.

Vandereycken, W., & Pierloot, R. (1983). The significance of subclassification in anorexia nervosa: A comparative study of clinical features in 141 patients. *Psychological Medicine, 13,* 543–549.

Van Strien, T., Frijters, J. E. R., Bergers, G. P. A., & Defares, P. B. (1986). The Dutch Eating Behavior Questionnaire (DEBQ) for assessment of restrained, emotional and external eating behavior. *International Journal of Eating Disorders, 5,* 295–315.

Vitousek, K. B., Daly, J., & Heiser, C. (1991). Reconstructing the internal world of the eating-disordered individual: Overcoming denial and distortion in self-report. *International Journal of Eating Disorders, 10,* 647–666.

Vitousek, K. B., & Ewald, L. (1993). Self-representation in the eating disorders: The cognitive perspective. In Z. V. Segal & S. J. Blatt (Eds.), *The self in emotional distress: Cognitive and psychodynamic perspectives* (pp. 221–257). New York: Guilford Press.

Vitousek, K., Ewald, L., Yim, L., & Manke, F. (1995). *Interpretation of ambiguous stimuli in the eating disorders: The influence of contextual cues.* Manuscript submitted for publication.

Vitousek, K. B., & Hollon, S. D. (1990). The investigation of schematic content and processing in eating disorders. *Cognitive Therapy and Research, 14,* 191–214.

Vitousek, K., & Manke, F. (1994). Personality variables and disorders in anorexia nervosa and bulimia nervosa. *Journal of Abnormal Psychology, 103,* 137–147.

Vitousek, K. B., & Orimoto, L. (1993). Cognitive-behavioral models of anorexia nervosa, bulimia nervosa, and obesity. In P. Kendall & K. Dobson (Eds.), *Psychopathology and cognition* (pp. 191–242). New York: Academic Press.

Vitousek, K., Orimoto, L., & Ewald, L. (1995). *Indirect assessment methods in the study of anorexia nervosa and bulimia nervosa.* Unpublished manuscript. University of Hawaii, Honolulu, Hawaii.

Walker, M. K., Ben-Tovim, D. I., Jones, S., & Bachok, N. (1992). Repeated administration of the adapted Stroop test: Feasibility for longitudinal study of psychopathology in eating disorders. *International Journal of Eating Disorders, 12,* 103–105.

Walsh, B. T. (1991). Psychopharmacological treatment of bulimia nervosa. *Journal of Clinical Psychiatry, 52S,* 34–38.

Wilfley, D. E., Agras, W. S., Telch, C. F., Rossiter, E. M., Schneider, J. A., Cole, A. G., Sifford, L., & Raeburn, S. D. (1993). Group cognitive-behavioral therapy and group interpersonal psychotherapy for the nonpurging bulimic individual: A controlled comparison. *Journal of Consulting and Clinical Psychology, 61,* 296–305.

Williamson, D. A., Kelley, M. L., Davis, C. J., Ruggiero, L., & Veitia, M. C. (1985). The psychophysiology of bulimia. *Advances in Behaviour Research and Therapy, 7,* 163–172.

Wilson, G. T. (1989). The treatment of bulimia nervosa: A cognitive-social learning analysis. In A. J. Stunkard & A. Baum (Eds.), *Perspectives in behavioral medicine* (pp. 73–98). Hillsdale, NJ: Erlbaum.

Wilson, G. T. (1991). The addiction model of eating disorders: A critical analysis. *Advances in Behaviour Research and Therapy, 13,* 27–72.

Wilson, G. T. (1993). Psychological and pharmacological treatment of bulimia nervosa: A research update. *Applied and Preventive Psychology: Current Scientific Perspectives, 2,* 35–42.

Wilson, G. T., & Fairburn, C. G. (1993). Cognitive treatments for the eating disorders. *Journal of Consulting and Clinical Psychology, 61,* 261–269.

Wilson, G. T., & Smith, D. (1989). Assessment of bulimia nervosa: An evaluation of the Eating Disorder Examination. *International Journal of Eating Disorders, 8,* 173–179.

Wolf, E. M., & Crowther, J. M. (1992). An evaluation of behavioral and cognitive-behavioral group interventions for the treatment of bulimia nervosa in women. *International Journal of Eating Disorders, 11,* 3–15.

Zotter, D. L., & Crowther, J. H. (1991). The role of cognitions in bulimia nervosa. *Cognitive Therapy and Research, 15,* 413–426.

Chapter 18

Conceptualizing the Cognitive Component of Sexual Arousal: Implications for Sexuality Research and Treatment

Tracy Sbrocco
David H. Barlow

The experience of sexual arousal is a complex interaction between cognitive, affective, behavioral, and physiological processes. The tangible psychological changes observed during sexual arousal (e.g., tumescence) provide a unique opportunity to examine the cognitive and affective mechanisms mediating it. As is evident from examining the table of contents of this book, cognitive concepts have become prominent in models of emotion and behavior.

Cognitive theory, initially developed by Beck to explain and treat depression (Beck, 1963, 1964, 1967), now forms a theoretical and empirical foundation for the development, maintenance, and treatment of a number of Axis I and II disorders and interpersonal problems. Implementation of cognitive theory as a foundation for the descriptive psychopathology of sexual dysfunctions is particularly valuable because an understanding of sexual functioning must take into consideration the individual's idiosyncratic reality and the social reality of sexual functioning. In this context, similar to the systematic bias observed in other psychiatric disorders (Beck & Weishaar, 1989, Chap. 1), we see disorder-specific cognitive vulnerability. Similarly, the etiological and maintenance mechanisms of such difficulties are more understandable. In particular, the reversion to more primitive processing mechanisms (Beck, Rush, Shaw, & Emery, 1979, p. 14) triggered by the person–environment interaction is placed in context. In addition, cognitive therapy for sexual dysfunctions provides a basis to address individuals' cognitive content and processing style. Equally important, the development of cognitive therapy, particularly in the area of couples and marital therapy

(Epstein & Baucom, 1989, Chap. 25), has direct applicability to the treatment of sexual dysfunctions.

Much has happened since cognitive therapy's inception 30 years ago. The speed of model development leads us to look backward and reformulate our model of sexual dysfunction (Barlow, 1986, 1988). Cognitive structures and processes receive an increased focus in this revised model of sexual dysfunction. In particular, understanding the etiology and maintenance of sexual dysfunctions requires examination of four critical areas: schematic vulnerability, skill deficits, negative outcome expectancies, and disengagement or withdrawal. Briefly, these constructs are related in the following manner. Cognitive structures that unite views of the self with unrealistic beliefs about sexual performance form the core psychopathology of sexual dysfunction. This self-schema may contribute to skills deficits and to the development of negative outcome expectancies for behavioral regulation in the sexual situation. As predicted by self-regulation theories, negative outcome expectancies may prompt task disengagement (either overt or covert disengagement) (cf. Carver & Scheier, 1988). In the following section we outline the five domains differentiating functional and dysfunctional responses to erotica. Next we discuss extension of our model through application of self-regulatory theory (Barlow, 1986, 1988). Lastly, we recommend directions for future research on schematic content and processing in sexual functioning, focusing on male sexual functioning. This is our area of expertise and, perhaps unfortunately, is represented by a greater body of literature.

THE RELATIONSHIP OF SEXUAL AROUSAL AND "ANXIETY"

During the second half of this century anxiety has been heralded as the cause of impaired sexual arousal. This represented a tremendous improvement over the Victorian conceptualization of sexual dysfunction as the result of "moral degeneracy" or over the Freudian view of sexual dysfunction as the representation of arrested psychosexual development (LoPiccolo, 1992). Early behaviorists posited that anxiety was the major cause of sexual dysfunction because anxiety reciprocally inhibited sexual arousal (e.g., Wolpe, 1958). Concurrent with the development of behavioral therapies, treatment for sexual disorders became directive and focused on anxiety reduction. Wolpe (1958) recommended the use of systematic desensitization in the treatment of sexual dysfunctions with the premise that anxiety inhibits sexual arousal and therefore the elimination of anxiety is the treatment goal. Masters and Johnson (1970) revolutionized the field of sex therapy with publication of *Human Sexual Inadequacy*. They too posited a central role for anxiety in the development and maintenance of sexual dysfunction, asserting performance anxiety and fear lay as the etiological basis. They further elucidated sexual anxiety by describing the process of "spectatoring," whereby individuals detach themselves from the sexual experience as though they were outside observers. And importantly, they presented sex as a skill to be learned. Kaplan (1977) similarly described anxiety as the root of sexual dysfunctions and extended the umbrella of anxious domains to include partner-demand characteristics.

Treatments based on these conceptualizations have focused, not surprisingly, on reducing anxiety in a sexual context. Masters and Johnson's method involves "sensate focus" and an "intercourse ban" to avoid further anxiety-laden attempts at intercourse. During this process arousal occurs through nongenital body massage. When erections occur spontaneously, the couple advances progressively to intercourse; thus, this technique resembles techniques of *in vivo* systematic desensitization. Such approaches to treatment based on anxiety reduction have had moderate success and it appears approximately 50–70% of patients show some immediate improvement (Cranston-Cuebas & Barlow, 1990). Psychological treatments have changed some over the past decade. Along with the development of cognitive-behavioral approaches, there has been an increasing focus on cognitions as etiological and maintaining factors in sexual dysfunction as well as more general relationship issues (LoPiccolo, 1992; Pryde, 1989). Unfortunately, there continues to be a paucity of treatment-outcome research on these innovations as well as basic psychopathology research on the nature of sexual dysfunction.

Persistence in the belief that anxiety inhibits sexual arousal continues, despite research during the past decade suggesting anxiety does not necessarily inhibit it. In fact, the effect of anxiety on sexual arousal depends largely on how anxiety is defined. That is, anxiety is a three-response system with cognitive, affective, and physiological components that can all be assessed and manipulated (Barlow, 1988). Our model of sexual dysfunction (Barlow, 1986) posits cognitive interference, fueled by the physiological arousal associated with anxiety, as responsible for sexual dysfunction (see Figure 18.1).

The nature of this cognitive interference in sexually dysfunctional individuals seems to revolve largely around focusing on or attending to a "task-irrelevant" context. More specifically, we have hypothesized that dysfunctionals are not focusing on erotic cues. Rather, dysfunctionals focus on nonerotic material, possibly performance-related or non-sex-related thoughts. This nonerotic focus of attention then becomes heightened by the physiological aspects of arousal. That is, arousal functions to narrow attention on task-irrelevant information resulting in further deterioration in sexual performance. Paralleling this process, sexually functionals' focus on erotic cues is enhanced by attentional narrowing, up to a point. Therefore, arousal generally facilitates performance in functional subjects.

This conceptualization is based on the observation of five fundamental differences in responding between sexually functional and dysfunctional subjects. These differences were manifested over a series of studies examining the interplay of anxiety and sexual arousal that resulted in the following observations: (1) Experimental induction of anxiety often facili-

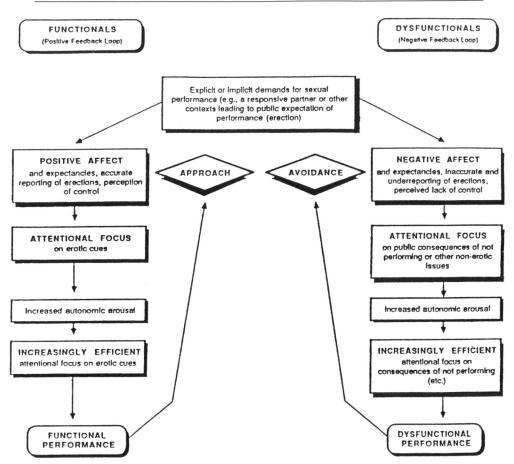

FIGURE 18.1. Model of functional and dysfunctional sexual performance. From Barlow (1986). Copyright 1986 by the American Psychological Association. Reprinted by permission.

tates sexual responding in individuals who are not already experiencing sexual difficulties. And, heightened arousal, up to a point, magnifies typical response patterns such that functional men experience increased arousal and dysfunctional men experience decreased arousal; (2) subjective report of arousal is accurate or overreported among functionals and underreported among dysfunctionals; (3) distraction from erotic cues decreases arousal in functionals and either has no effect or slightly enhances arousal among dysfunctionals; (4) performance demand facilitates responding among functional men and inhibits responding in dysfunctional men; and (5) dysfunctionals evidence greater negative affect pre- and postexposure to erotica. Thus, it appears, based on these results, that affective states and specific cognitive processes have consistent effects on sexual response. Yet it is currently unclear whether these basic differences are the cause of dysfunction or the consequence of the dysfunction. We first review research supporting the

sequence of the dysfunction. We first review research supporting the identification of these differentiating findings and then apply Carver and Scheier's
(1986, 1988) behavioral self-regulatory theory to tackle the questions of
etiology and maintenance of dysfunction in a refined model of sexual dysfunction.

Anxiety Facilitates Arousal

Several early reports ran contrary to the notion pinpointing anxiety as the
causal mechanism in sexual dysfunction (e.g., Bancroft, 1970; Ramsey, 1943;
Sarrel & Masters, 1982). These reports included nonsexual stimuli associated
with erectile response and sexual performance under threat of physical harm.
In addition, the very nature of paraphilias runs contrary to the premise that
anxiety inhibits sexual arousal, as sexual arousal among some paraphilics—
such as exhibitionists—is often associated with the threat of being caught
(Beck & Barlow, 1984). In one of the first studies examining anxiety and
sexual arousal in the laboratory, Hoon Wincze, and Hoon (1977) examined
sexual arousal in response to erotica pre- and postexposure to either a neutral or noxious (automobile accident) film clip. First, sexually functional
women viewed a 2-minute film sequence. Immediately following subjects
viewed an erotic film. Sexual arousal, assessed with vaginal plethysmogra-
phy, was significantly greater in those women who had been preexposed
to the anxiety-producing noxious film as opposed to the neutral film. Interestingly, when the order of the film types was reversed such that subjects
viewed the erotic films first, sexual arousal was lower following the anxiety producing segment. These results were replicated with males (Wolchik
et al., 1980).

At the time of the original Hoon et al. (1977) study, these results were
taken as evidence against Wolpe's (1958) contention that anxiety and sexual arousal are mutually inhibitory. However, Wolpe (1978) contended that
the anxiety exposure paradigm was an insufficient test of the reciprocal inhibition theory due to the paradigm's reliance on the carryover effects of
the noxious exposure. In response to this contention, a subsequent series
of studies by different investigators attempted to simultaneously induce anxiety and sexual arousal. Lange, Wincze, Zwiek, Feldman, and Hughes (1981),
operationalizing anxiety as sympathetic arousal, simultaneously induced anxiety and sexual arousal using injections of epinephrine hydrochloride. In a
single-blind study, subjects received either saline or epinephrine injections
before viewing erotic films. No differences in sexual responding between
the placebo and epinephrine groups were noted thus providing further support for the notion that sympathetic activation does not necessarily inhibit
sexual arousal in the presence of erotica.

A series of studies in our lab support these findings. Barlow, Sakheim,
and Beck (1983) employed a repeated measures design using these two shock
threat conditions and a no-shock condition with functional males. In this

paradigm, shock threat is utilized to induce anxiety. Subjects in the contingent shock threat condition were told there was a 60% chance they would receive a shock if they did not achieve the average level of erection achieved by previous subjects. In the noncontingent threat, subjects were told that the chance they would receive a shock remained 60%; however, this chance of shock was unrelated to their level of erection or any other response. The results indicated that noncontingent shock threat increased sexual arousal compared with the no-shock condition, a finding that confirmed the results of earlier investigations. However, even the demand condition (contingent shock threat) increased sexual responding and, in fact, this condition produced the highest overall level of tumescence (see Figure 18.2).

These results were partially replicated with the addition of dysfunctional males by J. G. Beck, Barlow, Sakheim, and Abrahamson (1987). Functionals evidenced greater tumescence in the noncontingent shock condition. However, arousal in the contingent shock condition was not elevated over control arousal. Unfortunately, with only eight subjects per group, this study may have not had enough power to adequately evaluate these differences were they to exist. Dysfunctionals, on the other hand, evidenced significantly less tumescence in both shock conditions compared to the control condition.

It becomes obvious, in examining the methods used to operationalize the construct anxiety, that a concise definition of anxiety is imperative (J. G. Beck & Barlow, 1984). The results discussed thus far suggest that the physiological component of anxiety is associated with no decrement or an increase in sexual arousal for functionals and a decrement in responding for dysfunctionals.

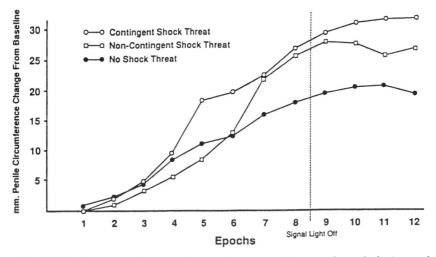

FIGURE 18.2. Mean penile circumference change per 15-second epoch during each of three conditions: No-shock threat, noncontingent shock threat, and contingent shock threat. From Barlow, Sakheim, and Beck (1983). Copyright 1983 by the American Psychological Association. Reprinted by permission.

Control of Performance and Performance Demand

Performance demand manipulations in experiments on sexual arousal are similar to instructions to enhance erectile response in experiments on voluntary control of sexual arousal (Cranston-Cuebas & Barlow, 1990). An examination of capacity to voluntarily control erectile response suggests functionals can voluntarily increase their erectile responding to erotica or fantasy when given instruction to do so (Bancroft & Mathews, 1971; Laws & Rubin, 1969). Others (e.g., Henson & Rubin, 1971; Mavissakalian, Blanchard, Abel, & Barlow, 1975) have also demonstrated voluntary inhibition of erectile responding. Mahoney and Strassberg (1991) address functional males' ability to control their arousal in experiments evaluating subjects' ability to fake preferences for arousing stimuli. Their results provide support for functional subjects' ability to control their arousal and, importantly, note that this response depends on attendance to experimental stimuli. Dysfunctionals, too, appear able to suppress their erections in the presence of erotica (J. G. Beck, Barlow, & Sakheim, 1982). While functionals readily reported cognitive strategies they had employed, dysfunctionals evidenced little awareness that they had been successful nor could they report the strategies they had used. Similarly, dysfunctionals often underreport level of erection (Abrahamson, Barlow, Sakheim, Beck, & Athanasiu, 1985b; Bruce, Cerny, & Barlow, 1986; Sakheim, 1984) and subjective arousal (Sakheim, Barlow, Abrahamson, & Beck, 1987; Morokoff & Heiman, 1980).

Operationalization of the concept of performance demand is also important. This term refers to the cognitive aspects of anxiety under conditions in which individuals believe they are challenged to achieve some standard. Various methodologies are used to operationalize this concept, both directly and indirectly. For example, the contingent shock threat described earlier represents a direct manipulation of performance demand, while observation of one's own genital feedback (Sakheim et al., 1984) discussed subsequently represents a less direct manipulation. Several studies have attempted to manipulate performance demand. In two early studies (Farkas, Sine, & Evans, 1979; Lang et al., 1981) with functional males no differences were found between high-demand and low- or no-demand instruction sets. Dysfunctional men, however, demonstrated a different pattern when given high-demand versus low-demand instructions (Heiman & Rowland, 1983). That is, dysfunctionals evidence lower levels of tumescence during the high- relative to the low-demand condition.

In an attempt to extend these findings by manipulating attentional focus in addition to performance demand, J. G. Beck, Barlow, and Sakheim (1983) examined the interactive effects of self-focused versus partner-focused attention across three levels of partner arousal (high, low, and ambiguous). Under conditions of high partner arousal, functional males evidenced greater responding under partner-focused compared to self-focused instruction sets.

Conversely, dysfunctional males displayed lower levels of tumescence in the high partner arousal condition with partner-focused versus self-focused instructions. Abrahamson, Barlow, Beck, Sakheim, and Kelly (1985) replicated these findings. Results from J. G. Beck et al. (1983) and a replication by Abrahamson, Barlow, Beck, et al. (1985) point out that functionals and dysfunctionals reacted differently to pressure to respond sexually when attending to high partner arousal. In addition, functionals reported this experience as arousing whereas dysfunctionals found it nonarousing. Although thought content is not directly addressed in these studies, results of a recent study examining thought listing in response to erotica (Bach, Sbrocco, Weisberg, Weiner, & Barlow, 1993) suggest dysfunctionals experience more negative internal thoughts in response to erotica. It is not difficult to understand why dysfunctionals would not be aroused concurrently with negative, deprecatory self-statements during sexual performance demand conditions.

Sakheim, Barlow, Beck, and Abrahamson (1984) provide additional support to the notion that directed focus and performance demand interact. Functional males viewed three levels of erotic film clips while their genitals were either covered or uncovered. Uncovered genitals in the slightly arousing film decreased erectile responding, but facilitated tumescence during the highly arousing stimulus. The authors suggest attentional focus on aroused genitals provides additional erotic cues, whereas focus on limited genital response may induce performance concerns.

Based on differential responding between functionals and dysfunctionals in response to performance demands, it has been concluded that concerns labeled variously as "performance demand," "fear of inadequacy," "spectatoring," and the like are all forms of situation-specific, task-irrelevant, cognitive activities that prevent dysfunctionals from task-relevant processing of stimuli in the sexual context. Similarly, this process represents dysfunctionals' disengagement from an erotic focus. We turn now to studies directly manipulating distraction in the context of erotica.

Distraction and Sexual Arousal

Geer and Fuhr (1976) were one of the first groups to conduct an empirical examination of the effects of distraction on sexual arousal using a dichotic listening paradigm. As subjects increased their attention to the distracting task, their remaining attention available to focus on the erotic passage diminished and corresponding decrements in sexual arousal occurred. These findings have been replicated using a different stimulus modality (Farkas et al., 1979). Thus these studies suggest that the competing cognitive tasks result in significant decrements in physiological sexual arousal. Abrahamson, Barlow, Sakheim, et al. (1985) reported findings that indicated distraction might differentially affect the sexual arousal of functional and dysfunctional males. Replicating earlier findings of decrements in tumescence for functionals, the authors did not find a corresponding effect for

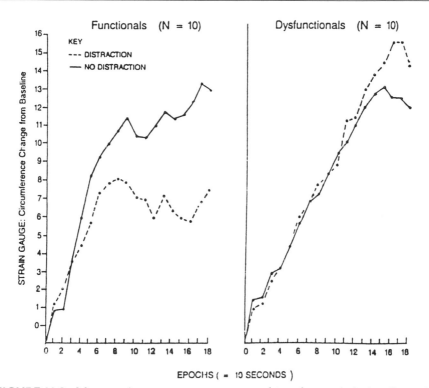

FIGURE 18.3. Mean strain gauge response across subjects by epoch during distraction and no distraction: sexually functional versus sexually dysfunction subjects. From Abrahamson, Barlow, Sakheim, Beck, and Athanasiou (1985). Copyright 1985 by the Association for Advancement of Behavior Therapy. Reprinted by permission.

dysfunctionals. These results are presented in Figure 18.3. In fact, dysfunctionals showed a nonsignificant increase in tumescence. The authors speculated that whereas functionals were diverted from erotic cues by the distraction, dysfunctional subjects' attention may have already been focused on nonerotic thoughts (e.g., performance concerns). Thus, the distracting task shifted dysfunctionals' attention away from one distractor onto another resulting in no appreciable change in tumescence.

J. G. Beck et al. (1987) evaluated the interaction of autonomic arousal and cognitive interference. They presented functional males with four noncontingent shock conditions and used a sentence recognition task afterwards to examine attentional focus. As shown in Figure 18.4, the results revealed that shock threat decreased erectile responding under the half tolerance and tolerance condition. Yet levels of tumescence returned to normal under the twice tolerance threat to a level near the no-shock condition. Conversely, attention on the sentence completion task mirrored this response. That is, the better subjects did on the sentence recognition task, the lower their sexual arousal.

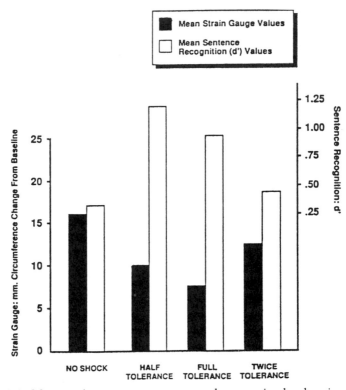

FIGURE 18.4. Mean strain guage response averaged across stimulus duration, and mean sentence recognition values, during four shock threat conditions. From J. G. Beck, Barlow, Sakheim, and Abrahamson (1987). Copyright 1987 by the Society for Psychological Research. Reprinted by permission.

In a study designed to examine the effect of anxiety without a distractor, Jones, Bruce, and Barlow (1986) used this paradigm with functionals and dysfunctionals minus the sentence completion task. Sexually functional males evidenced increasing levels of arousal as intensity of shock threat increased up to full tolerance level where it asymptotes (see Figure 18.5). Actually, functionals evidence greatest arousal at half tolerance while arousal in the other conditions seemed similar (no shock, full tolerance, and twice tolerance) thus suggesting anxiety is facilitatory only at certain levels. Dysfunctionals, on the hand, evidence lowest responding in the half tolerance condition compared to the other conditions. It is curious that when the functionals are at their best, the dysfunctionals are at their worst.

Abrahamson, Barlow, and Abrahamson (1989) reported similar differential response to different types of distractors. Subjects were distracted by a neutral (nonsexual) distractor and a performance sexual distractor while watching erotica. Under the neutral distraction condition, subjects judged the width and length of a line in comparison to a standard line viewed earlier.

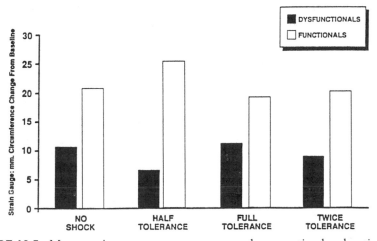

FIGURE 18.5. Mean strain gauge responses, averaged across stimulus duration, during four shock threat conditions. From Jones, Bruce, and Barlow (1986). Reprinted by permission of the authors.

For the sexual distractor subjects viewed live genital feedback from a video camera focused on their genitals. During this feedback, performance demand was manipulated by having subjects estimate their level of erection and whether their tumescence was sufficient for intercourse. Functional males showed significantly greater levels of tumescence under the genital feedback relative to neutral distraction and a control condition. However, dysfunctional males evidenced significantly lower levels of tumescence with the sexual distractor. Viewing the sexual distractor also as a performance demand complicates the interpretation of this study. Initially, dysfunctionals may have performed more poorly because they had negative expectancies regarding their ability to achieve an erection or because they did not process these cues and effectively withdrew from the situation (or both). However, this study is somewhat confounded because dysfunctionals were viewing less erotic cues. That is, functional individuals not only experienced greater tumescence, they viewed greater tumescence compared to their dysfunctional counterparts. Simply put, the dysfunctionals' erotic cues were less arousing. Still, this study suggests neutral distraction interferes with functionals and dysfunctionals in a similar manner.

In examining distraction, the etiology of this phenomenon is of most importance. Until recently it was not clear whether distraction duplicates dysfunctionals' "natural" distracting process or whether dysfunctionals' natural detracting process continued and therefore was not affected by the task. Examining task performance in a recent study suggests that when subjects perform equally well or attend equally (as measured by reaction time and correct response) to a distracting task, tumescence does not differ between functional and dysfunctional groups (Weisberg, Weiner, et al., 1994). And, tumescence is less than what would be expected for functional performance. Thus, suggesting when subjects attended equally to a distracting task, functional performance matched dysfunctional performance and functional performance suffered. To examine attention less obtrusively, future studies should examine memory for film and task events to further explain attentional processes and differences in functional and dysfunctional subjects. It is hypothesized that without a distraction manipulation, memory for erotica would be greater for functionals compared to dysfunctionals. Furthermore, tapping the domain for which dysfunctional memory is expected to be greater than functional memory will provide clues about where functionals' attentional focus lies.

Constructs labeled variously as performance demand, fear of inadequacy, spectatoring, and so forth are all forms of situation-specific, task-irrelevant, cognitive activities that "distract" dysfunctional individuals from task-relevant processing of stimuli in the sexual context. However, while these activities seem to be associated with dysfunctional performance, it may be more helpful to examine why dysfunctionals are not focusing on erotica.

Affect and Sexual Arousal

Thus far, few studies have examined the impact of affect (other than "anxiety") on sexual responding. To our knowledge, in addition to Wolchik's study (Wolchik et al., 1980) described earlier, only two studies have examined the impact of affect manipulations on sexual arousal. Mitchell et al. (1992) provided dysfunctional males with a positive versus negative affect manipulation operationalized as music. Subjects evidence greater tumescence in the positive versus negative or neutral affect condition. Meisler and Carey (1991) used elation and depression mood inductions to preexpose subjects before an erotic film. They report a trend toward decreased subjective responding initially and longer time until maximum arousal following depressive mood induction. However, no differences in tumescence were noted. Interestingly, tumescence during erotica was predictive of posterotica affect, independent of preerotica affect. Thus individuals' affective state was in accord with current physiological responding (or another aspect of this experience). More commonly, other investigations have included affective self-report measures in a variety of laboratory paradigms as dependent variables. Both pre- and postexposure to erotica there is evidence for higher dysphoria among dysfunctionals (e.g., Abrahamson, Barlow, Sakheim, et al., 1985; Abrahamson et al., 1989; Beck & Barlow, 1986a, 1986b; Heiman & Rowland, 1983).

In summary, the results of several studies provide support for five areas in which the responding of sexually functional and dysfunctional males differs. Descriptively, these factors are related meaningfully in a model of sexual dysfunction (Barlow, 1986) shown in Figure 18.1. A key feature of this model is the proposition that it is actually cognitive interference, a distraction process, that is the mechanism of action through which many experiences act to inhibit sexual responsivity. This process, when combined with increased autonomic arousal, leads to the inhibition of sexual arousal through a facilitated distraction effect. Thus, it is not autonomic arousal alone that inhibits arousal. As such, this model shares several similarities with current models of social and other evaluative anxieties that emphasize the role of cognitive interference in the dysfunctional performance. We turn now to such a model, a model of self-regulation, to understand how and why these differences may exist.

COGNITIVE REGULATION OF SEXUAL AROUSAL

Understanding the process with the aid of self-regulatory theory provides increased specificity regarding constructs and mechanisms of action hypothesized in the model of sexual dysfunction presented in Figure 18.1. Further, this refinement may facilitate the conceptualization of etiology and developmental psychopathology. In the following section we outline this conceptualization focusing on four key areas: schematic vulnerability, skill deficit, outcome expectancies, and disengagement. A schematic depiction of the framework adapted from Carver and Scheier (1988) can be found in Figure 18.6.

A presupposition of this model of sexual functioning is that sexual behavior, like all human behavior, is regulated in a system of feedback control (see Carver & Scheier, 1981, 1986, 1988). The process of behavioral regulation involves people using reference points for ensuing behavior. Reference points consist of personal goals, standards, and intentions that are both short term and long term. These goals and desired outcomes can be conceptualized as schematic content. As people engage in tasks, they self-attend and monitor their actions with regard to their standards (Carver & Scheier, 1988). When necessary, they adjust their behavior to conform to the desired goals and outcomes. This behavioral adjustment is basic to self-regulation and operates through feedback control. Generally, the process of behavioral regulation operates smoothly. During sexual activity, conflict may arise due to contextual or environmental disruptions (e.g., uninterested partner) and competing reference values. For example, a man with difficulty obtaining an erection may experience anxiety because he believes his partner will be angry and disappointed. The rising anxiety functions as a warning signal to induce behavioral adjustment.

We believe most individuals can adjust their behavior (e.g., shift positions to increase stimulation). That is, we are operating under the premise that most individuals experience varying degrees of discrepancy in their desired arousal and experienced arousal. And, most individuals make appropriate adjustments. Yet, several factors may interfere with discrepancy adjustment and therefore have implications for understanding sexual dys-

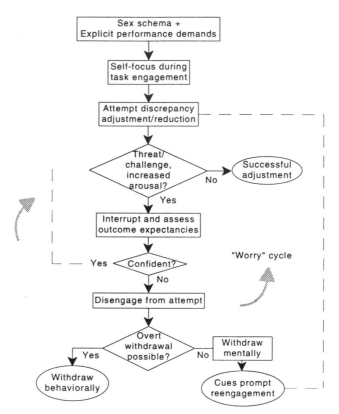

FIGURE 18.6. A self-regulatory model of sexual arousal. Model depicts an integrated conceptualization of mechanisms accounting for functional and dysfunctional performance. From Carver and Scheier (1988). Copyright 1988 by Harwood Academic Publishers. Adapted by permission.

functions. These factors include schematic content, skill deficit, negative outcome expectancies, and disengagement or avoidance. The first two factors may be considered primary variables while the latter two are secondary factors. Each is explicated below with reference to empiric literature.

Schematic Content

The present discussion on schema will be guided by two basic assumptions. First, sexually dysfunctional individuals develop organized cognitive structures (schemas) around issues of sexuality and implications for the self that influence their thoughts, affect, and behavior. Second, the operation of these self-schemas can help account for the persistence of erectile dysfunction in the context of self-regulation. Ample evidence from other areas of psychopathology indicates that biases in information processing are related to the maintenance of depressive and anxiety disorders.

Sexual self-schemas, which include standards, expectations, and self-implications for sexual behavior, are often unrealistic and inaccurate. For example, it is not uncommon for men to believe they can have multiple sequential ejaculations. As well, this belief set and these standards are exposed to little new information that is correct or realistic. Therefore, there is often little accommodation and assimilation of new accurate information into these schemas. The conceptualization that individuals' beliefs about sex are paramount in directing their behavior is similar to John Gagnon's (Gagnon, 1990; Gagnon, Rosen, & Leiblum, 1982; Gagnon & Simon, 1987) scripting perspective used to explain sexual behavior in its cultural context. This perspective emphasizes that, despite similar physiological functioning, there is often little similarity in the meaning of sexual behavior in different cultures.

The idea that beliefs about sex direct behavior is particularly important in examining the etiology of sexual dysfunctions (Lavender, 1985). Inaccurate or distorted schemas may function as a vulnerability factor for the development of a sexual dysfunction. This includes the self-implications of an inability to regulate. Such implications may increase anxiety and further impair regulation. For example, imagine a man who holds the following belief: "A real man can have an erection whenever and wherever." The consequence of not completing this goal may seem catastrophic. Such a discrepancy in behavior and expectation may be perceived as extremely threatening and by that impair regulation. In addition, this process impairs problem solving because there is little room in the rigid schema for dealing with this difficulty because "it is not supposed to happen."

It is important to note that functional individuals are equally disposed to subscribing to normatively distorted views about their sexual functioning. The terms "impotent" or "rigid" provide anecdotal evidence of the association of sexual difficulties with negative qualities. However, we postulate that the meaning of the dysfunction will also be unique for dysfunctionals compared to others. That is, while the more superficial content is almost universally endorsed, the intensity and personal relevance of sex-related schema may distinguish dysfunctionals from their peers. An important reminder is to examine both the cultural- and cohort-specificity of such schemas. For example, we may know something about older adults' views of sex in the 1970s yet there is a good possibility older adults in the 1990s will have different viewpoints.

Although little has been written directly about dysfunctionals' view of themselves, numerous clinical accounts suggest that men with erectile dysfunctions view themselves as "less than men" (e.g., Zilbergeld, 1992). Even the term "impotence" suggests societies' view that a man without an erection is not a "real man." Beyond clinical and anecdotal data, Byrne and colleagues have demonstrated that erotophobia is associated with later sexual difficulties (Byrne & Schulte, 1990). Erotophobia–erotophilia is "the disposition to respond to sexual cues along a negative–positive dimension of affect and evaluation" (Fisher, Byrne, White, & Kelley, 1988, p. 123).

Erotophobia is a cognitive set, presumably learned in childhood, characterized by the association of certain erotic cues and behaviors with negative affect (e.g., guilt). As well, cross-sectional research from our lab suggests dysfunctionals are more erotophobic than their functional counterparts (Jones, Carpenter, Bruce, & Barlow, 1987; Sbrocco, Weiner, & Barlow, 1992). Besides reacting more negatively to erotic cues, dysfunctionals appear more likely to endorse inaccurate information about sex. Baker and de Silva (1989) investigated the relationship between belief in the myths described by Zilbergeld (1978) and sexual dysfunction among men. Dysfunctional men evidence a significantly greater degree of belief for myths about sex (Baker & de Silva, 1989).

Skill Deficit

Behavioral skill deficits are intertwined with the notion that dysfunctionals may have beliefs and attitudes about sex that predispose them to have difficulty becoming aroused. In particular, discrepancy adjustment may be difficult due to skill deficiency. This may be due to lack of experience or practice, or, as described above, it also may be the direct result of the sexual schemas (erotophobia) that hold certain behaviors to be "taboo." For example, take the common scenario of a woman who is nonorgasmic during intercourse. If she refuses to engage in self-stimulation or receive partner stimulation because this is not "okay" and she "should" be able to have an orgasm the "right way" (coitus), it is likely her dysfunction will remain. Here, her beliefs about sexual behavior impede her from attempting behaviors that would likely help her become orgasmic.

Self-report, as discussed in relation to erotophobia, suggests dysfunctionals endorse a limited sexual behavioral repertoire. This limitation may be conceptualized as both a skill and a knowledge deficit. Such a deficit would make dysfunctionals less adroit at discrepancy adjustment. Of greatest interest is research indicating that this disposition is associated with deficits in sex-specific behavioral responses including learning about sex in an academic setting and effective contraceptive use (Allgier, 1983; Gerrard & Reis, 1989; Goldfarb, Gerrard, Gibbons, & Plank, 1988; Fisher, Byrne, & White, 1983; Byrne & Schulte, 1990). This evidence bears on the possibility, discussed above, that erotophobic individuals are at risk for developing a dysfunction because their cognitive schema does not allow for accommodation and assimilation of new information nor does it provide them with a repertoire of behavioral responses to increase arousal.

Kelly and Strassberg (1990) found anorgasmic women, in addition to reporting more negative attitudes toward masturbation, greater sex guilt, and greater endorsement of sex myths, specifically reported discomfort in communicating with their partner about sexual activities that might increase their arousal or lead to orgasm such as direct coital stimulation. Little of this research has been directly extended to dysfunctionals. Yet, the focus of sex therapy involves helping clients modify their beliefs about sex and teaching behaviors facilitating arousal and indirectly supports the notion that dysfunctionals are skill deficient.

A more formal assessment of self-proscribed behaviors for functionals and dysfunctionals has yet to be examined. Similarly, it would be important to continue to determine the predictive usefulness of this difference in much the same way as Byrne and Schulte (1990). That is, if we know erotophobic individuals engage in certain types of behaviors less frequently (a diathesis), can we show they are at risk for developing a dysfunction? And, can we use such information to predict treatment outcome? For example, learning that oral sex is dangerous or forbidden may make one vulnerable to developing a sexual dysfunction and, additionally, individuals holding less rigid views about behaviors proscribed in sex therapy may do better.

Skill differences have been noted in the lab. As reviewed earlier, laboratory evidence suggests that while dysfunctional males can adjust their arousal according to demand to increase their tumescence they were less aware of this process and generally were unable to describe the strategies they used to make these adjustments (J. G. Beck et al., 1982).

The question remains about whether the absent skills represent a skill deficiency precipitating development of a dysfunction or if they are the result of the sexual dysfunction. To some extent, this appears unlikely particularly considering the tie to the dispositional construct erotophobia. Yet, this phenomenon may result from task disengagement which is covered later. Nevertheless, this question requires prospective examination.

Negative Outcome Expectancies

A third factor contributing to a sexual dysfunction is negative outcome expectancies regarding discrepancy adjustment. Individuals unable to successfully adjust their behavior will begin to predict failure. As described above, the inability to adjust successfully or regulate behavior may be the result of several factors. According to behavioral regulation theory, negative outcome expectancies, regardless of their source, promote disengagement from the task (cf., Carver & Scheier, 1988). Consequently, the expectancy of failure becomes enough to maintain the dysfunction. Thus, it is important to view the development of a dysfunction as a process where a key part of the process is the development of negative expectancies regarding one's ability to mediate arousal to meet one's needs and goals. This likely develops after unsuccessful attempts to mediate arousal.

Recent results from our lab suggest dysfunctionals, compared to their functional counterparts, report more negative internal thought listings in response to erotica (Bach et al., 1993). These thoughts could be conceptualized as indicators of negative outcome expectancies as the thoughts represented subjects' report of self-relevant failure- or fear-associated predictions. In addition, no differences were found between the number of positive thoughts endorsed by the groups.

Conceptualization of negative outcome expectancies may be relevant within the context of several existing paradigms including those that create such demands either explicitly or implicitly and those that heighten focus of attention and by that could make such expectancies salient. As well, the studies reviewed earlier suggest dysfunctional males respond poorly to laboratory paradigms including "performance concerns." Presumably performance demand for dysfunctional individuals increases the chances an individual would predict failure as they have the added pressure of external demands, whereas functional individuals do not predict failure—they have no reason to.

Interestingly, a recent study using a misattribution paradigm provides the strongest evidence to date that manipulating expectancies can greatly affect sexual response (Cranston-Cuebas, Barlow, Mitchell, & Athanasiou, 1993). In a within-subjects design, functional and dysfunctional male subjects viewed erotic films followed by the ingestion of each of three placebo pills. Subjects were given an inert substance and told this would enhance, detract, or not affect their erection. Surprisingly, as shown in Figure 18.7, functional individuals exhibited a reverse placebo response, responding with increased tumescence to the detraction manipulation (see Figure 18.7). Tumescence in the detraction condition was greater than responding in the enhancement or control conditions for which there were no differences. Dysfunctional individuals, however, responded with a direct placebo effect exhibiting decreased tumescence to the detraction condition. Tumescence did not differ in the enhancement and control conditions. Arousal during the detraction condition was lower than tumescence in the enhancement and control condition. Interestingly, despite differences in tumescence, there were no differences in subjective arousal across the three conditions for both functionals and dysfunctionals. In addition, a majority of the subjects (70% of the functionals, 60% of the dysfunctionals) believed the "active" pills had no effect on their erectile response. Functionals believed the enhancement and detraction pills had 8% and 13.5% control, respectively, over their tumescence. Dysfunctional subjects reported 9% control for enhancement and 24% control for detraction.

The results of this study illustrate two important steps in behavioral regulation: discrepancy monitoring and outcome expectancies. Applying a self-regulatory model to these results, it appears that functionals would only seek to reduce discrepancy in the detraction condition. That is, they have essentially been provided with feedback that they will not be aroused enough and they then use their skills to reduce the probability of this anticipated discrepancy. It is here they notice or have their attention focused on the potential for a discrepancy. In response to this "threat" or challenge, they regulate their behavior, that is, they increase tumescence. Functionals have the skills, positive outcome expectancies, and confidence to effect change. It is important to note that engagement in discrepancy adjustment hinges on the notion that most males in U.S. culture have a somewhat distorted

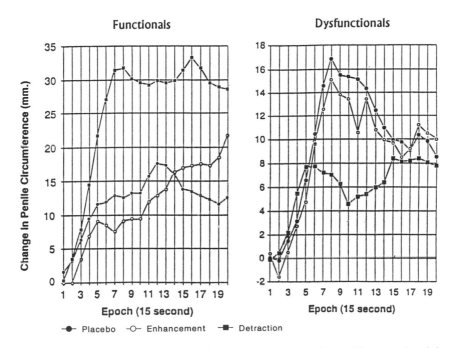

FIGURE 18.7. Mean change in penile circumference across subjects (functional and dysfunctional) by epoch across three conditions (placebo, enhancement, distraction). From Cranston-Cuebas, Barlow, Mitchell, and Athanasiou (1993). Copyright 1993 by the American Psychological Association. Reprinted by permission.

sexual self-schema and thus would find decreased tumescence to be a "bad" thing. The enhancement condition, on the other hand, provides a very different set of circumstances for the functional individual. There is less "threat" to attend to discrepancy because no discrepancy is expected—they have been told they will get aroused and they always get aroused.

Applying the same type of rationale to dysfunctional individuals' performance, the detraction pill likely magnifies their typical response process characterized by an increased salience in negative outcome expectancies and decreased confidence in their ability to perform. The detraction pill would not challenge dysfunctionals as it did the functionals. Rather, this condition would represent confirmation of their status quo, that is, their negative expectancies. Therefore they have little reason to even try to respond. In fact, they may not be task engaged at all. An enhancement manipulation would only increase tumescence if dysfunctional individuals changed their outcome expectancies such that they believed this change could occur and had the skills to adjust arousal.

An interesting issue is whether changing outcome expectancies is sufficient to break the negative feedback cycle. It is easy to imagine only temporary improvement if skills and core cognitions are not dealt with. This phenomenon likely represents the temporary "cure" sometimes experienced by individuals at the start of treatment. In summary, dysfunctional individuals have little confidence in their ability to become aroused. This is not unlike predicting failure for any activity if you are not making headway.

Avoidance: Covert and Overt Disengagement

The fourth factor characterizing dysfunctional sexual arousal is task disengagement. Two aspects of disengagement are important in understanding the etiology and maintenance of sexual dysfunctions. First, disengagement results from an inability to regulate behavior and therefore can be characterized as a secondary factor. That is, it is not a primary or vulnerability factor like an erotophobic schema. Second, disengagement also contributes to the maintenance of the problem.

Task disengagement is a natural response for individuals doubting their ability to cope and expecting failure (Carver & Scheier, 1988). The probability of disengagement increases in the presence of physiological arousal which increases the salience of the negative cognitions. For individuals in a sexual situation, immediate behavioral withdrawal may manifest itself as "giving up" after losing an erection and eventually as decreased frequency of sexual behavior.

In the sexual situation, behavioral disengagement is not always possible due to such things as social constraints and hierarchical goals that make the impact of disengagement "catastrophic" (see Carver & Scheier, 1985). Consequently, disengagement may be covertly expressed through self-distraction or off-task thinking. In addition, covert disengagement may be difficult to sustain due to the contextual cues that prompt task engagement. Reengagement prompts reexperiencing the cycle of anxiety, negative outcome expectancies, doubt, and disengagement. This cycle, described by Carver and Scheier (1988) as self-deprecatory rumination, is similar to the construct of self-focus used by other theorists (Sarason, 1975; Wine, 1982). We will return to a conceptualization of self-focus in the sex literature following a review of empirical data on disengagement.

To our knowledge, overt withdrawal and avoidance have received little attention in the literature. Operationalizing overt withdrawal as ceasing task engagement, we examined subjects' retrospective reports of ceasing to try to obtain an erection, that is, "quitting," when they lost their erection during partner-related sexual behavior. Ninety percent of men seeking help for erectile dysfunction reported they quit. Interestingly, men were fairly equally distributed in their reported response to quitting. Approximately half ceased sexual behavior altogether while the others reported focusing on pleasuring their partner to climax. However, no data are available on functionals' response to difficulty. Interestingly, preliminary results for a study underway where functional and dysfunctional men are asked to either fantasize about a successful or unsuccessful sexual situation provides indirect evidence of this avoidance (Weisberg, Sbrocco, & Barlow, 1994).

Thus far, all of the dysfunctional males have refused to participate in the unsuccessful fantasy while none of the functionals have objected. In fact, functionals become equally aroused to fantasies incorporating erectile difficulty. The implication being, dysfunctionals avoid engaging in a behavior for which they have "no chance" and negative expectancies. In fact, a primary treatment component for erectile dysfunction is to teach men to lose their erection and regain it (e.g., Zilbergeld, 1992).

Data from our lab suggest dysfunctional individuals attempt intercourse less frequently, controlling for partner availability. In addition, retrospective report suggests frequency before the development of the dysfunction is similar to functional's frequency. While this may seem documentation of the obvious, it is important to provide empirical evidence of behavior that behavioral regulation theory conceptualizes as withdrawal and avoidance.

SELF-FOCUSED ATTENTION, DISTRACTION, AND TASK ENGAGEMENT

Most empirical evidence regarding focus of attention suggests the mechanisms outlined in the model but is currently not sufficient to conclude with any certainty what is occurring in the "black box." In essence, an integrated model of sexual arousal and sexual dysfunction illustrates three points or processes at which to examine attentional focus. These stages, illustrated in Figure 18.8, include initial task engagement or orientation to the task, intermediary task engagement focused on discrepancy adjustment, and sustained task engagement or disengagement (see Figure 18.8).

Functional task engagement begins with attention to erotica followed by discrepancy adjustment and sustained attention to erotica and task engagement. Dysfunctional individuals, however, take a different path. There is reason to believe that dysfunctionals, at least for a time, focus on erotic stimuli. However, their inability (or perceived inability) to regulate arousal results in off-task thinking and eventually withdrawal, overtly or covertly. We hypothesize, in order to understand attentional focus, researchers must define the stage they are examining. In addition to stage of engagement and functional status, the chronicity or severity of the dysfunction is expected to influence this process. We suspect, the more experience individuals have with failure, the less they try to regulate, and therefore, they spend little time in the initial stages. At its extreme, this is reflected in avoiding sex altogether. The conceptualization of sexual arousal as a process has important implications for refining our definitions of terms in sexuality research including the constructs of distraction and self-focus. What follows is an attempt to clarify use of these terms and, more importantly, to define the phenomena they purport to characterize by drawing on the self-regulatory aspects of our model.

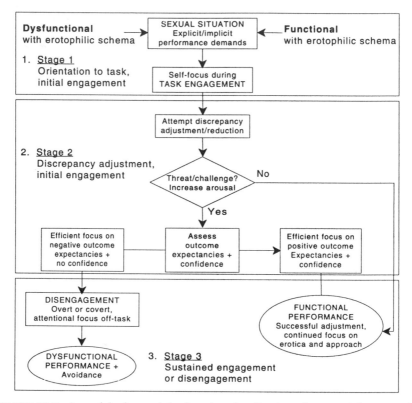

FIGURE 18.8. A model of sexual dysfunction: implications for examining attentional processes.

Defining Self-Focus

As Carver and Scheier (1988) and others (cf. Ingram, 1990) point out, the term "self-focus" can be potentially misleading and must be carefully operationalized. Self-focus is involved somewhat in both functional and dysfunctional task engagement. Therefore, it is important to define self-focus incorporating a more general definition (Ingram, 1990) and to define it capturing the construct as it has been used within the area of sex research.

Generally, self-focus within the context of sex research refers to the process by which an individual attends to information that originates from within and concerns the self. It is defined as a process and by its content. The content is hypothesized to concern negative affect and negative self-statements or performance-related concerns rather than positive affect and an erotophilic focus. The process refers to mechanisms by which the focus becomes self-deprecation rather than erotophilia. Behavioral regulation provides etiological and maintenance mechanisms for this process beginning with discrepancy adjustment. Both functionals and dysfunctionals attempt to adjust their behavior. However, due to a multitude of reasons, the result is an inability to regulate behavior for the dysfunctional individual. This process, by definition, can be described in terms of task engagement. Thus, it seems important to consider defining task engagement as attention to erotica. Task disengagement is characterized by both the process of becoming disengaged and the content of the cognitive activity (be it self-focused on self-deprecatory statements or "non-sex"-related thoughts).

In our view, the difference between facilitation and dysfunction depends not on the presence or absence of self-focus per se, but on a difference in the processes taking place in the person. The individual with favorable expectancies remains "functionally" task engaged, even when highly anxious and highly self-focused. As a result, the phenomenology of this person may be conceptualized as task focus rather than self-focus. Yet, from a self-regulatory framework, self-focus is implicit in task focus (Carver, Blaney, & Scheier, 1979; Scheier & Carver, 1983). That is, in order to monitor behavior in task performance, one must be focused on oneself. For the person whose performance is deteriorating, the self-focus is on different aspects of the self. This person's attention is focused on perceived deficits, salient doubts, and the possible larger ramifications of being unable to proceed toward his or her goal. In many ways, this conceptualization parallels that used in research on test anxiety suggesting facilitation occur for individuals if their expectancies are favorable (Carver, Peterson, Follansbee, & Scheier, 1983; Rich & Woolever, 1992). That is, subjects about to take a test are all equally physiologically aroused. However, only those with doubts perform poorly (assuming they know the material, of course). In summary, self-focus in the sex literature has often been used as an "either–or" construct where dysfunctionals are conceptualized as "self-focused" on performance concerns at the expense of erotic cues. It may be helpful to characterize the nature of the self-focus by defining not only the affective valence and intensity but the context of the focus as task engagement or task disengagement. The idea being, as described above, both groups may attempt task engagement. Functionals focus on erotic cues and dysfunctionals focus off task after trying to engage and regulate their behavior.

Defining Distraction

The term "distraction" has been used in the sex literature to describe several phenomena. As reviewed earlier, distraction has also been used as a dependent variable in laboratory paradigms examining sexual arousal. Generally, distraction refers to attentional processes diverted away from the "correct" attentional focus (i.e., erotic cues). Mechanisms of action underlying dysfunctional performance have focused on increased self-focused attention whereby negative performance-related concerns become salient. This process has been conceptualized as "distraction" and, at times, this definition implies that distraction is deliberate or purposeful. Similarly, at first glance, this definition suggests that if we could prevent distraction, functional performance would result. Dysfunctional individuals may appear distracted at four points or during four processes: initial task engagement, discrepancy adjustment, disengagement, and reengagement prompted by situational cues. Thus, indicators of distraction may include the self-performance concerns during initial task engagement, off-task thinking during disengagement, or rumination during reengagement. Behavioral regulation suggests that while performance concerns likely distract individuals from an erotic focus, this dysfunctional task engagement is the result of these processes.

Thus distraction in the existing literature may be synonymous with both ineffective task engagement and task disengagement. Ineffective engagement refers to the process of behavioral regulation by which individuals initially focus on erotic cues, attempt to adjust their behavior, meet with negative outcome expectancies, and so forth. This process may represent what is typically referred to as a focus on performance concerns. The term "distraction" is commonly used to indicate that attention is diverted from erotica. We must be careful to examine the etiological underpinnings of this phenomenon rather than circularly attributing it to distraction. While this difference in definition is subtle, it highlights etiological mechanisms. Similarly, distraction may be a label for disengagement. There is no doubt that a focus of attention away from erotica would interfere with sexual arousal. What is key is the process by which individuals exhibit this disengagement. Thus, it may be more helpful to define disengagement as an off-task focus. Distraction, therefore, may be a process or the by-product of this dysfunctional focus rather than defined as a primary operational procedure.

The distraction paradigms described earlier are important in that they provide grounds for an analogue of sexual dysfunction. We have evidence that distraction differentially affects sexual arousal with dysfunctionals showing no change or slight improvement when distracted. Functional males experience a decrement in tumescence inversely proportional to the level of a distracting task. That is, the more distracting the task, the less the arousal. Presumably, this occurs as the result of limitations on the information-processing system (e.g., the bottleneck effect). As distraction increases, attention to erotica decreases. Dysfunctionals, however, are not affected by distraction during laboratory exposure to erotica (Abrahamson, Barlow, Sakheim, et al., 1985).

It is important to emphasize that while distraction mimics sexual dysfunctionals' processing, this does not imply causality for distraction, per se, as the primary mechanism of action. Studies manipulating distraction suggest that functional subjects who are distracted look like dysfunctional subjects. It seems important to emphasize that the dysfunctional may focus on erotic cues; however, the processing of these cues is not arousing. There is little doubt that distraction interferes with processing of erotic cues and that performance concerns (etc.) would function to draw one's attention away from them. However, these points are secondary to ineffective self-regulation. The key issue is how to characterize the processing of cues including etiological and maintenance mechanisms. It may be more helpful to conceptualize dysfunctionals' process of task engagement as ineffective and/or as disengaged rather than distracted, thereby highlighting mechanisms of action. As well, a definition of the content of this engagement or disengagement is equally important.

SUMMARY AND FUTURE DIRECTIONS

In general, sex researchers need to improve basic methodology, examine etiological/maintenance mechanisms, and empirically examine treatment components and treatment outcome. Improvements in basic methodology would include better operationalization of constructs such as anxiety and distraction, incorporation of validity measures, and, perhaps most importantly, a focus on the status of task engagement. Many studies to this point have not adequately operationalized affect. In addition, studies generally have examined one affect at the exclusion of other affects or affective dimensions. Consequently, most findings regarding affect exist without convergent or divergent validity. In addition, little has been done to operationalize physiological arousal (besides tumescence) whether by psychophysiological means or report of physical symptoms.

Research over the past decade has functioned to differentiate the sexual responding of sexually functional and dysfunctional individuals. Now it is time to extend these findings by focusing on etiological and maintenance mechanisms. The etiology of male and female sexual arousal disorders arises from application of self-regulatory models to the descriptive model of sexual dysfunction. Unrealistic and/or maladaptive beliefs about sexual behavior and one's definition of self based on these beliefs function as a diathesis for sexual disorders. Converging evidence on the existence and operation of self-schemas in sexual dysfunction exists. However, further information is needed. Conventions for documenting the existence of schema (Vitousek & Hollon, 1991) suggest building evidence from a variety of "suggestive-but-not-sufficient" indicators. Methods and analyses derived from cognitive science should prove more informative in the study of cognitive operations and processes in sexual dysfunction. For example, it is worth exploring whether negative information about sex is more elaborately encoded and more readily retrieved by dysfunctional versus functional individuals. In addition, inclusion of dysphoric and positive affect induction studies should further elucidate differential responding of functionals and dysfunctionals. These types of questions must be conceptualized in the context of the stage of processing or regulation being examined. Cognitions, affect, and behavior for dysfunctionals at earlier stages of initiation may be reflected in increasing performance concerns, movements to increase arousal, mild negative affect, and, similar to functionals, somewhat of an erotic focus. However, examination of information processing at a much later point, such as disengagement, may present a very different picture.

The next step would be experimentally demonstrating the process by which the negative schemas impact behavior in sexual situations. Here we would expect decrements in problem solving. That is, dysfunctionals would lack the ability to describe how they might increase their arousal when experiencing decrements. Dysfunctional men can adjust their level of arousal under certain conditions, yet they are unable to report how they carried out this adjustment. On the other hand, functional men readily report their means of action. Poor skill development and problem solving necessary to adjust arousal set up individuals for failure and the development of negative outcome expectancies. Another hypothesis is that self-report of perceived arousal differs depending on the individual's stage of processing. Similarly, this skill difference should be observed in nonclinical populations among those higher on the dimension of erotophobia.

As described earlier, treatment grew out of a belief that anxiety reduction is key. Based on the conceptualization presented, we would argue it is not relaxation or sensate focus techniques (at least globally) that are most effective. Rather, it is strategies that (1) directly impact beliefs about sex, the original sexual schema, (2) build skills, (3) impact negative outcome expectancies, and (4) encourage engagement despite difficulty or "imperfections." Therefore sex therapy is largely a manner of dealing with an individual and his or her beliefs about sex. Without changing such core beliefs it is difficult to proceed. For example, it would be senseless to simply encourage an individual who has failed repeatedly to keep trying "no matter what." Similarly, an individual in treatment may no longer lose his erection yet steadfastly maintain the belief that it is catastrophic to lose it. This individual would be viewed as "at risk" for relapse unless the core catastrophic cognitions are dealt with. This example illustrates the importance of multiple outcome indicators. While existing techniques and sex therapy likely do many if not all the things mentioned above, systematic evaluation of treatment components—both efficacy and mechanisms of action—is needed.

A model functions heuristically to conceptualize treatment components and to identify important treatment outcome variables. Similarly, a model enables us to conceptualize laboratory paradigms designed to manipulate the experience of functionals within the lab to produce dysfunctional responses. The distraction paradigms have shown that withdrawal or inattention to erotic cues impairs performance. In particular, manipulating information and provision of false feedback may be useful in inducing negative expectancies for functionals, though it is likely such manipulations need to be used repeatedly with the laboratory session to mimic the same type of experience. As well, changes over the course of treatment should be observed with dysfunctionals.

In summary, several areas are worth pursuing. Following from the model we have presented, we recommend research on schematic content, schematic processing, skill deficits, and patterns of engagement and withdrawal. As in any area of psychopathology, information on the course of a disorder is imperative not only for treatment, but ultimately for prevention. In the area of sexual dysfunctions we have little understanding of the empirical basis or the mechanisms of action for various treatment modalities.

A primary goal in the area of sexuality research is to further develop an empirically based model of sexual dysfunction, and, in so doing, provide an empirical basis to evaluate current treatment strategies and modify/develop new techniques if needed. Cognitive therapy provides a firm theoretical basis from which to draw both research and treatment techniques. Techniques from marital therapy are obviously relevant as well as individual methods. The complexity of sexual behavior in our culture makes a cognitive focus germane to the area of human sexuality. Today, we are fortunate to have the tools to both sharpen this focus and to offer help once we have that focus.

ACKNOWLEDGMENTS

The opinions or assertions contained herein are the private ones of the authors and are not to be construed as official or reflecting the views of the Department of Defense or the Uniformed Services University of the Health Sciences.

REFERENCES

Abrahamson, D. J., Barlow, D. H., & Abrahamson, L. S. (1989). Differential effects of performance demand and distraction on sexually functional and dysfunctional males. *Journal of Abnormal Psychology, 98,* 241–247.

Abrahamson, D. J., Barlow, D. H., Beck, J. G., Sakheim, D. K., & Kelly, J. P. (1985). The effects of attentional focus and partner responsiveness on sexual responding: Replication and extension. *Archives of Sexual Behavior, 14,* 361–371.

Abrahamson, D. J., Barlow, D. H., Sakheim, D. K., Beck, J. G., & Athanasiou, R. (1985). Effects of distraction on sexual responding in functional and dysfunctional men. *Behavior Therapy, 16,* 503–515.

Allgier, A. R. (1983). Informational barriers to contraception. In D. Byrne & W. A. Fisher (Eds.), *Adolescents, sex, and contraception* (pp. 143–169). Hillsdale, NJ: Erlbaum.

Bach, A. K., Sbrocco, T., Weisberg, R., Weiner, D. N., & Barlow, D. H. (1993, November). *Sexually functional and dysfunctional males: Categorization of cognitive responses to erotica.* Paper presented at the Association for Advancement of Behavior Therapy, Atlanta, GA.

Baker, C. D., & de Silva, P. (1989). The relationship between male sexual dysfunction and belief in Zilbergeld's myths: An empirical investigation. *Sexual and Marital Therapy, 3,* 229–238.

Bancroft, J. (1970). Disorders of sexual potency. In O. Hill (Ed.), *Modern trends in psychosomatic medicine* (pp. 246–259). New York: Appleton-Century-Crofts.

Bancroft, J., & Mathews, A. M. (1971). Autonomic correlates of penile erection. *Journal of Psychosomatic Research, 15,* 159–167.

Barlow, D. H. (1986). Causes of sexual dysfunction: The role of anxiety and cognitive interference. *Journal of Consulting and Clinical Psychology, 54,* 140–148.

Barlow, D. H. (1988). *Anxiety and its disorders: The nature and treatment of anxiety and panic.* New York: Guilford Press.

Barlow, D. H., Sakheim, D., & Beck, J. G. (1983). Anxiety increases sexual arousal. *Journal of Abnormal Psychology, 92,* 49–54.

Beck, A. T. (1963). Thinking and depression. *Archives of General Psychiatry, 9,* 324–333.

Beck, A. T. (1964). Thinking and depression: 2. Theory and therapy. *Archives of General Psychiatry, 10,* 561–571.

Beck, A. T. (1967). *Depression: Clinical, experimental, and theoretical aspects.* New York: Hoeber. (Reprinted as *Depression: Causes and treatment.* Philadelphia: University of Pennsylvania Press, 1972).

Beck, A. T., Rush, A. J., Shaw, B. F., & Emery, G. (1979). *Cognitive therapy of depression.* New York: Guilford Press.

Beck, A. T., & Weishaar, M. (1989). Cognitive therapy. In A. Freeman, K. M. Simon, L. E. Beutler, & H. Arkowitz (Eds.), *Comprehensive handbook of cognitive therapy* (pp. 21–36). New York: Plenum Press.

Beck, J. G., & Barlow, D. H. (1984). Current conceptualizations of sexual dysfunction: A review and an alternative perspective. *Clinical Psychology Review, 4,* 363–378.

Beck, J. G., & Barlow, D. H. (1986a). The effects of anxiety and attentional focus on sexual responding: I. Physiological patterns in erectile dysfunction. *Behaviour Research and Therapy, 24,* 9–17.

Beck, J. G., & Barlow, D. H. (1986b). The effects of anxiety and attentional focus on sexual responding: II. Cognitive and affective patterns in erectile dysfunction. *Behaviour Research and Therapy, 24,* 19–26.

Beck, J. G., Barlow, D. H., & Sakheim, D. (1982, August). *Sexual arousal and suppression patterns in functional and dysfunctional men.* Paper presented at the annual convention of the American Psychological Association, Washington, DC.

Beck, J. G., Barlow, D. H., & Sakheim, D. (1983). The effects of attentional focus and partner arousal on sexual responding in functional and dysfunctional men. *Behaviour Research and Therapy, 21,* 1–8.

Beck, J. G., Barlow, D. H., Sakheim, D. K., & Abrahamson, D. H. (1987). Shock threat and sexual arousal: The role of selective attention, thought content, and affective states. *Psychophysiology, 24,* 165–172.

Bruce, T. S., Cerny, J. A., & Barlow, D. H. (1986, November). *Spectatoring operationalized: Its influence on sexually functional and dysfunctional men.* Paper presented at the annual convention of the Association for Advancement of Behavior Therapy, New York.

Byrne, D., & Schulte, L. (1990). Personality dispositions as mediators of sexual responses. In J. Bancroft, C. M. Davis, & D. Weinstein (Eds.), *Annual Review of Sex Research* (pp. 93–118). Lake Mills, IA: The Society for the Scientific Study of Sex.

Carver, C. S., Blaney, P. H. & Scheier, M. (1979). Reassertion and giving up: The interactive role of self-directed attention and outcome expectancy. *Journal of Personality and Social Psychology, 37,* 1859–1870.

Carver, C. S., Peterson, L. M., Follansbee, D. J., & Scheier, M. F. (1983). Effects of self-directed attention on performance and persistence among persons high and low in test anxiety. *Cognitive Therapy and Research, 7,* 333–354.

Carver, C. S., & Scheier, M. F. (1981). *Attention and self-regulation: A control–theory approach to human behavior.* New York: Springer-Verlag.

Carver, C. S., & Scheier, M. F. (1985). Self-consciousness, expectancies, and the coping process. In T. M. Field, P. McCabe, & N. Schneiderman (Eds.), *Stress and coping* (pp. 305–330). Hillsdale, NJ: Erlbaum.

Carver, C. S., & Scheier, M. F. (1986). Functional and dysfunctional responses to test anxiety: The interaction between expectancies and self-focused attention. In R. Schwarzer (Ed.), *Self-related cognitions in anxiety and motivation* (pp. 111–141). Hillsdale, NJ: Erlbaum.

Carver, C. S., & Scheier, M. F. (1988). A control–process perspective on anxiety. *Anxiety Research, 1,* 17–22.

Carver, C. S., & Scheier, M. F. (1991) A control-process perspective on anxiety. In R. Schwarzer & R. A. Wicklund (Eds.), *Anxiety and self focus attention* (pp. 3–8). Chur, Switzerland: Hardwood Academic Press.

Cranston-Cuebas, M., & Barlow, D. H. (1990). Cognitive and affective contributions to sexual functioning. In J. Bancroft, C. M. Davis, & D. Weinstein (Eds.), *Annual review of sex research* (pp. 119–162). Lake Mills, IA: The Society for the Scientific Study of Sex.

Cranston-Cuebas, M., Barlow, D. H., Mitchell, W., & Athanasiou, R. (1993). Differential effects of misattribution on sexually functional and dysfunctional men. *Journal of Abnormal Psychology, 102,* 525–533.

Epstein, N., & Baucom, D. H. (1989). Cognitive therapy. In A. Freeman, K. M. Simon, L. E. Beutler, & H. Arkowitz (Eds.), *Comprehensive handbook of cognitive therapy* (pp. 491–513). New York: Plenum Press.

Farkas, G., Sine, L. F., & Evans, I. M. (1979). The effects of distraction,, performance demand, stimulus explicitness, and personality on objective and subjective measures of male sexual arousal. *Behaviour Research and Therapy, 17,* 25–32.

Fisher, W. A., Byrne, D., & White, L. A. (1983). Emotional barriers to contraception. In D. Byrne & W. A. Fisher (Eds.), *Adolescents, sex, and contraception* (pp. 207–239). Hillsdale, NJ: Erlbaum.

Fisher, W. A., Byrne, D., White, L. A., & Kelley, K. (1988). Erotophobia-erotophophilia as a dimension of personality. *Journal of Sex Research, 25,* 123–151.

Gagnon, J. H. (1990). The explicit and implicit use of the scripting perspective in sex research. In J. Bancroft, C. M. Davis, & D. Weinstein (Eds.), *Annual review of sex research* (pp. 1–44). Lake Mills, IA: The Society for the Scientific Study of Sex.

Gagnon, J. H., Rosen, R. C., & Leiblum, S. R. (1982). Cognitive and social aspects of sexual dysfunction: Sexual scripts in sex therapy. *Journal of Sexual and Marital Therapy, 8,* 44–56.

Gagnon, J. H., & Simon, W. (1987). The scripting of oral genital sexual conduct. *Archives of Sexual Behavior, 16,* 1–25.

Geer, J. H., & Fuhr, R. (1976). Cognitive factors in sexual arousal: The role of distraction. *Journal of Consulting and Clinical Psychology, 44,* 238–243.

Gerrard, M., & Reis, T. J. (1989). Retention of contraceptive and AIDS information in the classroom. *Journal of Sex Research, 26,* 315–323.

Goldfarb, L., Gerrard, M., Gibbons, F. X., & Plante, T. (1988). Attitudes toward sex, arousal, and the retention of contraceptive information. *Journal of Personality and Social Psychology, 55,* 634–641.

Heiman, J. R., & Rowland, D. L. (1983). Affective and physiological sexual response patterns: The effects of instructions on sexually functional and dysfunctional men. *Journal of Psychosomatic Research, 27,* 105–116.

Henson, D. E., & Rubin, H. G. (1971). Voluntary control of eroticism. *Journal of Applied Behavior Analysis, 4,* 37–44.

Hoon, P., Wincze, J., & Hoon, E. (1977). A test of reciprocal inhibition: Are anxiety and sexual arousal in women mutually inhibitory? *Journal of Abnormal Psychology, 86,* 65–74.

Ingram, R. E. (1990). Self-focused attention in clinical disorders: Review and a conceptual model. *Psychological Bulletin, 107,* 156–176.

Jones, J. C., Bruce, T. J., & Barlow, D. H. (1986, November). *Effects of four levels of "anxiety" on the sexual arousal of sexually functional and dysfunctional men.* Paper presented at the annual convention of the Association for the Advancement of Behavior Therapy, Chicago.

Jones, J. C., Carpenter, K., Bruce, T. J., & Barlow, D. H. (1987, November). *Sexual attitudes and affective responding in sexually functional and dysfunctional men.* Paper presented at the annual convention of the Association for the Advancement of Behavior Therapy, Boston.

Kaplan, H. S. (1977). *The new sex therapy.* New York: Brunner/Mazel.

Kelly, M. P., & Strassberg, D. S. (1990). Attitudinal and experiential correlates of anorgasmia. *Archives of Sexual Behavior, 19,* 165–177.

Lange, J. D., Wincze, J. P., Zwick, W., Feldman, S., & Hughes, P. (1981). Effects of demand for performance, self-monitoring of arousal, and increased sympathetic nervous system activity on male erectile response. *Archives of Sexual Behavior, 10,* 443–463.

Lavender, A. D. (1985). Societal influences on sexual dysfunctions: The clinical sociologist as sex educator. *Clinical Sociology Review, 3,* 129–142.

Laws, D. R., & Rubin, H. G. (1969). Instructional control of an autonomic response. *Journal of Applied Behavioral Analysis, 2,* 93–99.

LoPiccolo, J. (1992). Postmodern sex therapy for erectile failure. In R. C. Rosen & S. R. Leiblum (Eds.), *Erectile disorders: Assessment and treatment* (pp. 172–199). New York: Guilford Press.

Mahoney, J. M., & Strassberg, D. S. (1991). Voluntary control of male sexual arousal. *Archives of Sexual Behavior, 20,* 1–16.

Masters, W., & Johnson, V. (1970). *Human sexual inadequacy.* Boston: Little, Brown.

Mavissakalian, M., Blanchard, E. B., Abel, G. G., & Barlow, D. H. (1975). Responses to complex erotic stimuli in homosexual and heterosexual males. *British Journal of Psychiatry, 126,* 252–257.

Meisler, A. W., & Carey, M. P. (1991). Depressed affect and male sexual arousal. *Archives of Sexual Behavior, 20,* 541–554.

Mitchell, W. B., Brown, T., Barlow, D. H., Wackett, A., Rozalewycz, J., Sbrocco, T., & Weiner, D. (1992, November). *The effects of affect on male sexual dysfunction.* Paper presented at the Association for Advancement of Behavior Therapy, Boston.

Morokoff, P. J., & Heiman, J. R. (1980). Effects of erotic stimuli on sexually functional and dysfunctional women: Multiple measures before and after therapy. *Behaviour Research and Therapy, 18,* 127–137.

Pryde, N. A. (1989). Sex therapy in context. *Sexual and Marital Therapy, 4,* 215–227.

Ramsey, G. (1943). The sexual development of boys. *American Journal of Psychology, 56,* 217.

Rich, A. R., & Woolever, D. K. (1992). Expectancy and self-focused attention: experimental support for the self-regulation model of test anxiety. *Journal of Social and Clinical Psychology, 7,* 246–259.

Sakheim, D. K. (1984). *Waking assessment of erectile potential: The validation of a laboratory procedure to aid in the differential diagnosis of psychogenic and organic impotence.* Unpublished doctoral dissertation, State University of New York at Albany.

Sakheim, D. K., Barlow, D. H., Abrahamson, D. J., & Beck, J. G. (1987). Distinguishing between organogenic and psychogenic erectile dysfunction. *Behaviour Research and Therapy, 25,* 379–390.

Sakheim, D. K., Barlow, D. H., Beck, J. G., & Abrahamson, D. (1984). The effect of an increased awareness of erectile cues on sexual arousal. *Behaviour Research and Therapy, 22,* 151–158.

Sarason, L. G. (1975). Anxiety and self-preoccupation. In L. G. Sarason & C. D. Spielberger (Eds.), *Stress and anxiety* (Vol. 2, pp. 27–44). New York: Wiley.

Sarrel, P. M., & Masters, W. H. (1982). Sexual molestation of men by women. *Archives of Sexual Behavior, 11,* 117–131.

Sbrocco, T., Weiner, D., & Barlow, D. (1992, November). *Behavioral subtypes of dysfunctional males: Preliminary results and treatment implications.* Paper presented at the Association for Advancement of Behavior Therapy, Boston.

Scheier, M. F., & Carver, C. S.(1983). Self-directed attention and the comparison of self with standards. *Journal of Experimental Social Psychology, 10,* 205–222.

Vitousek, K. B., & Hollon, S. H. (1991). The investigation of schematic content and processing in the eating disorders. *Cognitive Therapy and Research, 29,* 71–83.

Weisberg, R., Sbrocco, T., & Barlow, D. H. (1994, November). *Imagery ability in male sexual arousal: Work in progress.* Paper presented at the Association for Advancement of Behavior Therapy, San Diego, CA.

Weisberg, R., Weiner, D., Sbrocco, T., Brown, T., Bach, A., & Barlow, D. H. (1994, November). *Attention allocation and anxiety in sexually functional and dysfunctional males.* Paper presented at the Association for Advancement of Behavior Therapy, San Diego, CA.

Wine, J. D. (1982). Evaluation anxiety: A cognitive-attentional construct. In H. W. Krohne & L. Laux (Eds.), *Achievement, stress, and anxiety* (pp. 207–219). Washington, DC: Hemisphere.

Wolchik, S. A., Beggs, V., Wincze, J. P., Sakheim, D. K., Barlow, D. H., & Mavissakalian, M. (1980). The effects of emotional arousal on subsequent sexual arousal in men. *Journal of Abnormal Psychology, 89,* 595–598.

Wolpe, J. (1958). *Psychotherapy by reciprocal inhibition.* Stanford, CA: Stanford University Press.

Wolpe, J. (1978). Comments on "A test of reciprocal inhibition" by Hoon, Wincze & Hoon. *Journal of Abnormal Psychology, 87,* 452–454.

Zilbergeld, B. (1978). *Male sexuality.* New York: Bantam Books.

Zilbergeld, B. (1992). *The new male sexuality.* New York: Bantam Books.

Chapter 19

When Bad Things Happen to Rational People: Cognitive Therapy in Adverse Life Circumstances

Stirling Moorey

THE PARADOX OF EMOTIONAL DISTRESS

One of Beck's major contributions to the field of psychopathology has been the recognition that "thought disorder" is not restricted to psychosis: Patients with neurotic conditions show characteristic distortions in their thinking patterns (Beck, 1963). In pervasive disorders of mood, such as depression and generalized anxiety, these distorted thought patterns are prevalent and involve systematic errors in the processing of information available from the outside world. The objective environment of someone with an emotional disorder is often far less aversive than it seems to the sufferer. Beck describes the paradox of depression well in his 1967 text:

> There is . . . an astonishing contrast between the depressed person's image of himself and the objective facts. A wealthy man moans that he doesn't have the financial resources to feed his children. A widely acclaimed beauty begs for plastic surgery in the belief that she is ugly. An eminent physicist berates himself "for being stupid."

> Despite the torment experienced as the result of these self-debasing ideas, the patients are not readily swayed by objective evidence or by logical demonstration of the irrationality of these ideas. Moreover, they often perform acts that seem to enhance their suffering. The wealthy man puts on rags and publicly humiliates himself by begging for money to support himself and his family. A clergyman with an unimpeachable reputation tries to hang himself because "I'm the world's worst sinner." A scientist whose work has been confirmed by numerous independent investigators, publicly "confesses" that his discoveries were a hoax.

This discrepancy between external reality and the depressed person's internal reality results from a consistent bias in information processing. In depression there is a pervading negative view of the self, the world, and the future: the well known cognitive triad (Beck, 1967). In generalized anxiety there is a similar bias in the interpretation of the world, but here the self is seen as vulnerable, the world as dangerous, and the future as unpredictable (Blackburn & Davidson, 1990). In Beck's theory disorders of mood that persist across many situations are maintained by the cognitive apparatus preventing disconfirming evidence from becoming available to the sufferer through the distortion of incoming information. In other emotional disorders, such as panic or hypochondriasis, the cognitive model is slightly different. Certain beliefs predispose to the episodic anxiety seen in these disorders. Patients who experience panic attacks may often have beliefs that physical symptoms are indicative of an impending catastrophe (e.g., palpitations are a sign of a heart attack). Here maladaptive beliefs lead to misinterpretations of specific physical symptoms, rather than a general tendency to think in a distorted way about the world.

In this chapter I will be primarily concerned with depression and generalized anxiety. Beck's model holds well for the patients described above, for whom there is a dramatic gulf between their objective circumstances and their subjective experience, but what if the person's life situation is realistically stressful? Losing your job at an age when you have little chance of further employment, facing the death of a loved one, or developing a serious illness like cancer are likely to generate realistic negative thoughts. These thoughts may be accurate representations of a depressing situation. We know that stressful life events may precipitate depression (Brown, Harris, & Copeland, 1977) and that ongoing stress such as critical comments from a spouse may increase the risk of relapse (Hooley, Orley, & Teasdale, 1986).

One test of the robustness of Beck's cognitive therapy is the extent to which it can contribute to depression associated with negative life circumstances. The negative thoughts verbalized by these patients may reflect an accurate appraisal of their surroundings. Even if these thoughts are distorted, it could be argued that they are often part of a natural sequence of reactions to stress, part of a natural process of grieving. Adverse life events therefore pose two problems for standard cognitive therapy:

1. How does cognitive therapy deal with realistic negative thoughts? Are there perhaps times when life really is so hard on someone that we can talk about anxiety or depression being a "rational" response to an appalling situation? And if this is the case, can we really expect to help by using a therapy based on the premise that anxious and depressed thinking is illogical?

2. How does cognitive therapy deal with a process of adjustment? Cognitive models of depression and anxiety are essentially steady state models, but people's reactions to loss and trauma are often part of a continuing ad-

justment process. Can cognitive therapy meet the challenge of adjustment disorders?

In this chapter I will address these two problems, with particular reference to people suffering from cancer, and will consider the extent to which cognitive therapy can be applied to the emotional distress experienced by this group of patients. I hope to show that Beck's theory and therapy do, in fact, have a great deal to offer patients facing real life difficulties, and that working with them can be both challenging and rewarding.

EMOTIONAL DISORDERS IN PATIENTS WITH CANCER

The psychiatric morbidity associated with cancer is now well documented. Studies of outpatients and inpatients in North America with various types of cancer have shown that 34–44% (Farber, Weinerman, & Kuypers, 1984; Derogatis et al., 1983) meet DSM-III-R criteria for psychiatric disorder (adjustment disorder being the most common diagnosis with anxiety and depression the next most common). Despite recent advances many cancers still have a high mortality, and, although public perception has changed, cancer is still seen as a terrifying diagnosis. Much of the psychological distress is associated with fear of death. Even those given a good prognosis are faced with an uncertain future and the possibility of recurrence. Most patients go through a period of numbness and shock immediately after diagnosis which is followed by a range of emotional reactions including anger, depression, and fear. Similar adjustment reactions occur with each new stage of the disease—starting treatment, recurrence, and terminal illness. It seems that most of the psychological morbidity occurs around these times of crisis. Silberfarb and Greer (1982) reported recurrence to be associated with more psychological disturbance than diagnosis. It is not only the threat to survival that is stressful. The treatments used in cancer can produce very distressing side effects: mastectomy is associated with body image difficulties, low self-esteem, and sexual problems, which can persist for as long as 2 years after the operation (Maguire et al., 1978; Morris, Greer, & White, 1977). Chemotherapy also produces substantial psychological morbidity (Maguire, Tait, Brooke, & Selwood, 1980). Patients face the prospect of months of treatment that can make them ill with recurrent nausea, hair loss, and fatigue. Women who perceived their coping efforts to be ineffective against side effects experienced greater distress. Radiotherapy, while causing fatigue and listlessness, does not seem to cause as much psychiatric disturbance as surgery or chemotherapy (Wallace, Priestman, Dunn, & Priestman, 1993).

In advanced cancer, physical symptoms of the disease itself become important. Pain, immobility, nausea, and breathlessness all contribute to emotional distress. Although developments in palliative care and the hospice movement have made the terminal phase of the disease more bearable, there is still significant psychological morbidity.

DEPRESSIVE REALISM

The extent of emotional distress in patients with cancer is, therefore, well established, but could it be that this distress is largely realistic and rational? Traditionally cognitive therapists have asserted that there is no such thing as a rational depression: Sadness is not depression. Burns (1979), for instance, distinguishes between the two states thus: "Sadness is a normal emotion created by realistic perceptions that describe a negative event involving loss or disappointment in an undistorted way. Depression is an illness that always results from thoughts that are distorted in some way" (p. 205). For instance, following the death of a loved one we might think, "I lost him/her and I will miss the companionship and love we shared." This accurate appraisal would lead to feelings of sadness and loss. If we think, "I'll never be happy again. It's not fair," the appraisal includes distortions such as overgeneralization, arbitrary inference, and making unrealistic demands on the world. This interpretation will lead to depression.

In adopting this stance, cognitive therapy is being true to its roots in stoic philosophy. Epictetus (1983) addresses the issue of illness and death:

> Illness interferes with the body, not with one's faculty of choice, unless that faculty of choice wishes it to. Lameness interferes with the limb, not with one's faculty of choice. Say this at each thing that happens to you, since you will find that it interferes with something else, not with you. (p. 327)

> What upsets people is not things themselves but their judgements about the things. For example, death is nothing dreadful (or else it would have appeared dreadful to Socrates), but instead the judgement about death that is dreadful — that is what is dreadful. (p. 326)

In direct opposition to this view that depression comes from distorted judgments, even in the face of illness and death, is the idea that, in fact, the depressive has a more accurate view of reality than the rest of us (Alloy & Abramson, 1979). This idea also has a distinguished pedigree. Freud alluded to the depressive's apparently realistic self-image in *Mourning and Melancholia* (Freud, 1917/1984). Concerning the depressed person's tendency to make severely critical comments about himself Freud (1917/1984, p. 255) remarked,

> It is merely that he has a keener eye for the truth than other people who are not melancholic. When in his heightened self-criticism he describes himself as petty, egoistic, dishonest, lacking in independence . . . it may be, so far as we know, that he has come pretty near to understanding himself; we only wonder why a man has to be ill before he can be accessible to truth of this kind.

These observations are consistent with Freud's doleful comment that "much will be gained if you succeed in transforming your hysterical misery into common unhappiness" (cited in Daintith & Isaacs, 1989).

The concept of depressive realism is Beck's theory turned on its head. It is the rest of us who are seeing the world in a distorted way by putting a positive gloss on suffering. Alloy and Abramson (1979) reported a series of experiments in which they compared depressed college students and non-depressed controls on a task. The task involved pressing or not pressing a button, and as feedback either receiving or not receiving a green light. Subjects were asked to estimate the degree of contingency between the task and the outcome, that is, how frequently did the light come on in response to the button being pressed. The actual contingency was manipulated experimentally. All subjects were accurate at contingencies set at 25%, 50%, and 75%, but when there was no connection between the two events the depressives were more accurate. However, this was in very special circumstances and the subjects were not clinically depressed. Vazquez (1987) showed that if the response was a sign showing a negative self-referent statement such as "My problems are unsolvable," and the actual contingency was 0%, the depressed students were no longer more accurate, but they were if the sign showed a non-self-referent statement such as "Problems of human beings will never be solved." Other studies with depressed psychiatric patients have shown that depressives tend to underestimate positive reinforcement. Taking the studies together there is not much evidence to suggest that clinically depressed patients really see the world more accurately than the rest of us.

In conclusion, there seems to be evidence that most of us exhibit a slight positive bias in the way we see the world. With lowering of mood this bias changes and the lower the mood the more likely it is that there will be negative distortions of information. Clinically depressed patients have a distorted, unrealistic view of the world. It is, therefore, conceivable that patients with serious illnesses like cancer demonstrate distorted cognitions when they become depressed. No studies have yet been carried out comparing cognitive factors in the depression of patients with and without physical illness. There would therefore seem to be room for interventions that identify the distortions in the thinking of people in adverse life situations, to help them appraise the situation more accurately and thus enhance their problem solving.

THE PROCESS OF ADJUSTMENT

Individuals' appraisals of negative life events are not static. Most people recognize that in response to a major change in one's life circumstances there has to be a period of adjustment, during which a variety of cognitive interpretations and emotional responses occur. Kübler-Ross (1970) was one of the first to describe the stages of adjustment to terminal illness. Barraclough

(1994) summarizes the cancer patient's progression through various emotional stages:

1. Shock, numbness, or disbelief on first learning the truth; the bad news seems too much to be taken in. This may be called the stage of denial and usually lasts no more than a few days.
2. Acute distress as the full reality dawns: anxiety, anger, bargaining, and protest, often lasting several weeks.
3. Depression and despair which may also last several weeks.
4. Gradual adjustment and acceptance, often taking several months.

There has been a tendency by some writers to reify these stages, but clinically it is clear that patients do not conform to a set pattern. Some show acceptance from the very beginning, while others may show delayed reactions, only demonstrating distress well after the initial diagnosis. Yet other patients exhibit denial throughout their illness (Greer, 1992). The empirical evidence for the stage theory is not great (Silver & Wortman, 1991). Other writers have conceptualized the adjustment process differently. Horowitz (1986) postulates two oscillating phases: one of "overmodulated" emotions where avoidance and denial are manifest, and another of "undermodulated" emotions where overwhelming feelings are experienced. While the exact nature of the adjustment process is a matter of debate, there is general agreement that some form of processing of the cognitive and emotional significance of adverse life events is necessary, and that this takes time. Psychoanalysts refer to this as "working through" (Sandler, Dare, & Holder, 1970), while more cognitively oriented writers have referred to it as "emotional processing" (Rachman, 1980). Horowitz suggests that a major life event challenges our view of the world, and that to come to terms with this we must readjust our internal working models or "schemas" to fit with this new information. The more dramatic the life event—such as a bereavement or a threat to life—the greater the discrepancy between the new information and existing schemas, and the greater the task of assimilating the new information.

Beck's cognitive model of emotional disorder has been developed with stable emotional states such as clinical anxiety and depression in mind. It describes the fixed cognitive patterns seen in these disorders. The basic model does, of course, contain an interaction between the underlying cognitive schemas and adverse life events. Underlying assumptions about the self and the world develop during childhood as a result of formative experiences. In adult life the assumptions are usually latent or mildly valent until a critical life event occurs—a traumatic event with idiosyncratic meaning. Classically depression is triggered by a loss event. In this model little attention is paid to the *process* of change in self-image. The previously held model of the self as competent, lovable, and worthwhile is simply replaced by another model of the self as incompetent, unlovable, and worthless. This state shift can in fact be viewed as an arrest of the process of assimilation of new information from the critical life event. Because assumptions are rigid, absolutistic, and global, the flexibility is not available to allow emotional processing in patients who develop full-blown depression or generalized anxiety.

Studies of people in difficult life situations have shown that a high proportion of the emotional distress experienced is part of a process of adjustment. In cancer patients various studies using DSM-IV criteria have shown a level of psychological morbidity around 50%. A formal psychiatric diagnosis, usually anxiety or depression, is present in 20% of patients with cancer, while 30% receive a diagnosis of adjustment disorder. Table 19.1 shows the DSM-IV criteria for adjustment disorder.

The relationship between adjustment disorder and diagnoses such as generalized anxiety disorder and major depressive disorder remains unclear. The distinction is partly one of time and also one of severity. But it is possible for a diagnosis of adjustment disorder to be made if the full criteria for another diagnosis are not fulfilled and the patient is suffering in response to a significant life event. To diagnose adjustment disorder it has to be judged that the individual is going through a process that will eventually lead to adaptive adjustment. This is crystal ball gazing. A proportion of these patients will go on to develop major depressive disorder, dysthymia, or generalized anxiety disorder.

Clearly if a process of adjustment is ongoing, formal cognitive therapy may be inappropriate. As Freud (1917/1984, p. 252) pointed out in *Mourning and Melancholia,* mourning involves "grave departures from the normal attitude to life" but we would not think of labeling it as pathological or "treating" it. A supportive relationship in which the patient is helped to ventilate feelings will probably be sufficient to facilitate adjustment. However, there are two areas where cognitive techniques may still be useful in adjustment. Firstly, excessive distorted thinking may cause unnecessary distress (e.g., inappropriate guilt) and may be legitimately addressed. Secondly, maladaptive beliefs may influence the process of adjustment and so prevent it from proceeding. Williams et al. (1995) have suggested that beliefs relating to emotional expression may be associated with the development of posttraumatic stress disorder after major trauma.

There is some evidence that cognitive therapy may contribute something more than simple supportive therapy in patients with adjustment reactions. In a recent trial of cancer patients with adjustment reactions who were referred for therapy, we randomly allocated subjects to either 8 weeks of adjuvant psychological therapy (APT; Moorey & Greer, 1989) or nondirective counseling. Change between baseline and 8-week assessment showed significant differences between the treatments. APT produced more change than counseling in fighting spirit, hopelessness, anxiety, and a measure of coping with cancer. Change between baseline and assessment at 4 months showed that these effects had persisted for fighting spirit, anxiety, and the Cancer Coping Questionnaire, but not for hopelessness.

TABLE 19.1. DSM-IV Criteria for Adjustment Disorder

A. The development of emotional or behavioral symptoms in response to an identifiable stressor(s) occurring within 3 months of the onset of the stressor(s).

B. These symptoms or behaviors are clinically significant as evidenced by either of the following:
   (1) marked distress that is in excess of what would be expected from exposure to the stressor
   (2) significant impairment in social or occupational (academic) functioning.

C. The stress-related disturbance does not meet the criteria for another specific Axis I disorder and is not merely an exacerbation of a preexisting Axis I or Axis II disorder.

D. The symptoms do not represent Bereavement.

E. Once the stressor (or its consequences) has terminated, the symptoms do not persist for more than an additional 6 months.

Note. From American Psychiatric Association (1994, p. 626). Copyright 1994 by the American Psychiatric Association. Reprinted by permission.

An examination of the proportion of patients meeting the entry criteria at 8 weeks and at 4 months revealed that the majority of patients (100% APT, 82% counseling) scored > 8 on anxiety at baseline. In the APT group this fell to 48% at 8 weeks and 29% at 4 months. In the counseling group the changes were considerably less: 68% at 8 weeks and 71% at 4 months still met the inclusion criteria for anxiety.

The area of adjustment is one that has not been covered fully by Beck's cognitive theory and is a fruitful area for research. In the next section I will consider how cognitive techniques may be applied to "rational" emotional disorders and to adjustment disorders.

COGNITIVE THERAPY FOR "REALISTIC" ANXIETY AND DEPRESSION: SOME CLINICAL SUGGESTIONS

Mrs. A was a 50-year-old woman referred for treatment of a depression secondary to her cancer. She had suffered from polymyalgia rheumatica for 20 years. In the last few years this had grown worse, and she was becoming increasingly limited in her physical activities. She gave up work because if she carried out any moderately strenuous task she experienced great pain. The previous year she had been found to have cancer of the breast which was treated with excision and radiotherapy. Following this she became depressed but refused to admit it to herself. She got no pleasure out of life, found it difficult to make decisions, could not concentrate, and had disturbed sleep and appetite. She was highly self-critical and saw her inability to do what she used to do as a failure. In fact, she saw herself as a complete failure. Although she had grown to accept that she was depressed, she still thought she ought to do the things other people were doing, despite her physical and mental illness.

This woman's initial interpretation of her situation was accurate:

"Because of my disability I cannot do the things I used to do."

According to the cognitive model this would be expected to induce feelings of sadness. But she then imposed demands on herself about how she *should* be managing:

"I should be doing more to look after the house and my husband."

And she then overgeneralized from this to make negative, global predictions about the future and her ability to cope:

"I can't cope."
"I'm a failure."

The more she looked around her the more she found evidence for her deficiencies which compounded her depressed state. This patient had, over the years of living with her illness, developed the belief that she must always cope and never show any weakness, and further, that if she expressed her negative feelings or looked to others for support she was a burden and a failure. The stress of cancer, together with a deterioration in her physical mobility, had made her feel naturally sad, but her assumption meant: (1) She could not express this sadness to anyone; (2) she perceived her distress and disability as signs of failure.

Therapy consisted of a combination of antidepressant medication and cognitive therapy. The therapist explained how much of her thinking was distorted by her depressive illness. She was given behavioral assignments that encouraged her to do the things she was still capable of doing but had given up because of her depression. She learned to recognize her frequent "should" statements and gradually learned to challenge them with more constructive thoughts. Rather than challenge the realistic thoughts about the loss, the therapist actually encouraged her to express these thoughts and feelings and helped her distinguish this realistic sadness from depression.

This case demonstrates how an apparently "rational" response to a negative life situation can still be amenable to cognitive therapy, if attention is paid to what distorted thinking may be present. It also demonstrates the role of beliefs in blocking the normal process of adjustment. In this case, the patient's belief that she must always fight on and that showing distress was a sign of weakness prevented her from acknowledging the reality of the gradual loss of her mobility. If she had been able to ventilate feelings she may have been able to work through the sadness and loss without it becoming depression. What follows are some practical suggestions on how to apply cognitive and behavioral techniques in situations where negative automatic thoughts initially appear realistic and the response of depression or anxiety a rational one. Although derived largely from work with cancer patients and their relatives, this schema is equally applicable to bereavement, other losses, and some posttraumatic states.

Recognizing and Facilitating the Adjustment Process

The therapist should first establish if the patient's emotional distress is part of an adjustment process. If this is the case it may not be appropriate to intervene with formal cognitive therapy. In liaison settings patients can sometimes be referred simply because they are experiencing emotional distress or are manifesting tearfulness or overt anger. These reactions may be transient reactions to bad news, or side effects of treatment or other changing circumstances. The symptomatology in these cases may be as severe as a depressive illness or anxiety state, but the affective disturbance is part of the continuing task of coming to terms with the recent life event. A cognitive-behavioral intervention is not needed in an adjustment reaction of this kind, because what appears to be a very low mood one day may have lifted by the next. For example, a patient with cancer may experience severe anticipatory anxiety prior to a checkup, but as soon as the results of investigations show the person is clear of disease the anxiety disappears.

In a study that evaluated the effectiveness of a cognitive-behavioral intervention in cancer, patients were screened using a self-report measure of anxiety and depression (the Hospital Anxiety and Depression Scale; Zigmond & Snaith, 1983) within 3 months of diagnosis or first recurrence. Seventy-eight percent scored within the clinical range for anxiety at initial assessment, but by the time they received therapy (1–2 weeks later) this had dropped to 47% (Greer et al., 1992). Cross-sectional assessments may, therefore, pick up a high percentage of patients whose distress will remit spontaneously in a short time. It is not always possible to predict which patients will continue to have problems with adjustment, and it is therefore difficult to know when to intervene and when to let nature take its course. The time since the adverse life event is obviously one factor to take into account. Evidence of changing emotions—for example, from depression to anger—may indicate that the adjustment process is still continuing. A third factor to consider is the degree of distortion in the patient's appraisal of the situation. In these cases simple supportive, nondirective measures may be enough. Indeed, introducing a problem-focused approach too early could conceivably interrupt emotional processing.

The psychological problems experienced by some patients in response to a critical life event seem to make most sense if understood as the result of an interruption of the process of adjustment to that life event. This applies particularly to traumas or losses that can shatter the equilibrium of an individual's life. Murray-Parkes (1965) has divided abnormal grief reactions into two categories: arrested grief and chronic unresolved grief. From a cognitive perspective it is interesting to ask what might be the factors that predispose to these abnormal grief reactions and to the analogous states of incomplete processing seen in posttraumatic stress disorder. It is possible that certain basic assumptions may influence the process of coming to terms with trauma, either by preventing the emotional expression necessary to engage in processing (causing arrested grief) or by preventing the completion of the process (causing chronic grieving). Williams, Hodgkinson, Josephs, and Yule (1995) have suggested that the belief that it is weak or unacceptable to show strong feelings may prevent emotional processing following a trauma and predispose to posttraumatic stress disorder.

Mrs. A believed that she should not burden anyone with her troubles and insisted on trying to cope alone. This prevented her from sharing her thoughts and feelings with her husband, which might have both allowed some appropriate grieving for her lost independence and activity, and also encouraged reality testing of her distorted cognitions about being useless. Some evidence suggests that cancer patients are more likely to suppress negative emotions (Greer & Morris, 1975), so it is possible that facilitating emotional expression may have an important part to play in any psychological intervention with this group of patients (Moorey & Greer, 1989). Basic assumptions concerning the desirability or safety of expressing emotions would seem to be related to delayed or arrested grieving over loss or incomplete processing of trauma. If we consider chronic grieving, another set of beliefs are implicated that relate to accepting the loss and moving on to reconstructing one's life. The following two case examples illustrate how beliefs can trap one in a state of chronic grieving.

> Mrs. B's mother had died from breast cancer 9 years ago. Through all that time Mrs. B had never really come to terms with her mother's death. She would frequently think about how much she missed her, and had become markedly phobic of anything connected with cancer or illness. She could not watch any television programs associated with hospitals or medicine. She had crying spells precipitated by illness-related cues, and was very scared of developing cancer herself. It appeared that she had always been very close to her mother and, being the youngest in the family, was somewhat protected. The mother was successfully treated for breast cancer, but after a disease-free period of several years developed brain metastases and died. In the last few days before her death the patient had been kept away from her mother's bedside because the family thought she would not be able to cope. She had consequently never completed her grief: She was still troubled by intrusive negative images of her mother looking weak and ill and could not access positive, happy memories of her.
>
> As the therapist explored the patient's beliefs about the mother's death it became clear that Mrs. B blamed herself for the death. The previous year they had been on a picnic and the daughter had acci-

dentally hit her mother on the head when shutting the trunk of her car. She was convinced that this blow had caused the recurrence of cancer, and her guilt had prevented her from sharing thoughts with anyone. This myth that a blow can cause the development of a cancer is not that rare and even exists in other cultures. Sharing her guilty secret and testing the reality of her attribution with appropriate information from the therapist allowed her to see that her belief was erroneous. She immediately felt a tremendous sense of relief and burst into tears saying, "I feel better for knowing I didn't kill her, but I also feel very sad, because now I have to really say good-bye to her." She subsequently successfully employed self-directed exposure to the negative memories as used in guided mourning (Mawson, Marks, Ramm, & Stern, 1981) and over just a few weeks managed to complete the process of grieving that had been incomplete for so long. This is a dramatic example of how correcting a mistaken belief can be the key to unlock the door to experiencing painful emotions in a different way that allows them to be worked through.

The second case illustration also covers the subject of guilt over a lost loved one, but this time it is a form of survivor guilt, associated with the belief that creating a new life for oneself is in some way being disloyal to the lost person.

Mrs. C was a 40-year-old teacher whose husband had died of leukemia a year previously. While he was ill she discovered a breast lump that was found to be malignant. She had to face the diagnosis and treatment while preparing for her husband's death. Some months later she became clinically depressed. She felt that she had not really been able to deal with her own illness because she had been too busy coping with his. Now she felt low in mood, lacking in motivation, and unable to get any pleasure from life. When, as an intervention to help motivate her to engage in therapy, the therapist asked her if her husband would want her to be so unhappy she affirmed that he would! She believed that he would genuinely not want her to enjoy life without him. It emerged that he had been somewhat older than she and had sought to guide and control her. When he was dying he had asked her never to remarry. She now had the belief that if she reconstructed her life without him and achieved happiness she would be being disloyal. This idea that happiness equals disloyalty is not uncommon in the bereaved. Therapy for this patient involved examining her husband's motivation for trying to control her life from beyond the grave and understanding how this might derive from his own vulnerability and his way of coping with impending death. It also required challenging the cultural myth about honoring deathbed promises. Over eight sessions the patient was able to acknowledge some of her husband's less desirable qualities and express her anger at his controlling attitude toward her. It was with a mixture of guilty rebellion and liberation that she finally lit a bonfire in the garden—he had never allowed her to do this when he was alive.

These two cases show how morbid grief, a condition on the surface requiring support, empathy, and cathartic expression of emotions, can still benefit from a Beckian cognitive approach. Maladaptive beliefs can both arrest and prolong adjustment reactions, and the recognition and revision of these beliefs can allow the adjustment process to commence or progress.

Identifying and Challenging Cognitions

Of course, the core of any therapy using Beck's approach with patients facing adverse life circumstances is going to be identifying negative automatic thoughts and restructuring them. Naming thinking errors, correcting faulty thinking through guided discovery in the session, and challenging cognitions in the thought diary and behavioral experiments are all as applicable in patients with serious real life problems as with any other patients. The therapist must be willing to explore what might on the surface appear to be understandable distress and ask what might be distorted in the patient's perceptions of his or her situation. Guilt and self-blame are reactions that have already been discussed and are often very readily dealt with using cognitive techniques. The search for meaning in the face of negative events provides a fertile ground for the germination of negative causal attributions. Someone or something must be to blame. So the patient may make an internal attribution and blame him- or herself inducing guilt, or may make an external attribution and blame others. In cancer, anger can be directed at family, doctors and nurses, or God. While in some cases helping patients to ventilate anger can be therapeutic, in other cases direct challenging of the faulty inferences is necessary (Moorey & Greer, 1989).

One of the most common distortions encountered is overgeneralization. The sense of helplessness and hopelessness felt as a direct consequence of serious illness, loss of a loved one, or some other disaster can sometimes generalize to the whole of life. Rather than realistically appraising a loss that is serious but nonetheless only part of one's life, it seems that everything is lost. This reaction in cancer patients has been labeled a "helpless/hopeless" adjustment style (Moorey & Greer, 1989). For instance, patients undergoing radiotherapy may conclude that because they are too tired to do things now they will *never* regain their energy; because their physical disability prevents them from enjoying their usual activities there is *nothing* they can enjoy. Overgeneralization may be compounded by all-or-nothing thinking; for example, "Unless I can do everything I used to do, there's no point in doing anything." This will then prevent patients from investigating new ways of getting pleasure or success that might be less tiring than previous activities. Details of how standard cognitive therapy techniques can be applied to cancer patients can be found in Moorey and Greer (1989). In using these techniques with patients in real difficulties it is important to emphasize the role of empathy. Patients must feel that you understand why they are so distraught and that they have a right to see things the way they do. Many will have had plenty of people tell them to fight and pull themselves together. Beck's emphasis on a collaborative nature of cognitive therapy provides the ideal medium for working with these patients. Psychodynamic approaches can make patients feel the therapy is distant and cold when they want the human contact at a time of great need. Nondirective counseling, which is widely practiced with these sorts of adjustment reactions, allows the patient to feel understood and then validated, but it may not be enough to help them develop coping strategies. Other cognitive approaches, which are more confrontational, like rational emotive therapy, may leave patients feeling persecuted. Beck's collaborative empiricism allows for sufficient empathy for the patients to feel understood, together with a joint participation in problem solving.

Exploring "Realistic" Negative Thoughts

While not easy to perform, it is not difficult to see how standard cognitive therapy techniques can be applied to thoughts that show characteristic thinking errors (see Table 19.2). But what about negative thoughts that are realistic interpretations of the situation in which people find themselves? The worrying thoughts a cancer patient has often relate to a realistic possibility of death; a bereaved person who ruminates about no one ever being able to *replace* the loved one is correct; a posttraumatic stress disorder patient may more accurately assess the risk of being attacked in certain parts of the city than we do. What can Beck's cognitive therapy offer these types of thoughts? They may in fact be the most frequent negative automatic thoughts reported by these patients and swamp the more obviously distorted ones. I think there is a pragmatic and a radical solution to deal with them. The pragmatic solution is to accept the thoughts and help the patient to develop appropriate coping strategies. The radical solution is to seek the deeper meaning behind the negative automatic thoughts, to search for more cognitive distortions.

Identifying the Personal Meaning of "Realistic" Negative Cognitions

The radical approach to these negative thoughts adopts one of Beck's fundamental maxims: "Don't make assumptions." All too often our own empathic (sympathetic) response to people in horrendous circumstances means that we assume we know what they mean. Take, for instance, the subject of death. If someone experiences frequent, distressing intrusive thoughts about their impending death we are inclined to feel for them and we understand that their psychological pain is perfectly natural. But what are they

TABLE 19.2. Working with Realistic Negative Automatic Thoughts

1. Identify the personal meaning of the thoughts.
2. Challenge underlying distortions.
3. Identify and solve problems.
4. Encourage appropriate emotional expression.
5. Examine the usefulness of the negative automatic thoughts.
6. Teach distraction strategies.
7. Use activity scheduling to enhance personal control.
8. Plan for the future.
9. Schedule worry/grief.

distressed by? For everyone death will have a special meaning. For one person it might be the implied pain and suffering, for another the lingering helplessness; a single man may fear dying alone; a young mother may fear for the consequences of her death for her children. Your emotional response as a therapist to the dying patient's psychic pain may have more to do with your own attitude toward death than an accurate understanding of the patient.

The idiosyncratic nature of our response to universal phenomena is well evidenced by hypochondriacal patients. The personal meaning of illness and death can be very specific and sometimes even bizarre. Usually it will have some origin in patients' past experience which has influenced the way they construct the world. For instance, a patient with chronic health anxiety, despite having varied fluctuating physical symptoms, always feared they were signs of cancer. When asked to associate to the idea of cancer he had an image of himself alone in a hospital bed "cut off and disconnected." At the age of 4 he had been looked after by a next-door neighbor for a short time while his mother was in hospital having a baby. He developed an ear infection that was left untreated until his mother came home. Because of this he had to be admitted to the hospital for several weeks. He described "shaming" himself by screaming every time his mother left after visiting. Initially the therapist thought that these experiences had led to a straightforward fear of abandonment, but further questioning revealed that for this patient cancer was always incurable and therefore meant that it radically and irrevocably altered your life. For him once you became a cancer patient you were inevitably a different person and this was his deepest fear—losing his identity and becoming disconnected.

By not making assumptions the therapist can tap into the personal meaning of the negative situation. At the very least this promotes accurate empathy and aids the therapeutic alliance. It often does more than this. The underlying meaning may be distorted and potentially can be challenged by standard cognitive therapy techniques. In other cases, the underlying meaning may indicate a real problem that can be addressed. Finally, disclosing underlying meaning, although painful, may facilitate further the process of adjustment. To illustrate these three outcomes I will consider ruminations about death in patients with terminal cancer.

On one level intrusive images or thoughts about death are perfectly natural in these circumstances, but in some patients they do not seem to be part of a process of anticipatory grieving and they may be associated with extreme distress. In this case looking for the personal meaning of death can be very helpful. Worrying in these circumstances is no different from worrying in any others. Borkovec (Borkovec & Inz, 1990) has suggested that worry in generalized anxiety disorder may be an avoidance of aversive imagery. In some terminally ill patients worry about apparently trivial things may serve the function of helping avoid painful images about death itself. Fear and ruminations about death may in themselves contain distortions. Past experiences of death may induce fears that it will be painful or lingering; although this may sometimes occur, modern palliative care means that pain can be effectively controlled and the process of death does not have to be terrible (Cassidy, 1991). Identifying these fears and giving basic education about pain control can markedly reduce anxiety. This fear is also amenable to problem solving: The patient can be put in touch with the palliative care team and the specific worries can be discussed openly. The patient can be encouraged to ask the team questions directly related to the fears.

Once the aspects of dying that cause distress are identified they are often amenable to some sort of problem-solving intervention. For instance, if a patient has not had contact with a relative for many years following a family dispute there may be a sense of dying with unfinished business — establishing contact again and even a reconciliation gives the patient a sense of completion. These problem-solving strategies give the dying patient a feeling that he or she is still making a contribution. Actions as simple as making a will can induce a sense of self-efficacy.

One of the most distressing encounters for anyone working with cancer patients is that with a young mother with terminal illness. For her the meaning of death will normally have implications for her family. Thoughts such as "they won't be able to cope without me" can be challenged using cognitive techniques.

As the meaning of death is elucidated it inevitably provokes strong emotional reactions. This can become part of the process of anticipatory grieving for one's own death.

Pragmatic Solutions to Bypass Negative Automatic Thoughts

It may not always be appropriate to work in the way described above, and even if this more radical approach is adopted there will be times when patients will want to get on with life rather than think about their negative situation. In this case a more pragmatic approach based on Beck's cognitive theory is possible. Here, rather than challenging the negative automatic thoughts, strategies are developed to distract from them and indirectly challenge some of their implications.

The first step requires the patients to accept the maladaptive nature of the negative thoughts. While the thoughts may be accurate, they are not necessarily helpful. Worries about what might happen in the future and ruminations about a past loss both prevent you from living in the present. Realistic negative automatic thoughts can sometimes promote problem solving or be part of a process of adjustment, but if they seem to disrupt the person's life and have a repetitive, ruminative quality they are in effect maladaptive. Looking at the advantages and disadvantages of the negative thinking can prove a useful exercise, while Socratic questioning can be used to direct the patients to the effect of their ruminations on their ability to enjoy the areas of life that are open to them and the effect on relationships with family and friends. Two options can be put to the patient. For instance, a patient with a terminal illness has the choice of ruminating about the inevitability of death or living the life that remains to the full. Aaron T. Beck (personal communication, 1986) has succinctly put it: "You cannot control your death, but you can control your life." Recording negative thoughts can help to establish just how much of the time is devoted to unconstructive thinking and how much time is available for constructive engagement with life.

Once the patients are able to see how this wastes the time that is available to them they are usually willing to look at how to use distraction techniques to reduce negative thinking. The techniques used will depend on the patient. Sometimes scheduling time for worry or grieving can be helpful. This not only has the effect of freeing time for more constructive activity, but also may make the time spent on negative thinking more productive in terms of problem solving or effective grieving. Activity scheduling can be an effective tool in helping to distract, to enhance self-efficacy, and to increase a sense of personal control. It can also help to reverse the circle of helplessness.

Many patients, finding they are unable to carry out tasks they previously found easy, give up altogether. They generalize their lack of control in one area of their life to the whole of their life. This process can be reversed: Finding an area of life that can be controled generates a more general sense of control. So it is possible that finding small activities that give the patient a feeling of mastery induce a sense of control over the disease. Activities that give the patient the feeling that he or she is still alive and contributing can be particularly helpful.

For instance, a patient with carcinoid syndrome had spent 15 years fighting recurrences of the disease with numerous operations. Each time he made a rapid recovery and returned to his old self as soon as possible. When he took longer over his recovery from his most recent operation he became initially frustrated and then depressed. He thought that if he could not be cheerful and cope without any help from others he was useless. He believed his family would be better off without him because he was useless and a burden to them. The therapist encouraged the patient to engage in some small activities that could be helpful to his family and at the same time asked him to test his belief by asking them if they did indeed feel they would be better off if he were dead. The response was a very moving, open display of affection from his grown-up children that they had not been able to show before. This convinced him that he was valued and needed and led to a marked improvement in his mood.

CONCLUSIONS

The recognition that emotional disorders show characteristic thinking errors is one of Beck's major contributions to psychiatry, and from this observation an effective set of clinical interventions has been developed. Cognitive therapy is clearly at its most effective and most straightforward when it is dealing with people who have objectively favorable external circumstances. Here it is possible to make use of a large amount of disconfirming evidence from the patient's surroundings. Cognitive therapy is not so straightforward when the patient has objectively negative surroundings. This is in some respects analogous to the challenge presented by personality disorders, where the usual recourse to past experiences of validation or periods of high self-esteem is not open to the therapist. Interestingly, the clinical approach presented here also has some similarities in its use of more emotion-focused strategies: In personality disorder these techniques promote schematic restructuring, in adjustment disorders emotional processing. More work is needed to understand the role of cognitive factors in the adjustment process, and the way in which standard cognitive therapy might be modified to facilitate adjustment.

Despite these modifications, the therapy described here remains rooted in a cognitive model. It is still possible to apply Beck's cognitive therapy to patients who at first sight have realistically negative automatic thoughts. It is a tribute to Beck's theoretical and clinical insight that the cognitive model is sufficiently broad to cover depression and anxiety reactions to truly negative situations.

REFERENCES

Alloy, L. B., & Abramson, L. Y. (1979). Judgements of contingency in depressed and non-depressed college students: Sadder but wiser? *Journal of Experimental Psychology: General, 108,* 441–485.

American Psychiatric Association. (1994). *Diagnostic and statistical manual of mental disorders* (4th ed.). Washington, DC: Author.

Barraclough, J. (1994). *Cancer and emotion: A practical guide to psycho-oncology.* Chichester, UK: Wiley.

Beck, A. T. (1963). Thinking and depression: 1. Idiosyncratic content and cognitive distortions. *Archives of General Psychiatry, 9,* 324–333.

Beck, A. T. (1967). *Depression: Causes and treatment.* Philadelphia: University of Pennsylvania Press.

Blackburn, I. M., & Davidson, K. M. (1990). *Cognitive therapy for depression and anxiety: A practitioner's guide.* Oxford, UK: Blackwell.

Borkovec, T. D., & Inz, J. (1990). The nature of worry in generalised anxiety disorder: A predominance of thought activity. *Behaviour Research and Therapy, 28,* 153–158.

Brown, G. W., Harris, T., & Copeland, J. R. (1977). Depression and loss. *British Journal of Psychiatry, 130,* 1–18.

Burns, D. D. (1979). *Feeling good: The new mood therapy.* New York: Morrow.

Cassidy, S. (1991). Terminal care. In M. Watson, (Ed.) *Cancer patient care: Psychosocial treatment methods.* Cambridge, UK: BPS Books and Cambridge University Press.

Daintith, J., & Isaacs, A. (Eds.) (1989). *Medical quotes: A thematic dictionary.* Oxford, UK: Market House Books.

Derogatis, L. R., Morrow, G. R., Fetting, J., Penman, D., Piasetsky, S., Schmale, A. M., Henrichs, M., & Carnicke, D. L. M. (1983). The prevalence of psychiatric disorder among cancer patients. *Journal of the American Medical Association, 249,* 751–757.

Epictetus. (1983). Encheiridion. In N. White (Trans.), *The handbook of Epictetus.* Indianapolis: Hackett Publishing.

Farber, J. M., Weinerman, B. H., & Kuypers, J. A. (1984). Psychosocial distress in oncology out-patients. *Journal of Psychosocial Oncology, 2,* 109–118.

Freud, S. (1984). Mourning and melancholia. In *On metapsychology: The theory of psychoanalysis.* London: Penguin. (Original work published 1917)

Greer, S. (1992). The management of denial in cancer patients. *Oncology, 6,* 33–40.

Greer, S., Moorey, S., Baruch, J. D. R., Watson, M., Robertson, B., Mason, A., Rowden, L., Law, M. G., & Bliss J. M. (1992). Adjuvant psychological therapy for cancer patients: A prospective randomised trial. *British Medical Journal, 304,* 675–680.

Greer, S., & Morris, T. (1975). Psychological attributes of women who develop breast cancer: A controlled study. *Journal of Psychosomatic Research, 19,* 147–153.

Hooley, J. M., Orley, J., & Teasdale, J. D. (1986). Levels of expressed emotion and relapse in depressed patients. *British Journal of Psychiatry, 148,* 642–647.

Horowitz, M. J. (1986). *Stress response syndromes.* Northvale, NJ: Aronson.

Kübler-Ross, E. (1970). *On death and dying.* London: Tavistock.

Maguire, G. P., Lee, E. G., Bevington, D. J., Kucherman, C., Crabtree, R. J., & Cornell, C. E. (1978). Psychiatric problems in the first year after mastectomy. *British Medical Journal, 281,* 963–965.

Maguire, G. P., Tait, A., Brooke, M., & Selwood, R. (1980). Psychiatric morbidity and physical toxicity associated with mastectomy. *British Medical Journal, 281,* 1179–1180.

Mawson, D., Marks, I. M., Ramm, L., & Stern. R. S. (1981). Guided mourning for morbid grief. *British Journal of Psychiatry, 138,* 185–193.

Moorey, S., & Greer, S. (1989). *Psychological therapy for patients with cancer: A new approach.* Oxford, UK: Heinemann Medical.

Morris, T., Greer, H. S., White, P. (1977). Psychological and social adjustment to mastectomy: A 2 year follow-up to study. *Cancer, 40,* 2381–2387.

Murray-Parkes, C. (1965). Bereavement and mental illness, part II: A classification of bereavement reactions. *British Journal of Medical Psychology, 38,* 13–26.

Rachman, S. (1980). Emotional processing. *Behaviour Research and Therapy, 18,* 51–60.

Sandler, J., Dare, C., & Holder, A. (1970). Basic psychoanalytic concepts: IX. Working through. *British Journal of Psychiatry, 117,* 617–621.

Silberfarb, P. M., & Greer, S. (1982). Psychological concomitants of cancer: Clinical aspects. *American Journal of Psychotherapy, 36,* 470–478.

Silver, R. C., & Wortman, C. B. (1991). Coping with undesirable life events. In A. Monat & R. Lazarus (Eds.), *Stress and coping: An anthology* (3rd ed., pp. 279–364). New York: Columbia University Press.

Vazquez, C. (1987). Judgement of contingency: Cognitive biases in depressed and non depressed subjects. *Journal of Personality and Social Psychology, 52,* 419–431.

Wallace, L. M., Priestman, S. G., Dunn, J. A., & Priestman, T. J. (1993). The quality of life of early breast cancer patients treated by two different radiotherapy regimens. *Clinics of Oncological Radiotherapy & Radiology, 5,* 228–233.

Williams, R. M., Hodgkinson, P., Joseph, S., & Yule, W. (1995). Attitudes to emotion, crisis support and distress 30 months after the capsize of a passenger ferry disaster. *Crisis Intervention, 1,* 209–214.

Zigmond, A. S., & Snaith, R. P. (1983). The Hospital Anxiety and Depression Scale. *Acta Psychiatrica Scandinavica, 67,* 361–370.

Chapter 20

Treating Substance Use Disorders with Cognitive Therapy: Lessons Learned and Implications for the Future

Bruce S. Liese
Robert A. Franz

For several years we have been providing cognitive therapy to individuals with substance use disorders and developing a model for understanding and treating these disorders[1] (Beck, Wright, Newman, & Liese, 1993; Liese, 1993, 1994a, 1994b; Liese & Beck, in press; Liese & Chiauzzi, 1995; Wright, Beck, Newman, & Liese, 1992). Our work has taught us many lessons about cognitive therapy and substance abuse. In this chapter we discuss these lessons and outline our theory and treatment of substance abuse. We hope that our work will lead to more effective treatment strategies and empirical validation of our model.

The development of psychological treatments for substance use disorders is an important undertaking. During a recent 1-year period, 3.4 million Americans sought outpatient treatment for substance use disorders and another 437,000 were admitted to inpatient treatment facilities (Narrow, Regier, Rae, Manderscheid, & Locke, 1993). While the number of individuals who have actually sought treatment for substance use disorders is large, the potential number of additional individuals who might benefit from addiction treatment services is staggering. Recent large-scale epidemiological studies have estimated that between 17% and 26% of Americans have abused or been dependent on psychoactive substances during their lifetimes (Anthony & Helzer, 1991; Kessler et al., 1994). Given these high prevalence rates, effective treatments are certainly needed. Unfortunately, psychotherapists (including cognitive therapists) have not traditionally perceived themselves as appropriate or capable providers of addiction treatment services. Conversely, addiction specialists have not traditionally viewed cognitive therapy as the optimal treatment for substance abuse.

This chapter will be divided into four sections: background, conceptualization, treatment, and implications for the future. In the background section we will outline advances in the areas of addictions and cognitive therapy over the past few decades. In the conceptualization section we will discuss the role of cognitive processes (e.g., schemas, basic beliefs, automatic thoughts, and cognitive distortions) in substance abuse. In the treatment section we will discuss how we have applied cognitive therapy to help patients with substance use disorders. Finally, we will offer suggestions (i.e., "lessons learned") regarding future applications of cognitive therapy to substance abuse.

BACKGROUND

The treatment of individuals with substance use disorders is extremely challenging. Despite sincere efforts to control their substance use, many individuals persist in self-destructive addictive behaviors. One frequently cited review (Hunt, Barnett, & Branch, 1971) reported that between 70% and 80% of persons who attempted to quit using alcohol, heroin, or nicotine relapsed within 1 year of treatment. Approximately two-thirds relapsed within the first 3 months following treatment. A more recent review of 68 alcoholism treatment outcome studies (Riley, Sobell, Leo, Sobell, & Klajner, 1987) found that only 34% of a total sample of 14,546 were able to abstain or engage in nonproblem drinking following treatment. Successful long-term treatment of substance use disorders has remained an uncertain proposition.

The Psychology of Addictions

Recent theory and research have greatly advanced the psychology of addictions. This work has provided clinicians with exciting ideas for developing new treatment strategies. For example, in their model, Marlatt and his colleagues (e.g., Brownell, Marlatt, Lichtenstein, & Wilson, 1986; Daley & Marlatt, 1992; Marlatt & Gordon, 1985, 1989) have identified important cognitive and behavioral determinants of relapse (e.g., high-risk situations, ineffective coping strategies). Their work has inspired many others to develop innovative relapse prevention strategies.

Prochaska, DiClemente, and Norcross have developed a transtheoretical model of change (Prochaska & DiClemente, 1986; Prochaska, DiClemente, & Norcross, 1992; Prochaska, Norcross, & DiClemente, 1994) that has profoundly impacted perspectives on addictive behaviors. According to their model, individuals who abuse substances can be characterized as being in one of five stages of change: precontemplation, contemplation, preparation, action, or maintenance. Each of these stages is characterized by certain thoughts and beliefs. Precontemplators deny having problems related to substance abuse: "I don't need to make changes." Contemplators consider that they may have such problems: "I might benefit from changing." Those in the preparation stage are formulating strategies for change: "It's time for me to do something different." Individuals in the action stage have changed their behaviors for at least 24 hours: "I'm doing something good for myself." Those in the maintenance stage have succeeded at maintaining change for at least 6 months: "I'm no longer a drinker, smoker, or drug user." Prochaska, DiClemente, and Norcross explain that interventions are most effective when they match individuals' readiness to change.

Miller and his colleagues (e.g., Miller, 1983; Miller & Rollnick, 1991) extend the work of Prochaska, DiClemente, and Norcross by proposing strategies for motivational interviewing. In their important text, Miller and Rollnick (1991) challenge the widely held belief that all addicts are "in denial." Instead they propose that addicted individuals are ambivalent about their drug use. According to Miller and Rollnick, understanding that addicted individuals are "ambivalent" rather than labeling them as "in denial" contributes to an improved collaborative treatment environment.

A recent development in the field of addictions in the United States has been the introduction of harm reduction (Des Jarlais, 1995; Marlatt, Larimer, Baer, & Quigley, 1993; Marlatt & Tapert, 1993). Proponents of harm reduction view substance use on a continuum from harmless to harmful. Rather than providing a specific set of techniques, harm reduction offers a paradigm for guiding public policy and treating substance use disorders. Therapists who adopt harm reduction philosophies view even small harm-reducing steps as better than no steps. Harm reduction is compatible with cognitive therapy because both place strong emphasis on collaboration, empathy, respect, recognition of individual differences, and attention to personal beliefs. With its focus on individualized goal setting, harm reduction is another important advancement in the development of collaborative treatments of substance abuse.

The psychology of addictions is complicated by several factors: Individuals with substance use disorders comprise a heterogeneous group, they tend to be simultaneously involved in the use of multiple substances, and they tend to have coexisting psychological and psychiatric problems. These factors are discussed in the following paragraphs.

Contrary to stereotypes, individuals with substance use disorders comprise a diverse group. They differ in the substances they use, in their patterns of use, and in their personality and socioeconomic characteristics. The fourth edition of the *Diagnostic and Statistical Manual of Mental Disorders* (DSM-IV; American Psychiatric Association, 1994) lists 11 classes of substances associated with disorders of intoxication, withdrawal, abuse, and dependence (see Table 20.1). Each of these substances produces unique psychological, physiological, and behavioral changes in the user. In addition, many of these substances are capable of inducing transitory or permanent psychiatric symptoms such as anxiety, depression, delusions, hallucinations,

TABLE 20.1. DSM-IV Diagnoses for Major Psychoactive Substance Use

Substance	Intoxication	Withdrawal	Abuse	Dependence
Alcohol	×	×	×	×
Amphetamines	×	×	×	×
Caffeine	×			
Cannabis	×		×	×
Cocaine	×	×	×	×
Hallucinogens	×		×	×
Inhalents	×		×	×
Nicotine		×		×
Opioids	×	×	×	×
Phencyclidine	×		×	×
Sedatives, hypnotics, or anxiolytics	×	×	×	×

Note. Adapted from American Psychiatric Association (1994, p. 177). Copyright 1994 by the American Psychiatric Association. Adapted by permission.

cognitive impairment, insomnia, and fatigue during the phases of intoxication or withdrawal.

The specific problems of an individual primarily dependent on nicotine are likely to be quite different from those of a person dependent on opiates, although both individuals are substance dependent. A person who abuses cocaine may be an impoverished inner-city youth or a wealthy executive. A person dependent on alcohol may be a highly visible community leader or an anonymous homemaker. A person who abuses amphetamines may be a streetwise criminal or a university professor. Any person, under the "right" combination of circumstances and opportunities, has the potential to develop substance use problems.

Many individuals with substance use disorders use multiple psychoactive substances. For example, epidemiological studies have found that 19% of alcoholic men (vs. 7% of nonalcoholic men) and 31% of alcoholic women (vs. 5% of nonalcoholic women) either abuse or depend on one or more other drugs (Helzer & Pryzbeck, 1988). University-based studies have found that students presenting themselves to a counseling center for help with alcohol abuse or dependence are significantly more likely to use nicotine and cannabis than students without such problems (Ross & Tisdall, 1994).

Polysubstance use is more likely to occur in individuals who use illicit (vs. legal) substances. Persons who abuse THC, amphetamines, and cocaine have alcoholism prevalence rates of 36%, 62%, and 84%, respectively (Helzer & Pryzbeck, 1988). Overall, approximately half of all people who abuse or are dependent on illicit drugs also abuse or are dependent on alcohol (Anthony & Helzer, 1991).

A strong association between nicotine dependence and other addictive disorders has also been well established (Bien & Burge, 1990; Henningfield, Clayton, & Pollin, 1990; Istvan & Matarazzo, 1984). Between 75%

and 100% of individuals receiving treatment for chemical dependence use tobacco (Bobo, 1989; Kozlowski, Jelinek & Pope, 1986; Stark & Campbell, 1993). Unfortunately nicotine dependence tends to be downplayed in chemical dependence programs (Bobo & Gilchrist, 1983; Goldsmith & Knapp, 1993; Sobell, 1994).

Substance use disorders commonly coexist with psychiatric disorders. A recent large-scale population-based study found that alcohol and drug abuse and dependence were highly associated with antisocial personality disorder, mania, and schizophrenia (Anthony & Helzer, 1991; Helzer, Burnam, & McEvoy, 1991). The association between substance use disorders and affective disorders was not as pronounced, but persons with substance use disorders were still two to three times more likely than the general public to be diagnosed with dysthymia or major depression (Anthony & Helzer, 1991; Helzer & Pryzbeck, 1988). Overall, about 37% of persons with substance use disorders have coexisting Axis I disorders, while about 29% of persons with psychiatric disorders have coexisting problems with drugs or alcohol (Regier et al., 1990). As with polysubstance use, psychopathology is more prevalent in individuals who use illicit substances. For example, psychiatric disorders are far more prevalent in persons with cocaine and barbiturate use disorders than in persons with alcohol or cannabis use disorders (Regier et al., 1990).

Despite the high incidence of polysubstance use and psychiatric comorbidity, most individuals with substance use disorders have a single drug of choice and do not have coexisting psychiatric disorders. We see many such people in our practice, including individuals whose only addiction is to nicotine. We have also worked with numerous addicted individuals without psychiatric problems who use only alcohol, prescription drugs, marijuana, cocaine, and other illicit drugs.

Individuals with substance use disorders may become entangled in complex social, economic, legal, and health problems related to their substance use. They may face the disintegration of intimate relationships, loss of employment, arrest, and serious illness as a result of their problematic substance use. When individuals use illicit drugs, the potential consequences become even more serious as they engage in illegal behaviors to procure drugs. For example, one of our patients recently used $1,000 worth of crack cocaine in the 12 hours immediately preceding his therapy appointment. Barely coherent during his visit, this patient revealed that he had stolen the money to pay for this binge. To complicate matters, his life was in danger because he had stolen the money from a drug dealer known for retaliating against his enemies.

Substance abuse is currently a major political, economic, and social concern in the United States. Despite growing awareness of the health risks associated with substance use and despite billions of dollars spent fighting the "war on drugs," many people continue to smoke, drink, and abuse illicit drugs at an alarming cost to themselves and society. Most of these people eventually attempt to abstain from drugs, but unfortunately many fail and better treatment strategies are certainly needed.

Cognitive Therapy

Over the past 30 years cognitive therapy has undergone important changes and developments. In his earliest formulation of the cognitive model, Beck (1961, 1964) was primarily interested in understanding and treating depression. He described depression as resulting from pervasive negative beliefs about self, world, and future (the cognitive triad). These negative beliefs were seen as influencing the way depressed persons attended to and processed information. Systematic cognitive errors based on faulty information processing helped to maintain these negative beliefs, and therefore depression. Beck, Rush, Shaw, and Emery (1979) developed a therapy using cognitive and behavioral techniques by which depressed persons were able to identify, objectively evaluate, and change their negative beliefs, thereby relieving depression. Beck and his colleagues eventually adapted cognitive therapy to anxiety (Beck & Emery with Greenberg, 1985) and other psychiatric problems. Since the publication of a text on personality disorders (Beck, Freeman, & Associates, 1990), cognitive therapy has been applied to the treatment of substantially more chronic and complex disorders (e.g., Wright, Thase, Beck, & Ludgate, 1993). Given the chronic, pervasive nature of substance use disorders and their high association with psychopathology, it was only a matter of time before cognitive therapy would be applied to the treatment of substance abuse and dependence.

THE COGNITIVE CONCEPTUALIZATION
OF SUBSTANCE ABUSE

Cognitive therapy is based on a comprehensive personality theory that emphasizes the importance of beliefs and thought processes in mediating behaviors, emotions, and physiologic responses. The importance of the cognitive case conceptualization cannot be overstated: In order to *do* cognitive therapy, one must *think* like a cognitive therapist. If constructed carefully and accurately the case conceptualization enables the therapist to develop a thorough understanding of the complexity of the individual who abuses psychoactive substances. The case conceptualization provides both a framework for understanding the patient's problems and a basis for developing an appropriate treatment strategy. The most effective techniques may be of little value if applied to the wrong individual or in an untimely manner. In this section we first outline the basic cognitive model of substance abuse. We then present the cognitive developmental model of substance abuse, explaining how substance use problems are likely to develop.

The Basic Cognitive Model of Substance Abuse

We developed the basic cognitive model of substance abuse over several years, based on our clinical observations and discussions with thousands of addicted patients. In the usual tradition of cognitive therapy we began by asking patients such questions as: "What are your *automatic thoughts* when you use alcohol/drugs?" "What *basic beliefs* motivate you to use alcohol/drugs?" and "What goes through *your mind* when you continue to use in spite of the devastating consequences of your alcohol/drug use?"

Over time the answers to these questions provided the foundation for our theory. We hypothesized the existence of cognitive processes specific to substance use (e.g., anticipatory beliefs, relief-oriented beliefs, and permissive beliefs). We developed and revised numerous algorithms that seemed to represent the cognitive, behavioral, and affective patterns of patients with addictions. After gaining confidence in our algorithms we enlisted numerous experts in the field of addictions to scrutinize our model and provide feedback, leading to further revisions. The resulting basic cognitive model of substance abuse is presented in Figure 20.1.

Activating Stimuli

According to the basic cognitive model of substance abuse, individuals are most likely to engage in addictive behaviors following exposure to certain *activating stimuli*. Activating stimuli are idiosyncratic cues or triggers. Marlatt and Gordon (1985) were among the first to recognize the importance of activating stimuli. In fact, they coined the synonymous term "high-risk situation," defined as "any situation that poses a threat to the individual's sense of control and increases the risk of potential relapse" (p. 37). In the cognitive model it is hypothesized that particular stimuli are defined as activating when they trigger basic drug-related beliefs and automatic thoughts, leading to urges and cravings. Nothing is inherently risky about any particular activating stimulus; an activating stimulus for one individual may be innocuous for another.

In our model we distinguish between *internal* and *external* cues. This distinction is useful because it facilitates identification of situations that put individuals at risk for drug use. Internal stimuli are cues that occur *within* an individual, while external stimuli are cues that occur *outside* of an individual. Examples of common internal cues are emotions (e.g., anxiety, depression, boredom, anger, frustration, loneliness) and physical sensations (e.g., pain, hunger, fatigue, withdrawal symptoms). Examples of common *external cues* are interpersonal conflicts, availability of preferred substances, and task accomplishment (when drugs are used to celebrate).

Based on their study of 311 relapse episodes, Marlatt and his colleagues (Cummings, Gordon, & Marlatt, 1980) divided relapse situations into two broad categories: inter*personal determinants and intr*apersonal determinants.

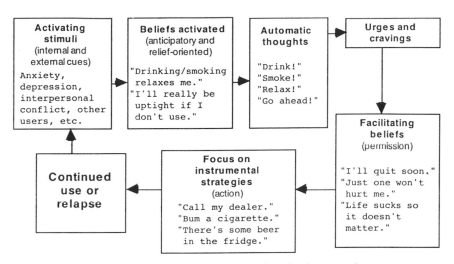

FIGURE 20.1. Basic cognitive model of substance abuse.

Within these two categories they found that three types of stimuli were most predictive of relapse: negative emotional states (35% of relapses in their sample), social pressure (20% of relapses), and interpersonal conflict (16% of relapses). Thus, 35% of relapses were attributable to what we have termed internal cues (negative emotional states) and approximately the same number of relapses were attributable to what we have termed external cues (social pressure and interpersonal conflict). We prefer to use the terms "internal" and "external" rather than "intrapersonal" and "interpersonal" because the concepts of internal and external seem more meaningful to our patients.

It is extremely important to understand that psychoactive substances provide *immediate regulation of mood states*. For example, alcohol and benzodiazapines provide immediate antianxiety effects; cocaine, amphetamines, nicotine, and caffeine provide immediate stimulation; and almost all drugs can be used as antiboredom agents. Most individuals addicted to drugs are dependent upon their *mood-regulating* effects. Though individuals may identify their high-risk situations as external (e.g., the availability of cigarettes), their ultimate goal in drug use is to regulate or modify their internal mood states (e.g., boredom, anxiety, anger, tension, frustration, depression). While most of our addicted patients report using drugs to remove unpleasant mood states, many explain that they also use drugs when they feel good. These individuals "celebrate" with drugs because they believe that they can turn *good* moods into *great* moods by using drugs. An important feature of cognitive therapy that makes it particularly appropriate for treating substance abuse is that it provides alternative cognitive strategies for mood regulation.

Beliefs Activated

According to the cognitive model of substance abuse, the most important difference between addicted and nonaddicted individuals is how they think. It is hypothesized that internal and external cues activate two types of drug-related basic beliefs — *anticipatory* and *relief-oriented* beliefs — that lead to automatic thoughts, urges, and cravings. Anticipatory beliefs involve predictions of gratification, increased efficacy, and heightened sociability following substance use. Examples include: "An ice cold beer will really hit the spot," "I'll be able to party all night if I start with a few lines of coke," and "Everything is more fun when I'm high." As people become dependent on drugs they develop relief-oriented beliefs, involving the expectation of relief from unpleasant physical and emotional states. Examples of relief-oriented beliefs include "Drinking/smoking relaxes me" or "I'll be really irritable if I don't drink/smoke." Typically persons with addictions have both anticipatory and relief-oriented beliefs, although either may be more salient for particular individuals.

Again it is important to emphasize the role of *mood regulation* in substance use and abuse. Individuals addicted to drugs tend to hold strong beliefs about the ability of drugs to regulate their moods. They accurately believe that some drugs will relieve their boredom, some drugs will help them to relax, and other drugs will give them an immediate burst of energy or make them feel powerful.

Automatic Thoughts

The activation of basic drug-related beliefs triggers automatic thoughts — brief, spontaneous cognitive processes (i.e., ideas or images) derived from individuals' substance-related beliefs. Typically, automated thoughts are abbreviated versions of corresponding basic beliefs. For example, if an individual believes "I'm going to have a nicotine fit if I don't smoke," the associated automatic thought might be "Smoke!" Similarly, if an individual believes "I can't have fun unless I'm drinking," the associated automatic thought might be "Relax!" or "Go ahead!" As previously mentioned, automatic thoughts may also take the form of mental images. Examples of mental images include lighting the first cigarette of the day, taking a deep hit from a joint, popping an ice cold beer, or feeling the warm rush following an intravenous heroin injection. The occurrence of automatic thoughts leads to urges and cravings.

Urges and Cravings

Urges and cravings are manifested as physical sensations, much like hunger or thirst. Patients have reported that they feel like they are "starving for a hit," "thirsty for a drink," or "dying for a smoke" when they experience particularly strong urges and cravings. The distinction between urges and cravings is subtle and we consider the two terms synonymous.

Individuals vary in the extent to which they experience urges and cravings. Their strength escalates during withdrawal from drugs as individuals continue to *think* about using substances while at the same time *not indulging* in substance use. Many individuals initially abstaining from drugs experience severe cravings because they ruminate about using drugs while resisting the desire to do so. Conversely, individuals freely indulging in drug use rarely experience strong cravings because they take drugs before their level of craving has an opportunity to escalate.

Facilitating Beliefs

The term "facilitating beliefs" is synonymous with "permission." Facilitating beliefs typically involve themes of entitlement, minimization of consequences, and justification. They also typically involve cognitive distortions that allow the user to ignore the negative effects of substance use. Examples of facilitating beliefs include "I deserve a drink" (entitlement); "Just one hit won't hurt me" (minimization of consequences); and "Life sucks, so it doesn't matter if I smoke" (justification). Individuals attempting to change addictive behaviors may have facilitating beliefs such as "Just one more" or "Eventually I'll quit." Such beliefs may undermine an individual's ability to tolerate urges and cravings. In fact, resisting an urge is a function of the relative strength of the urge on one hand, and the strength of facilitating beliefs on the other. Individuals with strong facilitating beliefs (e.g., "*Nobody* has *ever* died from smoking just one cigarette!") are likely to use drugs following slight urges. Conversely, individuals with weak or tentative facilitating beliefs (e.g., "*Maybe* I can have just one") can withstand stronger urges. In sum, the stronger the facilitating belief, the more likely it is that a person will succumb to urges and cravings.

Focus on Instrumental Strategies

Developing an action plan is essential to acquiring drugs. After individuals have granted themselves permission to use their attention shifts to procuring drugs. Instrumental strategies vary widely depending on the substance used and the person using. For example, if a person is addicted to nicotine, the instrumental strategy for obtaining the drug is simple: "A trip to the store," "Bum a cigarette," or "I may have some old [smokeable] butts in the ashtray." In contrast, instrumental strategies for obtaining illicit drugs might be difficult, complicated, and risky. The person attempting to procure cocaine, for example, may face the threat of arrest and physical harm.

Although many individuals who are addicted (especially to legal substances such as alcohol and nicotine) view their substance use as based on simple plans of action, most have elaborate strategies for acquiring their drugs of choice. One patient described using a particular convenience store to purchase gasoline. This store was located well out of her way home. On careful questioning she admitted that this convenience store sold discounted cigarettes by the carton. While this patient's short-term instrumental strategy for smoking was to reach for a cigarette, her long-term instrumental strategy involved stocking up on cigarettes purchased at the store where she "coincidentally" purchased gasoline. Marlatt and Gordon (1985) coined the term "apparently irrelevant decisions" to describe chains of "coincidental" behaviors that lead to high-risk situations.

Continued Use or Relapse

Following implementation of an instrumental strategy, individuals are likely to use their drugs of choice. Lapses may vary in severity from a single puff on a cigarette to a full-blown binge. *Any* substance use may become an activating stimulus for continued substance use. Lapses may trigger negative emotional states (e.g., depression over one's inability to abstain), interpersonal conflict (e.g., fighting with a spouse about the lapse), and social pressure to use (e.g., renewed contact with old "drinking buddies"). As discussed earlier, these states may put users at risk for complete relapses as they become caught in vicious circles of use and self-recrimination. In addition, such episodes may confirm basic beliefs, such as "I can't stop using," and may contribute to the development of new permissive beliefs, such as "I've used some, so I might as well keep using." Such all-or-nothing thinking is facilitated by myths and clichés like "One drink, one drunk" and "I've fallen off the bandwagon" (and presumably can't get up).

For these reasons we support total abstinence as a treatment goal for individuals dependent on psychoactive substances. Patients who successfully achieve abstinence are likely to develop new control beliefs such as "I can survive without using." When patients cannot successfully remain abstinent, however, we support harm reduction as a goal, where substance use is seen on a continuum (i.e., a "step-down" process rather than an all-or-nothing phenomenon). The benefits of a harm-reduction philosophy can be illustrated by one of our patients who was a heavy marijuana smoker. After a brief period of treatment this woman reported control over her marijuana use, except for the hours between putting her children to bed and going to sleep herself. Rather than insist on complete abstinence as a treatment goal (which probably would have resulted in her dropping out of treatment), we reinforced the positive progress she had made. Simultaneously we helped her to understand that her evening marijuana smoking was an effort to reduce her feelings of depression. We eventually taught this patient alternative cognitive depression-reduction strategies to replace marijuana smoking, which was actually contributing to her depression. In the past this same woman had dropped out of abstinence-oriented treatment programs because of their heavy handedness.

The Cognitive Developmental Model of Substance Abuse

Addictions are extremely complex processes characterized by deeply held, persistent, maladaptive beliefs. Over time we have been impressed by the quantity and complexity of beliefs associated with addictive behaviors. We have learned that maladaptive schemas and core beliefs are basic to addictive disorders. We have also become aware of numerous idiosyncratic drug-related beliefs, including anticipatory, relief-oriented, and facilitating beliefs. In order to treat patients who abuse drugs, we have necessarily become interested in the development of these related problematic beliefs.

Since the original formulation of our model (Beck et al., 1993), we have hypothesized a developmental model of substance abuse (Figure 20.2). This model places significant emphasis on learning processes rather than merely focusing on acute substance use episodes. The developmental model attends to early life experiences and the development of schemas and basic beliefs. It is hypothesized that drug-related beliefs are formed and maintained through the interaction of schemas, basic beliefs, and critical life experiences with psychoactive substances. It is important to note that the contents of schemas and basic beliefs are not initially drug related. Instead, individuals' schemas and basic beliefs about themselves, their personal worlds, other individuals, and their futures affect their attitudes toward drugs, alcohol, and other addictive substances. Thus, schemas and basic beliefs determine vulnerability to substance use problems.

Early Life Experiences

According to the cognitive developmental model, significant early life experiences make lasting impressions on individuals and result in the development of schemas, basic beliefs, and conditional beliefs. While significant early life experiences may include isolated incidents, it is the ongoing family, social, cultural, and financial circumstances that are central to the formation of schemas and basic beliefs. In the developmental model it is assumed that early *negative* life experiences lead to schemas and beliefs that make individuals vulnerable to the development of substance use problems. Examples of early negative life experiences include parents who model problematic substance use, environments where drugs or alcohol are prevalent, and the absence of validation from important others. Conversely, early *positive* life experiences are hypothesized to lead to schemas and beliefs that contribute to resilience against substance use problems. Examples of early positive life experiences include parents who model responsible substance use, secure personal relationships, supportive family, and validation from important others.

Development of Schemas, Basic Beliefs, and Conditional Beliefs

Schemas may be categorized into two major domains: lovability and adequacy. Lovability schemas involve basic beliefs about connectedness, self-

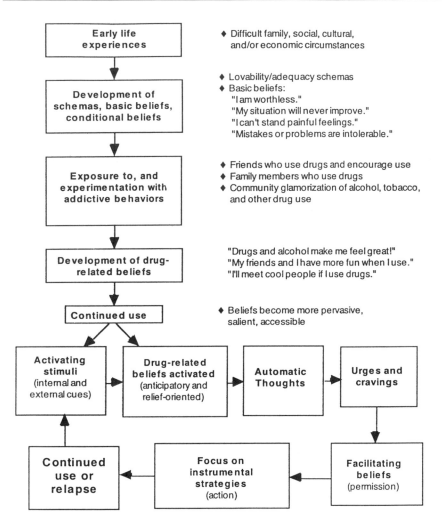

FIGURE 20.2. Cognitive-developmental model of substance abuse.

worth, and intimacy. Adequacy schemas involve beliefs about competence, success, and autonomy. As described above, negative life experiences contribute to the development of maladaptive schemas and basic beliefs that make individuals vulnerable to substance abuse. Examples of maladaptive basic beliefs include: "My situation will never improve," "I am worthless," "I can't stand painful feelings," and "Mistakes or problems are intolerable."

In early development, individuals' basic beliefs are not drug related. However, when individuals begin to use drugs as compensatory strategies (i.e., to cope with problems), they develop drug-related beliefs that become associated with maladaptive basic beliefs. For example, "I can't stand to be bored" becomes "Getting high is a great way to keep from getting bored."

Over time, beliefs become more deeply ingrained and more easily activated. In contrast, positive life experiences contribute to the development of adaptive basic beliefs: "My future is promising," "I am worthwhile," and "Painful feelings are endurable." It is assumed that these beliefs reduce individuals' vulnerability to substance abuse.

Early in life individuals also develop powerful conditional beliefs, which take the form of "If _____, then _____," where the first blank represents a condition and the second represents a consequence. Examples of conditional beliefs related to substance abuse include: "If I use drugs, then I'll be popular," "If I drink expensive alcohol, then I'll be respected," and "If I smoke cigarettes, I'll be one of the gang." Conditional beliefs may also be worded negatively: "If I don't use drugs I'll be seen as an outsider," and "If I don't smoke cigarettes, my friends will think I'm a wimp." Such conditional beliefs make individuals particularly vulnerable to social influence and the allure of drugs.

Exposure to and Experimentation with Addictive Behaviors

The development of substance use problems requires exposure to and experimentation with drugs. Most individuals begin experimenting with drugs (especially nicotine, alcohol, and marijuana) during youth and young adulthood. The decision to engage in early drug use is likely to be influenced by individuals' schemas, basic beliefs, and conditional beliefs. For instance, young people who feel particularly insecure or unlovable might be vulnerable to pressure from peers to engage in substance use. These individuals might receive instant validation from peers for using drugs. Rather than risking the shame of refusing, they are likely to accede to pressures to use drugs.

Individuals driven by perfectionistic beliefs may be vulnerable to the use of "power" drugs such as caffeine, nicotine, cocaine, and amphetamines that ostensibly improve their ability to perform longer and harder. Persons who believe that painful feelings or difficult situations are unmanageable are likely to use numbing, anxiolytic substances such as alcohol, marijuana, or barbiturates. By experimenting with and engaging in continued substance use, individuals further reinforce their maladaptive schemas, thus maintaining the vicious circle of problematic drug use.

Development of Drug-Related Beliefs

Specific drug-related beliefs are developed and maintained by continued drug use. For most individuals with substance use disorders, initial use provides a positive experience that becomes chronically sought. Positive substance use experiences result in, and reinforce, anticipatory beliefs (occurring early in the history of most addictive disorders), including: "Drugs and alcohol make me feel great!" "My friends and I have more fun when we use!"

and "I'll meet cool people if I use drugs." With continued use, relief-oriented beliefs may develop, including: "I need drugs to relax," and "I'll have a nicotine fit if I don't smoke a cigarette." Individuals with substance use disorders also develop facilitating beliefs that grant them permission to use. These include: "I've worked all day, and I deserve a drink," "I'm feeling really terrible, so it's all right this time," and "Just one more, then I'll quit."

Continued Use

With continued use, drug-related beliefs become more pervasive, salient, and accessible. As they are activated by an ever-increasing number of stimuli, these beliefs become increasingly automatic and available. Addicted individuals become trapped in vicious circles of drug use and belief reinforcement that escalate their addictions.

THE TREATMENT OF SUBSTANCE USE DISORDERS

There are five essential components in the cognitive therapy of substance abuse: the collaborative therapeutic relationship, the cognitive case conceptualization, structure, socialization, and cognitive-behavioral techniques. Each of these will be discussed in detail in this section.

Individuals with addictions may have a variety of personal concerns including interpersonal relationship problems, complex psychopathology, unstable lifestyles, poor insight, and coping skills deficits. Table 20.2 relates each component of cognitive therapy to the problems associated with substance use disorders (Liese, 1994b).

The Collaborative Therapeutic Relationship

The therapeutic relationship provides the foundation for all other aspects of substance abuse treatment. A genuine, open, respectful, collaborative relationship between therapist and patient increases the likelihood that the patient will remain engaged in treatment. Of course, such a relationship is essential to all psychotherapy. However, the active establishment of a positive therapeutic relationship is especially important in the treatment of substance abuse.

Many individuals with substance use disorders experience shame and alienation related to their substance use; today even cigarette smokers are chastised for their addiction. As a result, people with substance use disorders are likely to feel embarrassed about seeking help for their addictions and they may find it difficult to trust clinicians attempting to help them. The effects of stigma and shame can lead to significant distortions and underreporting of addictive behaviors and thoughts, which may ultimately undermine the treatment process.

TABLE 20.2. Problems Associated with Substance Use Disorders and Corresponding Components of Cognitive Therapy

Problems associated with substance use disorders	Components of cognitive therapy
Interpersonal relationship problems	Collaboration
Complex psychopathology	Case conceptualization
Unstable lifestyles	Structure
Poor insight	Socialization
Coping skills deficits	Specific techniques

Note. From Liese (1994, p. 19). Copyright 1994 by Harwood Academic Publishers. Reprinted by permission.

Some individuals with substance use disorders do not believe that non-users can meaningfully relate to them. These individuals are likely to view therapists as naive, and their mistrust might be reflected in subtle cues. For example, in a recent session one of our alcohol-dependent patients asked her therapist, "Are you in recovery?" The therapist (wishing to be honest with the patient) answered, "No." The patient responded, "Then you'll probably learn more from me than I will from you." The therapist was initially startled by this response but she quickly regained her composure and explored the meaning of the patient's response. In doing so, she discovered that the patient had been regularly criticized by family members for her drinking. As a result she became defensive when discussing her drinking with anyone. The therapist gently guided the patient to understand that she would not respond like the patient's family members. Therapists who are attentive and responsive to subtle cues are most likely to gain patients' confidence and collaboration.

The general psychotherapy processes of empathy, respect, and unconditional positive regard all contribute to a collaborative therapeutic environment. In addition, several specific cognitive therapy interventions increase collaboration, including eliciting agenda items from the patient, explicitly "checking out" clinical hypotheses with the patient, and obtaining feedback from the patient regarding reactions to therapy. When therapists use these interventions effectively, patients are less likely to feel threatened and more likely to openly participate in therapy. For example, therapists' regular requests for patients' feedback (i.e., inquiring about patients' responses to therapy) can help reduce doubts and suspicions by demonstrating therapists' willingness to openly listen.

As patients begin to trust their therapists, some attempt to enlist therapists in the role of "enabler." Rather than acting collaboratively (i.e., honestly), these patients may try to take advantage of therapists' genuine concern for them. For example, some patients have asked us to attest to their abstinence from drugs or attendance at Alcoholics Anonymous (AA) meetings, despite the fact that we could not validate their claims. In several cases we have discovered that these patients have falsified these and other claims. When such acts of dishonesty occur it is essential for the therapist to explore patients' views, thoughts, beliefs, and attitudes about the therapist and therapy.

Among the most significant barriers to collaboration are therapists' own negative thoughts and beliefs about addicted patients. Therapists who do not identify and challenge their own negative beliefs are likely to experience counterproductive negative feelings toward their patients. Even "enlightened" therapists occasionally find themselves having negative beliefs about their addicted patients. A list of some of these beliefs follows (with corresponding cognitive distortions in parentheses).

"Drug addicts are all the same!" (overgeneralization)
"Lapses and relapses are catastrophic!" (all-or-nothing thinking)
"This guy is a typical addict!" (labeling)
"After detox they all just relapse again!" (fortune telling)
"This patient thinks I'm stupid!" (mind reading)
"This feels like a waste of my time!" (emotional reasoning)

It is important for therapists to recognize patient behaviors likely to trigger their own negative beliefs. Such behaviors include, but are not limited to, missed appointments, substance use, dishonesty, superficial agenda items, defensiveness, and lack of apparent concern about substance use. When these behaviors occur, therapists are encouraged to reflect them back to patients directly and objectively (e.g., "You almost seem proud of your recent binge, rather than remorseful"). When patients are receptive to such interventions, therapists are encouraged to discuss the underlying beliefs leading to patients' behaviors. When patients respond defensively to therapists' observations, therapists are encouraged to respond empathetically, exploring the beliefs underlying the defensiveness (e.g., "You're calling me a liar!").

Given the high likelihood of lapses and other problematic behaviors it is helpful for therapists to *expect* to occasionally feel upset with some addicted patients. In response, therapists are encouraged to carefully identify, evaluate, and modify their counterproductive thoughts. The following is a list of some adaptive thoughts that may provide therapists relief from their own distress:

"My patient is struggling to overcome his or her addiction."
"My patient feels ambivalent about quitting drugs right now."
"My patient's relapse is not a reflection of me."
"When patients are dishonest it's likely that they are ashamed of the truth."
"A relapse is not the end of the world."
"We really *can* learn something from this relapse."

The Cognitive Case Conceptualization

As discussed earlier, the case conceptualization provides an essential framework for understanding patients and for developing and implementing appropriate treatment strategies. A comprehensive case conceptualization integrates information about the patient's early development, current life problems, stimulus situations, schemas, beliefs, automatic thoughts, emotions, and maladaptive behaviors. By gathering and integrating this information the therapist can address the history, development, and pervasiveness of the patient's substance use problem and related maladaptive beliefs. Data for the case conceptualization can be usefully divided into six categories: background information, presenting problems, psychiatric diagnoses, developmental profile, cognitive profile, and integration.

Background Information

In collecting background information, useful questions include the following:

- Tell me about your background; whatever you think is most important (e.g., your age, education, employment status).
- What is your current living situation and social support network (e.g., Do you live alone or with another substance user; are you homeless)?
- What drugs are popular/prevalent in your environment?

Unfortunately, background information is sometimes gathered early in therapy and then ignored during the course of treatment. It is optimal to collect background data briefly at the beginning of treatment and then collect more in-depth information as it is relevant to specific agenda items. For example, in the first session a therapist might ask some of the questions above. In a subsequent session the patient might present a marital problem as an agenda item. It might then be appropriate for the therapist to collect data about the patient's marriage, the role drugs have played in the marital problem, and the role marital problems have played in drug use.

Presenting Problems and Current Functioning

Assessment of presenting problems and current functioning involves understanding the patient's current difficulties and adaptation to substance use. Useful questions might include:

- What drugs do you currently use?
- What is your current pattern of use?
- What are the effects of your drug use?
- What chronic problems do you have as a result of using drugs (e.g., job-related problems, relationship difficulties)?

• Are there any current or pending crises in your life as a result of your drug use (e.g., loss of employment, marital separation, divorce, suicide ideation, health problems)?

Some problems will be presented by patients at the beginning of therapy. However, patients will typically admit to additional problems in subsequent sessions as their trust in the therapist increases. The structure of therapy (reviewed later) provides a means of organizing patients' presenting problems and current functioning.

Psychiatric Diagnoses

In the cognitive therapy of substance abuse it is extremely important to formulate psychiatric diagnoses, focusing on clinical syndromes (e.g., mood, anxiety, thought disorders) and personality disorders (e.g., antisocial and borderline disorders). Coexisting psychiatric problems have major implications for the development of therapeutic treatment plans, since substance use may function as self-medication for psychiatric problems. Useful questions to address include:

• What is your drug of choice (including alcohol and nicotine)?
• What other drugs do you use (including alcohol and nicotine)?
• What emotional problems or concerns have you experienced?
• How might drugs help you with, or contribute to, your emotional concerns?

Earlier in this chapter it was explained that individuals with substance use disorders tend to have coexisting psychiatric problems. During this part of the case conceptualization, therapists are encouraged to evaluate general psychiatric functioning. If a patient is discovered to have a coexisting disorder, cognitive therapy can be customized to address the other psychiatric symptoms.

In some patients, coexisting psychiatric disorders (e.g., depression, anxiety, mania) might not be apparent until patients have been abstinent from alcohol and drugs for several weeks or months. The symptoms of these underlying disorders potentially make patients vulnerable to future drug use and therefore these disorders should be evaluated and addressed as early in treatment as possible. As a case example, a patient addicted to cocaine recently presented herself to one of our therapists with pressured speech, irritability, crying spells, difficulty sleeping, racing thoughts, and labile emotions. She had been abstinent from cocaine (validated by urine testing) for several months. This patient continued to report strong cocaine urges and craving until she was successfully treated, with psychotherapy and pharmacotherapy, for bipolar disorder.

Developmental Profile

The developmental profile consists of a comprehensive history of the patient, including information from the following domains: family, social, educational, medical, psychiatric, and vocational. When data for the developmental profile have been collected carefully, therapists and patients are likely to gain important insights about the development of drug-related problems. Useful questions in the developmental profile include:

- Who in your family has used drugs (including alcohol and nicotine), and how did they use drugs (i.e., any problems associated with substance use)?
- How old were you when you first used any drugs?
- When did drugs become problematic for you?
- How did your drug problems develop?
- Have you ever lived with anyone who had emotional problems?
- What other significant events or traumas have occurred in your life that might be significant?

As discussed earlier, persons with substance use disorders typically have developmental experiences that predispose them to abuse substances. As these experiences are uncovered and reflected back to patients, they begin to *reconceptualize* their substance use. For example, rather than thinking "I need to use drugs to have fun" they learn to think "I use drugs to have fun because that's what others did in my family and community."

Cognitive Profile

The cognitive profile describes the thought processes associated with drug use. The cognitive profile consists of information about the individuals' activating stimuli, drug-related beliefs, automatic thoughts, and facilitating beliefs. In addition, the cognitive profile includes information about patients' basic beliefs and schemas. Useful questions for the cognitive profile include:

- What are your high-risk situations for substance use? In other words, when are you most likely to use drugs?
- What are your beliefs about your drug use?
- How do you give yourself permission to use drugs? In other words, how do you convince yourself that it is okay?
- What beliefs do you hold about yourself, other people, or the world that contribute to your drug use? For example, do you think, "Oh, I'll live to be a hundred years old, regardless of what I do"?
- What are the negative and positive consequences of your substance use? In other words, what are the desired and undesired effects of your drug use?

Most therapists find that synthesizing the cognitive profile is facilitated by using a visual representation of the cognitive model available with blank spaces for listing patients' idiosyncratic drug-related triggers, beliefs, thoughts, and behaviors (see Figure 20.3). Therapists are encouraged to repeatedly use the cognitive model to evaluate various episodes of use with various drugs at various times in therapy, rather than using the model only once or twice over the course of treatment. Even when the patient has been abstinent, the model can be used to understand past drug use and to avoid future use.

Integration of Cognitive and Developmental Profiles

The final component of the case conceptualization is critical. It involves the formulation of hypotheses about the development and maintenance of patients' problems, especially regarding substance abuse. These hypotheses involve relationships between life experiences, cognitive vulnerabilities, and compensatory strategies leading to problematic patterns of substance use. The integration of cognitive and developmental profiles leads to the development of appropriate treatment strategies. Useful questions for integration include:

- How does your drug use serve as a coping strategy for you?
- How motivated are you to change your addictive behaviors?
- How do your substance use and self-esteem impact each other?
- What treatment strategies will be most effective for you?
- What are your potential barriers to change?

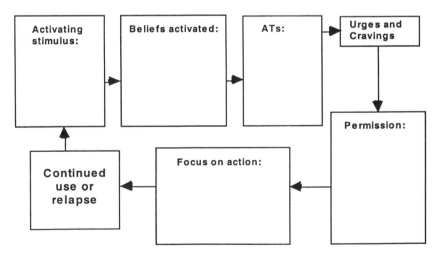

FIGURE 20.3. Cognitive model worksheet (completed with patient).

If the cognitive and developmental profiles are gathered carefully and synthesized accurately, the treatment process will be greatly facilitated.

Structure

Structure is essential to the cognitive therapy of substance abuse. The structure of a cognitive therapy session consists of eight elements: (1) setting the agenda, (2) mood check, (3) bridge from the last sessions, (4) discussion of current agenda items, (5) guided discovery, (6) capsule summaries, (7) homework assignments, and (8) summary and feedback from the patient. Some individuals with substance use problems lead highly unstable, chaotic lives. They may have health problems, intimate relationship difficulties, financial problems, and legal problems related to their substance use. Given these multiple problems patients may find it extremely difficult to focus on one problem at a time. The structure of cognitive therapy facilitates systematic problem definition and problem solving. The elements of a cognitive therapy session are discussed in the following sections.

Setting the Agenda

The first step in a cognitive therapy session is agenda setting, when the therapist asks: "What do you want to put on the agenda?" Agenda setting should result in a finite list of topics around which the remainder of the session is focused. Without an agenda, discussion is likely to drift to unproductive topics and irrelevant details. Setting an agenda encourages the patient to take an active, collaborative role in the therapeutic process and contributes to a sense of responsibility and control during therapy sessions. Setting an agenda may also be a first step toward teaching patients to identify and prioritize their problems and goals.

It is important to pay attention to patients' difficulties with setting the agenda. For example, patients frequently respond to therapists' requests for agenda items with statements such as: "I haven't given it much thought" and "Whatever you think is important." Such responses provide an excellent opportunity for therapists to foster collaboration by encouraging patients to generate their own items. A persistent inability to set an agenda might indicate other problems: low motivation, anxiety, depression, dependency, or lack of engagement in therapy. Patients who regularly defer agenda setting should be encouraged to focus on this as a therapeutic issue. In such cases the therapist might state: "It is difficult for you to generate agenda items; let's put *that* on the agenda and try to understand why it's so difficult."

Patients often list agenda items that seem unrelated to substance use (e.g., "I won $1,000 in the lottery last week"). However, an astute therapist can relate most issues to potential substance use. For example, relationship problems, boredom, financial difficulties, loneliness, depression, anxiety, homelessness, and even recent successes (e.g., winning the lottery) can all contribute to substance use.

While setting the agenda it is extremely important to inquire about recent urges, cravings, and substance use, and about upcoming high-risk situations. Patients should be taught, or "socialized," to regularly place these on the agenda. When these items are not placed on the agenda by the patient, it is essential that they be raised by the therapist early in the session.

Mood Check

As previously discussed, drugs provide powerful sources of mood regulation. Thus, a variety of positive and negative mood states can be important activating stimuli for substance use. To complicate matters, continued drug use leads to chronic mood problems. Depression, boredom, anxiety, and anger are particularly relevant to episodes of substance use. Therefore, it is important to assess patients' mood states at the outset of each session. The mood check can be accomplished simply by asking "How's your mood today?" If it is determined that a patient's mood is negative or problematic, the patient's mood is placed on the agenda for discussion.

It is common for persons with addictions to have difficulty identifying their moods. Vague descriptions such as "okay" or "neutral" are often given. These responses offer an excellent opportunity to teach patients mood recognition. The ability to recognize and label mood states is the first step in cognitive therapy mood management. When patients have chronic difficulties labeling their feelings, therapists are encouraged to provide them with a list of emotions from which to choose. It is important to attend to patients' feelings of despair and hopelessness. Depressed mood may lead to increased suicide risk, especially in patients with substance use problems.

Bridge from Previous Sessions

After checking the patient's mood it is important to bridge (i.e., review salient points) from previous sessions. Bridging provides continuity and helps ensure that important therapeutic issues are not forgotten or neglected. There are several ways to bridge between cognitive therapy sessions. One strategy is to simply ask the patient to reflect on what has been important from previous sessions. Another strategy is for the therapist to briefly review important issues. Reviewing homework (discussed below) is also an effective way of bridging between sessions.

When bridging from the last session the therapist should inquire about how the patient has used the cognitive model of substance abuse since the previous visit. Reviewing the model provides an excellent opportunity for both therapist and patient to refine the case conceptualization. The therapist, during the bridge, can test the degree to which previous learning has been retained. Issues raised during the bridge may also be placed on the agenda for extended discussion. As stated earlier, patients with substance use disorders may lead chaotic lives. Bridging helps patients to focus on important issues.

Discussion of Current Agenda Items

It is important to prioritize agenda items prior to discussing them. With only a finite number of minutes in a therapy session, patients will be best served by first discussing the most important agenda items. It is assumed that these are relevant to problematic substance use, including urges, cravings, and upcoming high-risk situations. Drug-related items should be given top priority, as they are directly related to potential future use.

It is important to remain focused on one agenda item at a time. Therapists and patients alike have a tendency to wander off the current topic, shifting from issue to issue. In order to remain focused it is recommended that the therapist regularly summarize agenda items and current issues. This should also facilitate the patient's sense of direction and productivity in sessions.

Guided Discovery

Guided discovery is basic to the effective delivery of cognitive therapy. In guided discovery therapists ask patients open-ended questions designed to objectively evaluate and examine relationships between schemas, beliefs, automatic thoughts, emotions, and behaviors. Rather than assuming correct answers, guided discovery is meant to stimulate patients' self-knowledge and independent thought. In guided discovery the therapist should explore specific hypotheses developed during the cognitive case conceptualization. The questioning process should be supportive, directive, and empathetic. In particular, therapists should encourage patients to explore their drug-related beliefs and automatic thoughts, reflect on related cognitive errors, and generate alternative ways of thinking in response to activating stimuli. Most patients prefer guided discovery to preaching, lecturing, or disputing. In fact, many of our patients have described frustration with traditional addiction treatment programs that primarily utilize such coercive techniques.

Capsule Summaries

Capsule summaries play an important role in cognitive therapy. Defined as therapists' reviews of central issues and themes, capsule summaries enable therapists to test hypotheses. At the same time, capsule summaries provide patients with objective feedback about themselves. They also help therapists and patients remain focused on agenda items. For example, a therapist might provide the following capsule summary to "John," who feels particularly depressed and lonely after 3 weeks of abstinence from cocaine:

> " John, you've been abstinent for 3 weeks. You expected to see more improvement in your life by now, and you are disappointed in the recovery process. You explain that you've been isolated for the past 3 weeks,

so you haven't received any emotional support. As you become increasingly bored, lonely, and depressed, drugs look more and more inviting. At times you've told yourself that you might be better off using drugs. Is this an accurate summary? [Patient responds affirmatively.] Then I can understand how you'd be having more urges and cravings."

Capsule summaries should be followed by additional questions, specific cognitive-behavioral interventions, or homework assignments. In the example above, follow-up questions might focus on John's reasons for isolating himself. A specific cognitive-behavioral intervention might be completion of a daily thought record (DTR) to address the emotional distress associated with John's isolation. And finally, homework might involve attending AA meetings over the next week and completing daily DTRs.

Capsule summaries should be made at least three times per cognitive therapy session. The first capsule summary should occur after the agenda has been set, the second at approximately midpoint in the session, and the third capsule summary should occur near the end of the session.

Homework Assignments

Homework is an essential feature of cognitive therapy, providing patients with opportunities to practice new skills, test maladaptive beliefs, and collect information between sessions. Homework assignments should be related to issues discussed in the current session in order to build on progress made in the session. Again, homework is most appropriately assigned following capsule summaries, when therapist and patient can focus on ways to continue and reinforce progress. Homework assignments might consist of standard cognitive or behavioral techniques (e.g., DTRs, advantages–disadvantages analyses, behavioral experiments, activity scheduling) and they may specifically relate to the development of drug-free lifestyles (e.g., attendance at AA meetings, talking to an AA sponsor, or spending time with drug-free friends). It is important to assign and begin homework early in sessions so that potential difficulties are identified and alternative strategies planned.

Patients seem to be more invested in homework when they understand its function in their lives. Thus, it is important for the therapist to explain the rationale for each homework assignment. Homework should be jointly formulated, so that patients feel a sense of control and responsibility for assignments. And finally, it is important for therapists to underscore the importance of homework by reviewing it in each session.

Feedback in the Therapy Session

It is important that therapists regularly check patients' perceptions of therapy by explicitly asking for feedback and by attending to important nonverbal cues. Questions such as "What are you getting out of this?" and "Why do you think I asked you that question?" may clarify potential miscommunication during cognitive therapy sessions. Feedback should also be obtained at the conclusion of sessions regarding what was learned, how patients feel about sessions, and how patients feel about the progress of therapy in general.

An excellent time for obtaining feedback is immediately after the patient emits a salient nonverbal cue (e.g., a frown, a sigh, rolling of the eyes, yawning). It is especially important to pay attention to changes in facial expressions, which are likely to reflect affective shifts. For example, if a patient smiles, the therapist may ask, "You just smiled. What was going through your mind right then?" The responses to such questions may provide the therapist with valuable information on the patient's feelings about, and understanding of, the session. Like capsule summaries, feedback should be elicited at least three times per session, even when sessions appear to be productive. When patients respond to feedback requests with generalizations, ambivalence, or ambiguous responses, follow-up questions are particularly important.

Socializing Patients to the Cognitive Model

In applying cognitive therapy to addictive behaviors, it is assumed that individuals have learned to think in ways that make them vulnerable to substance use. Thus, an important component of cognitive therapy is "socializing" (i.e., teaching) patients to develop "control" thoughts and beliefs that inhibit drug use. Perhaps the most important strategy for socializing patients is to reproduce the cognitive model (see Figures 20.1–20.3) and teach patients how each box relates to their drug use. Then, as homework, they can be asked to memorize the concepts in the boxes and apply each concept to their own situations and addictions. A common mistake made in the socialization process is to begin teaching the cognitive model prior to having a substantial conceptualization of the patient. When therapists prematurely teach patients about the cognitive model, they have difficulty relating the concepts to their own lives.

Cognitive-Behavioral Techniques

Literally hundreds of cognitive and behavioral techniques might be considered "cognitive therapy" (see, e.g., McMullin, 1986). In the cognitive therapy of substance abuse, a major goal in using techniques is to undermine *drug-related beliefs* and replace them with *control beliefs*.

Most individuals who abuse substances are ambivalent about their substance use. That is, they possess control beliefs that contradict their drug-related beliefs. These control beliefs reduce the likelihood of substance use. Examples of control beliefs include: "Smoking and drinking are killing me," "I need to quit using drugs!" and "I don't need drugs to have fun." In the active phase of drug use, control beliefs are not strong enough to predominate over drug-related beliefs. Thus, cognitive techniques are designed to weaken drug-related beliefs and bolster control beliefs. The most basic cognitive technique is guided discovery. Because it is fundamental to all cognitive therapy techniques, guided discovery was discussed earlier in this chapter. In the remainder of this section, some specific techniques of cognitive therapy will be described.

Identifying Drug-Related Beliefs and Control Beliefs

A basic cognitive therapy technique is to teach patients to use the cognitive therapy model to identify and modify drug-related beliefs and behaviors. As previously mentioned, patients are provided with worksheets outlining the basic cognitive model, with space provided for listing specific activating stimuli, beliefs, thoughts, and actions (see Figure 20.3). Patients are assisted in completing the worksheet, specifying their own activating stimuli, drug-related beliefs, and automatic thoughts. After each box is completed and patients have an increased understanding of their substance use, they are taught to use the same form to identify control beliefs, thoughts, and behaviors (see completed form in Figure 20.4).

Therapists are strongly encouraged to work collaboratively with patients to develop maximally accurate and useful control thoughts and beliefs. Some patients carry completed worksheets to help them remember control thoughts and beliefs.

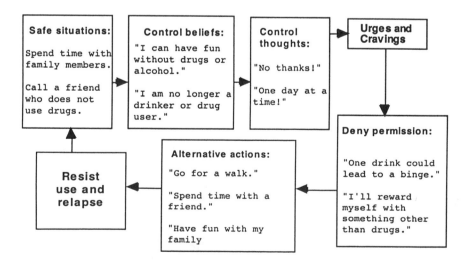

FIGURE 20.4. Cognitive model of control (completed with patient).

Advantages–Disadvantages Analysis

The advantages–disadvantages (A-D) analysis is another useful technique in the cognitive therapy of substance abuse. Patients with substance use disorders typically focus on the benefits of using, while minimizing the negative consequences. The A-D analysis guides the patient through an appraisal of the positive and negative consequences of substance use. At times the A-D analysis results in moving patients toward abstinence. At other times this technique simply helps therapists and patients to understand the continued appeal of addictive behaviors.

The A-D analysis begins with a blank four-cell matrix drawn by the therapist. Using guided discovery, the patient is helped to list the *advantages* and *disadvantages* of *using* and *not using* drugs in the appropriate cells of the matrix. The A-D analysis, when done properly, provides an objective and accurate view of the patient's substance use that can then be examined in an objective, rational fashion by the therapist and patient.

The following illustrates the A-D analysis of a patient discussing potential abstinence from alcohol (the completed matrix is presented in Figure 20.5):

THERAPIST: So you're not really sure if you want to stop drinking alcohol.

PATIENT: I guess not.

THERAPIST: Well, let's take a look at the potential advantages and disadvantages of your drinking. I'll draw this figure so we can keep track of your thoughts (*draws matrix*). On the horizontal axis we write "continued drinking" and "abstinence" and on the vertical axis we write "advantages" and "disadvantages."

PATIENT: Uh-huh.

THERAPIST: So what are the advantages of not drinking?

PATIENT: No hangovers.

THERAPIST: Anything else you can think of?

PATIENT: I might not miss so much work.

THERAPIST: Anything else?

PATIENT: I'll get my wife and boss off my back.

THERAPIST: What else?

PATIENT: I might save money.

THERAPIST: What else?

PATIENT: I'll stay out of jail if I don't drink and drive.

THERAPIST: Can you think of anything else?

PATIENT: I guess it'll be good for my health.

	Abstinence	**Continued drinking**
Advantages	• No hangovers • Won't miss work • Get my wife and boss off my back • Save money • Stay out of jail • Good for my health	• Hang out with my drinking buddies • Fall asleep easier • Helps me forget my problems
Disadvantages	• No contact with my old buddies • Trouble falling asleep • Can't forget my problems	• Hangovers • Miss work • Get nagged by my wife and boss • Spend lots of money • Could go to jail • Bad for my health

FIGURE 20.5. Advantages–disadvantages analysis.

THERAPIST: Anything else?

PATIENT: I can't think of anything.

THERAPIST: Okay. Now what are the advantages of drinking?

PATIENT: None, I guess.

THERAPIST: There must be some advantages or you wouldn't drink, right?

PATIENT: I guess. Let's see. It's what I do when I hang around with my buddies.

THERAPIST: Any other advantages?

PATIENT: It helps me fall asleep easier.

THERAPIST: What else?

[The discussion continues until all cells are complete.]

It is important to note that the A-D analysis has several goals. The most obvious of which is to help patients recognize that their drug use has negative consequences. However, another often overlooked goal is to help patients and therapists identify the advantages of using in order to find other alternative strategies for achieving the same advantages.

Three-Question Technique

The three-question technique is another method that uses guided discovery to examine patients' maladaptive thought processes. In this technique, therapists ask patients a series of three questions regarding substance-related beliefs and thoughts.

1. What is the evidence for your belief?
2. How else can you interpret the situation?
3. If the alternative interpretation is true, what are the implications?

For example, one patient who was abusing marijuana held the belief: "I can't relax without pot." We used the three-question technique to examine her belief:

1. *What is the evidence for that belief?* "I've never been able to come home at night and chill out without smoking a joint. I must need to smoke to relax, or I wouldn't do it so much, right?"
2. *How else can you interpret the situation?* "Well, I guess I've never tried very hard to go without smoking. Maybe it's just a habit. Actually, I have had a couple of nights when I couldn't cop any pot, and I did okay."
3. *If the alternative interpretation is true, what are the implications?* "I guess if it's just a habit and I have gone a couple of nights without pot, then I really don't need it. I suppose I can relax without a joint, I just never try too often."

As with the previous methods discussed, this technique should help patients to more objectively and realistically assess their beliefs about themselves and their drug use.

Daily Thought Record

The DTR helps patients objectively analyze automatic thoughts and feelings that potentially lead to drug use. The DTR consists of five columns for listing and describing situations, emotions, automatic thoughts, rational responses, and outcomes. In the first column, patients describe situations that place them at high risk for substance use. In the next column, associated automatic thoughts are listed and rated (from 0% to 100%) according to how much they are believed. Then, emotions associated with the situation are listed and rated for intensity (again, from 0% to 100%). Next, patients list possible rational responses and rate their belief in those responses. Finally, patients rerate their belief in the previously listed automatic thoughts and specify and rate the resulting change in their emotions. The DTR is especially useful for teaching patients to regulate their moods without drugs.

Since some patients initially have difficulty formulating rational responses, the following open-ended questions may be useful in generating such responses (Beck et al., 1993, p. 144):

1. What concrete, factual evidence supports or refutes your automatic thoughts and beliefs?
2. Are there other ways you could view this situation? Is there a blessing in disguise here?

3. What is the *worst* thing that could possibly happen? What is the *best* thing? What is most likely to *realistically* happen?
4. What constructive *action* can you take to deal with the situation?
5. What are the pros and cons of changing the way you view this situation?
6. What advice would you give your best friend in this situation?

At first, DTRs are completed in therapy sessions. When patients are able to effectively complete them on their own, however, DTRs are assigned as homework to be reviewed in later sessions. Used effectively, DTRs are powerful tools for helping patients see relationships between their thoughts, emotions, and behaviors.

In addition to the cognitive techniques described above, certain behavioral techniques are extremely useful in helping patients to either avoid or cope with external and internal activating stimuli. Two particularly effective behavioral techniques are weekly activity scheduling and communication skills training.

Weekly Activity Scheduling

In weekly activity scheduling, patients are provided with calendars where they record their activities on an hourly basis for 1 week (as homework). Therapists help patients examine completed calendars for typical high-risk and low-risk situations. This baseline assessment is used to plan future activities so that high-risk situations are minimized and low-risk situations are maximized. Follow-up activity schedules are used to evaluate patients' success at implementing proposed schedule changes. Success at planning and implementing substance-free activities contributes to patient satisfaction and self-efficacy and promotes the development of control beliefs and adaptive behaviors.

Communication Skills Training

Teaching patients to communicate effectively is an important behavioral technique. As mentioned earlier, one study of 311 relapse episodes found that 36% were due to interpersonal determinants: 20% related to social pressure, and 16% related to interpersonal conflict (Cummings, Marlatt, & Gordon, 1980). Many of these episodes may not have occurred if individuals had the skills (e.g., assertiveness) to solve interpersonal problems. In cognitive therapy, patients and therapists work collaboratively to establish such skills. Role playing, an important component of communications skills training, enables patients to acquire and practice new skills in a safe environment.

Cognitive Therapy and 12-Step Programs

Cognitive therapy is a highly integrative and collaborative endeavor. As such, every effort is made to facilitate the integration of cognitive therapy with other available addiction treatment services, including 12-step programs (such as AA and Narcotics Anonymous [NA]). Since some readers may not be fully knowledgeable about 12-step programs, they are briefly discussed here.

AA, NA, and other 12-step programs are mutual support groups with one requirement for membership: the desire to abstain from alcohol and drugs. Twelve-step programs have been labeled as such because members are encouraged to follow 12 steps to recovery.

In addition to following the 12 steps, members are encouraged to attend meetings regularly, be supportive of other members, seek help when relapse is imminent, and study the basic text of AA ("The Big Book"; Alcoholics Anonymous World Services, 1976). The spiritual dimension (not necessarily religious) is considered a key aspect of recovery; members are encouraged to identify a higher power. They are also encouraged to gain a greater knowledge of themselves and their relationships with others. Twelve-step programs do not solicit members, promote religion, provide social services, accept money or advertising, offer psychotherapy, engage in research, or take attendance. As a result, it is difficult to quantify the effects of 12-step programs.

Certain slogans and themes from 12-step programs have relevance to cognitive therapy. For example the Serenity Prayer, which is central to the 12-step tradition, seems to reflect the essence of CT:

> *Grant me the serenity to accept the things I cannot change,*
> *The courage to change the things I can,*
> *And the wisdom to know the difference.*

Cognitive therapists who treat addicted patients are strongly encouraged to learn about 12-step programs. One strategy for doing so is to discuss 12-step programs with patients who have benefited from them. Another strategy is to read resources published by 12-step programs (e.g., "The Big Book").

TEN LESSONS LEARNED AND IMPLICATIONS FOR THE FUTURE

Over the past few years we have learned numerous lessons about the cognitive therapy of substance abuse. In this section we review 10 of these lessons. Our goals are to encourage cognitive therapists to work effectively with addicted patients and share what we have learned.

Lesson 1: Become knowledgeable about psychoactive drugs, addictive behaviors, and traditional treatment modalities. When first beginning to treat addicted patients, most cognitive therapists are naive about drugs and the "drug culture." For example, they may not realize the powerful physiologic effects of cocaine, marijuana, alcohol, nicotine, and other psychoactive agents. They may not be aware of the "seductive" sociocultural context within which drug use takes place. Furthermore, they may not be familiar with predominant treatment modalities (e.g., inpatient and 12-step programs).

In treating addicted patients it is important to learn as much as possible about psychoactive drugs, addictive behaviors, and traditional drug treatment modalities. An excellent learning strategy is to study professional journals, textbooks (e.g., Beck et al., 1993; Marlatt & Gordon, 1985; Miller & Rollnick, 1991; Prochaska et al., 1994; Sobell & Sobell, 1993), and self-help books (e.g., Alcoholics Anonymous World Services, 1976; Burton, 1986; Daley, 1991; Dorsman, 1991; Ellis & Velten, 1992; Gorski, 1989; Miller & Munoz, 1976; Mooney, Eisenberg, & Eisenberg, 1992; Trimpey, 1989). Another *essential* strategy is to listen carefully to patients who have struggled with addictions (including cigarette smokers).

Lesson 2: Communicate and collaborate with other addiction treatment personnel. Numerous treatment resources are available to addicted individuals, including inpatient, outpatient, and self-help programs. Most personnel involved in these programs can be valuable resources to cognitive therapists working with addicted patients. Unfortunately, many psychotherapists underestimate the potential value of these individuals. Cognitive therapists are strongly encouraged to communicate and collaborate with these people whenever possible.

Lesson 3: Address the important role of drugs in mood regulation. Addicted individuals, like all other human beings, encounter a wide range of mood states: anger, happiness, boredom, joy, emptiness, sadness, loneliness, despair, anxiety. Drugs provide powerful methods for regulating these moods, and addicted patients become habituated to the immediate mood regulating effects of drugs. Even nicotine, within seconds after inhalation, can have a profound effect on individuals' moods. It is important to help addicted individuals understand that their drug use reflects their attempts to regulate even "good" moods (to transform them into "great" moods). Of course, given the mood regulating function of drugs, it is essential that therapists help patients develop alternative (cognitive) strategies for regulating mood states.

Lesson 4: Conceptualize and treat coexisting psychopathology. As discussed in the beginning of this chapter, acute and chronic psychiatric disorders (e.g., depression, anxiety, antisocial personality disorder) tend to coexist with addictive behaviors. It is extremely important for cognitive therapists to recognize, diagnose, and treat psychopathology that coexists with substance abuse. Specifically, therapists are encouraged to conceptualize patients carefully and accurately, and they are urged to apply appropriate psychological techniques to address psychiatric symptoms. Again, a major advantage of treating addicted patients with cognitive therapy is that cognitive therapy has been shown to be effective in the treatment of psychiatric disorders that coexist with addictions.

Lesson 5: Explore the development of patients' drug use problems. The historical context in which patients' addictions developed is important. Numerous factors may contribute to addictive disorders (e.g., growing up with parents who were addicted). Careful examination of the development and maintenance of patients' drug problems is often neglected by clinicians or, at the opposite extreme, focused on in excessive detail.

It is essential for cognitive therapists to conceptualize the development of their patients' addictions. In doing so, they can help patients develop new conceptualizations of their drug use. For example, many addicted individuals initially believe "I just use drugs to have fun. I don't really have a serious problem." By focusing on their parents' drug and alcohol histories, these same individuals can begin to view their own drug use as maladaptive. Furthermore, they can begin to see how they developed their own drug problems.

Lesson 6: Address therapeutic relationship problems. Therapeutic relationship problems are inevitable in the treatment of individuals with drug problems. Patients' drug-related beliefs and maladaptive behaviors are likely to trigger therapists' distress. This distress, in turn, is likely to trigger patients' mistrust of their therapists. Unfortunately, many of these problems go undetected. Unless therapeutic relationship problems are resolved, they are likely to hinder therapy (e.g., by resulting in premature termination).

Therapists need to recognize and discuss therapeutic relationship problems. Specifically, they are encouraged to be attentive to their own emotions (e.g., boredom, anger, confusion, frustration) and associated thoughts. They are encouraged to share concerns about the therapeutic relationship with patients and get patients' feedback about the therapeutic process on a regular basis. Most importantly, therapists are encouraged to maintain collaborative and empathetic attitudes as they conduct cognitive therapy with addicted patients.

Lesson 7: Confront patients appropriately and effectively. Addicted individuals may possess numerous maladaptive, self-defeating thoughts and behaviors (e.g., avoidance, denial, withdrawal, aggression). Some clinicians are reluctant to address or confront these because they believe "it's not nice" to do so. These clinicians think, "I don't want to make my patient feel bad."

Confrontation is an art. In treating patients with addictive disorders it is essential to identify and conceptualize patients' maladaptive coping strategies and reveal these to them. In addition, it is important to anticipate patients' reactions to such interventions and respond appropriately (i.e., listen carefully and keep an open mind when patients disagree with therapists' confrontations).

Lesson 8: Stay focused in sessions. Severely addicted individuals tend to live disorganized, chaotic lives. Thus, some psychotherapy sessions may become unfocused and disorganized. When this occurs, sessions may become diluted and both therapist and patient may feel unfulfilled.

In order to help patients whose lives are disorganized, it is important to provide some structure in psychotherapy. All ingredients of cognitive therapy structure are potentially therapeutically and diagnostically useful. Cognitive therapy sessions should be agenda driven (i.e., focused on what the patient is motivated to work on) and therapists should regularly check on the extent to which agenda items are successfully addressed.

Lesson 9: Use cognitive therapy techniques appropriately and sparingly. In many psychotherapy encounters there is a silent conspiracy, wherein therapists and patients search for quick, easy solutions to complex problems. Patients may be looking for panaceas while clinicians may be looking for "silver bullets." When this occurs, both have been deceived by the lure of simple and effective-appearing techniques. Unfortunately, change-oriented techniques may take inappropriate precedence over insight-oriented techniques.

Therapists are encouraged to avoid "technolatry," or the worship of techniques (Mahoney, 1991). Alternatively, therapists are urged to apply techniques only as they are appropriate to patients' problems and readiness to change. It is important to understand that an accurate case conceptualization takes precedence over change strategies (since change strategies should be guided by an accurate case conceptualization). Most importantly, when a specific technique doesn't work for a particular patient, or when a patient doesn't complete assigned homework, it is important for the therapist to strive to understand the patient's problem with the technique or homework.

Lesson 10: Don't give up on addicted patients. Throughout this chapter we have emphasized the difficult nature of the cognitive therapy of substance abuse. In practice we have discovered that most therapists, at times, become overwhelmed with the breadth and depth of their addicted patients' problems. But we have also learned to expect *positive* surprises; people with addictions generally have strong underlying desires to overcome their addictions.

This brings us to, perhaps, the most important lesson of all: Don't give up on addicted patients! In working with addicted patients, even if no apparent cognitive or behavioral changes are evident during the course of therapy, patients are likely to eventually benefit from the lessons they learn in cognitive therapy.

NOTE

1. The fourth edition of the *Diagnostic and Statistical Manual of Mental Disorders* (DSM-IV; American Psychiatric Association, 1994) classifies substance abuse and dependence as substance use disorders. In this chapter we use these terms and the term "addiction" interchangeably.

REFERENCES

Alcoholics Anonymous World Services. (1976). *Alcoholics Anonymous* ("The Big Book"; 3rd ed.). New York: Author.

American Psychiatric Association. (1994). *Diagnostic and statistical manual of mental disorders* (4th ed.). Washington, DC: Author.

Anthony, J. C., & Helzer, J. E. (1991). Syndromes of drug abuse and dependence. In L. Robins & D. Regier (Eds.), *Psychiatric disorders in America: The Epidemiological Catchment Area Study* (pp. 116–154). New York: Free Press.

Beck, A. T. (1961). A systematic investigation of depression. *Comprehensive Psychiatry, 2*, 163–170.

Beck, A. T. (1964). Thinking and depression: 2. Theory and therapy. *Archives of General Psychiatry, 10*, 561–571.

Beck, A. T., Emery, G., with Greenberg, R. L. (1985). *Anxiety disorders and phobias: A cognitive perspective.* New York: Basic Books.

Beck, A. T., Freeman, A., & Associates. (1990). *Cognitive therapy of personality disorders.* New York: Guilford Press.

Beck, A. T., Rush, A. J., Shaw, B. F., & Emery, G. (1979). *Cognitive therapy of depression.* New York: Guilford Press.

Beck, A. T., Wright, F. D., Newman, C. F., & Liese, B. S. (1993). *Cognitive therapy of substance abuse.* New York: Guilford Press.

Bien, T. H., & Burge, R. (1990). Smoking and drinking: A review of the literature. *International Journal of the Addictions, 25*, 1429–1454.

Bobo, J. K. (1989). Nicotine dependence and alcoholism epidemiology and treatment. *Journal of Psychoactive Drugs, 21*, 323–329.

Bobo, J. K., & Gilchrist, L. D. (1983). Urging the alcoholic to quit smoking cigarettes. *Addictive Behaviors, 8*, 297–305.

Brownell, K. D., Marlatt, G. A., Lichtenstein, E., & Wilson, G. T. (1986). Understanding and preventing relapse. *American Psychologist, 41*, 765–782.

Burton, D. (1986). *The American Cancer Society's 'Freshstart': 21 days to stop smoking.* New York: Pocket Books.

Cummings, C., Gordon, R. J., & Marlatt, G. A. (19808). Relapse: Prevention and prediction. In W. R. Miller (Ed.), *The addictive behaviors: Treatment of alcoholism, drug abuse, smoking, and obesity* (pp. 291–321). Oxford, UK: Pergamon Press.

Daley, D. C. (1991). *Kicking addictive habits once and for all: A relapse prevention guide.* Lexington, MA: Lexington Books.

Daley, D. C., & Marlatt, G. A. (1992). Relapse prevention: Cognitive and behavioral interventions. In J. Lowinson, R. Ruiz, R. Millman, & J. Langrod (Eds.), *Substance abuse: A comprehensive textbook* (2nd ed., pp. 533–542). Baltimore, MD: Williams & Wilkins.

Des Jarlais, D. C. (1995). Editorial: Harm reduction—A framework for incorporating science into drug policy. *American Journal of Public Health, 85,* 10–12.

Dorsman, J. (1991). *How to quit drinking without AA: A complete self-help guide.* Newark, DE: New Dawn.

Ellis, A., & Velten, E. (1992). *Rational steps to quitting alcohol.* Fort Lee, NJ: Barricade Books.

Goldsmith, R. J., & Knapp, J. (1993). Towards a broader view of recovery. *Journal of Substance Abuse Treatment, 10,* 107–111.

Gorski, T. T. (1989). *Understanding the twelve steps.* New York: Prentice Hall.

Helzer, J. E., Burnam, M. A., & McEvoy, L. T. (1991). Alcohol abuse and dependence. In L. Robins & D. Regier (Eds.), *Psychiatric disorders in America: The Epidemiological Catchment Area Study* (pp. 81–115). New York: Free Press.

Helzer, J. E., & Pryzbeck, T. R. (1988). The co-occurrence of alcoholism with other psychiatric disorders in the general population and its impact on treatment. *Journal of Studies on Alcohol, 49,* 219–224.

Henningfield, J. E., Clayton, R., & Pollin, W. (1990). Involvement of tobacco in alcoholism and illicit drug use. *British Journal of Addictions, 85,* 279–292.

Hunt, W. A., Barnett, L. W., & Branch, L. G. (1971). Relapse rates in addiction programs. *Journal of Clinical Psychology, 27,* 455–456.

Istvan, J., & Matarazzo, J. D. (1984). Tobacco, alcohol, and caffeine use: A review of their interrelationships. *Psychological Bulletin, 95,* 301–326.

Kessler, R. C., McGonagle, K. A., Zhao, S., Nelson, C. B., Hughes, M., Eshleman, S., Wittchen, H., & Kendler, K. S. (1994). Lifetime and 12-month prevalence of DSM-III-R psychiatric disorders in the United States: Results from the National Comorbidity Survey. *Archives of General Psychiatry, 51,* 8–19.

Kozlowski, L. T., Jelinek, L. C., & Pope, M. A. (1986). Cigarette smoking among alcohol users: A continuing and neglected problem. *Canadian Journal of Public Health, 77,* 205–207.

Liese, B. S. (1993). The KUFP five-visit quit smoking program: An office-based smoking cessation protocol. *Kansas Medicine, 94,* 294–298.

Liese, B. S. (1994a). Psychological principles of substance abuse: A brief overview. *Comprehensive Therapy, 20,* 125–129.

Liese, B. S. (1994b). Brief therapy, crisis intervention, and the cognitive therapy of substance abuse. *Crisis Intervention, 1*(1), 11–29.

Liese, B. S., & Beck, A. T. (in press). Back to basics: Fundamental cognitive therapy skills for keeping drug-dependent individuals in treatment. In J. J. Boren, L. S. Onken, & J. D. Blaine (Eds.), *Beyond the therapeutic alliance: Keeping drug dependent individuals in treatment* [National Institute on Drug Abuse Monograph]. Washington, DC: U.S. Government Printing Office.

Liese, B. S., & Chiauzzi, E. (1995). Alcohol and drug abuse. In *Home Study Self-Assessment Program* [Monograph No. 189]. Kansas City, KS: American Academy of Family Physicians.

Mahoney, M. J. (1991). *Human change processes: The scientific foundations of psychotherapy.* New York: Basic Books.

Marlatt, G. A., & Gordon, J. R. (1985). *Relapse prevention: Maintenance strategies in the treatment of addictive behaviors.* New York: Guilford Press.

Marlatt, G. A., & Gordon, J. R. (1989). Relapse prevention: Future directions. In M. Gossop (Ed.), *Relapse and addictive behavior* (pp. 278–291). London: Routledge.

Marlatt, G. A., Larimer, M. E., Baer, J. S., & Quigley, L. A. (1993). Harm reduction for alcohol problems: Moving beyond the controlled drinking controversy. *Behavior Therapy, 24,* 461–504.

Marlatt, G. A., & Tapert, S. F. (1993). Harm reduction: Reducing the risks of addictive behaviors. In J. Baer, G. Marlatt, & R. McMahon (Eds.), *Addictive behaviors across the lifespan* (pp. 243–273). Newbury Park, CA: Sage.

McMullin, R. E. (1986). *Handbook of cognitive therapy techniques.* New York: Norton.

Miller, W. R. (1983). Motivational interviewing with problem drinkers. *Behavioral Psychotherapy, 1,* 147–172.

Miller, W. R., & Munoz, R. F. (1976). *How to control your drinking.* Englewood Cliffs, NJ: Prentice-Hall.

Miller, W. R., & Rollnick, S. (1991). *Motivational interviewing: Preparing people to change addictive behavior.* New York: Guilford Press.

Mooney, A.M., Eisenberg, A., & Eisenberg, H. (1992). *The recovery book.* New York: Workman.

Narrow, W. E., Regier, D. A., Rae, D. S., Manderscheid, R. W., & Locke, B. Z. (1993). Use of services by persons with mental and addictive disorders: Findings from the National Institute of Mental Health Epidemiological Catchment Area Program. *Archives of General Psychiatry, 50,* 95–107.

Prochaska, J. O., & DiClemente, C. C. (1986). Toward a comprehensive model of change. In W. R. Miller & N. Heather (Eds.), *Treating addictive behaviors: Processes of change* (pp. 3–27). New York: Plenum Press.

Prochaska, J. O., DiClemente, C. C., & Norcross, J. C. (1992). In search of how people change: Applications to addictive behaviors. *American Psychologist, 47,* 1102–1114.

Prochaska, J. O., Norcross, J. C., & DiClemente, C. C. (1994). *Changing for good.* New York: William Morrow.

Regier, D. A., Farmer, M. E., Rae, D. S., Locke, B. Z., Keith, S. J., Judd, L. L., & Goodwin, F. K. (1990). Comorbidity of mental disorders with alcohol and other drug abuse: Results from the Epidemiological Catchment Area (ECA) Study. *Journal of the American Medical Association, 264,* 2511–2518.

Riley, D. M., Sobell, L. C., Leo, G. I., Sobell, M. B., & Klajner, F. (1987). Behavioral treatment of alcohol problems: A review and a comparison of behavioral and non-behavioral studies. In W. Cox (Ed.), *Treatment and prevention of alcohol problems: A resource manual* (pp. 73–116). New York: Academic Press.

Ross, H. E., & Tisdall, G. W. (1994). Alcohol use and abuse in a university psychiatric health service: Prevalence and patterns of comorbidity with other psychiatric problems. *Journal of Alcohol and Drug Education, 39,* 63–74.

Sobell, L. C. (1994, November). *Treatment implications and outcomes: What we can learn from studying naturally recovering alcohol abusers.* Paper presented at the National Institute on Alcohol Abuse and Alcoholism Symposium on Alcohol and Tobacco: From Basic Science to Policy, San Diego, CA.

Sobell, M. B., & Sobell, L. C. (1993). *Problem drinkers: Guided self-change treatment.* New York: Guilford Press.

Stark, M. J., & Campbell, B. K. (1993). Drug use and cigarette smoking in applicants for drug abuse treatment. *Journal of Substance Abuse Treatment, 5,* 175–181.

Trimpey, J. (1989). *The small book.* Lotus, CA: Lotus Press.

Wright, F. D., Beck, A. T., Newman, C. F., & Liese, B. S. (1992). Cognitive therapy of substance abuse: Theoretical rationale. In L. S. Onken, J. D. Blaine, & J. J. Boren (Eds.) *Behavioral treatments for drug aause and dependence* (NIDA Research Monograph No. 137, DHHS Publication No. 93-3684, pp. 123–146). Washington, DC: U.S. Government Printing Office.

Wright, J. H., Thase, M. E., Beck, A. T., & Ludgate, J. W. (Eds.). (1993). *Cognitive therapy with inpatients: Developing a cognitive milieu.* New York: Guilford Press.

Chapter 21

Emotional Disorders in Youth

Philip C. Kendall
Melissa J. Warman

In recent years, cognitive theories have been central in the efforts of the world's mental health professionals to understand, treat, and advance our knowledge of the affective disorders. Clearly one of the most seminal theories is that offered by Aaron T. Beck (e.g., Beck, 1976). Relatedly, Beck's cognitive therapy for depression (Beck, Rush, Shaw, & Emery, 1979) has become one of the most well-validated and widely applied treatment approaches. Of particular interest for our present undertaking, Beck has not only shaped the study and treatment of adult psychopathology, but he has also had a profound influence on child psychopathology research and the practice and evaluation of child therapy.

The purpose of this chapter is to illustrate the impact of Beck's theory on child psychopathology research and the practice and evaluation of child psychotherapy. His landmark works have prompted the critical question of whether or not depression occurs in youth and have opened the door to other theoretical and research investigations, such as the distinction between cognitive distortion and cognitive deficiency (Kendall, 1985) in child psychopathology and psychotherapy. As a result of Beck's theories there have been many efforts to assess, investigate, and treat depression. Furthermore, his distinction between depression as a mood, a symptom, and a syndrome has advanced assessment procedures and research investigations, and his content–specificity hypothesis has helped our understanding of the similarities and differences among and between depressed and anxious youth. Beck's provision of specifiable treatment strategies and procedures for the remediation of depressed mood has had a significant impact, while the utility of a manual-based treatment, allowing for greater transportability, has been another major contribution that has influenced methodological considerations in subsequent studies with children. Areas in need of future research also highlight Beck's far-reaching contribution in our attempts to better understand and treat emotionally distressed youth. It is our hope that the present chapter expresses our acknowledgment and appreciation for his profound influence on our field of study.

THE NATURE OF DEPRESSION AND ANXIETY IN YOUTH

Beck (e.g., 1967, 1976; Beck et al., 1979) placed cognitive processing square-ly at the center of the clinical research arena. His cognitive theory asserts that differences in cognitive content determine and maintain psychopathol-ogy (Beck, 1976) and that, furthermore, systematic biases are introduced in information processing. It is this faulty information-processing system that is associated with affective, behavioral, motivational, and physiologi-cal symptoms of anxiety and depression (Clark, Beck, & Brown, 1989).

Following Beck, Ingram and Kendall (Kendall, 1985, 1991; Ingram & Kendall, 1986, 1987; Kendall & Ingram, 1987, 1989) elaborated on the theoretical model of information processing that guides the approach. They described cognition as divided into four elements: (1) cognitive struc-tures, (2) cognitive content (propositions), (3) cognitive operations, and (4) cognitive products. Cognitive structures can be considered the way in which information is organized and represented in memory and is based on an individual's experiences in the world. Following repeated experiences within a particular context, a person anticipates the experience and this gets represented in the cognitive structures. The combination of cognitive con-tent and structure forms what Beck (1967) has referred to as cognitive schema, the focus of research for depressive disorders. This schema creates a frame of reference from which each individual develops his or her own unique view of him- or herself, others, the environment, and the world. This process affects what an individual perceives, recalls, and prioritizes as important. It is through schemas that an individual interprets the world and derives meaning accordingly.

Schemas, according to Clark et al. (1989), provide an economical sys-tem for processing information. Information consistent with existing schemas is encoded while inconsistent information is disregarded (Greenberg, Vaz-quez, & Alloy, 1988). However, when psychopathology is present, it is the-orized that the schemas that are activated are maladaptive, with a resulting systematic bias in information processing that takes the form of errors such as overgeneralization, arbitrary inference, selective abstraction, magnification–minimization, dichotomous thinking, and personalization (Beck, 1967; Beck et al., 1979). With psychopathology, the errors may persist even when there is contradictory evidence. Cognitive theory asserts that each disorder has a specific cognitive profile as evident in dysfunctional schemas, automatic thoughts, and biased interpretations (Beck, 1976).

Cognitive theory and subsequent research addressed cognitive distor-tions in information processing associated with emotional distress. Concur-rently, researchers were studying cognitive deficiencies in children with attention-deficit disorders. The similarity of the topic, as well as the differ-ences in the types of cognitive information-processing errors, led to a series of studies examining cognitive distortion versus cognitive deficiencies in child-hood psychopathology.

Cognitive Distortion versus Cognitive Deficiency

With cognitive dysfunction as a major focus for research and therapy, it is critical to recognize that all cognitive dysfunction is not the same, and that an understanding of the nature of the dysfunction for specific disorders has important implications for treatment. Theory and research (e.g., Kendall, 1985, 1991, 1993) have supported an important distinction in child psychopathology between cognitive deficiencies and cognitive distortions.

Cognitive deficiencies describe a lack of or insufficient amount of cognitive activity in situations where such mental activity would be useful to the child's adjustment. The absence of problem solving, planning, and perspective taking may be manifested as a result of insufficient cognitive activity and is also associated with a lack of verbal mediation and self-control (Fuhrman & Kendall, 1986). In comparison, *cognitive distortion* is not a result of a lack of processing activity, but is a consequence of an active but inaccurate thinking process. In other words, cognitive processing is taking place, but the thinking is in some way distorted (Kendall & MacDonald, 1993).

Kendall and MacDonald (1993) postulated that there are several important social and cognitive information-processing factors that must be considered, and that the differentiation between cognitive deficiencies and cognitive distortions is one of the more useful guides when working with children. They hypothesized that the distinction could be linked to the behavioral distinction between undercontrolled (externalizing) disorders and overcontrolled (internalizing) disorders (Achenbach, 1966). For example, attention-deficit/hyperactivity disorder, a disorder characterized by undercontrolled, externalizing, acting-out problems, involves deficiencies such as a lack of internally mediated self-control and a failure to use mediational skills. Psychopathology that involves overcontrolled or internalizing problems such as depression and anxiety can be conceptualized as a misinterpretation of environmental demands along with negative self-evaluations. A closer look at related research is informative.

Depression

Depression in children is a serious disorder that necessitates clinical attention (Cantwell, 1985; Kovacs, 1985). Central to Beck's (1967, 1976) theory is that depressed individuals are characterized by a tendency to distort information so that it corresponds to their more negative views of self, world, and future (Garber, Quiggle, & Shanley, 1990). This hypothesized relationship has received empirical support. There is also evidence to support that the cognitive dysfunctions found in depressed children are distortions similar to those found in depressed adults (Kovacs & Beck, 1977). Cognitive models of adult depression stress the influence of negative self-perceptions on the initiation and continuation of adult depression, while negative self-evaluation is also a common distortion evident in depressed children. Research on the cognitive characteristics of depressed children and adolescents has found distortions in attributions, self-evaluation, and perceptions of past and present events.

Cognitive distortions have been shown to be characteristic of different populations of depressed children, including outpatient, nonclinical, and inpatient samples. Kaslow, Rehm, Pollack, and Siegel (1988) reported that depressed clinical children had more depressogenic attributions than did nondepressed clinical children or nonclinical children. Leitenberg, Yost, and Carroll-Wilson (1986), in an effort to measure in children the four types of cognitive errors offered in Beck's model for adults (i.e., catastrophizing, overgeneralizing, personalizing, or selective abstraction), developed the Children's Negative Cognitive Error Questionnaire (CNCEQ). For the most part, children from a normal sample did not endorse any of the four errors, while children who reported depression on the Children's Depression Inventory (CDI; Kovacs, 1981) endorsed each of the four errors significantly more often.

Other researchers (Kaslow, Rehm, & Siegel, 1984; McGee, Anderson, Williams, & Silva, 1986) have also reported cognitive distortions in nonclinical populations of children whose scores on a measure of self-reported depression were elevated. In both studies, children who self-reported depressive symptomatology on the CDI evaluated their performance more negatively than did the children who did not self-report depressive symptomatology. In the McGee et al. (1986) report, the Wechsler Intelligence Scale for Children–Revised (WISC-R; Wechsler, 1974) was used as an objective measure of ability, and the depressed children did not score significantly lower. The results are consistent with the notion that a relationship exists between depressive symptomatology and distortions in self-perception.

The relationship between cognitive distortion and depression has been reported in studies of inpatient samples of children as well (e.g., Haley, Fine, Marriage, Moretti, & Freeman, 1985). Haley et al. (1985) utilized the Cognitive Bias Questionnaire for Children (CBQC; Haley et al., 1985), which was developed following Beck's (1967) view that depressed individuals interpret the world through cognitive distortions, such as a negative view of self. The outcome indicated that depressed children displayed this distortion in self-appraisal whereas the nondepressed children did not.

Inpatient depressed children in a study by Asarnow and Bates (1988) also exhibited cognitive distortions in self-evaluations. The depressed youth reported lower perceptions of their general self-worth, scholastic competence, athletic abilities, and physical appearance. On measures of IQ, achievement, and social status, the depressed children were no less competent than their nondepressed peers.

Fuhrman and Kendall (1986) investigated the relationship between cognitive tempo and a variety of behavioral and emotional problems in children. The Matching Familiar Figures Test (MFFT; Kagan, 1966) was used to operationalize cognitive deficiencies and was given to 150 children between the ages of 6 and 11. Their parents completed the Child Behavior Checklist (CBCL; Achenbach, 1978; Achenbach & Edelbrock, 1979). Fuhrman and Kendall (1986) found a significant relationship between cognitive deficiencies and hyperactivity but did not find a significant relationship between cognitive tempo and depression in children. The results suggested that the cognitive disturbance associated with depressed youth was not deficiencies in processing.

To further examine the nature of the cognitive disturbance among depressed children and, more specifically, to determine whether childhood depression was associated with cognitive distortion *or* cognitive deficiency, Kendall, Stark, and Adam (1990) designed a study with children in grades 3–6 who were diagnosed as depressed by the Schedule for Affective Disorders and Schizophrenia for School-Age Children (K-SADS; Puig-Antich & Ryan, 1986) and the Children's Depression Inventory (CDI; Kovacs, 1981). The depressed children, with their hypothesized bias toward negative self-evaluation, did in fact evaluate themselves significantly more negatively than did their nondepressed peers. Their self-ratings were then compared to ratings by the classroom teacher to examine if the depressed children were in fact lacking in ability or distorting their self-ratings. Teachers' blind ratings showed no significant difference between the evaluations of depressed and nondepressed children—a finding that gives credence to the notion that the cognitive views of the depressed children were distorted regarding their abilities. At the same time there was no evidence for deficiencies on a problem-solving task. Results indicated that the depressed children displayed distortions in cognition, but did not demonstrate a cognitive deficiency when compared to nondepressed children. Overall, these findings support the notion that cognitive distortion, but not cognitive deficiencies (Kendall, 1985), characterizes the nature of the cognitive disturbance in childhood depression.

Overall, the cognitive processes involved in childhood depression indicate difficulties that take the form of distortions rather than deficiencies in processing. Across different samples of depressed children, it has been shown that their evaluation of themselves, their performance, and their self-worth are lower than their nondepressed counterparts, and also lower than an objective evaluator, such as a teacher.

Anxiety

Cognitive theories have influenced not only the study of depression, but also research concerning anxiety in children. However, the role of cognitive dysfunction in childhood anxiety has not been as extensively researched. Beck (1976) offered his understanding for anxiety disorders in adults; he concluded that anxiety prompts adults to misinterpret internal and environmental cues in a way that results in an increase in their anxiety. Anxious adults also tend to have a biased view of the degree of danger presented in a given situation and their own vulnerability (Beck & Emery, 1985). Beck's theories have shaped and guided research with children as well. For instance, one model suggests that anxious children's cognitive processing is characterized by cognitive distortions that involve unrealistic concerns about self-evaluation, evaluation by others, and the probability of negative consequences (Kendall et al., 1992a).

Much of the existing literature on cognitive factors in childhood anxiety has focused on nonclinical samples of children with specific fears, as opposed to children diagnosed with an anxiety disorder. Zatz and Chassin (1983) found that test-anxious children had distorted perceptions of their own abilities as they did not significantly differ in ability from the nonanxious children on objective measures of performance. Prins (1985) considered cognitive processing in children from a nonclinical sample before an anxiety-provoking dental situation. Children with the highest dental anxiety had self-speech that was more negative than that of children with lower concerns.

Studies investigating cognitive dysfunction in children diagnosed with an anxiety disorder are rare, indicating the need for increased research in this area. Studies are needed to better understand the cognitive processing that occurs when children with an anxiety disorder are exposed to potentially distressing situations or tasks. Do children diagnosed with an anxiety disorder tend to distort, focus on self-evaluation, and perceive increased threat in the environment, as suggested by their self-talk?

Further Investigations of Depression in Children

Once beyond the question of whether or not depression occurs in youth, there have been and continue to be many efforts to further our understanding of mood disorder in youth. For example, differences have been found concerning depression in children, adolescents, and adults but, unlike in adults, studies of prepubertal children have not shown consistent sex differences in the prevalence of major depression (Carlson & Cantwell, 1979; Kashani, Cantwell, Shekim, & Reid, 1982). Some differences have been found between depressed boys and girls that have not been seen in adults. For instance, associations between depression and characteristics such as unpopularity and somatic complaints appear to be higher and more consistent among girls than boys (Jacobsen, Lahey, & Strauss, 1983; Kazdin, Sherick, Esveldt-Dawson, & Rancurello, 1985).

Other research with depression in children (Kovacs, 1983), for example, has found that after dysphoric mood, social withdrawal distinguished depressed from nondepressed children, yet social withdrawal is not an essential criteria in DSM-III-R (American Psychiatric Association, 1987) or DSM-IV (American Psychiatric Association, 1994), thus indicating the need for further investigation. At the same time, many similarities between depression in adults and children have been found in terms of cognitive attributes such as attributional style, locus of control, hopelessness, and cognitive distortion (Haley et al., 1985; Kaslow et al., 1984; Kendall et al., 1990).

Even the self-report assessment of depression has been advanced, due largely to Beck's landmark contributions. As with adults, one of the most common assessment techniques has been the use of self-reports. Self-report is critical, because the essential symptoms of depression involve self-perceptions along with subjective evaluations of personal feelings.

With regard to youth, the most widely used and researched measure is the CDI (Kovacs, 1981) — an adaptation of the Beck Depression Inventory (BDI; Beck, Ward, Mendelson, Mock, & Erbaugh, 1961) used with adults. The 27-item CDI taps the cognitive, affective, and behavioral signs of depression. Reviews of the measurement of depression in youth (e.g., Kendall, Cantwell, & Kazdin, 1989) routinely identify the CDI as the most often-used and studied measure.

Distinctions between Depression as a Mood, a Symptom, and a Syndrome

The syndrome of depression in children is not a transient phenomenon that occurs only at developmentally appropriate times. Rather, depression is an actual disorder that requires clinical attention. Even though the episodes remit, they generally last longer than previously believed and they tend to recur (Kovacs et al., 1984). In addition, depression may lead to major interferences in normal development (Puig-Antich et al., 1985).

Beck brought to light the conceptual distinctions between depression as a mood, a symptom, and a syndrome. Since depression is a widely used term, there is much ambiguity with its usage. The word "depression" when used as an individual symptom can indicate a sad mood, unhappiness, or feeling miserable. This understanding of depression indicates a dysphoric mood, only one aspect of a depressive syndrome or a depressive disorder. Depressive symptoms may be fleeting or connected to specific events, but in other cases they may be part of a disorder.

The term "depression" can also refer to a clinical syndrome that entails more than just a sad or dysphoric mood, but changes in psychomotor, cognitive, and motivational areas (Kendall, Cantwell, & Kazdin, 1989). Generally the term "syndrome" is used to indicate a set of symptoms that reliably co-occur (Carlson & Cantwell, 1981). At the same time, depression can signify a disorder where a depressive syndrome is present along with some degree of functional impairment in important areas of life and a specified duration that exceeds a more transient course (Kendall et al., 1989).

As a result, the use of the term "depression" has important implications since it can be a symptom such as being sad, a syndrome that would be a constellation of signs and symptoms that cluster together, or a nosologic category that would be established based on careful diagnostic procedures. For depression to be a nosologic category, other potential diagnostic categories need to be assessed and excluded if the criteria are not met.

Beck's theories stimulated research on depression, resulting in the acceptance of and distinction between the concepts of depression as a symptom, a syndrome, and a disorder. A major development has come with the recognition of the need for specific criteria that began with adults and has been extending more and more toward children and adolescents. There have even been attempts to develop sets of criteria specifically for the diagnosis of depression in children (Cantwell, 1983) and important questions are being asked as to whether or not there is a need for different diagnostic criteria for depressive syndromes at different ages (Kendall et al., 1989). Multivariate studies of child symptoms suggest that there may be developmental differences and that depressive symptoms may be differentially organized based on age and gender (Achenbach & Edelbrock, 1983).

Methodological Suggestions in Light of Beck's Distinction

Kendall, Hollon, Beck, Hammen, and Ingram (1987) provided guidelines for studies that rely solely on self-report devices to define experimental groups of "depressed" subjects. It has been suggested that adult participants be assessed during at least two time periods, once when initially selected and once right before the experiment. This procedure addresses the issue of stability as well as the actual status of the participant immediately preceeding participation. Furthermore, multiple screenings reduce the likelihood of assigning someone to the "depressed" group based on a transient mood fluctuation (Kendall & Flannery-Schroeder, 1995). Even though most depression inventories have relatively high test–retest reliability, a significant proportion of participants change classification when retested even only days after the initial assessment (Hatzenbuehler, Parpal, & Matthews, 1983). On a related note, Tennen, Hall, and Affleck (1995) and Kendall and Flannery-Schroeder (1995) argue against the use of a self-report short form because assignment of subjects to groups is known to be less reliable with short as compared to the full form. Although the literature on childhood depression is less well developed than that with adult participants, the issues pertinent to self-report assessment are nevertheless relevant.

According to Kendall and Flannery-Schroeder (1995), the failure to use a structured interview in research that compares groups that differ in diagnostic status could negatively affect the sensitivity, specificity, and validity of the diagnoses. As a result, distinctions between the terms "depression," "depression as a syndrome," "dysphoria," and "major depressive disorder" are easily lost (Tennen et al., 1995) Therefore, methodology that entails multimethod measurement of both syndromal and nosologic depression offers the most credible diagnostic statements (Kendall et al., 1987). Studies with depressed children will benefit from application of structured diagnostic interviews to make determinations of the presence of disorders.

Another important methodological consideration that brings to light the distinction between depression as a symptom, syndrome, or nosological category is the use of cut-off scores to form groups. This process is complicated by the fact that cut-off scores vary between studies, making it difficult to compare results (Tennen et al., 1995). Kendall et al. (1987) argue for consistent cut scores in studies of childhood depression

Differentiating between Anxiety and Depression

According to Beck (1976), the cognitive model of psychopathology describes each condition in terms of its specific cognitive content. The theory offers that cognitions are influential in the onset and maintenance of emotional disorders and that different disturbances have different themes or cognitive content. This conceptualization became known as the content–specificity hypothesis and has been the focus of much research with adults (Beck, Brown, Steer, Eidelson, & Riskind, 1987; Beck, Riskind, Brown, & Steer, 1988; Clark et al., 1989; Greenberg & Beck, 1989; Hollon, Kendall, & Lumry, 1986; Ingram, Kendall, Smith, Donnell, & Ronan, 1987; Ronan, Kendall, & Rowe, 1994).

According to the cognitive model, persons who suffer from depression and anxiety have different cognitions about themselves, their world, and their future. The Cognition Checklist (CCL; Beck et al., 1987), developed to measure the frequency of automatic thoughts, includes cognitions related to danger, characteristic of anxiety disorders (Beck & Emery, 1985), along with cognitions related to depression. Beck et al. (1987) found that patients who had received a diagnosis of depression based on DSM-III criteria reported higher levels of cognitions concerning loss, while those patients with a diagnosis of an anxiety disorder endorsed more threat-related cognitions. These results support the content–specificity hypothesis that the content representative of anxiety and depression can be distinguished. Furthermore, according to Kendall and Chansky (1991), cognitive content may be useful in differentiating childhood disorders: imagery and automatic thoughts of the depressed youth center around the theme of self-deprecation, loss, and negative attitudes about the past and the future, while the themes of anxiety disorders center around danger, threat, and exaggerated anticipation of harm (Beck et al., 1987).

According to Watson and Kendall (1989), there are important differences between anxiety and depression when considering emotions and the appraisal processes. As a result of these differences, the depressed child is inclined toward ignoring positive information and processing negative information concerning the self. Furthermore, the appraisals made about events that are personally relevant are generally negative, global, and absolutistic. Kendall and Ingram (1987, 1989) suggested that depressive affect seems most closely associated with self-referent, definitive, past-oriented cognitions of sadness, failure, and loss. The anxious child, in contrast, selectively processes information that involves threat or danger and makes appraisals that involve uncertainty and anticipation.

Few studies exist that examine cognitive distortion in clinical samples of anxious children. In one report, Ronan et al. (1994) described the development of a questionnaire (Negative Affectivity Self-Statement Questionnaire; NASSQ) to measure the anxious and/or depressive self-talk of 7–15-year-old children. In general, there was support for the content–specificity hypothesis Beck proposed for adults. In the 7–10-year-old sample, depression-only but not anxious-only subjects were found to have significantly higher scores on the depression-specific items than controls. Similarly, for the 11–15-year-olds, the depression-specific self-statements were found to discriminate between depression-only subjects and control subjects but not between anxious-only subjects and controls. Also, the anxiety-specific items discriminated between anxiety-only but not depression-only subjects and controls. These findings are consistent with prior research reports using adult populations that have found specificity for separate anxious and depressive cognition (Greenberg & Beck, 1989; Ingram et al., 1987).

Stark, Humphrey, Laurent, Livingston, and Christopher (1993) studied anxiety and depression in youth and used a multigate assessment (Kendall et al., 1987) that began with a questionnaire and then proceeded to a semistructured interview. Stark et al. (1993) reported that negative perceptions about the self, the world, and the future differentiated depressed from anxious children and concluded that the findings lent support to the notion that the two disorders can be distinguished by unique cognitive processes. The researchers also reported behavioral and family profiles that differentiated the groups.

Jolly and Dykman (1994), in a study that contrasted the cognitive content and cognitions of 162 inpatient adolescents, found that self-reports of depressive symptoms were significantly predicted by both specific depressive cognitions and general cognitions, while specific anxiety cognitions did not significantly predict depressive symptoms. Self-reported anxiety symptoms were significantly predicted by specific anxiety cognition and general cognition, but were not predicted by specific depressive cognition. These results again support the content–specificity hypothesis (Beck, 1976), in this instance among adolescents.

Overall, the cognitive model of depression (Beck, 1967, 1976) has been supported not only for the content–specificity for depression-relevant stimuli but also for its consistency across the self, world, and future. Since depression and anxiety have been related in studies of psychopathology, studies that have examined just one of the disorders have probably confounded the two conditions, both within subjects and within measures. Nevertheless, the studies that have examined both depression and anxiety have shown processing differences between depressed and anxious adults and children

(Beck et al., 1987; Beck, Riskind, Brown, & Sherrod, 1986; Greenberg & Beck, 1989; Hammen & Zupan, 1984; Jolly & Dykman, 1994; Stark et al., 1993).

Although research indicates that depressive and anxious states are correlated and may share some common features, the very fact that the correlation is not perfect suggests that there are unique mechanisms for each disorder and therefore there are important differences. Furthermore, establishing these differences has theoretical, methodological, empirical, assessment, and treatment implications (Kendall & Ingram, 1989). In order to understand the potential cognitive differences and similarities, depression and anxiety must be examined in an unconfounded manner, separating each state in the same study to best help children in distress.

THE TREATMENT OF EMOTIONAL DYSPHORIA IN YOUTH

It is again interesting to note that it was Beck who facilitated the investigation of whether or not depression occurs in youth. Currently, there is not only evidence that children can and do develop various forms of depressive disorder (e.g., Kovacs et al., 1984), but also there have been efforts to investigate the efficacy of different methods to treat it.

Overall, interest is growing in the treatment of childhood disorders involving cognitive distortions. In the past, much attention had been focused on treating externalizing problems, such as those evident in attention-deficit/hyperactivity disorder (Barkley, 1990) and impulsive behavior (Kendall & Braswell, 1993). For these conditions, the goal was typically to inhibit behavior and train the use of cognitive processing—to put thought between stimulus and response. Unlike the treatments for externalizing conditions, the goal of treatment with depressed or anxious children is to identify the distorted processing, aid in modification of distorted thinking, and teach new coping strategies (Kendall, Kortlander, Chansky, & Brady, 1992).

It is critical to understand the effect of sustained and untreated depression on the self-confidence and social functioning of children. Childhood is a vital time for the development of personal views (or schema) concerning the self, the world, and the future. Beck has suggested that it is these negative beliefs that increase the likelihood of later episodes of depression, and even if the episodes subside, these distorted views persist and result in inflexible attitudes and a maladaptive coping style. As a consequence, children will likely be unable to test alternative explanations and will find it difficult to make attributions to external causes when it is in fact appropriate to do so. It is clear that early intervention may alter the prognosis and result in substantial benefits to the functioning of potentially depressed children (Thase, 1990).

Beck et al. (1979) described the goal of cognitive therapy as the relief of distress, which is accomplished by focusing on inflexible misinterpretations, self-defeating behavior, and maladaptive attitudes. Nevertheless, Beck considers both science and emotion and writes that the therapist must also be understanding of the patient's intense sadness and should encourage the expression of these feelings as he or she identifies dysfunctional cognitions. He also sees the need to detail how emotions relate to cognitive processes and how cognitive therapy actually uses many emotional techniques as it attempts to interweave emotion with the modification of cognitions. This is especially the case with therapeutic interventions for depression, since linkages must be made between negative emotions and existing beliefs and assumptions, in order for treatment to be effective. Clients must know they can be themselves, which means experiencing any emotions they may need, without the risk of being invalidated or told to think happy thoughts. The client is in no way encouraged to hide his or her feelings, while the therapist encourages the client to explore underlying attitudes.

Shaped by the cognitive model of depression, cognitive therapy uses a set of general therapeutic methods individually suited to the child's specific problem within the framework of his or her depression. Cognitive therapy is active (grounded in "collaborative empiricism"; Beck et al., 1979; Hollon & Beck, 1979), structured, and time limited and is based on the rationale that an individual's emotions and actions are regulated by the way he or she perceives and processes the world. Current cognition is based on schemas (attitudes that are economically developed from past experiences), and while they often make day-to-day processing more efficient, if they are maladaptive, then assumptions can result in pathological thinking. Cognitive therapy techniques therefore are designed to enumerate and test the specific misconceptions in the current context.

The therapy process begins with self-monitoring automatic thoughts trying to understand the connections between cognition, emotion, and behavior. This process is followed by consideration of the evidence for and against the "distorted" cognitions with the goal of replacing them with more realistic alternatives. Other treatment strategies include self-control skills that involve rewarding more and punishing less, self-monitoring of events that could refute distorted thinking, self-evaluation, and assertiveness training. With children specifically, other components include the development of more adaptive social skills and more functional and less distorted perceptions (Stark, Rouse, & Livingston, 1991). The intervention teaches youth with distorted processing to identify their dysfunctional cognitions and modify or replace them with more adaptive ones through a process of empirical testing and logical analysis (Kendall, Chansky, et al., 1992; Kendall et al., 1992b; Rush, Beck, Kovacs, & Hollon, 1977) to determine the evidence for and against the distorted cognition. Therapeutic efforts require that the content of the distorted processing be identified and that opportunities be established, in the form of behavioral tasks, to test and modify these distortions, along with teaching rational skills and a new coping style.

It is interesting to note that Beck laid the groundwork for interventions with depressed children. His contribution is apparent in the treatments employed by Stark (1990) and Reynolds (Reynolds & Coats, 1986). Stark (1990) extended Beck's principles to help depressed children. According to Stark (1990), cognitive, self-control, and behavioral techniques are necessary for effective treatment of depression in youth. Cognitive procedures include problem solving, cognitive restructuring, and modeling. Self-monitoring and self-evaluation constitute some of the self-control techniques, while the behavioral skills entail teaching assertiveness, social skills, and relaxation exercises. Exposure is a critical component of treatment as well, so as to allow mastery to extend outside of the therapy setting.

Another interesting parallel between Beck's approach with adults and the treatment of depression in youth offered by Stark (1990) is an emphasis on emotion. Both treatments focus on the importance of the therapeutic relationship which centers on warmth, trust, open communication, and an empathic understanding of the child's sadness. Interventions that target affect are getting increased attention within cognitive therapy for children. Youth are taught to label feelings, acknowledging that they exist on a continuum, and they are encouraged to identify these emotions within themselves. The cognitive techniques start with restructuring automatic thoughts to examining themes that emerge that are indicative of dysfunctional cognition. Over time, the child gains ability in identifying and modifying his or her thoughts and affect.

Cognitive restructuring for children is based on Beck's approach (1979) which involves four strategies: (1) "What's the evidence?" (2) "What are the alternative ways of looking at it?" (3) "What if?" and (4) behavioral assignments to test the underlying structures (Stark, 1990). The goal of cognitive therapy with children is changing their cognitive structures, especially the central or core structures, which then alter the way the child derives meaning from the world (Stark, 1990).

The cognitive-behavioral model represents the consideration of various aspects of the child's environment integrating both internal and external aspects. Children and adolescents are in the process of developing ways to view their world. Consequently, cognitive-behavioral therapy helps to discourage the maintenance of dysfunctional schemas with the goal of constructing a new schema through which the child can identify and solve problems. A beneficial intervention focuses on creating behavioral experiences coupled with emotional involvement, while at the same time attending to the cognitive activities of the child. Work with children often involves the therapist and child sharing important experiences and the therapist guiding the youngster's attributions about prior behavior, along with his or her expectations for future behavior. Therefore (consistent with Beck, 1967, 1976), the youngster is shaped to develop a cognitive structure for future events that incorporates adaptive skills and appropriate cognition, which combines to produce adaptive functioning.

Manualized Treatment

Cognitive therapy has remained focused on the methods of science as the means to examine treatment effectiveness. Research has focused on highly controlled studies with adequate control groups and long-term follow-ups. Beck was among the first to develop a manual-based treatment—a task once thought to be impossible but essential for controlled evaluations. The manual (Treatment Manual; Beck, Rush, & Kovacs, 1975, as cited in Beck et al., 1979) has permitted and facilitated the transportability of the treatment from setting to setting. In a similar manner, Stark and associates developed a manualized treatment for depressed youth (see Stark & Kendall, 1996), and prepared a workbook for youth to follow as they progress through the treatment (Stark et al., 1996).

The development of treatment manuals facilitated the development and widespread use of cognitive interventions. Research demonstrated that cognitive therapy can be an effective short-term treatment for depressed outpatients. Furthermore, since manual-based cognitive therapy is a short-term treatment modality, it is available to a wider population of children and adults.

Outcome Research

Available research validates the use of both cognitive and behavioral therapies with outpatient unipolar depressed adults (see Chapters 4, 6, 12, and 14, this volume). Nevertheless, only a handful of studies have been reported on the posttreatment effects of the full cognitive-behavioral therapy with depressed children, even though clinically significant levels of depression seem to have manifestations similar to those found in adults (Kovacs & Beck, 1977).

Reynolds and Coats (1986) compared a cognitive-behavioral intervention and a relaxation intervention with a waiting-list control condition. Thirty moderately depressed adolescents were randomly assigned to the three conditions. The two interventions met twice weekly for 5 weeks. Both the cognitive-behavioral and the relaxation training interventions, compared with the waiting-list control condition, produced significant reductions in depression symptoms according to self-reports and clinical ratings. These treatment effects were maintained at a 5-week follow-up, along with reductions in anxiety and improvements in academic self-concept. Nevertheless, it is important to note that participants were not formally diagnosed using a structured diagnostic interview and this limits the assessment of other concomitant psychopathology as well as the duration of the depressive disorder. The small sample size may have precluded the determination of differences between the active treatments if such differences did in fact exist. Finally, it was not clear which specific factors are critical for treatment of depression, so future research should determine essential elements for a successful therapeutic intervention.

Stark, Reynolds, and Kaslow (1987) assigned 29 moderately to severely depressed children (aged 9–12 years) to self-control, behavioral problem solving, or waiting-list conditions. At posttreatment and at an 8-week followup, the self-control and behavioral problem-solving conditions produced significant reductions in depression for moderately depressed children using self-report and clinical interviews, in comparison with the waiting-list subjects. It was noted by these researchers that children would have been aided by a cognitive intervention as well, since some children displayed a negative information-processing style.

Lewinsohn, Clarke, Hops, and Andrews (1990) evaluated the efficacy of a cognitive-behavioral group intervention for depressed adolescents with and without parental participation. In addition, they wanted to assess the stability of the gains 24 months following treatment. Fifty-nine high school students between the ages of 14 to 18 who met DSM-III criteria for depression were randomly assigned to one of three conditions. One condition involved teaching both the parents and the adolescents skills for relaxation, controlling depressive thoughts, and improving communication and social skills; another group involved only the parents; and the final group was a waiting-list. Results indicated that treated subjects compared to the waiting-list group improved significantly on measures of depression and the improvements were maintained 2 years following the end of treatment. Nevertheless, the absence of control conditions does not allow the possibility to be ruled out that the results were due, in part, to other influences.

The clearest evidence for the specific effects of a cognitive-behavioral treatment emerged in a study reported by Stark et al. (1991) with 24 depressed children in grades 4–7 assigned to cognitive-behavioral therapy or to traditional counseling. Both interventions lasted 24–26 sessions over 3.5 months and were conducted in small groups. The cognitive-behavioral treatment was a more broad-band intervention than in previous studies and included self-control, social skills, and cognitive restructuring components. At posttreatment, cognitive-behavioral therapy produced greater improvements in depression and reductions in depressive cognitions than did traditional counseling. However, the long-term effects of cognitive-behavioral therapy has not yet been documented since treatment gains were not maintained at the 7-month follow-up.

Although these controlled studies provide an encouraging start in this area of research, there are limitations (e.g., reliance on self-report measures). It is evident that more research is needed, with increased comparison conditions, greater use of clinical cases, and long-term follow-ups. As is apparent in the data on depressed adults, a major contribution of cognitive-behavioral therapy may be its potency to prevent relapse (see Chapter 14; this volume).

A LOOK TO THE FAMILY

It is often argued, but rarely investigated, that family functioning has an important influence on child psychopathology. As the influence of the family on child adjustment and disorders receives more attention, it is important to keep in mind that these children are likely to have a parent that is depressed (Gotlib & Hammen, 1992). According to Billings and Moos (1983), families with a depressed parent are generally less expressive and cohesive, put less importance on developing independence, and tend to have more conflict. This reality may worsen the symptomatology found in children that come from such homes. In light of this possibility, it would be helpful to assess and address family functioning so as to provide the most comprehensive interventions for children.

Furthermore, parents are often used as the source of information to assess depression in children. Though this clearly offers advantages, there are potential problems in interpretation. Some studies (Forehand, Lautenschlager, Faust, & Graziano, 1986; Griest, Wells, & Forehand, 1979) have shown that maternal perceptions of child adjustment and functioning are related to maternal psychopathology, suggesting that data provided by parents cannot be seen as solely a reflection of the child's state (Kendall et al., 1989).

The critical role of the family in a child's life goes without question. However, research addressing child psychopathology in terms of an interaction between family factors and the cognitive functioning of the child is far from complete. Exactly what contributes to vulnerability in children is not clear and still needs investigation. Some studies have been conducted in this area (e.g., Stark et al., 1991) and they suggest that dysfunctional cognition and behavior displayed by depressed children are often produced and maintained by patterns established in the family. Stark et al. (1991) stress the need to involve the child's family in treatment thus allowing the family to construct new rules and ways of communicating that could help to modify the child's depressive cognitive processing and interpersonal behavior. Additional research is needed to separate the child's maladaptive thinking from the dysfunctional family patterns that oftentimes maintain the maladaptive system.

Along these lines, Hammen, Burge, and Adrian (1991), in a study of 92 children of unipolar, bipolar, medically ill, and normal mothers found a significant temporal association between mother and child diagnoses and that most children who experienced a major depressive episode did so in close proximity to maternal depression. Jaenicke et al. (1987) reported that the children of depressed mothers had lower self-esteem, less positive self-schemas, and a more negative attributional style than the children of non-depressed and of mothers who were medically ill. Jaenicke et al. (1987) suggested that maternal factors may contribute to vulnerability through which the depressive self-schema emerge.

Stark, Humphrey, Crook, and Lewis (1990, as cited in Stark, 1990) examined the perceptions of mothers with those of their children who were depressed, anxious, or normal as diagnosed on the K-SADS (Puig-Antich & Ryan, 1986). Children also completed the Self-Report Measure of Family Functioning (SRMFF-C; Stark et al., 1990). Results indicated that there were significant disturbances in the perceived family environments of children with depression or anxiety and the greatest dysfunction was found in families with a depressed child. Therefore, family interaction once again may be implicated in child functioning. Depressed children reported the highest levels of overt conflict and, as a consequence, it needs to be determined where the source of the conflict is as well as its direction, so as to better understand how to intervene at the level of the family (Stark, 1990). Furthermore, as Stark (1990) noted, if the parent conflict is addressed to the child, the message may be one of rejection and this could promote a negative view of the self.

Forehand, McCombs, and Brody (1987) reviewed 31 studies on the relationship between parental depressive state and four types of child behavior problems with three samples: depressed parents, clinic-referred children, and nonproblem parents and children. Results indicated that in 55% of the measures, there was a negative relationship between parental depressive state and child functioning and this occurred more often in clinically depressed parents. Studies like this indicate the need for more research within the family as well as research that considers factors that place children at risk or protect them from the depressed state of parents.

Finally, research and subsequent treatments must be extended to involve the family since the child's depressogenic thinking and actions may be maintained by familial interaction. With a focus on the family, cognitive therapy could be effectively applied with parents (e.g., Howard & Kendall, 1996, in press) and could be extended for preventive purposes, so as to target families at risk. It is not out of the realm of possibilities to consider widespread application of cognitive principles to the modification of depressive conditions as a valued part of parent training.

REFERENCES

Achenbach, T. M. (1966). The classification of children's psychiatric symptoms: A factor analytic study. *Psychological Monographs, 80*(Whole No. 165).

Achenbach, T. M. (1978). The Child Behavior Profile: I. Boys aged 6–11. *Journal of Consulting and Clinical Psychology, 46,* 478–488.

Achenbach, T. M., & Edelbrock, C. S. (1979). The Child Behavior Profile: II. Boys aged 6–11 and girls aged 6–11 and 12–16. *Journal of Consulting and Clinical Psychology, 47,* 223–233.

Achenbach, T. M., & Edelbrock, C. S. (1983). *Manual for the Child Behavior Checklist and Review Child Behavior Profile.* Burlington, VT: Department of Psychiatry, University of Vermont.

American Psychiatric Association. (1987). *Diagnostic and statistical manual of mental disorders* (3rd ed., rev.). Washington, DC: Author.

American Psychiatric Association. (1994). *Diagnostic and statistical manual of mental disorders* (4th ed.). Washington, DC: Author.

Asarnow, J. R., & Bates, S. (1988). Depression in child psychiatric inpatients: Cognitive and attributional patterns. *Journal of Abnormal Child Psychology, 16,* 601–616.

Barkley, R. A. (1990). *Attention-deficit hyperactivity disorder: A handbook for diagnosis and treatment* (2nd ed.). New York: Guilford Press.

Beck, A. T. (1967). *Depression.* New York: Harper & Row.

Beck, A. T. (1976). *Cognitive therapy and the emotional disorders.* New York: International Universities Press.

Beck, A. T., Brown, G., Steer, R., Eidelson, B., & Riskind, J. (1987). Differentiating anxiety and depression: A test of the cognitive content specificity hypotheses. *Journal of Abnormal Psychology, 96,* 179–183.

Beck, A. T., & Emery, G. (1985). *Anxiety disorders and phobias: A cognitive perspective.* New York: Basic Books.

Beck, A. T., Riskind, J. H., Brown, G., & Sherrod, A. (1986). *A comparison of likelihood estimates for imagined positive and negative outcomes in anxiety and depression.* Paper presented at the meeting of the Society for Psychotherapy Research, Wellsley, MA.

Beck, A. T., Riskind, J. H., Brown, G., & Steer, R. A. (1988). Levels of hopelessness in DSM-III disorders: A partial test of content specificity in depression. *Cognitive Therapy and Research, 12,* 459–469.

Beck, A. T., Rush, A. J., Shaw, B. F., & Emery, G. (1979). *Cognitive therapy of depression.* New York: Guilford Press.

Beck, A. T., Ward, C. H., Mendelson, M., Mock, J. E., & Erbaugh, J. K. (1961). An inventory for measuring depression. *Archives of General Psychiatry, 4,* 561–571.

Billings, A. G., & Moos, R. H. (1983). Comparisons of children of depressed and nondepressed parents: A social-environmental perspective. *Journal of Abnormal Child Psychology, 11,* 463–486.

Cantwell, D. P. (1983). Depression in childhood: Clinical picture and diagnostic criteria. In D. P. Cantwell & G. A. Carlson (Eds.), *Affective disorders in childhood and adolescence: An update* (pp. 3–18). New York: Spectrum.

Cantwell, D. P. (1985). Depressive disorders in children: Validation of clinical syndromes. *Psychiatric Clinics of North America, 8,* 779–792.

Carlson, G. A., & Cantwell, D. P. (1979). A survey of depressive symptoms in a child and adolescent psychiatric population. *Journal of the American Academy of Child Psychiatry, 18,* 587–599.

Carlson, G. A., & Cantwell, D. P. (1981). Diagnosis of childhood depression — A comparison of Weinberg and DSM-III criteria. *Journal of the American Academy of Child Psychiatry, 21,* 247–250.

Clark, D. A., Beck, A. T., & Brown, G. (1989). Cognitive mediation in general psychiatric outpatients: A test of the content–specificity hypothesis. *Journal of Personality and Social Psychology, 56,* 958–964.

Forehand, R., Lautenschlager, G. J., Faust, J., & Graziano, W. G. (1986). Parents perceptions and parent–child interactions in clinic-referred children: A preliminary investigation of the effects of maternal depressive moods. *Behaviour Research and Therapy, 24,* 73–75.

Forehand, R., McCombs, A., & Brody, G. H. (1987). The relationship between parental depressive mood states and child functioning. *Advances in Behaviour Research and Therapy, 9,* 1–20.

Fuhrman, M. J., & Kendall, P. C. (1986). Cognitive tempo and behavioral adjustment in children. *Cognitive Therapy and Research, 10,* 45–51.

Garber, J., Quiggle, N., & Shanley, N. (1990). Cognition and depression in children and adolescents. In R. E. Ingram (Ed.), *Contemporary psychological approaches to depression: Theory, research, and treatment* (pp. 87–115). New York: Plenum Press.

Gotlib, I. H., & Hammen, C. L. (1992). *Psychological aspects of depression: Toward a cognitive-interpersonal integration.* Chichester, UK: Wiley.

Greenberg, M. S., & Beck, A. T. (1989). Depression versus anxiety: A test of the content–specificity hypothesis. *Journal of Abnormal Psychology, 98,* 9–13.

Greenberg, M. S., Vazquez, C. V., & Alloy, L. B. (1988). Depression versus anxiety: Differences in self- and other-schemata. In L. B. Alloy (Ed.), *Cognitive processes in depression* (pp. 109–142). New York: Guilford Press.

Griest, D., Wells, K. C., & Forehand, R. (1979). An examination of predictors of maternal perceptions of maladjustment in clinic-referred children. *Journal of Abnormal Psychology, 88,* 277–281.

Haley, G. M. T., Fine, S., Marriage, K., Moretti, M. M., & Freeman, R. J. (1985). Cognitive bias and depression in psychiatrically disturbed children and adolescents. *Journal of Consulting and Clinical Psychology, 53,* 535–537.

Hammen, C., Burge, D., & Adrian, C. (1991). Timing of mother and child depression in a longitudinal study of children at risk. *Journal of Consulting and Clinical Psychology, 59,* 341–345.

Hammen, C., & Zupan, B. A. (1984). Self-schemas, depression, and the processing of personal information in children. *Journal of Experimental Child Psychology, 37,* 598–608.

Hatzenbuehler, L. C., Parpal, M., & Matthews, L. (1983). Classifying college students as depressed or nondepressed using the Beck Depression Inventory: An empirical analysis. *Journal of Consulting and Clinical Psychology, 51,* 360–366.

Hollon, S. D., & Beck, A. T. (1979). Cognitive therapy of depression. In P. C. Kendall & S. D. Hollon (Eds.), *Cognitive-behavioral interventions: Theory, research, and procedures* (pp. 153–204). New York: Academic Press.

Hollon, S. D., Kendall, P. C., & Lumry, A. (1986). Specificity of depressotypic cognitions in clinical depression. *Journal of Abnormal Psychology, 95,* 52–59.

Howard, B., & Kendall, P. C. (1996). *Cognitive-behavioral family therapy for anxious children: Therapist manual.* (Available from Workbooks, 208 Llanfair Road, Ardmore, PA 19003)

Howard, B., & Kendall, P. C. (in press). Cognitive-behavioral family therapy for anxiety-disordered children: A multiple-baseline evaluation. *Cognitive Therapy and Research.*

Ingram, R. E., & Kendall, P. C. (1986). Cognitive clinical psychology: Implications of an information processing perspective. In R. E. Ingram (Ed.), *Information processing approaches to clinical psychology* (pp. 3–21). Orlando, FL: Academic Press.

Ingram, R. E., & Kendall, P. C. (1987). The cognitive side of anxiety. *Cognitive Therapy and Research, 11,* 523–537.

Ingram, R. E., Kendall, P. C., Smith, T. W., Donnell, C., & Ronan, K. (1987). Cognitive specificity in emotional distress. *Journal of Personality and Social Psychology, 53,* 734–742.

Jacobsen, R. H., Lahey, B. B., & Strauss, C. C. (1983). Correlations of depressed mood in normal children. *Journal of Abnormal Child Psychology, 11,* 29–40.

Jaenicke, C., Hammen, C., Zupan, B., Hiroto, D., Gordon, D., Adrian, C., & Burge, D. (1987). Cognitive vulnerability in children at risk for depression. *Journal of Abnormal Child Psychology, 15, 559–572.*

Jolly, J. B., & Dykman, R. A. (1994). Using self-report data to differentiate anxious and depressive symptoms in adolescents: Cognitive content specificity and global distress. *Cognitive Therapy and Research, 18, 25–37.*

Kagan, J. (1966). Reflection–impulsivity: The generality and dynamics of conceptual tempo. *Journal of Abnormal Psychology, 71, 17–24.*

Kashani, J. H., Cantwell, D. P., Shekim, W. O., & Reid, J. C. (1982). Major depressive disorder in children admitted to an impatient community mental health center. *American Journal of Psychiatry, 139, 671–672.*

Kaslow, N. J., Rehm, L. P., Pollack, S. L., & Siegel, A. W. (1988). Attributional style and self-control behavior in depressed and nondepressed children and their parents. *Journal of Abnormal Child Psychology, 16, 163–175.*

Kaslow, N. J., Rehm, L. P., & Siegel, A. W. (1984). Social and cognitive correlates of depression in children: A developmental perspective. *Journal of Abnormal Child Psychology, 12, 605–620.*

Kazdin, A. E., Sherick, R. B., Esveldt-Dawson, K., & Rancurello, M. D. (1985). Nonverbal behavior and childhood depression. *Journal of the American Academy of Child Psychiatry, 24, 303–309.*

Kendall, P. C. (1985). Toward a cognitive-behavioral model of child psychopathology and a critique of related interventions. *Journal of Abnormal Child Psychology, 13, 357–372.*

Kendall, P. C. (1991). Guiding theory for treating children and adolescents. In P. C. Kendall (Ed.), *Child and adolescent therapy: Cognitive-behavioral procedures* (pp. 3–34). New York: Guilford Press.

Kendall, P. C. (1993). Cognitive-behavioral therapies with youth: Guiding theory, current status, and emerging developments. *Journal of Consulting and Clinical Psychology, 61, 235–247.*

Kendall, P. C., & Braswell, L. (1993). *Cognitive-behavioral therapy for impulsive children* (2nd ed.). New York: Guilford Press.

Kendall, P. C., Cantwell, D. P., & Kazdin, A. E. (1989). Depression in children and adolescents: Assessment issues and recommendations. *Cognitive Therapy and Research, 13, 109–146.*

Kendall, P. C., & Chansky, T. E. (1991). Considering cognition in anxiety-disordered children. *Journal of Anxiety Disorders, 5, 167–185.*

Kendall, P. C., Chansky, T. E., Kane, M., Kim, R., Kortlander, E., Ronan, K. R., Sessa, R., & Siqueland, L. (1992). *Anxiety disorder in youth: Cognitive-behavioral interventions.* Needham, MA: Allyn & Bacon.

Kendall, P. C., & Flannery-Schroeder, E. C. (1995). Rigor, but not rigor mortis, in depression research. *Journal of Personality and Social Psychology, 68, 892–894.*

Kendall, P. C., Hollon, S. D., Beck, A. T., Hammen, C. H., & Ingram, R. E. (1987). Issues and recommendations regarding use of the Beck Depression Inventory. *Cognitive Therapy and Research, 11, 289–299.*

Kendall, P. C., & Ingram, R. E. (1987). The future for cognitive assessment of anxiety: Let's get specific. In L. Michelson & M. Ascher (Eds.), *Anxiety and stress disorders: Cognitive-behavioral assessment and treatment* (pp. 89–104). New York: Guilford Press.

Kendall, P. C., & Ingram, R. E. (1989). Cognitive-behavioral perspectives: Theory and research on depression and anxiety. In P. C. Kendall & D. Watson (Eds.), *Anxiety and depression: Distinctive and overlapping features* (pp. 27–49). New York: Academic Press.

Kendall, P. C., Kane, M., Howard, B., & Siqueland, L. (1989). *Cognitive-behavioral treatment for anxious children: Treatment manual.* (Available from P. C. Kendall, Department of Psychology, Temple University, Philadelphia, PA 19122)

Kendall, P. C., Kortlander, E., Chansky, T., & Brady, E. (1992). Comorbidity of anxiety and depression in youth: Implications for treatment. *Journal of Consulting and Clinical Psychology, 60,* 869–880.

Kendall, P. C., & MacDonald, J. P. (1993). Cognition in the psychopathology of youth, and implications for treatment. In K. S. Dobson & P. C. Kendall (Eds.), *Psychopathology and cognition* (pp. 387–427). San Diego: Academic Press.

Kendall, P. C., Stark, K. D., & Adam, T. (1990). Cognitive deficit or cognitive distortion in childhood depression. *Journal of Abnormal Child Psychology, 18,* 255–270.

Kovacs, M. (1981). Rating scales to assess depression in school-aged children. *Acta Paedopsychiatrica, 46,* 305–315.

Kovacs, M. (1983, October 12–15). *DSM-III: The diagnosis of depressive disorders in children: An interim appraisal.* Paper presented at the American Psychiatric Association Invitational Workshop, DSM III: An Interim Appraisal, Washington, DC.

Kovacs, M. (1985). The natural history and course of depressive disorders in childhood. *Psychiatric Annals, 15,* 387–389.

Kovacs, M., & Beck, A. T. (1977). An empirical-clinical approach toward a definition of childhood depression. In J. G. Schulterbrandt & A. Raskin (Eds.), *Depression in childhood: Diagnosis, treatment, and conceptual models* (pp. 1–25). New York: Raven Press.

Kovacs, M., Feinberg, T. L., Crouse-Novack, M., Paulauskas, S. L., Pollack M., & Finkelstein, R. (1984). Depressive disorder in childhood: II. A longitudinal study of the risk for a subsequent major depression. *Archives of General Psychiatry, 41,* 643–649.

Leitenberg, H., Yost, L. W., & Carroll-Wilson, M. (1986). Negative cognitive errors in children: Questionnaire development, normative data and comparisons between children with and without self-reported symptoms of depression, low self-esteem, and evaluation anxiety. *Journal of Consulting and Clinical Psychology, 54,* 528–536.

Lewinsohn, P. M., Clarke, G. N., Hops, H., & Andrews, J. (1990). Cognitive-behavioral treatment for depressed adolescents. *Behavior Therapy, 21,* 385–401.

McGee, R., Anderson, J., Williams, S., & Silva, P. (1986). Cognitive correlates of depressive symptoms in 11-year old children. *Journal of Abnormal Child Psychology, 14,* 517–524.

Prins, P. J. M. (1985). Self-speech and self-regulation of high and low anxious children in the dental situation: An interview study. *Behavioral Research and Therapy, 23,* 641–650.

Puig-Antich, J., Lukens, E., Davies, M., Goetz, D., Brennan-Quattrock, J., & Todak, G. (1985). Psychosocial functioning in prepubertal major depressive disorders: I. Interpersonal relationships during the depressive episode. *Archives of General Psychiatry, 42,* 500–507.

Puig-Antich, J., & Ryan, N. (1986). *Schedule for Affective Disorders and Schizophrenia for School-Aged Children.* Pittsburgh, PA: Western Psychiatric Institute and Clinic.

Reynolds, W. M., & Coats, K. I. (1986). A comparison of cognitive-behavioral therapy and relaxation training for the treatment of depression in adolescents. *Journal of Consulting and Clinical Psychology, 54,* 653–660.

Ronan, K., Kendall, P. C., & Rowe, M. (1994). Negative affectivity in children: Development and validation of a self-statement questionnaire. *Cognitive Therapy and Research, 18,* 509–528.

Rush, A. J., Beck, A. T., Kovacs, M., & Hollon, S. (1977). Comparative efficacy of cognitive therapy and pharmacotherapy in the treatment of depressed outpatients. *Cognitive Therapy and Research, 1,* 17–37.

Stark, K. (1990). *Childhood depression: A school-based intervention.* New York: Guilford Press.

Stark, K. D., Humphrey, L. L., Laurent, J., Livingston, R., & Christopher, J. (1993). Cognitive, behavioral, and family factors in the differentiation of depressive and anxiety disorders during childhood. *Journal of Consulting and Clinical Psychology, 61,* 878–886.

Stark, K. D., & Kendall, P. C. (1996). *Treating depressed children: Therapist manual for "Taking ACTION."* (Available from Workbooks, 208 Llanfair Road, Ardmore, PA 19003)

Stark, K. D., Kendall, P. C., McCarthy, M., Stafford, M., Barron, R., & Thomeer, M. (1996). *Taking ACTION: A workbook for overcoming depression.* (Available from Workbooks, 208 Llanfair Road, Ardmore, PA 19003)

Stark, K. D., Reynolds, W. M., & Kaslow, N. J. (1987). A comparison of the relative efficacy of self-control therapy and a behavioral problem-solving therapy for depression in children. *Journal of Abnormal Child Psychology, 15,* 91–113.

Stark, K. D., Rouse, L. W., & Livingston, R. (1991). Treatment of depression during childhood and adolescence: Cognitive-behavioral procedures for the individual and family. In P. C. Kendall (Ed.), *Child and adolescent therapy: Cognitive-behavioral procedures* (pp. 165–206). New York: Guilford Press.

Tennen, H., Hall, J. A., & Affleck, G. (1995). Rigor, rigor mortis, and conspiratorial views of depression research. *Journal of Personality and Social Psychology, 68,* 895–900.

Thase, M. (1990). Major depression in adulthood. In M. Hersen & C. G. Last (Eds.), *Handbook of child and adult psychopathology: A longitudinal perspective* (pp. 51–66). New York: Pergamon Press.

Watson, D., & Kendall, P. C. (1989). Understanding anxiety and depression: Their relation to negative and positive affective states. In P. C. Kendall & D. Watson (Eds.), *Anxiety and depression: Distinctive and overlapping features* (pp. 3–26). San Diego: Academic Press.

Wechsler, D. (1974). *Manual for the Wechsler Intelligence Scale for Children—Revised.* New York: Psychological Corporation.

Zatz, S., & Chassin, L. (1983). Cognitions of test anxious children. *Journal of Consulting and Clinical Psychology, 51*(4), 526–534.

Epilogue

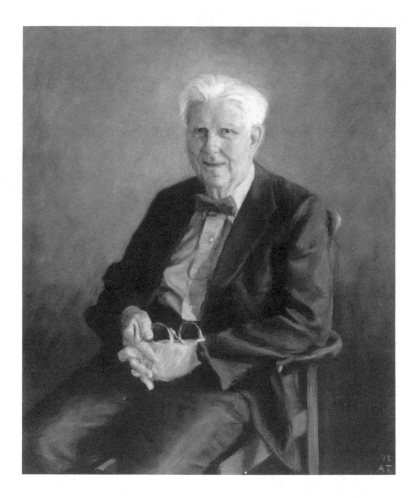

Cognitive Therapy and Aaron T. Beck

Paul M. Salkovskis

There are a range of cognitive theories of psychopathology, each of which have contributed to the approach called cognitive therapy or cognitive-behavioral therapy. The contribution of Aaron T. Beck stands out; when those involved in psychological treatment refer to cognitive therapy, they almost invariably mean Beck's cognitive therapy. Is this really justified? After all, however prodigious his capacity for theoretical and clinical creativity (and prodigious it is), he cannot have devised all that is encompassed here in this book. Nevertheless, not one of the authors in this book would quarrel with the notion that they are working on outgrowths of Beck's approach, and in most instances this involves a continuing relationship with Beck himself. For example, a few weeks before writing this I received a letter from Beck, commenting on an article he had read in a recent journal. He was responding to the writer and soliciting comments from me and three others in the field. The article had caught his imagination, and he noted some of its implications and then wanted to discuss them. I found myself excited and provoked by his comments; I mostly agreed with them but disagreed with some; I exchanged e-mail with the author, and considered writing something on the topic myself. And then I realized, he's done it again! At 75 he's still pushing forward the frontiers, not just of cognitive therapy, but of understanding, and he's firing others up with his enthusiasm.

THE BACKGROUND OF AARON T. BECK

Marjorie Weishaar has written the definitive guide to the life and contribution of Aaron T. Beck (Weishaar, 1993). In that book she describes his childhood, which was far from tranquil. What is notable is that he had to confront adversity, in different forms, and sometimes suffered negative psychological consequences as a result. It is telling that he not only overcame these difficulties, but used them as a stimulus to greater efforts. It seems likely that some of his brilliant clinical and theoretical insights also came from his personal experiences of sadness, anxiety, and feelings of abandonment and from his understanding (and dealing with) blood injury fears, fear of suffocation, tunnel phobia, public speaking fears, and anxiety about health.

Some basic facts: Aaron Temkin Beck was born on July 18th, 1921, in Providence, Rhode Island. His parents had met in the United States, but were originally from the Ukraine. Although his early schooling was interrupted by a life-threatening illness, he rapidly overcame this problem and ended up a year ahead of his peer group. At Hope High School he edited the school newspaper. At Brown University, he majored in English and political science. He was associate editor of the *Brown Daily Herald,* and received a number of honors and awards, including Phi Beta Kappa, the Francis Wayland Scholarship, the Bennet Essay Award, and the Gaston prize for oratory. After graduating magna cum laude in 1942, he went to Yale Medical School to begin his career in medicine. He served a rotating internship, followed by a residency in pathology at the Rhode Island Hospital. Although interested in psychiatry as a subject, he was attracted to the precision of neurology, a quality he saw to be completely lacking in psychiatry. However, during his residency in neurology, he found himself intrigued by some of the recent developments as he performed the required rotation in psychiatry. He decided to stay in psychiatry, as a fellow at the Austin Riggs Center at Stockbridge, Massachusetts, where he gained substantial experience in conducting long-term psychotherapy. During this period of his life, he married Phyllis Whitman; they now have four children and eight grandchildren.

During the Korean War he volunteered at the Valley Forge Army Hospital, where he was Assistant Chief of Neuropsychiatry. He was board-certified in psychiatry in 1953, and became an instructor in psychiatry at the University of Pennsylvania Medical School in 1954, where his research work began in earnest. He has remained there ever since; he is currently University Professor Emeritus of Psychiatry. Since 1959 he has directed funded research investigations into the psychopathology and treatment of depression, suicide, anxiety disorders, panic disorder, alcoholism, drug abuse, and personality disorders. His work is currently supported by a 10-year MERIT award from the National Institute of Mental Health. He is known and honored throughout the world, and serves or has served on numerous editorial boards and panels. He has been formally honored by many organizations and academic institutions, including Brown University, the American Psychopathological Association, the American Psychiatric Association, the American Psychological Association, the Royal College of Psychiatrists, Albert Einstein College of Medicine, New York Academy of Medicine, Harvard University, and the American Association of Suicidology (to name just a few!). These awards only reflect his achievements. His real achievement is greater still, and lies in the impact of cognitive theory and cognitive therapy on people suffering from psychological distress, and on those who can, as a result of Beck's work, offer them real hope and help.

THE ORIGINS OF COGNITIVE THERAPY

The origins of cognitive therapy are to be found in the combination of Beck himself and his theory—these are separate but interacting factors. Like Freud's, Beck's theory began as a general hypothesis of the links between the environment, the person, and his or her emotion and motivation. He explored ways in which the balance between and within these factors could become disturbed and result in emotional problems and disorders. But how did he arrive at the cognitive theory?

His career in psychiatry began with psychoanalysis. He was attracted to psychoanalysis because it offered a way of viewing the whole range of human experience and problems. However, from time to time, he wanted to challenge the authority of psychoanalysis. He suggested to his colleagues that some of the psychoanalytic formulations were farfetched; their response was that the problem lay in his resistance to these ideas rather than the theory itself. He accepted that this was possible, thinking "maybe my mind is really blind to this." This subsequently seemed to be so; his resistance to the psychoanalytic approach was largely broken down by his own analysis; at this stage, he became almost evangelical, and began to conduct research into psychoanalytic theory of depression. He undertook this research because he wanted to speak to those who were outside psychoanalysis who needed persuading of its scientific value. In particular, he was seeking to influence those working in experimental psychology.

His theoretical position (what we now know as the original theory behind cognitive therapy) was developed as a direct consequence of this research. He used dream analysis to validate the notion that depression arose from retroflexed (self-directed) hostility, arising from wish fulfillment; depressed people really wished to degrade themselves, and the negative content of dreaming reflected wish fulfillment. The results of these studies were generally consistent with the psychoanalytic hypothesis he was following. In a subsequent study, he assessed the impact of task failure and success on self-esteem. He expected depressed people to react negatively to success. What he found was that success was followed by improved self-esteem and better performance on subsequent tasks; moreover, the depressed patients showed this positive effect more often than did nondepressed subjects. It seemed to him that his experimental findings indicated that depressed patients did not wish to fail. Rather, what they did was adjust their views of themselves to conform to their experience of failure. Instead of the findings he expected, his research indicated that the ideas expressed in dreams reflected the everyday, waking concerns of the person having them. He describes this in the following way:

When the other studies did not fit in, I went back to my dream studies and I thought "maybe there is a simpler explanation and that is that the person sees himself as a loser in the dream because he ordinarily sees himself as a loser." Since I was doing therapy at the same time, it became clear to me as I went into it that the dream themes were consistent with the waking themes. It seemed to me a simpler notion about the dreams was that they simply incorporated the person's self-concept. Well, if it is just a question of the person's self-concept, you don't have to invoke the notion of dreams being motivated. Dreams could simply be a reflection of the person's thinking. If you take motivation and wish fulfillment out of the dream, this undermines the whole motivational model of psychoanalysis. I started to look at the motivational model all the way through, and its manifestations in behaviors, everyday slips, and so on. It seemed to me that the motivational model did not hold. Once that collapsed and I inserted the cognitive model, I saw no need for the rest of the super-structure of psychanalytic thinking. (Aaron T. Beck, personal communication, November 1992)

On completion of his research on depression, Beck describes experiencing intense feelings of disorientation and distress. His basic assumptions about the nature of psychological functioning had been violated, leaving him the choice of explaining away and discounting the discrepant findings, or of radically rethinking his views on the psychology of emotion and emotional disorders.

It is characteristic of the man that he chose the latter course. He endured isolation, hostility, and rejection as a result of his decision to depart so radically from psychodynamic orthodoxy. It says something about the strength of his vision that he persevered in a way that could almost be described as dysfunctional — until you consider the result in terms of the influence of his work in research, theory, and clinical practice.

The story of the origins of cognitive therapy sets themes that are reflected in present day cognitive-behavioral approaches: the interplay between theory and research, a flexibility and responsiveness both to individuals and to research findings, and above all the importance of understanding the emotional meaning of events and situations from the perspective of the individual experiencing them. On occasion I have used videotapes of Beck conducting therapy as a way of introducing experienced clinicians to the practice of cognitive therapy. It is often commented that "he's not doing cognitive therapy" or "he's just telling the patient he understands." Just! This is one of the great strengths of cognitive therapy. At the heart of it is understanding, but there is much, much more. It is a framework that allows the therapist to understand, offer help, and enable the sufferer to take control of his or her life. It is difficult to do well, but it is possible to learn.

THE ORIGINATOR OF COGNITIVE THERAPY

Aaron T. Beck may have been professionally isolated when he first began developing cognitive therapy, but this state was by no means permanent.

Over the past three decades he has accumulated a host of students, collaborators, coworkers, and friends. This book contains chapters from a small sample of those who have been influenced both by his work and by him as a person. Several contributors to this book have commented in their personal reminiscences that Beck has always offered time, consideration, and close attention to very junior clinicians and researchers, sometimes to the mortification of those who thought themselves more worthy of his attention. David A. Clark (personal communication, 1995) refers to "Tim's interest in young researchers and therapists. I think there are many researchers like myself who owe a great debt to Tim for the opportunities and encouragement he has shown in the advancement of our careers." John Rush (personal communication, 1995) describes being a 4th-year resident and his delight that "Tim not only agreed to provide mentorship on a weekly basis, but also advised me on career decisions. He was eager to work with me." Rush goes on to talk about some advice that Beck offered: "I had been asked to consider the position of Chief Resident. Tim's advice was to request a position without a title. He said 'Titles don't do you any good, but they create a lot of work, which in itself is not particularly creative. Its better to have no title and an opportunity to do the research that you think is important than to have all the titles in the world.' " There just might be a clue there as to why he is interested in people who are doing things rather than people whose status defines them.

Christine Padesky (personal communication, 1995) refers to his openness and willingness to receive feedback from her when she was a beginning clinician in UCLA. In a teaching session, he had brought a videotape in which he conducted cognitive therapy with a depressed woman. "As I watched this illustration of therapy, I felt so disappointed. In the interview he did not help the client label automatic thoughts, begin a thought record, or even fill out an activity schedule. *My* automatic thought was 'this man has developed such a brilliant therapy, and yet he doesn't do it very well.' " As a result of this appraisal, Padesky felt able to role-play a therapist, thinking "surely I can do at least as well as he did on the videotape." This began a friendship and collaboration that continues to this day. Five years after the teaching session, Padesky was coteaching cognitive therapy workshops with Beck. The evening before a workshop in Houston, Beck proposed to show a videotape the next day, after which Chris would comment on how his interventions matched the therapy principles they were teaching. Realizing this was the same video, she fretted and tried to plan something positive to say about it the next day. When the video began, Chris was stunned. The same videotape now appeared to be a brilliant illustration of cognitive therapy. It was easy for her to see how Beck's quiet, skillful questioning led the patient to a clear conceptualization of her problems and gently guided her discovery of paths she could take to solve her own depression. Padesky realized that, as a new clinician, she had thought of cognitive therapy simply as a collection of techniques and procedures, without which she had previously been unable to recognize the therapy. With more experience she appreciated the way in which conceptualization and guided discovery form the cornerstones of cognitive therapy, and she notes that Beck values client ownership of discovery over dramatic therapeutic interventions that make the therapist look clever.

In 1990, Kathleen Mooney (personal communication, 1995) asked Beck what his hope and vision were for the future of cognitive therapy. His response was "I hope in 10 years it no longer exists as a school of therapy." He hoped that "what we call cognitive therapy (conceptualizations and treatment plans informed by research, collaboration, and guided discovery) will be taken for granted as the basics of all good therapy, just as Carl Rogers's principles of warmth, empathy, and genuine regard for patients were adopted as necessary basics of all therapy relationships."

THE IMPACT OF BECK AND COGNITIVE THERAPY

David Goldberg, Professor of Psychiatry at the Institute of Psychiatry, London, suggests that Beck "bears the same relationship to psychoanalysis that Gorbachev does to communism. Just as Gorbachev bloodlessly ended communism . . . vowing that all he was trying to do was to reform it, so Tim Beck has dealt a profoundly subversive blow to psychoanalysis while assuring us that all he has been trying to do is to expand the frontiers of psychotherapy" (personal communication, 1995). Goldberg suggests that Beck has had a particularly profound influence on British psychiatry, and has some ideas about why this may be. "The pragmatic British like cognitive therapy not because they agree with its theoretical premises, but because it works. The fact that the theory is reasonably concise—and has the added bonus of not being grossly improbable—was helpful, but by no means decisive." Jean Cottraux points to the influence of Beck on French psychiatry, Michael Linden about German psychology, and so on. Beck's influence has become global.

Even more remarkably, this influence is both theoretical and personal. The correspondence I received from the contributors to this book almost all refer to Beck's mentoring them, to his openness. Several have remarked on Beck listening intently to their ideas, making notes, then feeding back ideas in refined and inspired form. This ability to listen properly and extract the meaning from what is being said is, of course, the hallmark of cognitive therapy. Anyone who has seen treatment sessions conducted by Beck remark on the same thing with patients; his intentness and focus are coupled with a strong sense that he is not only listening but that he understands. His interventions make it plain that he does.

BECK'S ACHIEVEMENT

David Goldberg points out that Beck's career changed radically when he reached 50. "His publications, which had been running at a modest 1.7

papers per year through the '60s, now blossomed into an average of 10 papers per year, and he has maintained a staggering scientific output ever since. Twenty-nine publications before 50, over 300 afterwards. There has been no sign of any diminution in his amazing creativity. Between 1986 and 1991 (years that took Tim up to the age of 70), he produced the six most frequently cited papers in the psychological literature." A large part of his real achievement is to be found here, in this book. Not that he necessarily directly devised the specific techniques and theories described here (although, in many instances, he did, or at least significantly contributed to them). The crucial point is that, without Beck, a scientific cognitive approach would not have developed. The rate of development of cognitive theory and therapy has been unprecedented. Cognitive treatments have been developed and validated for the full range of psychological problems. The *acceptability* of the cognitive approach for both patients and therapists is related not only to its scientific foundations, but also to the basic humanity which underpins both theory and practice. Tim, these are just some of your achievements. I and the contributors to this book salute you and your vision.

REFERENCE

Weishaar, M. E. (1993). *Aaron T. Beck.* London: Sage.

BIBLIOGRAPHY

Beck has published over 350 articles. His 11 books are:

Beck, A. T. (1967). *The diagnosis and management of depression.* Philadelphia: University of Pennsylvania Press.

Beck, A. T. (1967). *Depression: Clinical, experimental, and theoretical aspects.* New York: Harper and Row.

Beck, A. T. (1967). *Depression: Causes and treatment.* Philadelphia: University of Pennsylvania Press.

Beck, A. T., Resnick, H. L. P., & Lettieri, D. J. (Eds.). (1974). *The prediction of suicide.* Bowie, MD: Charles Press.

Beck, A. T. (1976). *Cognitive therapy and the emotional disorders.* New York: International Universities Press.

Beck, A. T., Rush, A. J., Shaw, B. F., & Emery, G. (1979). *Cognitive therapy of depression.* New York: Guilford Press. (Also published Sussex, England, by Wiley, 1980)

Beck, A. T., & Emery, G., with Greenberg, R. L. (1985). *Anxiety disorders and phobias: A cognitive perspective.* New York: Basic Books.

Beck, A. T. (1988). *Love is never enough.* New York: Harper and Row.

Beck, A. T., Freeman, A., & Associates. (1990). *Cognitive therapy of personality disorders.* New York: Guilford Press.

Wright, J. H., Thase, M. E., Beck, A. T., & Ludgate, J. W. (Eds.). (1993). *Cognitive therapy with inpatients: The cognitive milieu.* New York: Guilford Press.

Beck, A. T., Wright, F. D., Newman, C. F., & Liese, B. S. (1993). *Cognitive therapy of substance abuse.* New York: Guilford Press.

Index